KAPLAN

MCAT®
Biology Review
2027–2028

Edited by Alexander Stone Macnow, MD

ACKNOWLEDGMENTS

Editor-in-Chief, 2027–2028 Edition
M. Dominic Eggert

Contributing Editors, 2027–2028 Edition
Ae-Ri Kim, PhD; Elizabeth Minten, MD PhD; Gregory J. Riviello, MA; Christopher Vestuto

Prior Edition Editorial Staff: Elisabeth Fassas, MD MSc

Published by Kaplan North America, LLC
1515 West Cypress Creek Road
Fort Lauderdale, Florida 33309

Printed in India.

ISBN: 979-8-3497-0111-5

10 9 8 7 6 5 4 3 2 1

TABLE OF CONTENTS

THE *KAPLAN MCAT REVIEW* TEAM

Alexander Stone Macnow, MD
Editor-in-Chief

Áine Lorié, PhD
Editor

Pamela Willingham, MSW
Editor

Derek Rusnak, MA
Editor

Melinda Contreras, MS
Kaplan MCAT Faculty

Mikhail Alexeeff
Kaplan MCAT Faculty

Samantha Fallon
Kaplan MCAT Faculty

Laura L. Ambler
Kaplan MCAT Faculty

Jason R. Selzer
Kaplan MCAT Faculty

Krista L. Buckley, MD
Kaplan MCAT Faculty

M. Dominic Eggert
Editor

Kristen L. Russell, ME
Editor

MCAT faculty reviewers: Elmar R. Aliyev; James Burns; Jonathan Cornfield; Alisha Maureen Crowley; Brandon Deason, MD; Nikolai Dorofeev, MD; Benjamin Downer, MS; Colin Doyle; Christopher Durland; Marilyn Engle; Eleni M. Eren; Raef Ali Fadel; Elizabeth Flagge; Adam Grey; Tyra Hall-Pogar, PhD; Justine Harkness, PhD; Scott Huff; Samer T. Ismail; Aeri Kim, PhD; Elizabeth A. Kudlaty; Kelly Kyker-Snowman, MS; Ningfei Li; John P. Mahon; Brandon McKenzie; Matthew A. Meier; Nainika Nanda; Caroline Nkemdilim Opene; Kaitlyn E. Prenger; Uneeb Qureshi; Bela G. Starkman, PhD; Michael Paul Tomani, MS; Nicholas M. White; Allison Ann Wilkes, MS; Kerranna Williamson, MBA; MJ Wu; and Tony Yu.

Thanks to Kevin Anderson; Rebecca Anderson; Jeff Batzli; Jurre Blom; Hari Priya Chandran; Eric Chiu; James Coleman; Deepika Devan; Tim Eich; Samantha Fallon; Tyler Fara; Owen Farcy; Dan Frey; Robin Garmise; Rita Garthaffner; Joanna Graham; Allison Gudenau; Allison Harm; Beth Hoffberg; Aaron Lemon-Strauss; Keith Lubeley; Diane McGarvey; Leonard Mendoza; Petros Minasi; Elizabeth Minten, MD, PhD; Beena P V; John Polstein; Deeangelee Pooran-Kublall, MD, MPH; Andrea Repole; Rochelle Rothstein, MD; Larry Rudman; Tor Sanden; Srividhya Sankar; Sylvia Tidwell Scheuring; Carly Schnur; Aiswarya Sivanand; Todd Tedesco; Karin Tucker; Bonnie Wang; Lee Weiss; Christina Wheeler; Kristen Workman; Amy Zarkos; and the countless others who made this book possible.

GETTING STARTED CHECKLIST

Getting Started Checklist

- ☐ Register for your free online assets: if you bought this book new as part of a set, scan the QR code on the front of the book set's slipcase and enter the unique code there; if you bought this book separately, instead go to **www.kaptest.com/moreonline**.
- ☐ Create a study calendar that ensures you complete content review and sufficient practice by Test Day!
- ☐ As you finish a chapter and the online practice for that chapter, check it off on the table of contents.
- ☐ Register to take the MCAT at **www.aamc.org/mcat.**
- ☐ Set aside time during your prep to make sure the rest of your application—personal statement, recommendations, and other materials—is ready to go!
- ☐ Take a moment to admire your completed checklist, then get back to the business of prepping for this exam!

PREFACE

And now it starts: your long, yet fruitful journey toward wearing a white coat. Proudly wearing that white coat, though, is hopefully only part of your motivation. You are reading this book because you want to be a healer.

If you're serious about going to medical school, then you are likely already familiar with the importance of the MCAT in medical school admissions. While the holistic review process puts additional weight on your experiences, extracurricular activities, and personal attributes, the fact remains: along with your GPA, your MCAT score remains one of the two most important components of your application portfolio—at least early in the admissions process. Each additional point you score on the MCAT pushes you in front of thousands of other students and makes you an even more attractive applicant. But the MCAT is not simply an obstacle to overcome; it is an opportunity to show schools that you will be a strong student and a future leader in medicine.

We at Kaplan take our jobs very seriously and aim to help students see success not only on the MCAT, but as future physicians. We work with our learning science experts to ensure that we're using the most up-to-date teaching techniques in our resources. Multiple members of our team hold advanced degrees in medicine or associated biomedical sciences, and are committed to the highest level of medical education. Kaplan has been working with the MCAT for over 50 years and our commitment to premed students is unflagging; in fact, Stanley Kaplan created this company when he had difficulty being accepted to medical school due to unfair quota systems that existed at the time.

We stand now at the beginning of a new era in medical education. As citizens of this 21st-century world of healthcare, we are charged with creating a patient-oriented, culturally competent, cost-conscious, universally available, technically advanced, and research-focused healthcare system, run by compassionate providers. Suffice it to say, this is no easy task. Problem-based learning, integrated curricula, and classes in interpersonal skills are some of the responses to this demand for an excellent workforce—a workforce of which you'll soon be a part.

We're thrilled that you've chosen us to help you on this journey. Please reach out to us to share your challenges, concerns, and successes. Together, we will shape the future of medicine in the United States and abroad; we look forward to helping you become the doctor you deserve to be.

Good luck!

Alexander Stone Macnow, MD
Editor-in-Chief
Department of Pathology and Laboratory Medicine
Hospital of the University of Pennsylvania

BA, Musicology—Boston University, 2008
MD—Perelman School of Medicine at the University of Pennsylvania, 2013

ABOUT THE MCAT

Anatomy of the MCAT

Here is a general overview of the structure of Test Day:

Section	Number of Questions	Time Allotted
Test-Day Certification		4 minutes
Tutorial (optional)		10 minutes
Chemical and Physical Foundations of Biological Systems	59	95 minutes
Break (optional)		10 minutes
Critical Analysis and Reasoning Skills (CARS)	53	90 minutes
Lunch Break (optional)		30 minutes
Biological and Biochemical Foundations of Living Systems	59	95 minutes
Break (optional)		10 minutes
Psychological, Social, and Biological Foundations of Behavior	59	95 minutes
Void Question		3 minutes
Satisfaction Survey (optional)		5 minutes

The structure of the four sections of the MCAT is shown below.

Chemical and Physical Foundations of Biological Systems	
Time	95 minutes
Format	• 59 questions • 10 passages • 44 questions are passage-based, and 15 are discrete (stand-alone) questions. • Score between 118 and 132
What It Tests	• Biochemistry: 25% • Biology: 5% • General Chemistry: 30% • Organic Chemistry: 15% • Physics: 25%

Critical Analysis and Reasoning Skills (CARS)	
Time	90 minutes
Format	• 53 questions • 9 passages • All questions are passage-based. There are no discrete (stand-alone) questions. • Score between 118 and 132
What It Tests	Disciplines: • Humanities: 50% • Social Sciences: 50% Skills: • *Foundations of Comprehension: 30%* • *Reasoning Within the Text: 30%* • *Reasoning Beyond the Text: 40%*
Biological and Biochemical Foundations of Living Systems	
Time	95 minutes
Format	• 59 questions • 10 passages • 44 questions are passage-based, and 15 are discrete (stand-alone) questions. • Score between 118 and 132
What It Tests	• Biochemistry: 25% • Biology: 65% • General Chemistry: 5% • Organic Chemistry: 5%
Psychological, Social, and Biological Foundations of Behavior	
Time	95 minutes
Format	• 59 questions • 10 passages • 44 questions are passage-based, and 15 are discrete (stand-alone) questions. • Score between 118 and 132
What It Tests	• Biology: 5% • Psychology: 65% • Sociology: 30%
Total	
Testing Time	375 minutes (6 hours, 15 minutes)
Total Seat Time	447 minutes (7 hours, 27 minutes)
Questions	230
Score	472 to 528

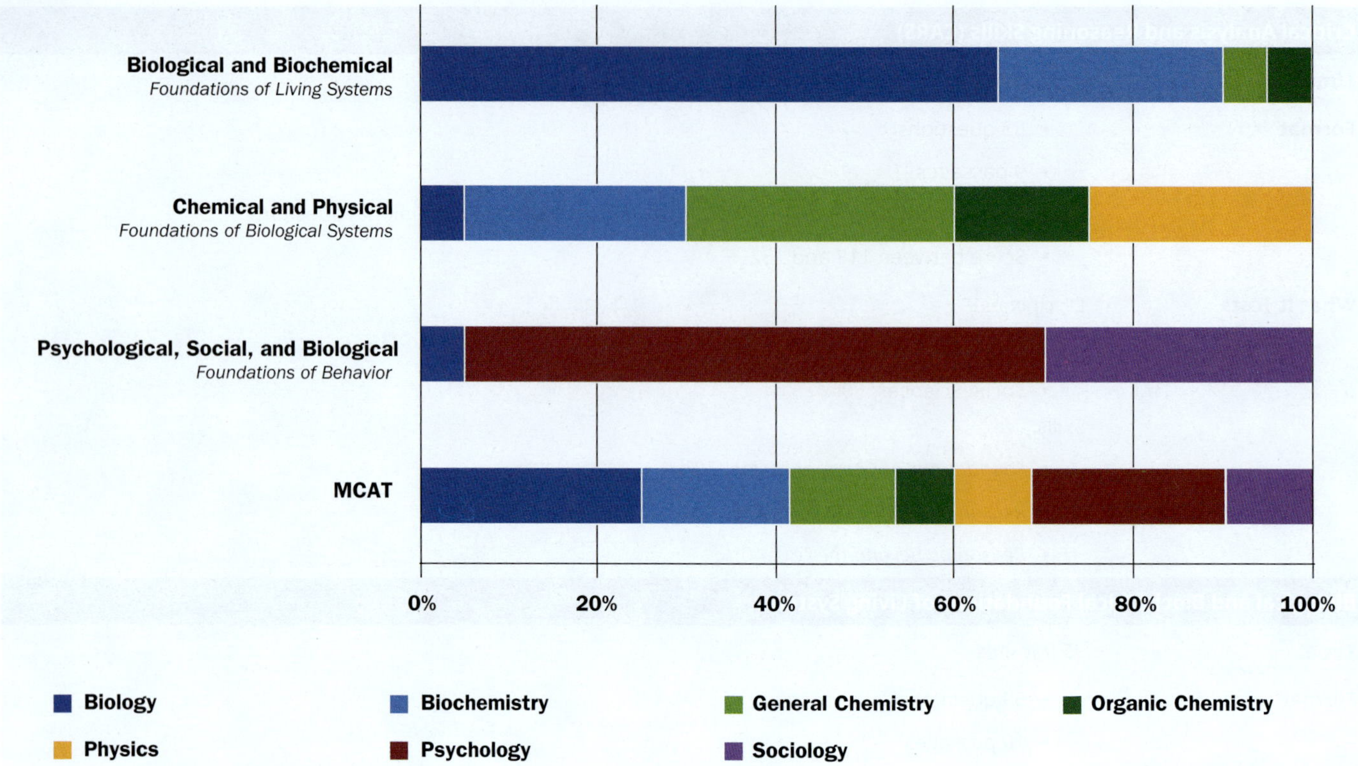

Scientific Inquiry and Reasoning Skills (SIRS)

The AAMC has defined four *Scientific Inquiry and Reasoning Skills* (SIRS) that will be tested in the three science sections of the MCAT:

1. *Knowledge of Scientific Concepts and Principles* (35% of questions)
2. *Scientific Reasoning and Problem-Solving* (45% of questions)
3. *Reasoning About the Design and Execution of Research* (10% of questions)
4. *Data-Based and Statistical Reasoning* (10% of questions)

Let's see how each one breaks down into more specific Test Day behaviors. Note that the bullet points of specific objectives for each of the SIRS are taken directly from the *Official Guide to the MCAT Exam*; the descriptions of what these behaviors mean and sample question stems, however, are written by Kaplan.

Skill 1: *Knowledge of Scientific Concepts and Principles*

This is probably the least surprising of the four SIRS; the testing of science knowledge is, after all, one of the signature qualities of the MCAT. Skill 1 questions will require you to do the following:

- Recognize correct scientific principles
- Identify the relationships among closely related concepts
- Identify the relationships between different representations of concepts (verbal, symbolic, graphic)
- Identify examples of observations that illustrate scientific principles
- Use mathematical equations to solve problems

At Kaplan, we simply call these Science Knowledge or Skill 1 questions. Another way to think of Skill 1 questions is as "one-step" problems. The single step is either to realize which scientific concept the question stem is suggesting or to take the concept stated in the question stem and identify which answer choice is an accurate application of it. Skill 1 questions are particularly prominent among discrete questions (those not associated with a passage). These questions are an opportunity to gain quick points on Test Day—if you know the science concept attached to the question, then that's it! On Test Day, 35% of the questions in each science section will be Skill 1 questions.

Here are some sample Skill 1 question stems:

- How would a proponent of the James–Lange theory of emotion interpret the findings of the study cited in the passage?
- Which of the following most accurately describes the function of FSH in the human menstrual cycle?
- If the products of Reaction 1 and Reaction 2 were combined in solution, the resulting reaction would form:
- Ionic bonds are maintained by which of the following forces?

Skill 2: *Scientific Reasoning and Problem-Solving*

The MCAT science sections do, of course, move beyond testing straightforward science knowledge; Skill 2 questions are the most common way in which it does so. At Kaplan, we also call these Critical Thinking questions. Skill 2 questions will require you to do the following:

- Reason about scientific principles, theories, and models
- Analyze and evaluate scientific explanations and predictions
- Evaluate arguments about causes and consequences
- Bring together theory, observations, and evidence to draw conclusions
- Recognize scientific findings that challenge or invalidate a scientific theory or model
- Determine and use scientific formulas to solve problems

Just as Skill 1 questions can be thought of as "one-step" problems, many Skill 2 questions are "two-step" problems, and more difficult Skill 2 questions may require three or more steps. These questions can require a wide spectrum of reasoning skills, including integration of multiple facts from a passage, combination of multiple science content areas, and prediction of an experiment's results. Skill 2 questions also tend to ask about science content without actually mentioning it by name. For example, a question might describe the results of one experiment and ask you to predict the results of a second experiment without actually telling you what underlying scientific principles are at work—part of the question's difficulty will be figuring out which principles to apply in order to get the correct answer. On Test Day, 45% of the questions in each science section will be Skill 2 questions.

Here are some sample Skill 2 question stems:

- Which of the following experimental conditions would most likely yield results similar to those in Figure 2?
- All of the following conclusions are supported by the information in the passage EXCEPT:
- The most likely cause of the anomalous results found by the experimenter is:
- An impact to a person's chest quickly reduces the volume of one of the lungs to 70% of its initial value while not allowing any air to escape from the mouth. By what percentage is the force of outward air pressure increased on a 2 cm^2 portion of the inner surface of the compressed lung?

Skill 3: *Reasoning About the Design and Execution of Research*

The MCAT is interested in your ability to critically appraise and analyze research, as this is an important day-to-day task of a physician. We call these questions Skill 3 or Experimental and Research Design questions for short. Skill 3 questions will require you to do the following:

- Identify the role of theory, past findings, and observations in scientific questioning
- Identify testable research questions and hypotheses
- Distinguish between samples and populations and distinguish results that support generalizations about populations
- Identify independent and dependent variables
- Reason about the features of research studies that suggest associations between variables or causal relationships between them (such as temporality and random assignment)
- Identify conclusions that are supported by research results
- Determine the implications of results for real-world situations
- Reason about ethical issues in scientific research

Over the years, the AAMC has received input from medical schools to require more practical research skills of MCAT test takers, and Skill 3 questions are the response to these demands. This skill is unique in that the outside knowledge you need to answer Skill 3 questions is not taught in any one undergraduate course; instead, the research design principles needed to answer these questions are learned gradually throughout your science classes and especially through any laboratory work you have completed. It should be noted that Skill 3 comprises 10% of the questions in each science section on Test Day.

Here are some sample Skill 3 question stems:

- What is the dependent variable in the study described in the passage?
- The major flaw in the method used to measure disease susceptibility in Experiment 1 is:
- Which of the following procedures is most important for the experimenters to follow in order for their study to maintain a proper, randomized sample of research subjects?
- A researcher would like to test the hypothesis that individuals who move to an urban area during adulthood are more likely to own a car than are those who have lived in an urban area since birth. Which of the following studies would best test this hypothesis?

Skill 4: *Data-Based and Statistical Reasoning*

Lastly, the science sections of the MCAT test your ability to analyze the visual and numerical results of experiments and studies. We call these Data and Statistical Analysis questions. Skill 4 questions will require you to do the following:

- Use, analyze, and interpret data in figures, graphs, and tables
- Evaluate whether representations make sense for particular scientific observations and data
- Use measures of central tendency (mean, median, and mode) and measures of dispersion (range, interquartile range, and standard deviation) to describe data
- Reason about random and systematic error

- Reason about statistical significance and uncertainty (interpreting statistical significance levels and interpreting a confidence interval)
- Use data to explain relationships between variables or make predictions
- Use data to answer research questions and draw conclusions

Skill 4 is included in the MCAT because physicians and researchers spend much of their time examining the results of their own studies and the studies of others, and it's very important for them to make legitimate conclusions and sound judgments based on that data. The MCAT tests Skill 4 on all three science sections with graphical representations of data (charts and bar graphs), as well as numerical ones (tables, lists, and results summarized in sentence or paragraph form). On Test Day, 10% of the questions in each science section will be Skill 4 questions.

Here are some sample Skill 4 question stems:

- According to the information in the passage, there is an inverse correlation between:
- What conclusion is best supported by the findings displayed in Figure 2?
- A medical test for a rare type of heavy metal poisoning returns a positive result for 98% of affected individuals and 13% of unaffected individuals. Which of the following types of errors is most prevalent in this test?
- If a fourth trial of Experiment 1 was run and yielded a result of 54% compliance, which of the following would be true?

SIRS Summary

Discussing the SIRS tested on the MCAT is a daunting prospect given that the very nature of the skills tends to make the conversation rather abstract. Nevertheless, with enough practice, you'll be able to identify each of the four skills quickly, and you'll also be able to apply the proper strategies to solve those problems on Test Day. If you need a quick reference to remind you of the four SIRS, these guidelines may help:

Skill 1 (**Science Knowledge**) questions ask:

- Do you remember this science content?

Skill 2 (**Critical Thinking**) questions ask:

- Do you remember this science content? And if you do, could you please apply it to this novel situation?
- Could you answer this question that cleverly combines multiple content areas at the same time?

Skill 3 (**Experimental and Research Design**) questions ask:

- Let's forget about the science content for a while. Could you give some insight into the experimental or research methods involved in this situation?

Skill 4 (**Data and Statistical Analysis**) questions ask:

- Let's forget about the science content for a while. Could you accurately read some graphs and tables for a moment? Could you make some conclusions or extrapolations based on the information presented?

Critical Analysis and Reasoning Skills (CARS)

The *Critical Analysis and Reasoning Skills* (CARS) section of the MCAT tests three discrete families of textual reasoning skills; each of these families requires a higher level of reasoning than the last. Those three skills are as follows:

1. *Foundations of Comprehension* (30% of questions)
2. *Reasoning Within the Text* (30% of questions)
3. *Reasoning Beyond the Text* (40% of questions)

These three categories of skills are tested through nine humanities- and social sciences-themed passages, with approximately 5 to 7 questions per passage. Let's take a more in-depth look into these three types. Again, the bullet points of specific objectives for each of the CARS are taken directly from the *Official Guide to the MCAT Exam*; the descriptions of what these behaviors mean and sample question stems, however, are written by Kaplan.

Foundations of Comprehension

Questions in this category will ask for basic facts and simple inferences about the passage; the questions themselves will be similar to those seen on reading comprehension sections of other standardized exams like the SAT® and ACT®. *Foundations of Comprehension* questions will require you to do the following:

- Understand the basic components of the text
- Infer meaning from rhetorical devices, word choice, and text structure

This covers a wide range of question skills (Summarize Text, Recognize Opinion, Paraphrase Detail, and Interpret Meaning), but finding the correct answer to all *Foundations of Comprehension* questions will follow from a basic understanding of the passage and the point of view of its author (and occasionally that of other voices in the passage). Because these questions tend to avoid digging too deeply into the passage, Kaplan calls these *surface* questions.

Here are some sample *Foundations of Comprehension* question stems:

- **Summarize Text**—The author's primary thesis in this passage is:
- **Recognize Opinion**—Based on the information in the second paragraph, which of the following is the most accurate summary of the opinion held by Schubert's critics?
- **Paraphrase Detail**—According to the passage, which of the following is FALSE about literary reviews in the 1920s?
- **Interpret Meaning**—The word "obscure" (paragraph 3), when used in reference to the historian's actions, most nearly means:

Reasoning Within the Text

While *Foundations of Comprehension* questions will usually depend on interpreting a single piece of information in the passage or understanding the passage as a whole, *Reasoning Within the Text* questions require more thought because they will ask you to identify the purpose of a particular piece of information in the context of the passage, or ask how one piece of information relates to another. *Reasoning Within the Text* questions will require you to:

- Integrate different components of the text to draw relevant conclusions

In other words, questions in this type often ask either *How do these two details relate to one another?* or *What else must be true that the author didn't say?* The CARS section will also ask you to judge certain parts of the passage or even judge the author. These questions, which fall under the *Reasoning Within the Text* skill, can ask you to identify authorial bias, evaluate the credibility of cited sources, determine the logical soundness of an argument, identify the importance of a particular fact or statement in the context of the passage, or search for relevant evidence in the passage to support a given conclusion. This category, which Kaplan refers to as *deep* questions because of their tendency to venture into the deep reasoning of the passage, encompasses the following skills: Describe Purpose, Evaluate Reasoning, and Make Deduction.

Here are some sample *Reasoning Within the Text* question stems:

- **Describe Purpose**—The author's discussion of the effect of socioeconomic status on social mobility primarily serves which of the following functions?
- **Evaluate Reasoning**—Which of the following facts is used in the passage as the most prominent piece of evidence in favor of the author's conclusions?
- **Make Deduction**—In putting together the argument in the passage, the author most likely assumes:

Reasoning Beyond the Text

The distinguishing factor of *Reasoning Beyond the Text* questions is in the title of the category: the word *Beyond*. Questions of this type, which make up a larger share of the CARS section than questions from either of the other two types, will always introduce a completely new situation that was not present in the passage itself; these questions will ask you to determine how one influences the other. *Reasoning Beyond the Text* questions will require you to:

- Apply or extrapolate ideas from the passage to new contexts
- Assess the impact of introducing new factors, information, or conditions to ideas from the passage

Because they always introduce ideas not discussed in the passage, Kaplan refers to these as *new info* questions. They test the following skills: Anticipate Response, Predict Outcome/Explanation, Imagine Example/Analogy, and Strengthen/Weaken Argument.

Here are some sample *Reasoning Beyond the Text* question stems:

- **Anticipate Response**—If a document were located that demonstrated Berlioz intended to include a chorus of at least 700 in his *Grande Messe des Morts*, how would the author likely respond?
- **Imagine Example/Analogy**—Which of the following is the best example of a "virtuous rebellion," as it is defined in the passage?
- **Predict Outcome/Explanation**—Extending the author's discussion of ancient Greek history, a conflict between a democracy and an oligarchy would most likely result in:
- **Strengthen/Weaken Argument**—Which of the following sentences, if added to the end of the passage, would most WEAKEN the author's conclusions in the last paragraph?

CARS Summary

Through the *Foundations of Comprehension* category of skills, the CARS section tests many of the reading skills you have been building on since grade school, albeit in the context of very challenging doctorate-level passages. But through the two other categories (*Reasoning Within the Text* and *Reasoning Beyond the Text*), the MCAT demands that you understand the deep structure of passages and the arguments within them at an advanced level. And, of course, all of this is tested under very tight timing restrictions: only 102 seconds per question—and that doesn't even include the time spent reading the passages.

Here's a quick reference guide to the three categories and 11 skills tested in CARS:

Foundations of Comprehension skills:

- Interpret Meaning: Use context to determine what a word/phrase from the passage is intended to communicate.
- Recognize Opinion: Identify what the author or someone else feels about a passage idea based on word choice or other context clues.
- Paraphrase Detail: Recognize a specific piece of information that is stated or strongly implied at one location in the passage.
- Summarize Text: Articulate the main idea of the passage or of a part of it.

Reasoning Within the Text skills:

- Describe Purpose: Identify why the author wrote the passage or a part of it.
- Evaluate Reasoning: Characterize logical connections between ideas in the passage.
- Make Deduction: Infer a claim that follows from multiple parts of the passage, such as an assumption in an argument.

Reasoning Beyond the Text skills:

- Anticipate Response: Identify what the author or someone else would feel/say/do about a new situation based on its similarities to passage ideas.
- Predict Outcome/Explanation: Apply causal reasoning or another connection from the passage to a new situation.
- Strengthen/Weaken Argument: Characterize the logical relationship between a new claim and arguments from the passage.
- Imagine Example/Analogy: Identify new examples of categories defined in the passage or analogies of passage concepts.

Scoring

Each of the four sections of the MCAT is scored between 118 and 132, with the median at approximately 125. This means the total score ranges from 472 to 528, with the median at about 500. Why such peculiar numbers? The AAMC stresses that this scale emphasizes the importance of the central portion of the score distribution, where most students score (around 125 per section, or 500 total), rather than putting undue focus on the high end of the scale.

Note that there is no wrong answer penalty on the MCAT, so you should select an answer for every question—even if it is only a guess.

The AAMC has released the 2022–2024 correlation between scaled score and percentile, as shown on the following page. It should be noted that the percentile scale is adjusted and renormalized over time and thus can shift slightly from year to year. Percentile rank updates are released by the AAMC around May 1 of each year.

Total Score	Percentile	Total Score	Percentile
528	100	499	46
527	100	498	42
526	100	497	39
525	100	496	36
524	100	495	34
523	99	494	31
522	99	493	28
521	98	492	25
520	97	491	23
519	96	490	21
518	95	489	18
517	94	488	16
516	92	487	14
515	91	486	12
514	89	485	11
513	87	484	9
512	84	483	8
511	82	482	6
510	79	481	5
509	77	480	4
508	74	479	3
507	71	478	2
506	68	477	2
505	65	476	1
504	62	475	1
503	58	474	<1
502	55	473	<1
501	52	472	<1
500	49		

Source: AAMC. 2025. *Summary of MCAT Total and Section Scores.* Accessed October 2025.
https://students-residents.aamc.org/mcat-research-and-data/percentile-ranks-mcat-exam

Further information on score reporting is included at the end of the next section (see *After Your Test*).

MCAT Policies and Procedures

We strongly encourage you to download the latest copy of *MCAT® Essentials*, available on the AAMC's website, to ensure that you have the latest information about registration and Test Day policies and procedures; this document is updated annually. A brief summary of some of the most important rules is provided here.

MCAT Registration

The only way to register for the MCAT is online. You can access AAMC's registration system at **www.aamc.org/mcat**.

The AAMC posts the schedule of testing, registration, and score release dates in the fall before the MCAT testing year, which runs from January into September. See the AAMC's website for the exact dates that registration opens each year. There is one standard registration fee, but the fee for changing your test date or test center increases the closer you get to your MCAT.

Fees and the Fee Assistance Program (FAP)

Payment for test registration must be made by American Express, Discover, MasterCard, or VISA. As described earlier, the fee for rescheduling your exam or changing your testing center increases as one approaches Test Day. In addition, it is not uncommon for test centers to fill up well in advance of the registration deadline. For these reasons, we recommend identifying your preferred Test Day as soon as possible and registering. There are ancillary benefits to having a set Test Day, as well: when you know the date you're working toward, you'll study harder and are less likely to keep pushing back the exam. The AAMC offers a Fee Assistance Program (FAP) for students with financial hardship to help reduce the cost of taking the MCAT, as well as for the American Medical College Application Service (AMCAS®) application. Further information on the FAP can be found at **www.aamc.org/students/applying/fap**.

Testing Security

On Test Day, you will be required to present a qualifying form of ID. Generally, a current driver's license or United States passport will be sufficient (consult the AAMC website for the full list of qualifying criteria). When registering, take care to spell your first and last names (middle names, suffixes, and prefixes are not required and will not be verified on Test Day) precisely the same as they appear on this ID; failure to provide this ID at the test center or differences in spelling between your registration and ID will be considered a "no-show," and you will not receive a refund for the exam.

During Test Day registration, other identity data collected may include: a digital palm vein scan, a Test Day photo, a digitization of your valid ID, and signatures. Some testing centers may use a metal detection wand to ensure that no prohibited items are brought into the testing room. Prohibited items include all electronic devices, including watches and timers, calculators, cell phones, and any and all forms of recording equipment; food, drinks (including water), and cigarettes or other smoking paraphernalia; hats and scarves (except for religious purposes); and books, notes, or other study materials. If you require a medical device, such as an insulin pump or pacemaker, you must apply for accommodated testing. During breaks, you are allowed access to food and drink, but not to electronic devices, including cell phones.

Testing centers are under video surveillance and the AAMC does not take potential violations of testing security lightly. The bottom line: *know the rules and don't break them.*

Accommodations

Students with disabilities or medical conditions can apply for accommodated testing. Documentation of the disability or condition is required, and requests may take two months—or more—to be approved. For this reason, it is recommended that you begin the process of applying for accommodated testing as early as possible. More information on applying for accommodated testing can be found at **www.aamc.org/students/applying/mcat/accommodations.**

After Your Test

When your MCAT is all over, no matter how you feel you did, be good to yourself when you leave the test center. Celebrate! Take a nap. Watch a movie. Get some exercise. Plan a trip or outing. Call up all of your neglected friends or message them on social media. Go out for snacks or drinks with people you like. Whatever you do, make sure that it has absolutely nothing to do with thinking too hard—you deserve some rest and relaxation.

Perhaps most importantly, do not discuss specific details about the test with anyone. For one, it is important to let go of the stress of Test Day, and reliving your exam only inhibits you from being able to do so. But more significantly, the Examinee Agreement you sign at the beginning of your exam specifically prohibits you from discussing or disclosing exam content. The AAMC is known to seek out individuals who violate this agreement and retains the right to prosecute these individuals at their discretion. This means that you should not, under any circumstances, discuss the exam in person or over the phone with other individuals—including us at Kaplan—or post information or questions about exam content to Facebook, Student Doctor Network, or other online social media. You are permitted to comment on your "general exam experience," including how you felt about the exam overall or an individual section, but this is a fine line. In summary: *if you're not certain whether you can discuss an aspect of the test or not, just don't do it!* Do not let a silly Facebook post stop you from becoming the doctor you deserve to be.

Scores are typically released approximately one month after Test Day. The release is staggered during the afternoon and evening, ending at 5 p.m. Eastern Standard Time. This means that not all examinees receive their scores at exactly the same time. Your score report will include a scaled score for each section between 118 and 132, as well as your total combined score between 472 and 528. These scores are given as confidence intervals. For each section, the confidence interval is approximately the given score ± 1; for the total score, it is approximately the given score ± 2. You will also be given the corresponding percentile rank for each of these section scores and the total score.

AAMC Contact Information

For further questions, contact the MCAT team at the Association of American Medical Colleges:

MCAT Resource Center
Association of American Medical Colleges
www.aamc.org/mcat
(202) 828-0600
www.aamc.org/contactmcat

HOW THIS BOOK WAS CREATED

The *Kaplan MCAT Review* project began shortly after the release of the *Preview Guide for the MCAT 2015 Exam*, 2nd edition. Through thorough analysis by our staff psychometricians, we were able to analyze the relative yield of the different topics on the MCAT, and we began constructing tables of contents for the books of the *Kaplan MCAT Review* series. A dedicated staff of 30 writers, 7 editors, and 32 proofreaders worked over 5,000 combined hours to produce these books. The format of the books was heavily influenced by weekly meetings with Kaplan's learning science team.

In the years since this book was created, a number of opportunities for expansion and improvement have occurred. This edition is the product of our largest revision since the series' creation more than a decade ago.

To better accommodate students who prefer learning visually, our six science titles have added more than 500 new images and updated more than a hundred existing figures. All of these new images were chosen by an expert team of MCAT faculty members, led by veteran teachers and tutors with advanced science or medical degrees. Our objective with these new images was not to add visual flair but to enhance student learning outcomes. Toward that end, our team of medical illustrators partnered with our MCAT experts to ensure scientific accuracy and relevance for the exam.

On top of this extensive science image expansion, we completely rewrote *Critical Analysis and Reasoning Skills Review* based on what we've learned from more than ten years of helping students improve on the CARS section in our classrooms. In addition to this collective experience, internal data suggests that our new approach is more effective at helping students get higher CARS scores. Our streamlined and simplified CARS strategies accompany an extended focus on the critical thinking skills tested on the exam, best embodied by our new Skillbuilder activities that enable targeted skill practice in a lower pressure setting.

These books were submitted for publication in January 2026. For any updates after this date, please visit www.kaptest.com/retail-book-corrections-and-updates.

If you have any questions about the content presented here, email KaplanMCATfeedback@kaplan.com. For other questions not related to content, email booksupport@kaplan.com.

Each book has been vetted through at least ten rounds of review. To that end, the information presented in these books is true and accurate to the best of our knowledge. Still, your feedback helps us improve our prep materials. Please notify us of any inaccuracies or errors in the books by sending an email to KaplanMCATfeedback@kaplan.com.

USING THIS BOOK

Kaplan MCAT Biology Review, and the other six books in the *Kaplan MCAT Review* series, bring the Kaplan classroom experience to you—right in your home, at your convenience. This book offers the same Kaplan content review, strategies, and practice that make Kaplan the #1 choice for MCAT prep.

This book is designed to help you review the biology topics covered on the MCAT. Please understand that content review—no matter how thorough—is not sufficient preparation for the MCAT! The MCAT tests not only your science knowledge but also your critical reading, reasoning, and problem-solving skills. Do not assume that simply memorizing the contents of this book will earn you high scores on Test Day; to maximize your scores, you must also improve your reading and test-taking skills through MCAT-style questions and practice tests.

Learning Objectives

At the beginning of each section, you'll find a short list of objectives describing the skills covered within that section. Learning objectives for these texts were developed in conjunction with Kaplan's learning science team, and have been designed specifically to focus your attention on tasks and concepts that are likely to show up on your MCAT. These learning objectives will function as a means to guide your study, and indicate what information and relationships you should be focused on within each section. Before starting each section, read these learning objectives carefully. They will not only allow you to assess your existing familiarity with the content, but also provide a goal-oriented focus for your studying experience of the section.

MCAT Concept Checks

At the end of each section, you'll find a few open-ended questions that you can use to assess your mastery of the material. These MCAT Concept Checks were introduced after numerous conversations with Kaplan's learning science team. Research has demonstrated repeatedly that introspection and self-analysis improve mastery, retention, and recall of material. Complete these MCAT Concept Checks to ensure that you've got the key points from each section before moving on!

Science Mastery Assessments

At the beginning of each chapter, you'll find 15 concept-focused multiple-choice questions. These are designed to help you assess your understanding of the chapter before you begin reading the chapter. Using the guidance provided with the assessment, you can determine the best way to review each chapter based on your personal strengths and weaknesses. Most of the questions in the Science Mastery Assessments focus on the first of the *Scientific Inquiry and Reasoning Skills* (*Knowledge of Scientific Concepts and Principles*), although there are occasional questions that fall into the second or fourth SIRS (*Scientific Reasoning and Problem-Solving* and *Data-Based and Statistical Reasoning*, respectively). You can complete each chapter's assessment in a testing interface in your online resources, where you'll also find a test-like passage set covering the same content you just studied to ensure you can also apply your knowledge the way the MCAT will expect you to!

Guided Examples with Expert Thinking

Embedded in each chapter of this book is a Guided Example with Expert Thinking. These examples will be located adjacent to the content that they are related to, and contain an MCAT-like scientific article as a passage. Read through the passage as you would on the real MCAT, referring to the Expert Thinking material to the right of the passage to clarify the key information you should be gathering from each paragraph. Read and attempt to answer the associated question once you have worked through the passage. There is a full explanation, including the correct answer, following the question given. These passages and questions are designed to help build your critical thinking, experimental reasoning, and data interpretation skills as preparation for the challenges you will face on the MCAT.

Sidebars

The following is a guide to the five types of sidebars you'll find in *Kaplan MCAT Biology Review:*

- **Bridge:** These sidebars create connections between science topics that appear in multiple chapters throughout the *Kaplan MCAT Review* series.
- **Key Concept:** These sidebars draw attention to the most important takeaways in a given topic, and they sometimes offer synopses or overviews of complex information. If you understand nothing else, make sure you grasp the Key Concepts for any given subject.
- **MCAT Expertise:** These sidebars point out how information may be tested on the MCAT or offer key strategy points and test-taking tips that you should apply on Test Day.
- **Mnemonic:** These sidebars present memory devices to help recall certain facts.
- **Real World:** These sidebars illustrate how a concept in the text relates to the practice of medicine or the world at large. While this is not information you need to know for Test Day, many of the topics in Real World sidebars are excellent examples of how a concept may appear in a passage or discrete (stand-alone) question on the MCAT.

What This Book Covers

The information presented in the *Kaplan MCAT Review* series covers everything listed on the official MCAT content lists. Every topic in these lists is covered in the same level of detail as is common to the undergraduate and postbaccalaureate classes that are considered prerequisites for the MCAT. Note that your premedical classes may include topics not discussed in these books, or they may go into more depth than these books do. Additional exposure to science content is never a bad thing, but all of the content knowledge you are expected to have walking in on Test Day is covered in these books.

Chapter Profiles, on the first page of each chapter, represent a holistic look at the content within the chapter, and will include a pie chart as well as text information. The pie chart analysis is based directly on data released by the AAMC, and will give a rough estimate of the importance of the chapter in relation to the book as a whole. Further, the text portion of the Chapter Profiles includes which AAMC content categories are covered within the chapter. These are referenced directly from the AAMC MCAT exam content listing, available on the testmaker's website.

You'll also see High-Yield badges scattered throughout the sections of this book:

In This Chapter

1.1 Amino Acids Found in Proteins High Yield

LEARNING OBJECTIVES

After Chapter 1.1, you will be able to:

These badges represent the top 100 topics most tested by the AAMC. In other words, according to the testmaker and all our experience with their resources, a High-Yield badge means more questions on Test Day.

This book also contains a thorough glossary and index for easy navigation of the text.

In the end, this is your book, so write in the margins, draw diagrams, highlight the key points—do whatever is necessary to help you get that higher score. We look forward to working with you as you achieve your dreams and become the doctor you deserve to be!

Studying with This Book

In addition to providing you with the best practice questions and test strategies, Kaplan's team of learning scientists are dedicated to researching and testing the best methods for getting the most out of your study time. Here are their top four tips for improving retention:

Review multiple topics in one study session. This may seem counterintuitive—we're used to practicing one skill at a time in order to improve each skill. But research shows that weaving topics together leads to increased learning. Beyond that consideration, the MCAT often includes more than one topic in a single question. Studying in an integrated manner is the most effective way to prepare for this test.

Customize the content. Drawing attention to difficult or critical content can ensure you don't overlook it as you read and re-read sections. The best way to do this is to make it more visual—highlight, make tabs, use stickies, whatever works. We recommend highlighting only the most important or difficult sections of text. Selective highlighting of up to about 10% of text in a given chapter is great for emphasizing parts of the text, but over-highlighting can have the opposite effect.

Repeat topics over time. Many people try to memorize concepts by repeating them over and over again in succession. Our research shows that retention is improved by spacing out the repeats over time and mixing up the order in which you study content. For example, try reading chapters in a different order the second (or third!) time around. Revisit practice questions that you answered incorrectly in a new sequence. Perhaps information you reviewed more recently will help you better understand those questions and solutions you struggled with in the past.

Take a moment to reflect. When you finish reading a section for the first time, stop and think about what you just read. Jot down a few thoughts in the margins or in your notes about why the content is important or what topics came to mind when you read it. Associating learning with a memory is a fantastic way to retain information! This also works when answering questions. After answering a question, take a moment to think through each step you took to arrive at a solution. What led you to the answer you chose? Understanding the steps you took will help you make good decisions when answering future questions.

Online Resources

In addition to the resources located within this text, you also have online resources awaiting you. If you purchased this book as part of a 7-book set, scan the QR code that appears on your slipcase (the illustrated box that originally contained the books) and enter your unique access code, which appears on a sticker on the front of that slipcase. If you purchased this book separately, book-specific resources are available at **www.kaptest.com/booksonline**. Make sure to log on and take advantage of free practice and access to other resources!

Please note that access to the online resources is limited to the original owner of this book.

STUDYING FOR THE MCAT

The first year of medical school is a frenzied experience for most students. To meet the requirements of a rigorous work schedule, students either learn to prioritize their time or else fall hopelessly behind. It's no surprise, then, that the MCAT, the test specifically designed to predict success in medical school, is a high-speed, time-intensive test. The MCAT demands excellent time-management skills, endurance, and grace under pressure both during the test as well as while preparing for it. Having a solid plan of attack and sticking with it are key to giving you the confidence and structure you need to succeed.

Creating a Study Plan

The best time to create a study plan is at the beginning of your MCAT preparation. If you don't already use a calendar, you will want to start. You can purchase a planner, print out a free calendar from the Internet, use a built-in calendar or app on one of your smart devices, or keep track using an interactive online calendar. Pick the option that is most practical for you and that you are most likely to use consistently. If you purchased this book new as part of a set, your online resources come with a study plan to space out your readings, chapter quizzes, full-length practice tests, and other study materials (see the previous page for how to log on).

Once you have a calendar, you'll be able to start planning your study schedule with the following steps:

1. **Fill in your obligations and choose a day off.**

   Write in all your school, extracurricular, and work obligations first: class sessions, work shifts, and meetings that you must attend. Then add in your personal obligations: appointments, lunch dates, family and social time, etc. Making an appointment in your calendar for hanging out with friends or going to the movies may seem strange at first, but planning social activities in advance will help you achieve a balance between personal and professional obligations even as life gets busy. Having a happy balance allows you to be more focused and productive when it comes time to study, so stay well-rounded and don't neglect anything that is important to you.

   In addition to scheduling your personal and professional obligations, you should also plan your time off. Taking some time off is just as important as studying. Kaplan recommends taking at least one full day off per week, ideally from all your study obligations but at minimum from studying for the MCAT.

2. **Add in study blocks around your obligations.**

   Once you have established your calendar's framework, add in study blocks around your obligations, keeping your study schedule as consistent as possible across days and across weeks. Studying at the same time of day as your official test is ideal for promoting recall, but if that's not possible, then fit in study blocks wherever you can.

   To make your studying as efficient as possible, block out short, frequent periods of study time throughout the week. From a learning perspective, studying one hour per day for six days per week is much more valuable than studying for six hours all at once one day per week. Specifically, Kaplan recommends studying for no longer than three hours in one sitting. Within those three-hour blocks, also plan to take ten-minute breaks every hour. Use these breaks to get up from your seat, do some quick stretches, get a snack and drink, and clear your mind. Although ten minutes of break for every 50 minutes of studying may sound like a lot, these breaks will allow you to deal with distractions and rest your brain so that, during the 50-minute study blocks, you can remain fully engaged and completely focused.

3. **Add in your full-length practice tests.**

   Next, you'll want to add in full-length practice tests. You'll want to take one test very early in your prep and then spread your remaining full-length practice tests evenly between now and your test date. Staggering tests in this way allows you to form a baseline for comparison and to determine which areas to focus on right away, while also providing realistic feedback throughout your prep as to how you will perform on Test Day.

When planning your calendar, aim to finish your full-length practice tests and the majority of your studying by one week before Test Day, which will allow you to spend that final week completing a final, brief review of what you already know. In your online resources, you'll find a sample study calendar to use as a starting point. This sample calendar may include more focus than you need in some areas, and less in others, and it may not fit your timeline to Test Day. You will need to customize your study calendar to your needs using the steps above.

The total amount of time you spend studying each week will depend on your schedule, your personal prep needs, and your time to Test Day, but it is recommended that you spend somewhere in the range of 300–350 hours preparing before taking the official MCAT. One way you could break this down is to study for three hours per day, six days per week, for four months, but this is just one approach. You might study six days per week for more than three hours per day. You might study over a longer period of time if you don't have much time to study each week. No matter what your plan is, ensure you complete enough practice to feel completely comfortable with the MCAT and its content. A good sign you're ready for Test Day is when you begin to earn your goal score consistently in practice.

How to Study

The MCAT covers a large amount of material, so studying for Test Day can initially seem daunting. To combat this, we have some tips on how to take control of your studying and make the most of your time.

Goal Setting

To take control of the amount of content and practice required to do well on the MCAT, break the content down into specific goals for each week instead of attempting to approach the test as a whole. A goal of "I want to increase my overall score by 5 points" is too big, abstract, and difficult to measure on the small scale. More reasonable goals are "I will read two chapters each day this week." Goals like this are much less overwhelming and help break studying into manageable pieces.

Active Reading

As you go through this book, much of the information will be familiar to you. After all, you have probably seen most of the content before. However, be very careful: Familiarity with a subject does not necessarily translate to knowledge or mastery of that subject. Do not assume that if you recognize a concept you actually know it and can apply it quickly at an appropriate level. Don't just passively read this book. Instead, read actively. Highlighting can be an excellent tool, but use it sparingly: highlighting every sentence isn't active reading, it's coloring. Frequently stop and ask yourself questions while you read (e.g., *What is the main point? How does this fit into the overall scheme of things? Could I thoroughly explain this to someone else?*). By making connections and focusing on the grander scheme, not only will you ensure you know the essential content, but you also prepare yourself for the level of critical thinking required by the MCAT.

Focus on Areas of Greatest Opportunity

If you are limited by only having a minimal amount of time to prepare before Test Day, focus on your biggest areas of opportunity first. Areas of opportunity are topic areas that are highly tested and that you have not yet mastered. You likely won't have time to take detailed notes for every page of these books; instead, use your results from practice materials to determine which areas are your biggest opportunities and seek those out. After you've taken a full-length test, make sure you are using your performance report to best identify areas of opportunity. Skim over content matter for which you are already demonstrating proficiency, pausing to read more thoroughly when something looks unfamiliar or particularly difficult. Begin with the Science Mastery Assessment at the beginning of each chapter. If you can get all of those questions correct within a reasonable amount of time, you may be able to quickly skim through that chapter, but if the questions prove to be more difficult, then you may need to spend time reading the chapter or certain subsections of the chapter more thoroughly.

Practice, Review, and Tracking

Leave time to review your practice questions and full-length tests. You may be tempted, after practicing, to push ahead and cover new material as quickly as possible, but failing to schedule ample time for review will actually throw away your greatest opportunity to improve your performance. The brain rarely remembers anything it sees or does only once. When you carefully review the questions you've solved (and the explanations for them), the process of retrieving that information reopens and reinforces the connections you've built in your brain. This builds long-term retention and repeatable skill sets—exactly what you need to beat the MCAT!

One useful tool for making the most of your review is the How I'll Fix It (HIFI) sheet. You can create a HIFI sheet, such as the sample below, to track questions throughout your prep that you miss or have to guess on. For each such question, figure out why you missed it and supply at least one action step for how you can avoid similar mistakes in the future. As you move through your MCAT prep, adjust your study plan based on your available study time and the results of your review. Your strengths and weaknesses are likely to change over the course of your prep. Keep addressing the areas that are most important to your score, shifting your focus as those areas change.

Section	Q #	Topic or skill	Why I missed it	How I'll fix it
Chem/Phys	*42*	*Nuclear chem.*	*Confused electron absorption and emission*	*Reread Physics Chapter 9.2*
Chem/Phys	*47*	K_{eq}	*Didn't know right equation*	*Memorize equation for* K_{eq}
CARS	*2*	*Paraphrase Detail*	*Didn't read "not" in answer choice*	*Slow down when finding match*
CARS	*4*	*Make Deduction*	*Forgot to research answer*	*Reread passage and predict first*

Where to Study

One often-overlooked aspect of studying is the environment where the learning actually occurs. Although studying at home is many students' first choice, several problems can arise in this environment, chief of which are distractions. Studying can be a mentally draining process, so as time passes, these distractions become ever more tempting as escape routes. Although you may have considerable willpower, there's no reason to make staying focused harder than it needs to be. Instead of studying at home, head to a library, quiet coffee shop, or another new location whenever possible. This will eliminate many of the usual distractions and also promote efficient studying; instead of studying off and on at home over the course of an entire day, you can stay at the library for three hours of effective studying and enjoy the rest of the day off from the MCAT.

No matter where you study, make your practice as much like Test Day as possible. Just as is required during the official test, don't have snacks or chew gum during your study blocks. Turn off your music, television, and phone. Practice on the computer with your online resources to simulate the computer-based test environment. When completing practice questions, do your work on scratch paper or noteboard sheets rather than writing directly on any printed materials since you won't have that option on Test Day. Because memory is tied to all of your senses, the more test-like you can make your studying environment, the easier it will be on Test Day to recall the information you're putting in so much work to learn.

CHAPTER 1

THE CELL

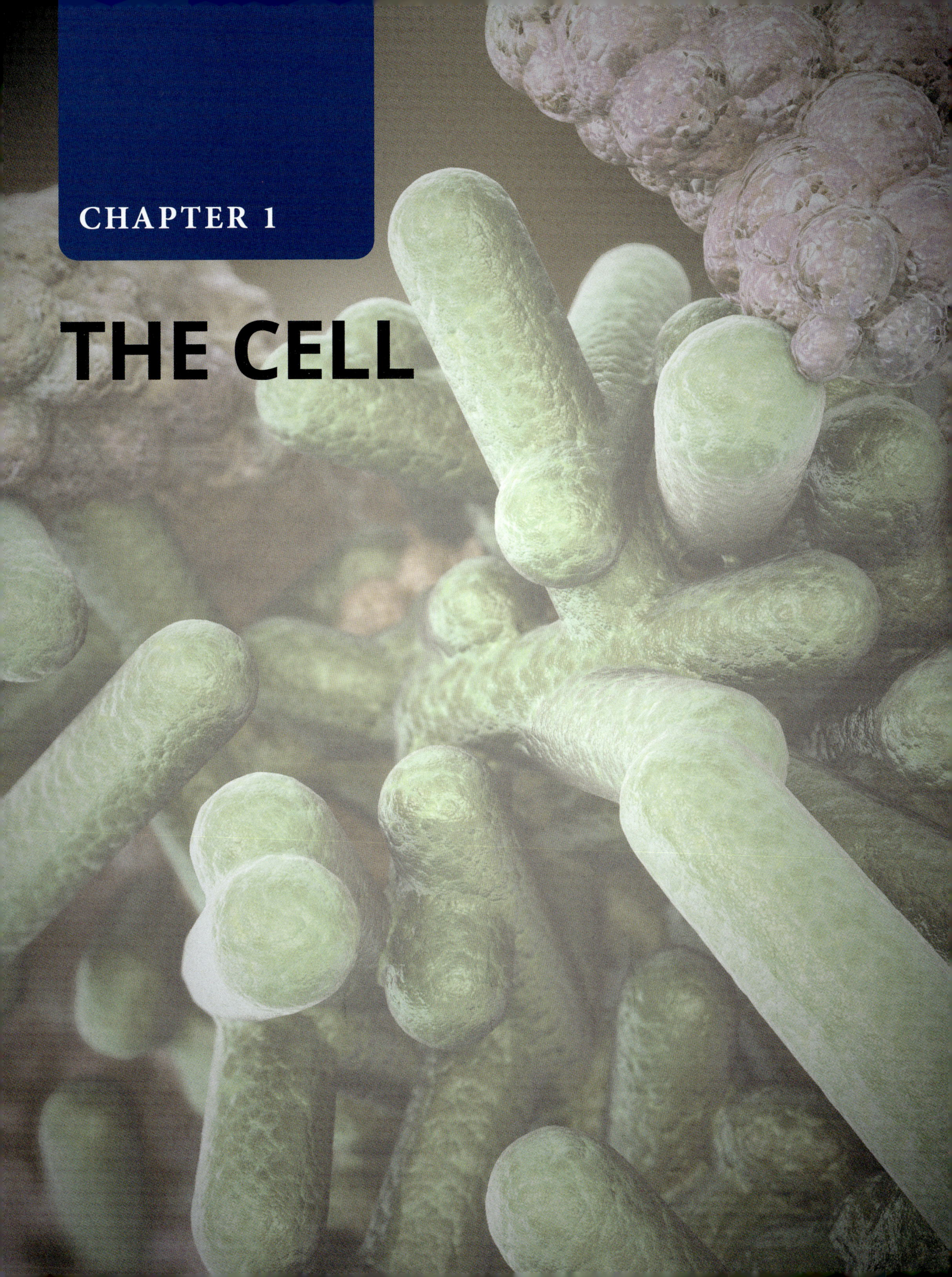

SCIENCE MASTERY ASSESSMENT

Every pre-med knows this feeling: there is so much content I have to know for the MCAT! How do I know what to do first or what's important?

While the high-yield badges throughout this book will help you identify the most important topics, this Science Mastery Assessment is another tool in your MCAT prep arsenal. This quiz (which can also be taken in your online resources) and the guidance below will help ensure that you are spending the appropriate amount of time on this chapter based on your personal strengths and weaknesses. Don't worry though—skipping something now does not mean you'll never study it. Later on in your prep, as you complete full-length tests, you'll uncover specific pieces of content that you need to review and can come back to these chapters as appropriate.

How to Use This Assessment

If you answer 0–7 questions correctly:

Spend about 1 hour to read this chapter in full and take limited notes throughout. Follow up by reviewing **all** quiz questions to ensure that you now understand how to solve each one.

If you answer 8–11 questions correctly:

Spend 20–40 minutes reviewing the quiz questions. Beginning with the questions you missed, read and take notes on the corresponding subchapters. For questions you answered correctly, ensure your thinking matches that of the explanation and you understand why each choice was correct or incorrect.

If you answer 12–15 questions correctly:

Spend less than 20 minutes reviewing all questions from the quiz. If you missed any, then include a quick read-through of the corresponding subchapters, or even just the relevant content within a subchapter, as part of your question review. For questions you answered correctly, ensure your thinking matches that of the explanation and review the Concept Summary at the end of the chapter.

1. Hyperbaric oxygen may be used as a treatment for certain types of bacterial infections. In this therapy, the patient is placed in a chamber in which the partial pressure of oxygen is significantly increased, increasing the partial pressure of oxygen in the patient's tissues. This treatment is most likely used for infections with:
   - **A.** obligate aerobic bacteria.
   - **B.** facultative anaerobic bacteria.
   - **C.** aerotolerant anaerobic bacteria.
   - **D.** obligate anaerobic bacteria.

2. Which of the following does NOT describe connective tissue cells?
   - **A.** They account for most cells in muscles, bones, and tendons.
   - **B.** They secrete substances to form the extracellular matrix.
   - **C.** In organs, they tend to form the stroma.
   - **D.** In organs, they provide support for epithelial cells.

3. Which of the following types of nucleic acid could form the genome of a virus?
   - **I.** Single-stranded RNA
   - **II.** Double-stranded DNA
   - **III.** Single-stranded DNA
   - **A.** I only
   - **B.** II only
   - **C.** I and II only
   - **D.** I, II, and III

4. The theory of spontaneous generation states that living organisms can arise from nonliving material. In 1859, Pasteur demonstrated that no organisms emerged from sterilized growth media, weakening the theory of spontaneous generation and supporting which tenet of cell theory?
   - **A.** All living things are composed of cells.
   - **B.** The cell is the basic functional unit of life.
   - **C.** Cells arise only from preexisting cells.
   - **D.** Cells carry genetic information in the form of DNA.

5. Mitochondrial DNA is:
   - **I.** circular.
   - **II.** self-replicating.
   - **III.** single-stranded.
   - **A.** I only
   - **B.** II only
   - **C.** I and II only
   - **D.** I, II, and III

6. Which of the following is NOT a function of the smooth endoplasmic reticulum?
   - **A.** Lipid synthesis
   - **B.** Poison detoxification
   - **C.** Protein synthesis
   - **D.** Transport of proteins

7. What is the main function of the nucleolus?
   - **A.** Ribosomal RNA synthesis
   - **B.** DNA replication
   - **C.** Cell division
   - **D.** Chromosome assembly

8. Which of the following organelles is surrounded by a single membrane?
   - **A.** Lysosomes
   - **B.** Mitochondria
   - **C.** Nuclei
   - **D.** Ribosomes

9. Which of the following is NOT a difference that would allow one to distinguish a prokaryotic and a eukaryotic cell?
   - **A.** Ribosomal subunit weight
   - **B.** Presence of a nucleus
   - **C.** Presence of a membrane on the outside surface of the cell
   - **D.** Presence of membrane-bound organelles

10. Which of the following does NOT contain tubulin?
    - **A.** Cilia
    - **B.** Flagella
    - **C.** Microfilaments
    - **D.** Centrioles

11. Herpes simplex virus (HSV) enters the human body and remains dormant in the nervous system until it produces an outbreak after exposure to heat, radiation, or other stimuli. Which of the following statements correctly describes HSV?
    - **A.** While it remains dormant in the nervous system, the virus is in its lytic cycle.
    - **B.** During an outbreak, the virus is in the lysogenic cycle.
    - **C.** Herpes simplex virus adds its genetic information to the genetic information of the cell.
    - **D.** The herpes simplex virus contains a tail sheath and tail fibers.

12. Resistance to antibiotics is a well-recognized medical problem. Which mechanisms can account for a bacterium's ability to increase its genetic variability and thus adapt itself to resist different antibiotics?
    - **I.** Binary fission
    - **II.** Conjugation
    - **III.** Transduction

    - **A.** I and II only
    - **B.** I and III only
    - **C.** II and III only
    - **D.** I, II, and III

13. A bacterial cell is noted to be resistant to penicillin. The bacterium is transferred to a colony that lacks the fertility factor, and the rest of the colony does not become resistant to penicillin. However, the penicillin-resistant cell has also started to exhibit other phenotypic characteristics, including secretion of a novel protein. Which of the following methods of bacterial recombination is NOT likely to account for this change?
    - **A.** Conjugation
    - **B.** Transformation
    - **C.** Transduction
    - **D.** Infection with a bacteriophage

14. In Alzheimer's disease, a protein called the amyloid precursor protein (APP) is cleaved to form a protein called β-amyloid. This protein has a β-pleated sheet structure and precipitates to form plaques in the brain. This mechanism of disease is most similar to which of the following pathogens?
    - **A.** Bacteria
    - **B.** Viruses
    - **C.** Prions
    - **D.** Viroids

15. After infection of a cell, a viral particle must transport itself to the nucleus in order to produce viral proteins. What is the likely genomic content of the virus?
    - **A.** Double-stranded DNA
    - **B.** Double-stranded RNA
    - **C.** Positive-sense RNA
    - **D.** Negative-sense RNA

Answer Key

1. **D** (See section 1.3)
2. **A** (See section 1.2)
3. **D** (See section 1.5)
4. **C** (See section 1.1)
5. **C** (See section 1.2)
6. **C** (See section 1.2)
7. **A** (See section 1.2)
8. **A** (See section 1.2)
9. **C** (See section 1.3)
10. **C** (See section 1.2)
11. **C** (See section 1.5)
12. **C** (See section 1.4)
13. **A** (See section 1.4)
14. **C** (See section 1.3)
15. **A** (See section 1.5)

The relevant section of the chapter to review for each question is given in parentheses after the correct answer. Detailed explanations can be found at the end of the chapter.

CHAPTER 1

THE CELL

In This Chapter

Introduction

The human body contains approximately 30 trillion cells, with bacterial cells slightly outnumbering eukaryotic cells, about 1.3 to 1 according to recent estimates. Our cells create tissues that form organs, and each cell serves a purpose, communicating and carrying out the reactions that make life possible.

The sheer number of cells that make up the human body is not nearly as impressive as the numerous functions these cells can perform—from the conduction of impulses through the nervous system that allows for memory and learning, to the simultaneous contraction of cardiac myocytes that pump blood through the entire human body. In order to understand the human organism as a whole and how the human body reacts to various pathogens, a thorough understanding of cell biology is required. It is not enough to simply memorize each part of the cell; the MCAT requires an understanding of how each cell structure carries out its functions and affects the entire organism.

CHAPTER PROFILE

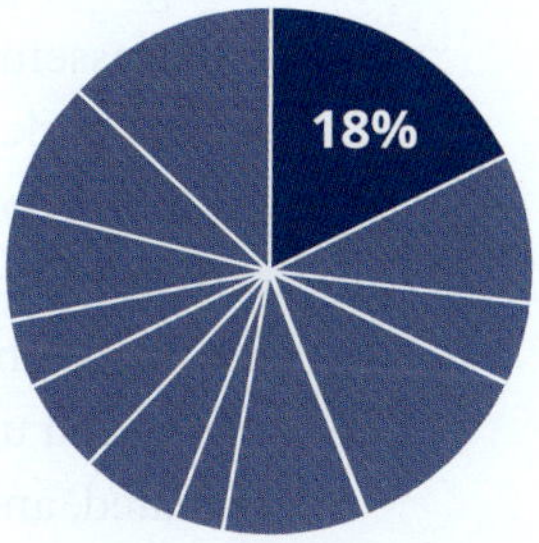

The content in this chapter should be relevant to about 18% of all questions about biology on the MCAT.

This chapter covers material from the following AAMC content categories:

1D: Principles of bioenergetics and fuel molecule metabolism

2A: Assemblies of molecules, cells, and groups of cells within single cellular and multicellular organisms

2B: The structure, growth, physiology, and genetics of prokaryotes and viruses

MCAT EXPERTISE

This chapter represents 18% of all biology questions you would see on Test Day. That makes the cell, specifically eukaryotic cell structure and function, one of the single highest-yield subjects within any of the review books. Make sure to work sufficient study of these materials into your study plan.

1.1 Cell Theory

LEARNING OBJECTIVE

After Chapter 1.1, you will be able to:

- Recall the four fundamental tenets of cell theory

Prior to the 1600s, organisms were perceived as being complete and inseparable into smaller parts. This was due in part to the inability to see smaller structures through simple optical instruments like magnifying glasses. In 1665, Robert Hooke assembled a crude compound microscope and tested its properties on a piece of cork. He noticed a honeycomb-like structure and compared the spaces within the cork to the small rooms of a monastery, known as cells. Because cork consists of desiccated nonliving cells, Hooke was not able to see nuclei, organelles, or cell membranes. In 1674, Anton van Leeuwenhoek was the first to view a living cell under a microscope. Later researchers noted that cells could be separated, and that each cell was a distinct structure. Further research indicated that tissues were made of cells, and the function of a tissue was dependent upon the function of the cells that make up the tissue. Two centuries later, in 1850, Rudolph Virchow demonstrated that diseased cells could arise from normal cells in normal tissues.

BRIDGE

Robert Hooke, who invented the first crude microscopes to look at cork, is also known for his characterization of springs. Hooke's law, $F = -kx$, describes the relationship between elastic force, the spring constant, and the displacement of a spring from equilibrium. While Hooke's law does not appear on the official MCAT content lists, the related topic of elastic potential energy, $U = \frac{1}{2}kx^2$, is testable content. This equation and other forms of energy are discussed in Chapter 2 of *MCAT Physics and Math Review*.

The original form of the **cell theory** consisted of three basic tenets:

- All living things are composed of cells.
- The cell is the basic functional unit of life.
- Cells arise only from preexisting cells.

Through advances in molecular biology, a fourth tenet has been added to the theory:

- Cells carry genetic information in the form of deoxyribonucleic acid (DNA). This genetic material is passed on from parent to daughter cell.

Cell theory has created an interesting dilemma with respect to viruses. Viruses are small structures that contain genetic material, but are unable to reproduce on their own. This violates the third and fourth tenets of the cell theory because virions can only replicate by invading other organisms and because they may use ribonucleic acid (RNA) as their genetic information. Therefore, viruses, discussed later in this chapter, are not considered living organisms.

MCAT CONCEPT CHECK 1.1

Before you move on, assess your understanding of the material with this question.

1. What are the four fundamental tenets of the cell theory?
   -
   -
   -
   -

BRIDGE

Solutions to concept checks for a given chapter in *MCAT Biology Review* can be found near the end of the chapter in which the concept check is located, following the Concept Summary for that chapter.

1.2 Eukaryotic Cells High Yield

LEARNING OBJECTIVES

After Chapter 1.2, you will be able to:

- Explain the importance of hydrogen peroxide to cellular function
- Identify the predominant proteins found in microfilaments, microtubules, and intermediate filaments
- Distinguish between the properties of different cytoskeletal structures
- Classify cell types as epithelial or connective tissue
- Recall the names and functions of cellular organelles:

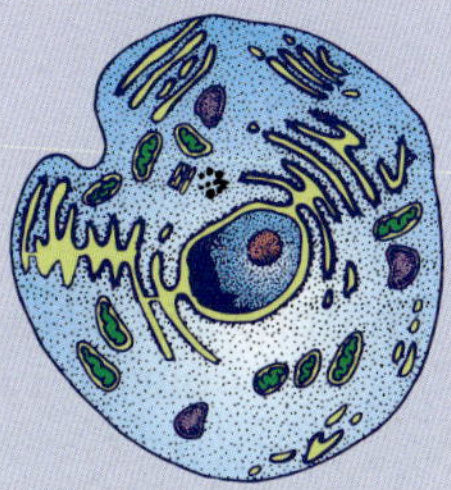

MCAT EXPERTISE

The "High-Yield" badge on this section indicates that the content is frequently tested on the MCAT.

The first major distinction we can make between living organisms is whether they are composed of prokaryotic or eukaryotic cells. Prokaryotic organisms are always single celled, while eukaryotic organisms can be unicellular or multicellular. Whereas **eukaryotic cells** contain a true nucleus enclosed in a membrane, **prokaryotic cells** do not contain a nucleus. The major organelles are identified in the eukaryotic cell in Figure 1.1.

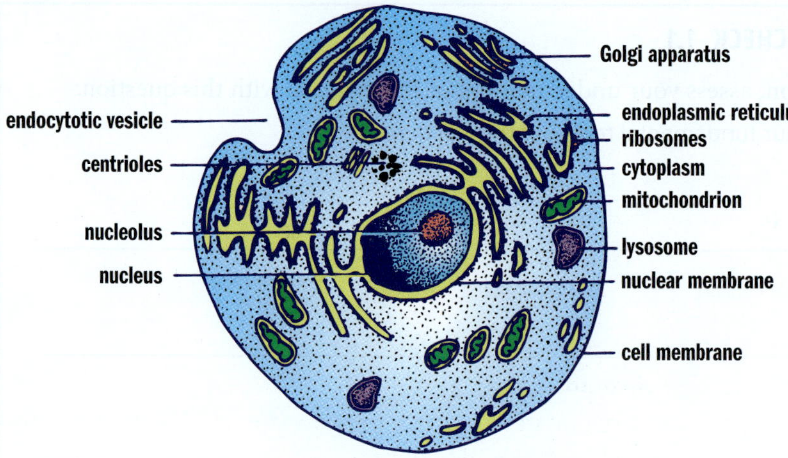

Figure 1.1 Eukaryotic Cell
Numerous membrane-bound organelles are found in the cytoplasm of a eukaryotic cell.

Membrane-Bound Organelles

Each cell has a membrane enclosing a semifluid cytosol in which the **organelles** are suspended. In eukaryotic cells, most organelles are membrane bound, allowing for compartmentalization of functions. Membranes of eukaryotic cells consist of a phospholipid bilayer, which can be seen in Figure 1.2. This membrane is unique in that its surfaces are hydrophilic, electrostatically interacting with the aqueous environments inside and outside of the cell, while its inner portion is hydrophobic, which helps to provide a highly selective barrier between the interior of the cell and the external environment. The cell membrane is such an important topic on the MCAT that an entire chapter—Chapter 8 of *MCAT Biochemistry Review*—is devoted solely to discussing the structure and physiology of biological membranes. The **cytosol** allows for the diffusion of molecules throughout the cell. Within the **nucleus**, genetic material is encoded in **deoxyribonucleic acid** (**DNA**), which is organized into **chromosomes**. Eukaryotic cells reproduce by **mitosis**, allowing for the formation of two identical daughter cells.

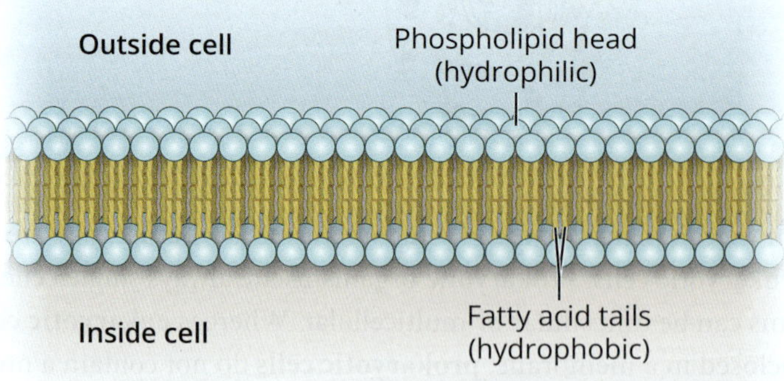

Figure 1.2 The Phospholipid Bilayer

The Nucleus

As the control center of the cell, the **nucleus** is the most heavily tested organelle on the MCAT. It contains all of the genetic material necessary for replication of the cell. The nucleus is surrounded by the **nuclear membrane** or **envelope**, a double membrane that maintains a nuclear environment separate and distinct from the cytoplasm. **Nuclear pores** in the nuclear membrane allow selective two-way exchange of material between the cytoplasm and the nucleus.

The genetic material (DNA) contains coding regions called **genes**. Linear DNA is wound around organizing proteins known as **histones**, and is then further wound into linear strands called **chromosomes**. The location of DNA in the nucleus permits the compartmentalization of DNA transcription separate from RNA translation. Finally, there is a subsection of the nucleus known as the **nucleolus**, where the **ribosomal RNA (rRNA)** is synthesized. The nucleolus actually takes up approximately 25 percent of the volume of the entire nucleus and can often be identified as a darker spot in the nucleus.

BRIDGE

The nuclear envelope creates two distinct environments within the cell because it separates the nucleus from the cytoplasm. This permits compartmentalization of transcription (the formation of hnRNA from DNA, which is subsequently processed to form mRNA) and translation (the formation of a peptide from mRNA). These processes are discussed in Chapter 7 of *MCAT Biochemistry Review*.

Mitochondria

Mitochondria, shown in Figure 1.3, are often called *the power plants of the cell*, in reference to their important metabolic functions. The mitochondrion contains two layers: the outer and inner membranes. The **outer membrane** serves as a barrier between the cytosol and the inner environment of the mitochondrion. The **inner membrane**, which is arranged into numerous infoldings called **cristae**, contains the molecules and enzymes of the electron transport chain. The cristae are highly convoluted structures that increase the surface area available for electron transport chain enzymes. The space between the inner and outer membranes is called the **intermembrane space**; the space inside the inner membrane is called the mitochondrial **matrix**. As described in Chapter 10 of *MCAT Biochemistry Review*, the pumping of protons from the mitochondrial matrix to the intermembrane space establishes the proton-motive force; ultimately, these protons flow through *ATP synthase* to generate ATP during oxidative phosphorylation.

REAL WORLD

The *serial endosymbiosis theory* attempts to explain the formation of some of the membrane-bound organelles; it posits that these organelles formed by the engulfing of one prokaryote by another and the establishment of a symbiotic relationship. In addition to mitochondria, chloroplasts in plant cells and organelles of motility (such as flagella) are believed to have originated from this process.

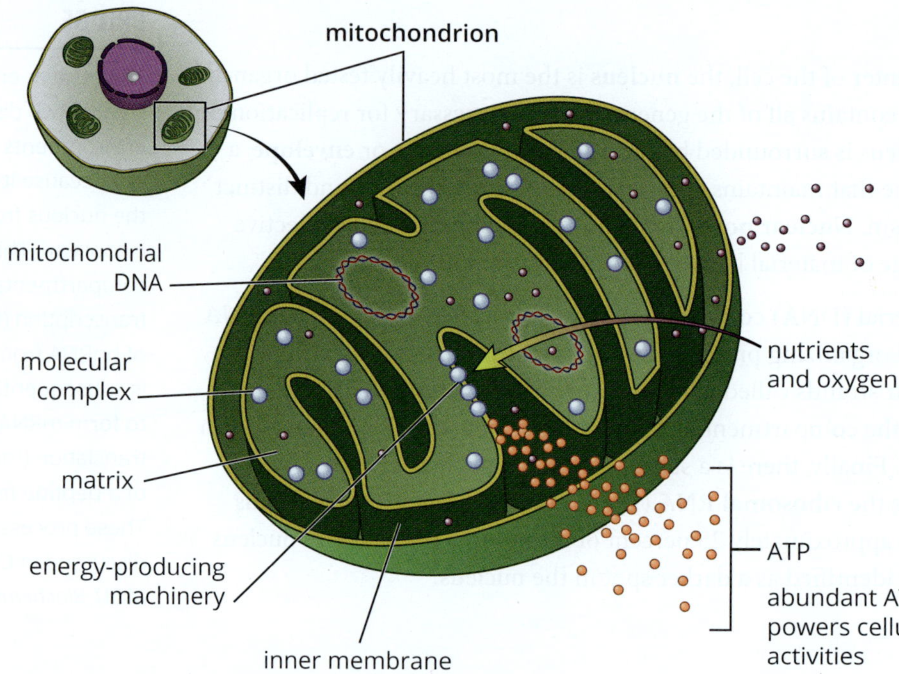

Figure 1.3 Mitochondrial Structure

Mitochondria are different from other parts of the cell in that they are semi-autonomous. They contain some of their own genes and replicate independently of the nucleus via binary fission. As such, they are paradigmatic examples of **cytoplasmic** or **extranuclear inheritance**—the transmission of genetic material independent of the nucleus. Mitochondria are thought to have originated when the engulfing of an aerobic prokaryote by an anaerobic prokaryote resulted in a symbiotic relationship.

In addition to keeping the cell alive by providing energy, the mitochondria are also capable of killing the cell by release of enzymes from the electron transport chain. This release kick-starts a process known as **apoptosis**, or programmed cell death.

Lysosomes

Lysosomes are membrane-bound structures containing hydrolytic enzymes that are capable of breaking down many different substrates, including substances ingested by endocytosis and cellular waste products. Lysosomes often function in conjunction with **endosomes**, which transport, package and sort cell material traveling to and from the membrane. Endosomes are capable of transporting materials to the *trans*-golgi, to the cell membrane, or to the lysosomal pathway for degradation. The lysosomal membrane sequesters these enzymes to prevent damage to the cell. However, release of these enzymes can occur in a process known as **autolysis**. Like mitochondria, when lysosomes release their hydrolytic enzymes, it results in apoptosis. In this case, the released enzymes directly lead to the degradation of cellular components.

KEY CONCEPT

Not all cells have the same relative distribution of organelles. Form will follow function. Cells that require a lot of energy for locomotion (such as sperm cells) have high concentrations of mitochondria. Cells involved in secretion (such as pancreatic islet cells and other endocrine tissues) have high concentrations of RER and Golgi apparatuses. Other cells, such as red blood cells, which primarily serve a transport function, have no organelles at all.

Endoplasmic Reticulum

The **endoplasmic reticulum** (**ER**) is a series of interconnected membranes that are actually contiguous with the nuclear envelope. The double membrane of the endoplasmic reticulum is folded into numerous invaginations, creating complex structures with a central lumen. There are two varieties of ER: smooth and rough. The **rough ER** (**RER**) is studded with **ribosomes**, which permit the translation of proteins destined for secretion directly into its lumen. On the other hand, the **smooth ER** (**SER**) lacks ribosomes and is utilized primarily for lipid synthesis (such as the phospholipids in the cell membrane) and the detoxification of certain drugs and poisons. The SER also transports proteins from the RER to the Golgi apparatus.

Golgi Apparatus

The **Golgi apparatus** consists of stacked membrane-bound sacs. Materials from the ER are transferred to the Golgi apparatus in vesicles. Once inside the Golgi apparatus, these cellular products may be modified by the addition of groups like carbohydrates, phosphates, and sulfates. The Golgi apparatus may also modify cellular products through the introduction of signal sequences, which direct the delivery of the product to a specific cellular location. After modification and sorting in the Golgi apparatus, cellular products are repackaged in vesicles, which are then directed to the correct cellular location. If the product is destined for secretion, the secretory vesicle merges with the cell membrane and its contents are released via **exocytosis**. The relationships between lysosomes, the ER, and the Golgi apparatus are shown in Figure 1.4.

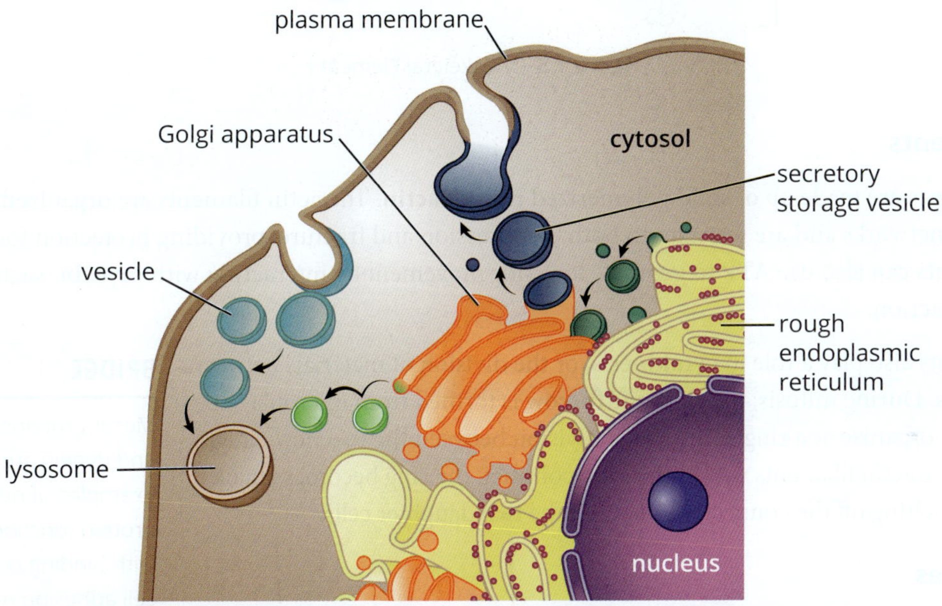

Figure 1.4 Lysosomes, the Endoplasmic Reticulum, and the Golgi Apparatus

Peroxisomes

Peroxisomes contain hydrogen peroxide. One of the primary functions of peroxisomes is the breakdown of very long chain fatty acids via β-oxidation. Peroxisomes participate in the synthesis of phospholipids and contain some of the enzymes involved in the pentose phosphate pathway, discussed in Chapter 9 of *MCAT Biochemistry Review*.

The Cytoskeleton

The **cytoskeleton**, shown in Figure 1.5, provides structure to the cell and helps it to maintain its shape. In addition, the cytoskeleton provides a conduit for the transport of materials around the cell. There are three components of the cytoskeleton: microfilaments, microtubules, and intermediate filaments.

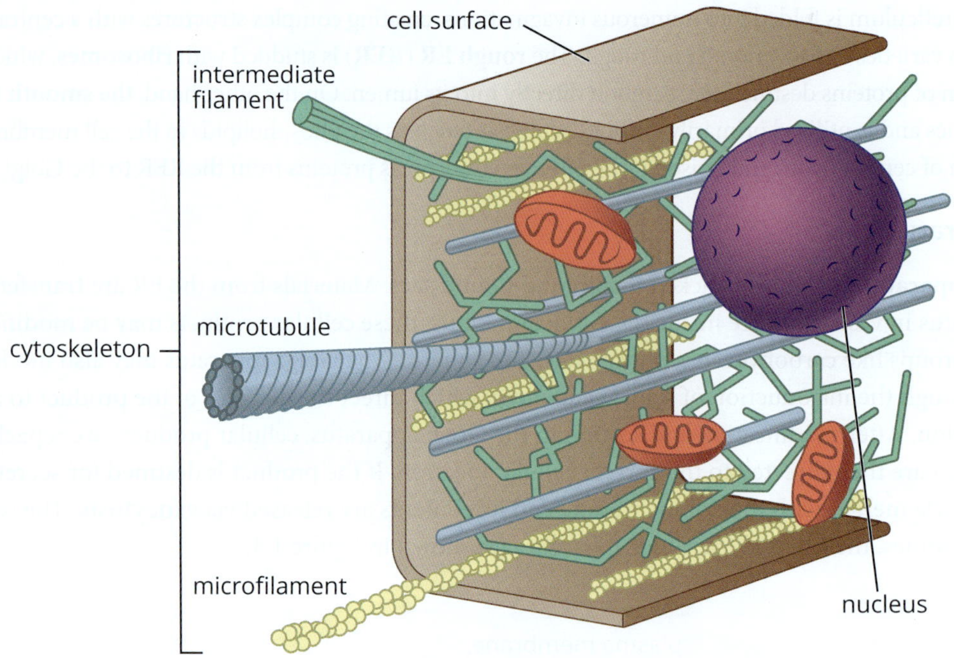

Figure 1.5 Cytoskeletal Elements

Microfilaments

Microfilaments are made up of solid polymerized rods of **actin**. The actin filaments are organized into bundles and networks and are resistant to both compression and fracture, providing protection for the cell. Actin filaments can also use ATP to generate force for movement by interacting with **myosin**, such as in muscle contraction.

Microfilaments also play a role in **cytokinesis**, or the division of materials between daughter cells. During mitosis, the **cleavage furrow** is formed from microfilaments, which organize as a ring at the site of division between the two new daughter cells. As the actin filaments within this ring contract, the ring becomes smaller, eventually pinching off the connection between the two daughter cells.

BRIDGE

Motor proteins like kinesin and dynein are classic examples of nonenzymatic protein function, along with binding proteins, cell adhesion molecules, immunoglobulins, and ion channels. Motor proteins often travel along cytoskeletal structures to accomplish their functions. Nonenzymatic protein functions are discussed in Chapter 3 of *MCAT Biochemistry Review.*

Microtubules

Unlike microfilaments, **microtubules** are hollow polymers of **tubulin** proteins. Microtubules radiate throughout the cell, providing the primary pathways along which motor proteins like ***kinesin*** and ***dynein*** carry vesicles.

Cilia and flagella are motile structures composed of microtubules. **Cilia** are projections from a cell that are primarily involved in the movement of materials along the surface of the cell; for example, cilia line the respiratory tract and are involved in the movement of mucus. **Flagella** are structures involved in the movement of the cell itself, such as the movement of sperm cells through the reproductive tract. Cilia and flagella share the same structure, composed of nine pairs of microtubules forming an outer ring, with two microtubules in the center, as shown in Figure 1.6. This is known as a **9 + 2 structure** and is seen only in eukaryotic organelles of motility. Bacterial flagella have a different structure with a different chemical composition, as discussed later in this chapter.

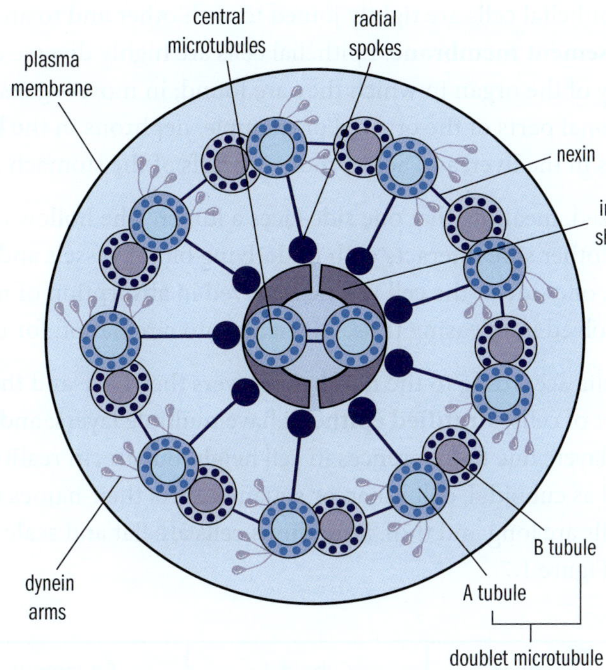

Figure 1.6 Cilium and Flagellum Structure
Microtubules are organized into a ring of 9 doublets with 2 central microtubules.

Centrioles are found in a region of the cell called the **centrosome**. They are the organizing centers for microtubules and are structured as nine triplets of microtubules with a hollow center. During mitosis, the centrioles migrate to opposite poles of the dividing cell and organize the mitotic spindle. The microtubules emanating from the centrioles attach to the chromosomes via complexes called **kinetochores** and exert force on the sister chromatids, pulling them apart.

Intermediate Filaments

Intermediate filaments are a diverse group of filamentous proteins, which includes keratin, desmin, vimentin, and lamins. Many intermediate filaments are involved in cell–cell adhesion or maintenance of the overall integrity of the cytoskeleton. Intermediate filaments are able to withstand a tremendous amount of tension, increasing the structural rigidity of the cell. In addition, intermediate filaments help anchor other organelles, including the nucleus. The identity of the intermediate filament proteins within a cell is specific to the cell and tissue type.

Tissue Formation

One of the unique characteristics of eukaryotic cells is the formation of tissues with division of labor, as different cells in a tissue may carry out different functions. For example, in the heart, some cells participate in the conduction pathways while others cause contraction; still others serve a supportive role like maintaining structural integrity of the organ. There are four tissue types: epithelial tissue, connective tissue, muscle tissue, and nervous tissue. While muscle and nervous tissue are considered more extensively in subsequent chapters, we explore epithelial and connective tissues below.

Epithelial Tissue

Epithelial tissues cover the body and line its cavities, providing a means for protection against pathogen invasion and desiccation. In certain organs, epithelial cells are involved in absorption, secretion, and sensation. To remain as one cohesive unit, epithelial cells are tightly joined to each other and to an underlying layer of connective tissue known as the **basement membrane**. Epithelial cells are highly diverse and serve numerous functions depending on the identity of the organ in which they are found; in most organs, epithelial cells constitute the **parenchyma**, or the functional parts of the organ. For example, nephrons in the kidney are composed of epithelial cells, and hepatocytes in the liver, and acid-producing cells of the stomach are epithelial cells.

Epithelial cells are often polarized, meaning that one side faces a lumen (the hollow inside of an organ or tube) or the outside world, while the other side interacts with underlying blood vessels and structural cells. For example, in the small intestine, one side of the cell will be involved in absorption of nutrients from the lumen, while the other side will be involved in releasing those nutrients into circulation for use in the rest of the body.

We can classify different epithelia according to the number of layers they have and the shape of their cells. **Simple epithelia** have one layer of cells; **stratified epithelia** have multiple layers; and **pseudostratified epithelia** appear to have multiple layers due to differences in cell height but are, in reality, only one layer. Turning to shape, cells may be classified as cuboidal, columnar, or squamous. As their names imply, **cuboidal** cells are cube-shaped and **columnar** cells are long and thin. **Squamous** cells are flat and scale-like. These classifications are organized and depicted in Figure 1.7.

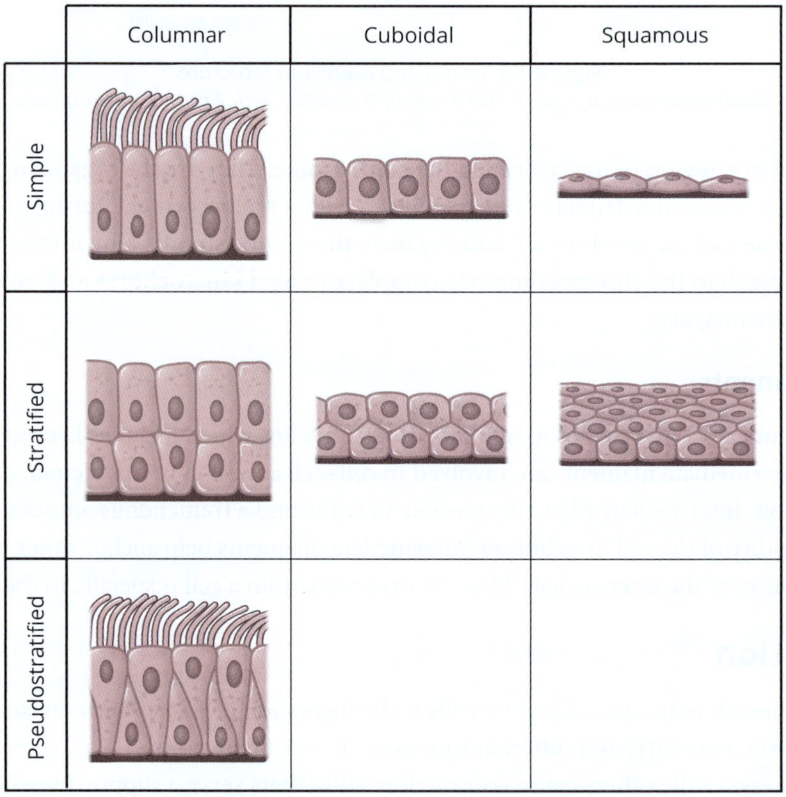

Figure 1.7 Epithelial Tissue Classifications

Connective Tissue

Connective tissue supports the body and provides a framework for the epithelial cells to carry out their functions. Whereas epithelial cells contribute to the parenchyma of an organ, connective tissues are the main contributors to the **stroma** or support structure. Bone, cartilage, tendons, ligaments, adipose tissue, and blood are all examples of connective tissues. Most cells in connective tissues produce and secrete materials such as collagen and elastin to form the **extracellular matrix**.

Microscopy

Microscopy is used to visualize small structures and cellular organisms. **Light microscopy** uses visible light and lenses to produce a magnified image. It is most suitable for visualizing specimens that are 200 nm or larger. **Confocal microscopy** is another method of visualizing small structures, but unlike light microscopy, it has increased optical resolution through the use of a spatial pinhole that blocks out-of-focus light to create sharper images. Because confocal microscopy can penetrate further into samples than light microscopy, confocal imaging can be used in conjunction with computer modeling to reconstruct three-dimensional images by arranging multiple images taken at different depths of the sample. Commonly, confocal microscopy is coupled with **immunohistochemistry**, where antibodies with fluorescent probes are used to label different subcellular components to better visualize the sample, allowing for better contrast resolution. **Scanning electron microscopes** use electrons instead of visible light to create an image, resulting in much higher resolution compared to light or even confocal microscopy. Samples are coated with a thin layer of a metal like gold, and a beam of electrons hit the surface and reflect, creating a topographical map of the cellular surface. In contrast, the electrons in **transmission electron microscopy** pass through the ultrathin sections of a specimen to create an image, and, due to better resolution, can visualize down to the subcellular structures within a cell. As a note, **fluorescence microscopy** is a general term that refers to any type of microscopy that uses fluorescence as a means of visualization.

MCAT CONCEPT CHECK 1.2

Before you move on, assess your understanding of the material with these questions.

1. Briefly describe the functions of each of the organelles listed below:
   - Nucleus:

     ___
   - Mitochondrion:

     ___
   - Lysosome:

     ___
   - Rough endoplasmic reticulum:

     ___
   - Smooth endoplasmic reticulum:

     ___
   - Golgi apparatus:

     ___
   - Peroxisome:

     ___

2. A child is diagnosed with an enzyme deficiency that prevents the production of hydrogen peroxide. What would the likely outcome be of such a deficiency?

____

3. What are the predominant proteins in each cytoskeletal element?
   - Microfilaments:

   ____

   - Microtubules:

   ____

   - Intermediate filaments:

   ____

4. How do the cytoskeletal structures of centrioles and flagella differ?

____

5. Classify each of the following cells as epithelial cells or connective tissue:
   - Fibroblasts, which produce collagen in a number of organs:

   ____

   - Endothelial cells, which line blood vessels:

   ____

   - α-cells, which produce glucagon in the pancreas:

   ____

   - Osteoblasts, which produce osteoid, the material that hardens into bone:

   ____

   - Chondroblasts, which produce cartilage:

   ____

1.3 Classification and Structure of Prokaryotic Cells

LEARNING OBJECTIVES

After Chapter 1.3, you will be able to:

- Compare and contrast archaea, bacteria, and eukaryotes
- Identify the three common bacterial shapes
- Explain the differences between gram-positive and gram-negative bacteria
- Detail the structural differences between eukaryotic and prokaryotic flagella
- Differentiate between the metabolic processes of aerobic and anaerobic bacteria

Prokaryotes are the simplest of all organisms and include all bacteria. Prokaryotes do not contain any membrane-bound organelles, and their genetic material is organized into a single circular molecule of DNA concentrated in an area of the cell called the **nucleoid region**. Despite the simplicity of prokaryotes, they are incredibly diverse, and knowledge of this diversity is essential for the study of medicine because many prokaryotes can cause infection. In fact, choosing the appropriate antibiotic to fight an infection requires knowledge about the basic structure of the bacteria causing the infection.

Prokaryotic Domains

There are three overarching domains into which all life is classified: Archaea, Bacteria, and Eukarya. Two of these—Archaea and Bacteria—contain prokaryotes. Initially, Archaea and Bacteria were classified together into the kingdom of Monera. However, modern genetics and biochemical techniques have indicated that the differences in the evolutionary pathways between Archaea and Bacteria are at least as significant as between either of these domains and Eukarya.

Archaea

Archaea are single-celled organisms that are visually similar to bacteria, but contain genes and several metabolic pathways that are more similar to eukaryotes than to bacteria. Historically, Archaea were considered **extremophiles**, in that they were most commonly isolated from harsh environments with extremely high temperatures, high salinity, or no light. More recent research has demonstrated a greater variety of habitats for these organisms, including the human body. Archaea are notable for their ability to use alternative sources of energy. While some are photosynthetic, many are chemosynthetic and can generate energy from inorganic compounds, including sulfur- and nitrogen-based compounds such as ammonia.

Due to the similarities of this domain to eukaryotes, it is hypothesized that eukaryotes and the Archaea share a common origin. Both eukaryotes and Archaea start translation with methionine, contain similar *RNA polymerases*, and associate their DNA with histones. However, Archaea contain a single circular chromosome, divide by binary fission or budding, and share a similar overall structure to bacteria. Interestingly, Archaea are resistant to many antibiotics.

Bacteria

All bacteria contain a **cell membrane** and **cytoplasm**, and some have **flagella** or **fimbriae** (similar to cilia), as shown in Figure 1.8. Because bacteria and eukaryotes often share analogous structures, it can be difficult to develop medicines that target only bacteria. However, in some cases, even seemingly similar structures have enough biochemical differences to allow the exclusive targeting of one kind of organism. For example, bacterial flagella and eukaryotic flagella are different enough that scientists are able to develop antibacterial vaccines that specifically target the bacterial flagellum. Also, many antibiotics target the bacterial ribosome, which is significantly smaller than the eukaryotic ribosome.

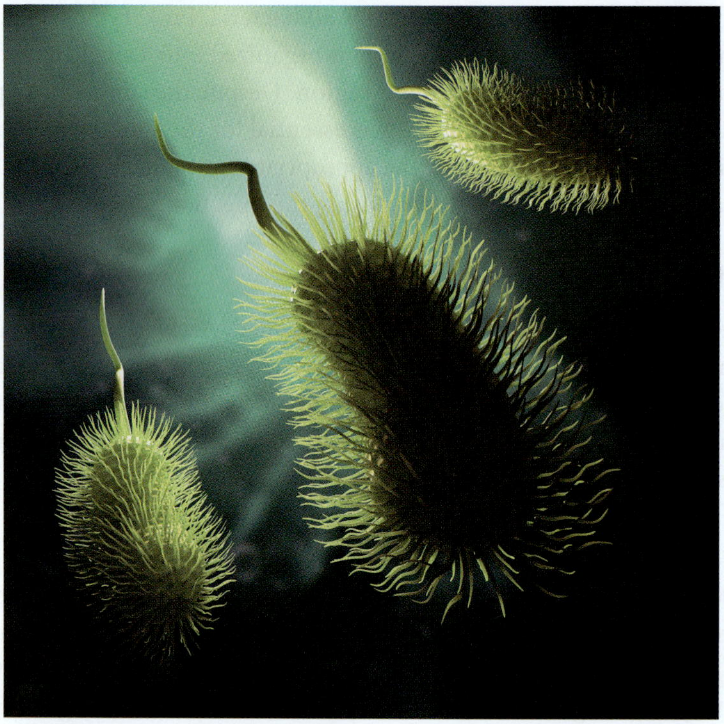

Figure 1.8 Prokaryotic Cell Specializations: Flagella and Fimbriae

There are approximately 5×10^{30} bacteria on Earth, outnumbering all of the plants and animals combined. As mentioned in the introduction to this chapter, bacteria outnumber human cells in the body by 10:1. The relationship between the human body and bacteria is complex. Some bacteria are **mutualistic symbiotes**, meaning that both humans and the bacteria benefit from the relationship. Examples include the bacteria in the human gut that produce vitamin K and biotin (vitamin B_7), and which also prevent the overgrowth of harmful bacteria. Other bacteria are **pathogens** or **parasites**, meaning that they provide no advantage or benefit to the host, but rather cause disease. Pathogenic bacteria may live intracellularly or extracellularly. For example, *Chlamydia trachomatis*, a common sexually transmitted infection, lives inside cells of the reproductive tract; *Clostridium tetani*, the cause of tetanus, lives outside of cells and produces toxins that enter the bloodstream.

REAL WORLD

Bacteria perform essential functions for human beings, including the production of vitamin K in the intestine. Vitamin K is required for production of the plasma proteins necessary for blood clotting. Newborn infants are not yet colonized by bacteria and cannot produce clotting factors, putting them at risk for hemorrhage. When babies are born, they are given an injection of vitamin K to aid in the production of clotting factors until they have been colonized with bacteria.

Classification of Bacteria by Shape

Classification of bacteria by shape provides scientists and pathologists (physicians who specialize in the identification and characterization of disease) a common language to talk about bacteria, as well as a way to identify different species of bacteria.

Most bacteria exist in one of three shapes, as shown in Figure 1.9. Spherical bacteria, known as **cocci**, include common pathogens such as *Streptococcus pyogenes*.

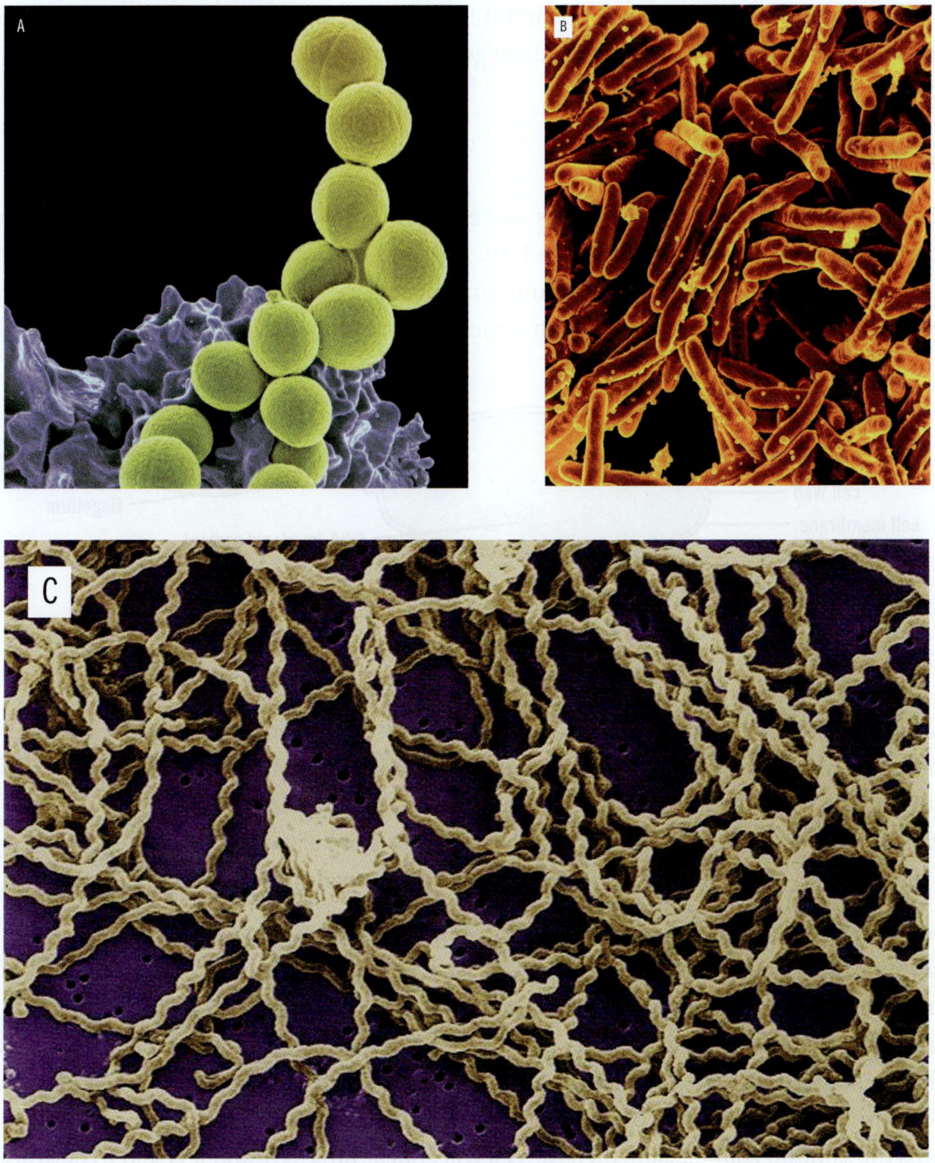

Figure 1.9 Prokaryotic Cell Shapes
(a) Cocci (Staphylococcus aureus), (b) Bacilli (Mycobacterium tuberculosis), (c) Spirilli (Leptospira interrogans)

Rod-shaped bacteria, like *Escherichia coli*, are known as **bacilli**. Finally, spiral-shaped bacteria, known as **spirilli**, include such species as *Treponema pallidum*, which causes syphilis.

Aerobes and Anaerobes

Some bacteria require oxygen for survival, while others do not. Bacteria that require oxygen for metabolism are termed **obligate aerobes**. Other bacteria that use fermentation, or some other form of cellular metabolism that does not require oxygen, are called **anaerobes**. There are different types of anaerobes. Anaerobes that cannot survive in an oxygen-containing environment are called **obligate anaerobes**; the presence of oxygen leads to the production of reactive oxygen-containing radicals in these species, which leads to cell death. Other bacteria can toggle between metabolic processes, using oxygen for aerobic metabolism if it

REAL WORLD

Very few pathogenic bacteria are spiral shaped. The three most common are:

- *Treponema pallidum*, the cause of syphilis
- *Borrelia burgdorferi*, the cause of Lyme disease
- *Leptospira interrogans*, the cause of Weil's disease

is present, and switching to anaerobic metabolism if it is not. These bacteria are called **facultative anaerobes**. Finally, **aerotolerant anaerobes** are unable to use oxygen for metabolism, but are not harmed by its presence in the environment.

Prokaryotic Cell Structure

One of the main differences between prokaryotes and eukaryotes is that prokaryotes lack a nucleus and membrane-bound organelles, as shown in Figure 1.10. Prokaryotes are also single-celled organisms, meaning that each cell must be able to perform all of the functions necessary for life on its own. However, prokaryotes may live in colonies with other cells and may signal these cells to share information about the environment.

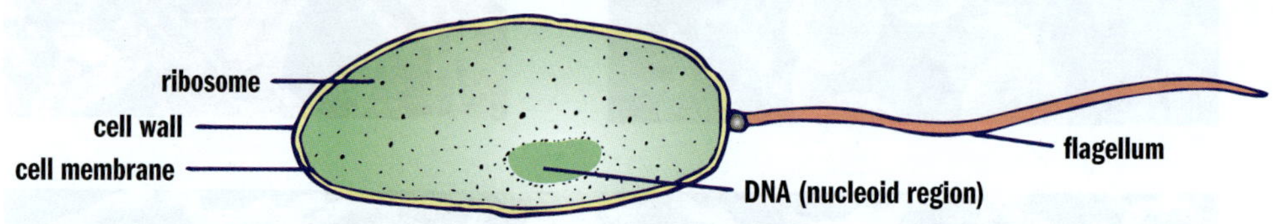

Figure 1.10 Prokaryotic Cell Structure

Cell Wall

Because prokaryotes do not form multicellular organisms, each bacterium is responsible for protecting itself from the environment. The **cell wall** forms the outer barrier of the cell. The next layer is the **cell membrane** (**plasma membrane**), which is composed of phospholipids, similar to that of a eukaryote. Together, the cell wall and the cell membrane are known as the **envelope**.

KEY CONCEPT

Bacteria contain a cell wall, the composition of which is different in gram-positive and gram-negative bacteria. Specific components of the cell wall can trigger an inflammatory response.

The cell wall both provides structure and controls the movement of solutes into and out of the bacterium. This allows the cell to maintain a concentration gradient relative to the environment. In bacteria, there are two main types of cell wall: gram positive and gram negative (see Figure 1.11). The type of cell wall is determined by the Gram staining process: a crystal violet stain, followed by a counterstain with a substance called *safranin*. If the envelope absorbs the crystal violet stain, it will appear deep purple, and the cell is said to be gram positive. If the envelope does not absorb the crystal violet stain, but absorbs the safranin counterstain, then the cell will appear pink-red, and it is said to be gram negative.

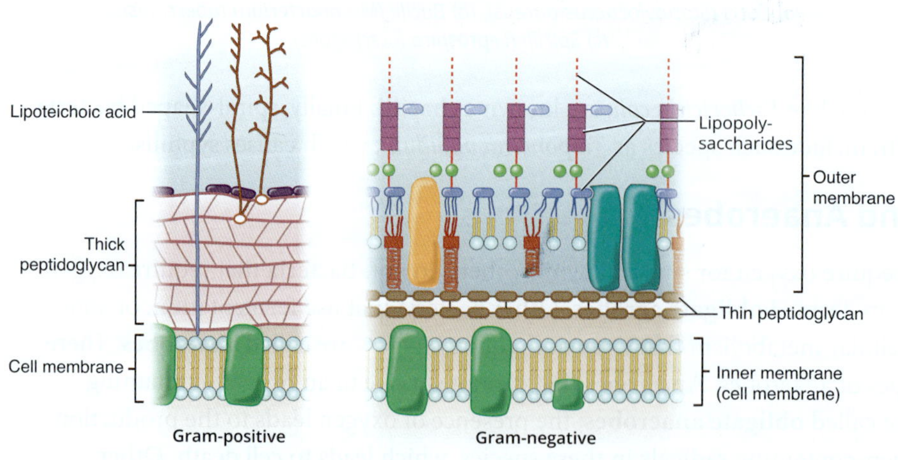

Figure 1.11 Prokaryotic Cell Envelope Types and Subsequent Structure

Gram-positive cell walls consist of a thick layer of **peptidoglycan**, a polymeric substance made from amino acids and sugars. In addition to its structural and barrier functions, the cell wall may also aid a bacterial pathogen by providing protection from a host organism's immune system. In addition to peptidoglycan, the gram-positive cell wall also contains **lipoteichoic acid**. It is not clear what role this acid serves for the bacterium, but the human immune system may be activated by exposure to these chemicals.

Gram-negative cell walls are very thin and also contain peptidoglycan, but in much smaller amounts. The peptidoglycan cell walls of these bacteria are adjacent to the cell membrane, and are separated from the membrane by the **periplasmic space**. In addition to the cell wall and cell membrane, gram-negative bacteria also have **outer membranes** containing phospholipids and **lipopolysaccharides**. Interestingly, lipopolysaccharides are the part of gram-negative bacteria that triggers an immune response in human beings; the inflammatory response to lipopolysaccharides is much stronger than the response to gram-negative-associated lipoteichoic acid.

REAL WORLD

The antibiotic penicillin targets the enzyme that catalyzes the cross-linking of peptidoglycan. If a gram-positive cell cannot cross-link its cell wall, it no longer serves as an effective barrier. The bacterium then becomes susceptible to osmotic damage and lyses. Most bacteria have developed resistance mechanisms to penicillin, although a few bacteria—including *Streptococcus pyogenes*, which causes strep throat and some skin infections, and *Treponema pallidum*, which causes syphilis—are still very sensitive to this antibiotic.

Flagella

Flagella are long, whip-like structures that can be used for propulsion; bacteria may have one, two, or many flagella, depending on the species. Flagella can be used to move toward food or away from toxins or immune cells. This ability of a cell to detect chemical stimuli and move toward or away from them is called **chemotaxis**. The flagella are composed of a filament, a basal body, and a hook, as shown in Figure 1.12. The **filament** is a hollow, helical structure composed of **flagellin**. The **basal body** is a complex structure that anchors the flagellum to the cytoplasmic membrane and is also the motor of the flagellum, which rotates at rates up to 300 Hz. The **hook** connects the filament and the basal body so that, as the basal body rotates, it exerts torque on the filament, which thereby spins and propels the bacterium forward. The overall structure of flagella is similar in both gram-positive and gram-negative bacteria, but there are slight differences due to the different physical structure and chemical composition of the envelope in gram-positive and gram-negative bacteria. Archaea also contain flagella, but the structure of their flagella is quite different from that of bacteria and is unlikely to be asked about on Test Day.

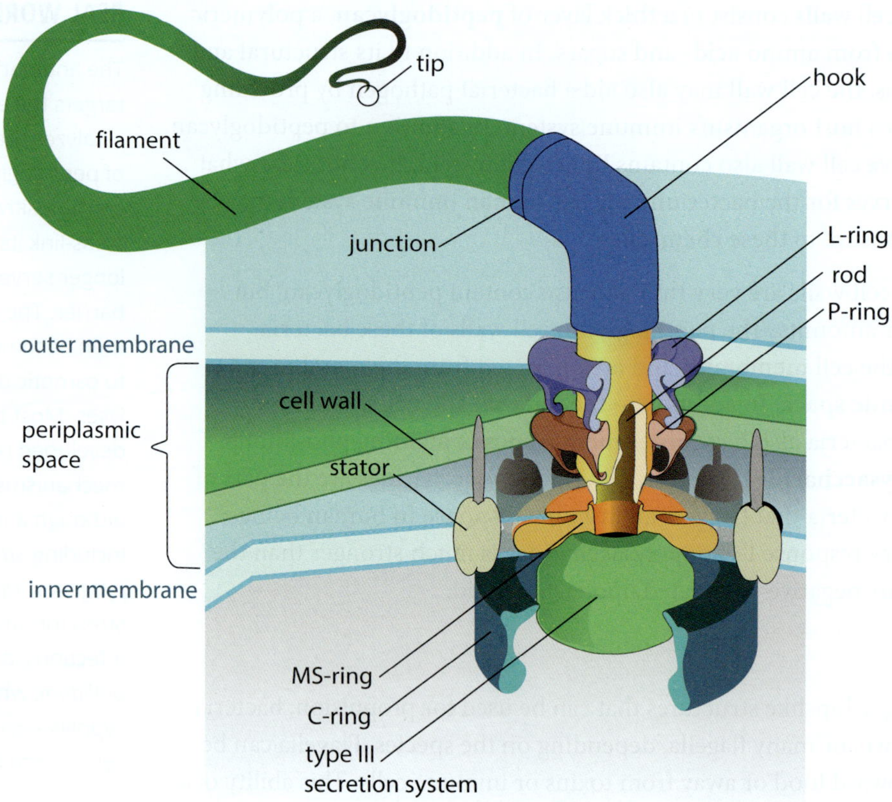

Figure 1.12 Prokaryotic Flagellum Structure
The hook connects the filament to the basal body (the complex structure of which is shown).

Other Organelles

As mentioned earlier, prokaryotes concentrate DNA in a region of the cell known as the nucleoid region, which does not contain a nuclear envelope. Prokaryotic DNA is carried on a single circular chromosome which can be found coiled around histone-like proteins in some bacteria. True histones are found in Archaea. In addition, DNA acquired from external sources may also be carried on smaller circular structures known as **plasmids**. Plasmids carry DNA that is not necessary for survival of the prokaryote—and therefore is not considered part of the genome of the bacterium—but may confer an advantage such as antibiotic resistance.

Prokaryotes lack several key organelles, such as mitochondria. Instead, the cell membrane is used for the electron transport chain and generation of ATP. Prokaryotes do contain a primitive cytoskeleton, but it is not nearly as complex as the one found in eukaryotes. Prokaryotes also contain ribosomes, but this ribosome is a different size from that found in eukaryotes: prokaryotic ribosomes contain 30S and 50S subunits, whereas eukaryotic ribosomes contain 40S and 60S subunits.

BRIDGE

The fact that prokaryotes and eukaryotes have different-sized ribosomes implies that they carry out protein synthesis in slightly different ways. These differences are highlighted in Chapter 7 of *MCAT Biochemistry Review*. This difference also allows us to target bacterial ribosomes with a number of antibiotics, including *tetracyclines*, *aminoglycosides*, and *macrolides*, while leaving the eukaryotic ribosome more or less unaffected.

MCAT CONCEPT CHECK 1.3

Before you move on, assess your understanding of the material with these questions.

1. In what ways are Archaea similar to bacteria? In what ways are Archaea similar to eukaryotes?
   - Similar to bacteria:

   ___

   - Similar to eukaryotes:

   ___

2. What are the three common shapes of bacteria?
   -

   ___

   -

   ___

   -

   ___

3. Compare and contrast the metabolisms of aerobic and anaerobic bacteria: (Note: Put "yes" or "no" in each box.)

	Oxygen Present		Oxygen Absent	
Type of Bacteria	**Can survive**	**Can carry out aerobic metabolism**	**Can survive**	**Can carry out anaerobic metabolism**
Obligate aerobe				
Facultative anaerobe				
Obligate anaerobe				
Aerotolerant anaerobe				

4. What difference between the envelopes of gram-positive and gram-negative bacteria make gram-positive bacteria more susceptible to antibiotics such as penicillin?

   ___

5. How do the structures of eukaryotic and prokaryotic flagella differ?
   - Eukaryotic:

   ___

   - Prokaryotic:

   ___

BIOLOGY GUIDED EXAMPLE WITH EXPERT THINKING

To investigate the collective resistance property of bacteria, co-colonization experiments were conducted. Eight-week-old female CD1 mice were infected intratracheally with chloramphenicol sensitive (Cm^S) pneumococci or an equivalent quantity of Cm^S:chloramphenicol resistant (Cm^R) pneumococci (1:1). One hour post-infection, mice were treated with one intraperitoneal injection of chloramphenicol (Cm) at a concentration of 75 mg kg^{-1}, followed by two additional doses spaced 5 hours apart. Control mice received vehicle injection only. Cm^R pneumococci are Cm resistant due to the expression of a resistance factor, chloramphenicol acetyltransferase (CAT).

Goal: investigate collective resistance of bacteria by comparing infection with one bacteria to a mixture of two bacteria

Experimental setup: Infect mice, then give intraperitoneal (IP) injections of chloramphenicol or vehicle only (vehicle is just the solvent without any antibiotic, probably saline)

Stable bacterial coexistence requires successful adjustment to several ecological constraints, such as limited resources and antibiotic concentration. To better quantify bacterial behavior under these conditions, in vitro population analysis was conducted.

Based on the experimental setup and this statement, collective resistance must be about the coexistence of bacterial types when only one is resistant to an antibiotic

Population analysis done to quantify collective resistance

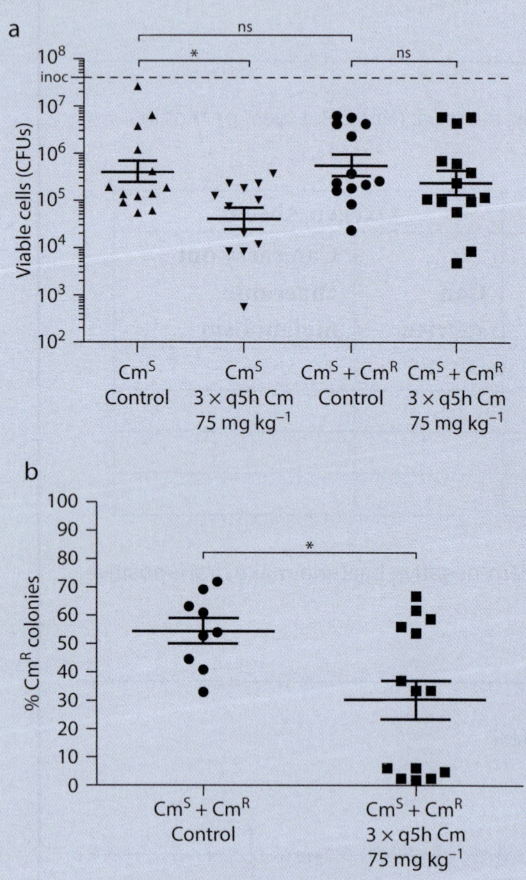

Figure 1 Mixed Culture Experiment. (a) Antibiotic stress on Cm^S alone and $Cm^S + Cm^R$ co-colonization condition. (b) Co-colonization colonies analysis of Cm^S to Cm^R ratio.

In figures always identify the variables and trends.

IVs: control or Cm administration, Cm^S or Cm^S/Cm^R bacteria

DVs: viable cells, percent Cm^R colonies

Trends: Cm^S bacteria have significantly fewer viable cells when treated with Cm. The percent of Cm^R colonies is significantly lower when Cm^S/Cm^R is treated with Cm.

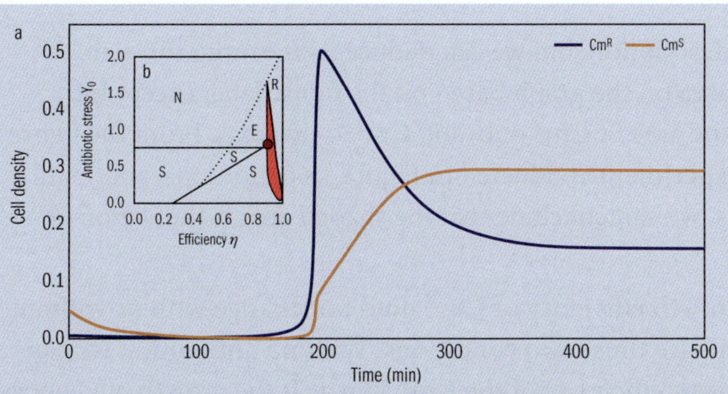

IVs: time, antibiotic stress

DVs: cell density, efficiency

Trends: highest cell density of Cm^R is at 200 min, Cm^S density levels off at 300 min. Based on the caption, the inner figure compares efficiency under several different conditions.

Figure 2 (a) Bacterial growth trajectories subject to antibiotic stress and resource competition. (b) Axes indicate co-colonization experiment parameters (efficiency refers to the growth rate efficiency of Cm^R cells). The dot indicates Figure 1 experiment antibiotic levels, with previous analysis establishing Cm^S only (area S), Cm^R only (area R), no bacterial growth (area N), and competition-induced extinction (area E, where Cm^S bacteria first outcompete Cm^R bacteria and are subsequently cleared by antibiotic).

Adapted from Sorg, R. A., Lin, L., Van Doorn, G. S., Sorg, M., Olson, J., Nizet, V., & Veening, J. W. (2016). Collective resistance in microbial communities by intracellular antibiotic deactivation. *PLoS Biology*, 14(12), e2000631.

Consider the following: For successful co-colonization with Cm^S, the growth efficiency of Cm^R must remain as a constant value in the presence or absence of antibiotic stress. Is this conclusion valid?

This question asks us to analyze a conclusion's validity. First, we must find where the key term is located in the passage. In this case, we are asked about growth efficiency, which can be found in the figure description of Figure 2(b). According to the description, growth efficiency is a reference to the growth rate of Cm^R, and is depicted as the x-axis of the graph. The conclusion given in the question stem states that the growth efficiency is unchanged by the presence of antibiotics. To determine if this conclusion is valid, we first need to decipher what the graph represents.

The figure description can be a rich source of crucial information. According to that same Figure 2(b) description, each area on the graph depicts a different outcome of Cm^S and Cm^R co-colonization. To ensure we're drawing valid conclusions, we should examine the graph one axis at a time. To analyze a graph, hold one variable constant first. Assume no antibiotics are present, meaning that the antibiotic stress is zero, looking at the x-axis along the zero line, as the growth efficiency of Cm^R decreases, the Cm^S strain starts to outcompete it. In fact, unless the growth efficiency of Cm^R is at its highest, the susceptible strain (Cm^S) will always outcompete Cm^R.

Now let's hold the same variable at a different level. Let us assume the antibiotic stress is high, so we'll look to the right side of the x-axis. Under those conditions, there's no growth of the susceptible strain at all. That makes sense, as the susceptible strain wouldn't be expected to survive the antibiotics. We can also see that, for this x-axis value, there's an area, E, where at slightly lower Cm^R growth efficiency, the susceptible strain outcompetes Cm^R, removing all protection, and then succumbs to the antibiotic. In fact, unless the growth efficiency of Cm^R is high, no bacteria will successfully grow. From these two observations, we can observe that the growth efficiency of the Cm^R strain has a large influence on how the co-colonized strain will grow.

The shaded area of Figure 2(b) is not explained in the figure description, but we can deduce its meaning through context. All the other possibilities already have a designated area on the graph based on the figure label except for successful co-colonization. Also, the shaded area is between the area of Cm^S only and Cm^R only areas. From the figure description, we also learned that the large dot indicates the experiment conducted in Figure 1's conditions, and Figure 1's experiment demonstrates successful co-colonization. Thus, we can conclude that the shaded area is the region of successful co-colonization of the two strains.

The conclusion presented in the question stem claims that growth efficiency of Cm^R does not change with or without the antibiotic presence. To assess this, we simply need to compare those two conditions. With no antibiotics, we can see that successful co-colonization only occurs when the growth efficiency of the Cm^R is at 1. If the growth efficiency is not that high, then the Cm^S strain will outcompete it. When we raise the antibiotic level to that of the red dot, we can see that if the growth efficiency remains at 1, the Cm^R bacteria will outcompete the Cm^S bacteria. In order for the two strains to coexist under antibiotic stress, the resistance strain's growth efficiency has to be lower than 1. Thus, we can reasonably argue that the conclusion is not valid.

1.4 Genetics and Growth of Prokaryotic Cells

LEARNING OBJECTIVES

After Chapter 1.4, you will be able to:

- Describe bacterial genetic recombination via transformation, conjugation, or transduction
- Recall the four phases of a bacterial growth curve and the major features of each phase:

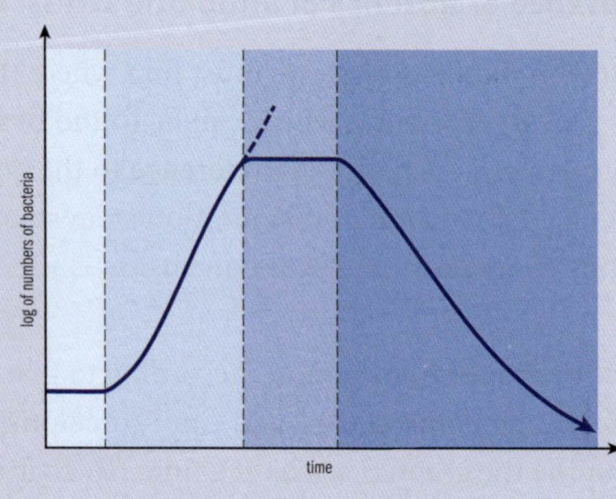

As we have seen, prokaryotic cells differ from eukaryotic cells both structurally and biochemically. Prokaryotes reproduce via asexual reproduction in the form of binary fission. In addition, prokaryotes are capable of acquiring and using genetic material from outside the cell.

Binary Fission

Binary fission, shown in Figure 1.13, is a simple form of asexual reproduction seen in prokaryotes. The circular chromosome attaches to the cell wall and replicates while the cell continues to grow in size. Eventually, the plasma membrane and cell wall begin to grow inward along the midline of the cell to produce two identical daughter cells.

Because binary fission requires fewer events than mitosis, it can proceed more rapidly. In fact, some strains of *E. coli* can replicate every 20 minutes under ideal growth conditions.

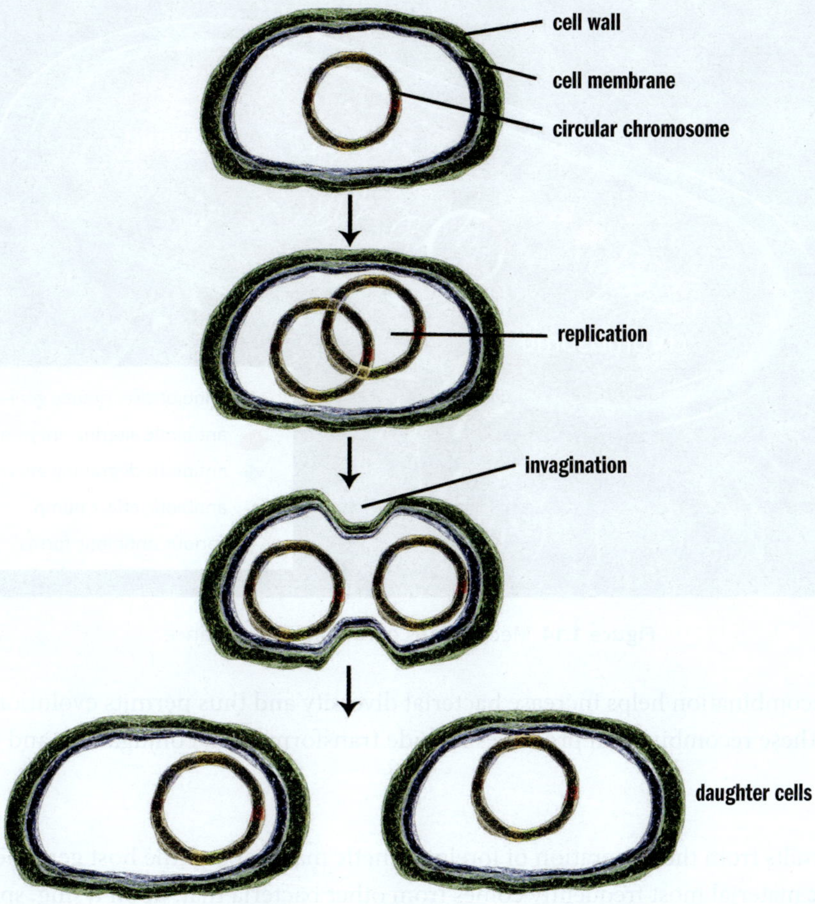

Figure 1.13 Stages of Binary Fission

Genetic Recombination

This single circular chromosome of a prokaryotic cell contains the information that is necessary for the cell to survive and reproduce. However, many bacteria also contain extrachromosomal (extragenomic) material known as **plasmids**. Plasmids often carry genes that impart some benefit to the bacterium, such as antibiotic resistance, some mechanisms of which are shown in Figure 1.14. Plasmids may also carry additional **virulence factors**, or traits that increase pathogenicity, such as toxin production, projections that allow attachment to certain kinds of cells, or features that allow evasion of the host's immune system. A subset of plasmids called **episomes** are capable of integrating into the genome of the bacterium.

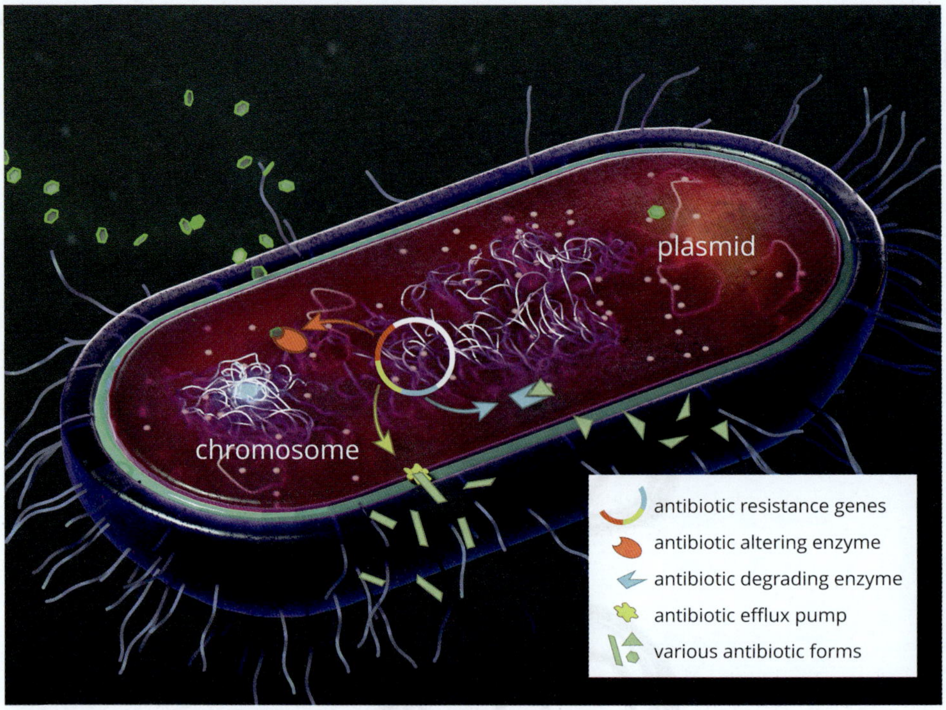

Figure 1.14 Mechanisms of Antibiotic Resistance

Bacterial genetic recombination helps increase bacterial diversity and thus permits evolution of a bacterial species over time. These recombination processes include transformation, conjugation, and transduction.

Transformation

Transformation results from the integration of foreign genetic material into the host genome (see Figure 1.15). This foreign genetic material most frequently comes from other bacteria that, upon lysing, spill their contents into the vicinity of a bacterium capable of transformation. Many gram-negative rods are able to carry out this process. The recipient bacterium must be in a state of **competence**, or a state in which extracellular DNA can be taken up, which can occur in environmental conditions such as starvation or high cell density, or induced in a laboratory via heat, electricity, or chemicals.

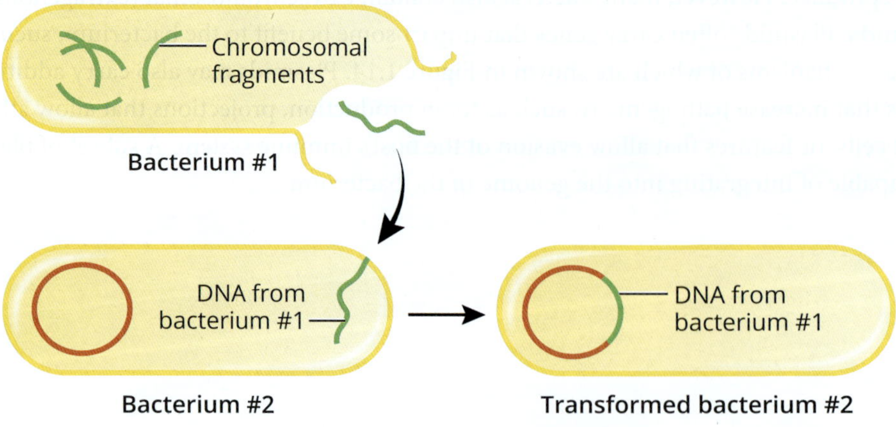

Figure 1.15 Bacterial Transformation

Specifically in research, bacteria can be induced to take up foreign genetic material like plasmids for the purpose of overexpressing a protein of interest that is not naturally expressed. A vial of competent bacterial cells are incubated with DNA and subsequently plated onto selective agar plates to grow colonies of the bacteria that took up the DNA. The selectivity of these plates result from two variables: the use of an antibiotic in the agar plate and a correlated antibiotic resistance gene in the plasmid. The logic goes as follows: If a strain of bacteria grows on the medium containing the antibiotic, then it has the antibiotic resistance gene. If it has the antibiotic resistance gene, then it must have taken up the plasmid containing the gene for the protein of interest.

The effectiveness of transformation, also known as **transformation efficiency**, can be calculated by counting the number of **colony forming units (CFUs)** and dividing it by the mass of DNA (usually measured in μg) added to the cells. If only a portion of the transformed cells are plated, this number is then multiplied by the ratio of the total volume of recovered cells to the plated volume for a final calculation of transformation efficiency, as expressed in Equation 1.1.

$$\frac{\text{CFU}}{\mu\text{g of DNA}} \times \frac{\text{total volume (mL)}}{\text{volume plated (mL)}} = \text{transformation efficiency}$$

Equation 1.1

Conjugation

Conjugation is the bacterial form of mating (sexual reproduction). It involves two cells forming a **conjugation bridge** between them that facilitates the transfer of genetic material. The transfer is unidirectional, from the **donor male** (+) to the **recipient female** (−). The bridge is made from appendages called **sex pili** that are found on the donor male. To form the pilus, bacteria must contain plasmids known as **sex factors** that contain the necessary genes. The best-studied sex factor is the **F (fertility) factor** in *E. coli*. Bacteria possessing this plasmid are termed F^+ cells; those without are called F^- cells. During conjugation the F^+ cell replicates its F factor and donates the copy to the F^- cell, converting it to an F^+ cell. This enables the cell obtaining the new plasmid to then transfer copies to other cells. This method of genetic recombination allows for rapid acquisition of antibiotic resistance or virulence factors throughout a colony because other plasmids can also be passed through the conjugation bridge. The process of conjugation is illustrated in Figure 1.16.

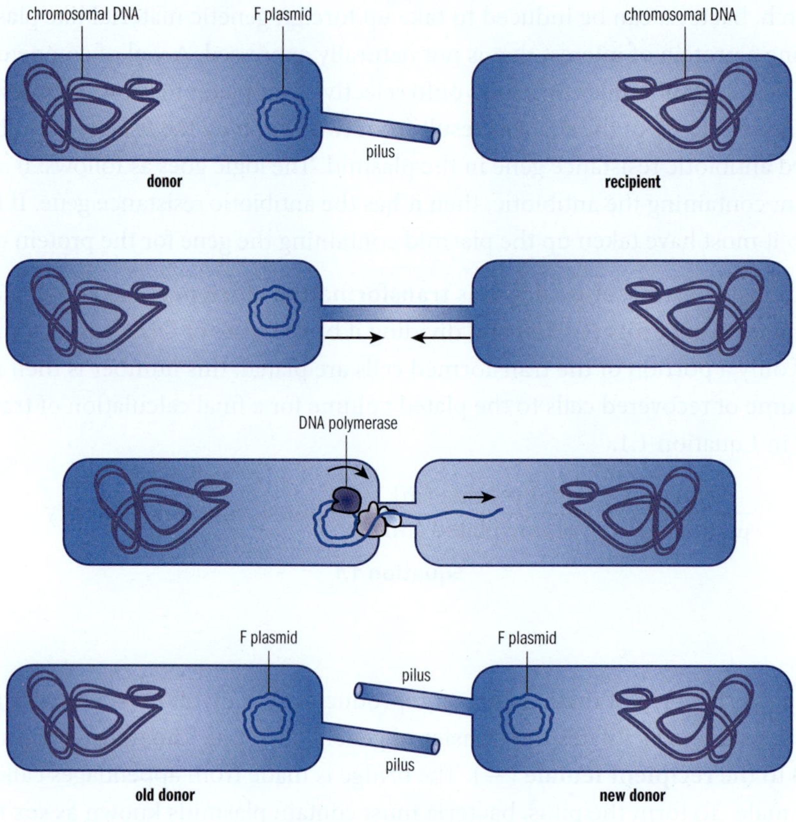

Figure 1.16 Bacterial Conjugation

The sex factor is a plasmid, but through processes such as transformation, it can become integrated into the host genome. In this case, when conjugation occurs, the entire genome replicates because it now contains the sex factor. The donor cell will then attempt to transfer an entire copy of its genome into the recipient; however, the bridge usually breaks before the full DNA sequence can be moved. Cells that have undergone this change are referred to by the abbreviation **Hfr** for **high frequency of recombination**.

Transduction

Transduction is the only genetic recombination process that requires a **vector**—a virus that carries genetic material from one bacterium to another. Viruses are obligate intracellular pathogens, which means that they cannot reproduce outside of a host cell. Because of this, **bacteriophages** (viruses that infect bacteria) can accidentally incorporate a segment of host DNA during assembly. When the bacteriophage infects another bacterium, it can release this trapped DNA into the new host cell. This transferred DNA can then integrate into the genome, giving the new host additional genes. The process of transduction is shown in Figure 1.17.

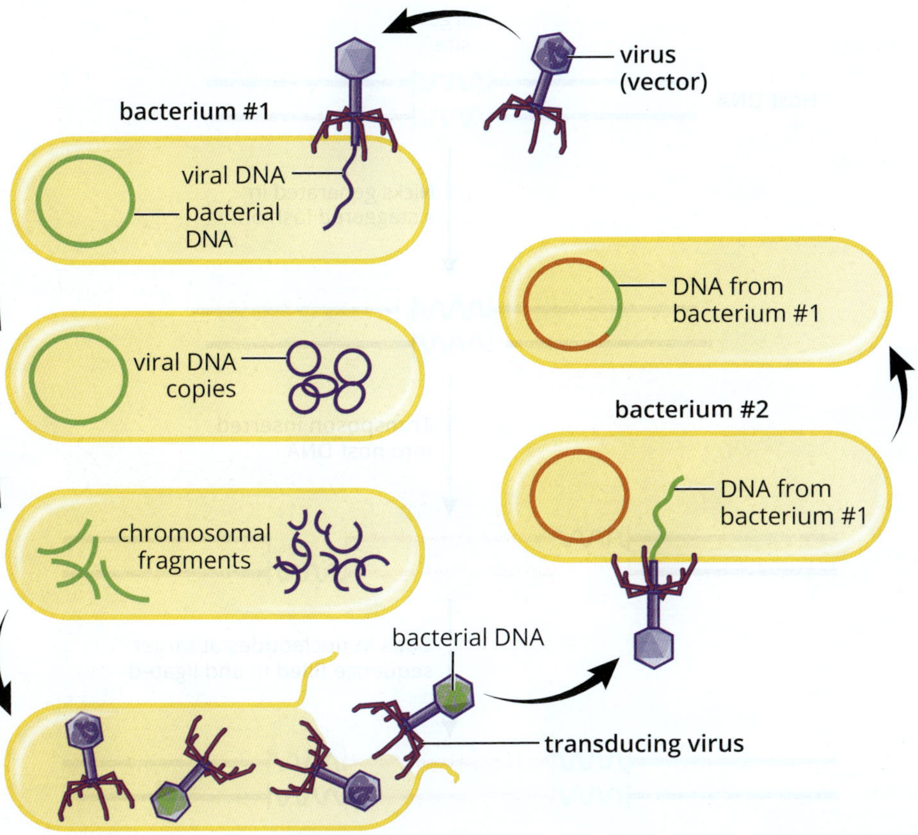

Figure 1.17 Bacterial Transduction

Transposons

Transposons are genetic elements capable of inserting and removing themselves from the genome. This process involves several enzymes to make staggered cuts in the DNA and remove/insert the transposons, as seen in Figure 1.18. This phenomenon is not limited to prokaryotes; it has been seen in eukaryotes as well. If a transposon is inserted within a coding region of a gene, that gene may be disrupted.

REAL WORLD

One of the biggest challenges a doctor faces is patient compliance with treatment, especially antibiotics. Many patients fail to complete an entire course of antibiotics, often discontinuing the treatment because they feel better. Unfortunately, this breeds antibiotic resistance by killing off the bacteria that are nonresistant and leaving behind bacteria that are more resistant. These resistant bacteria then reproduce, resulting in recurrence of the infection. Over time, this practice has led to bacteria that are resistant to multiple antibiotics, making common infections more difficult to treat.

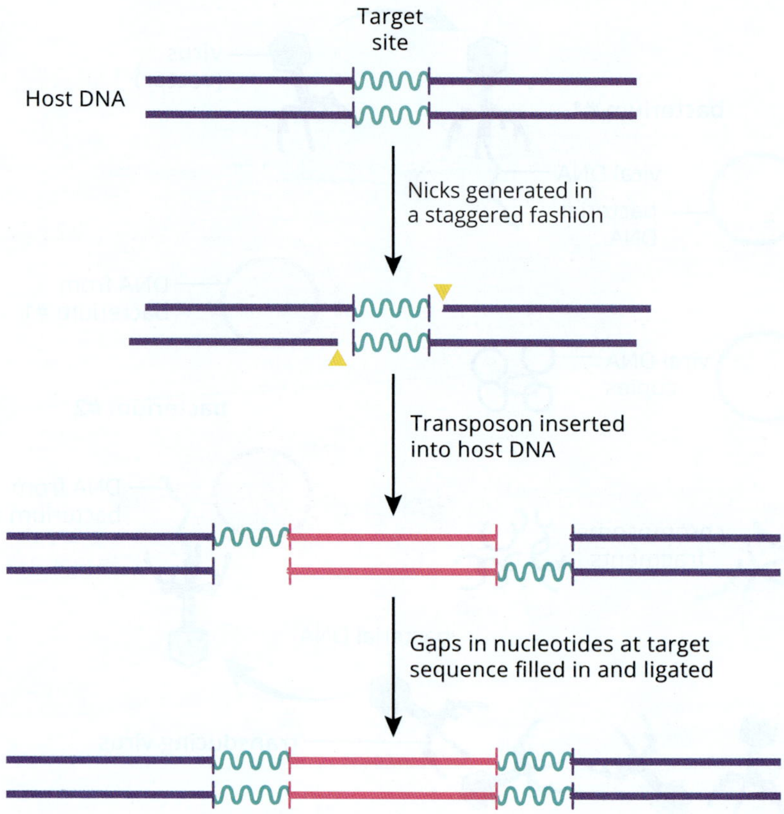

Figure 1.18 Transposon Insertion

Growth

As discussed previously, bacteria reproduce via binary fission. This implies that all of the bacteria are exactly the same in a local colony (assuming no mutations or genetic recombination), and that no bacteria are dividing faster than the others. Bacteria can be said to grow in a series of phases, as shown in Figure 1.19. In a new environment, bacteria first adapt to the new local conditions during the **lag phase**. As the bacteria adapt, the rate of division increases, causing an exponential increase in the number of bacteria in the colony during the **exponential phase**, also called the **log phase**. As the number of bacteria in the colony grows, resources are often reduced. The reduction of resources slows reproduction, and the **stationary phase** results. After the bacteria have exceeded the ability of the environment to support the number of bacteria, a **death phase** occurs, marking the depletion of resources.

BRIDGE

The bacterial growth curve is an example of a semilog plot. The fact that the *y*-axis is logarithmic means that a straight line (as seen during the exponential phase) actually represents an exponential increase in the number of bacteria, not a linear increase. Semilog and log–log plots are discussed in Chapter 12 of *MCAT Physics and Math Review*.

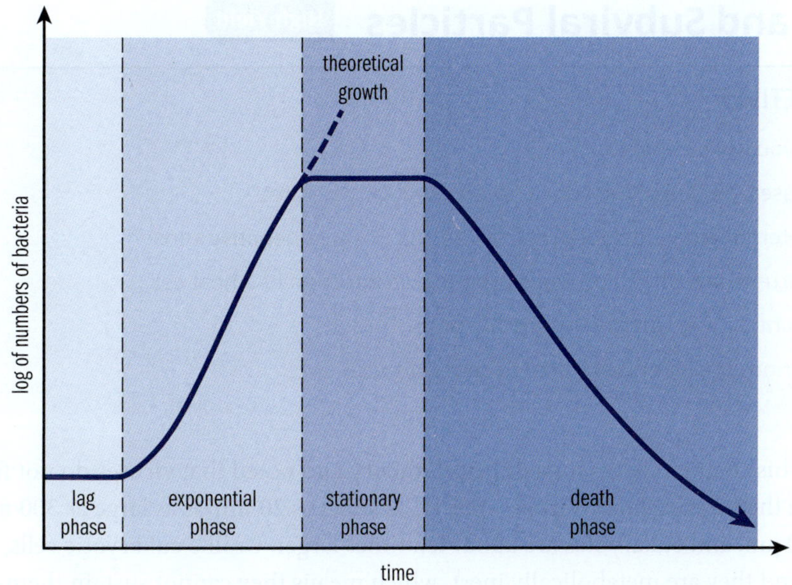

Figure 1.19 Bacterial Growth Curve

MCAT CONCEPT CHECK 1.4

Before you move on, assess your understanding of the material with these questions.

1. Briefly describe the three mechanisms of bacterial genetic recombination:

   - Transformation:

   - Conjugation:

   - Transduction:

   ---

2. What are the four phases of the bacterial growth curve? What are the features of each phase?

Phase	Features

1.5 Viruses and Subviral Particles High Yield

LEARNING OBJECTIVES

After Chapter 1.5, you will be able to:

- Explain why viruses are defined as "obligate intracellular parasites"
- Recall key virus terminology, including retrovirus and positive/negative sense
- Describe how viruses are able to produce progeny via infection of a host cell
- Compare and contrast the lytic and lysogenic cycles
- Describe how prions and viroids are able to cause disease

At the beginning of this chapter, we discussed the cell theory and noted that viruses do not fit the definition of living things because they are acellular. Viruses may be as small as 20 nm or as large as 300 nm. For reference, prokaryotes are 1–10 μm, and eukaryotes are about ten times larger. Unlike eukaryotic cells, viruses lack organelles and a nucleus, and they are metabolically inert, which means they cannot sustain themselves by making or harnessing energy from their environment. A model depicting viral structure can be seen in Figure 1.20.

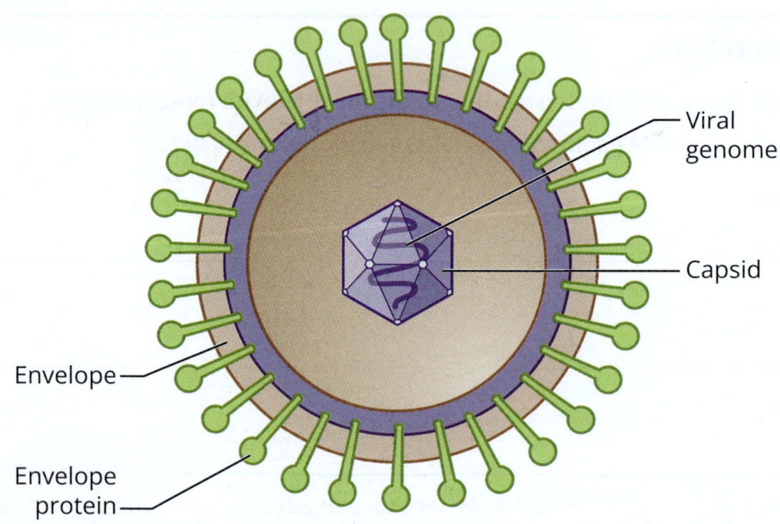

Figure 1.20 Virus Structure

Viral Structure

Viruses are composed of genetic material, a protein coat, and sometimes an envelope containing lipids. The genetic information may be circular or linear, single- or double-stranded, and composed of either DNA or RNA. The protein coat is known as a **capsid**, which may be surrounded by an envelope composed of phospholipids and virus-specific proteins. The envelope is very sensitive to heat, detergents, and desiccation; thus, enveloped viruses are easier to kill. On the other hand, viruses that do not have an envelope are more resistant to sterilization and are likely to persist on surfaces for an extended period of time.

Because viruses cannot reproduce independently, they are considered obligate intracellular parasites. Viruses must express and replicate genetic information within a **host cell** because they lack ribosomes to carry out protein synthesis. After hijacking a cell's machinery, a virus will replicate and produce viral progeny, called **virions**, which can be released to infect additional cells.

Bacteriophages are viruses that specifically target bacteria. They do not actually enter bacteria; rather, they simply inject their genetic material, leaving the remaining structures outside the infected cell. In addition to a capsid, bacteriophages contain a tail sheath and tail fibers, as shown in Figure 1.21. The **tail sheath** can act like a syringe, injecting genetic material into a bacterium. The **tail fibers** help the bacteriophage recognize and connect to the correct host cell.

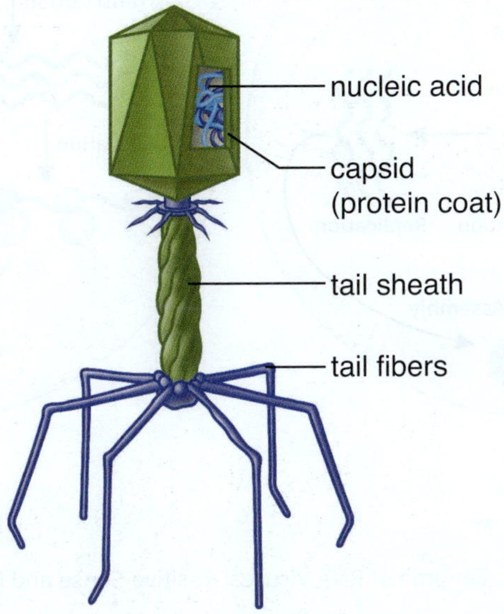

Figure 1.21 Structure of a Bacteriophage

Viral Genomes

Viral genomes come in a variety of shapes and sizes. Some are made of only a few genes, while others have several hundred. In addition, viral genomes may be made of either single- or double-stranded DNA or RNA.

Single-stranded RNA viruses may be positive sense or negative sense (see Figure 1.22). **Positive sense** implies that the genome may be directly translated to functional proteins by the ribosomes of the host cell, just like mRNA. **Negative-sense** RNA viruses are a bit more complicated: the negative-sense RNA strand acts as a template for synthesis of a complementary strand, which can then be used as a template for protein synthesis. Negative-sense RNA viruses must carry an **RNA-dependent RNA polymerase (RdRp)** in the virion to ensure that the complementary strand is synthesized.

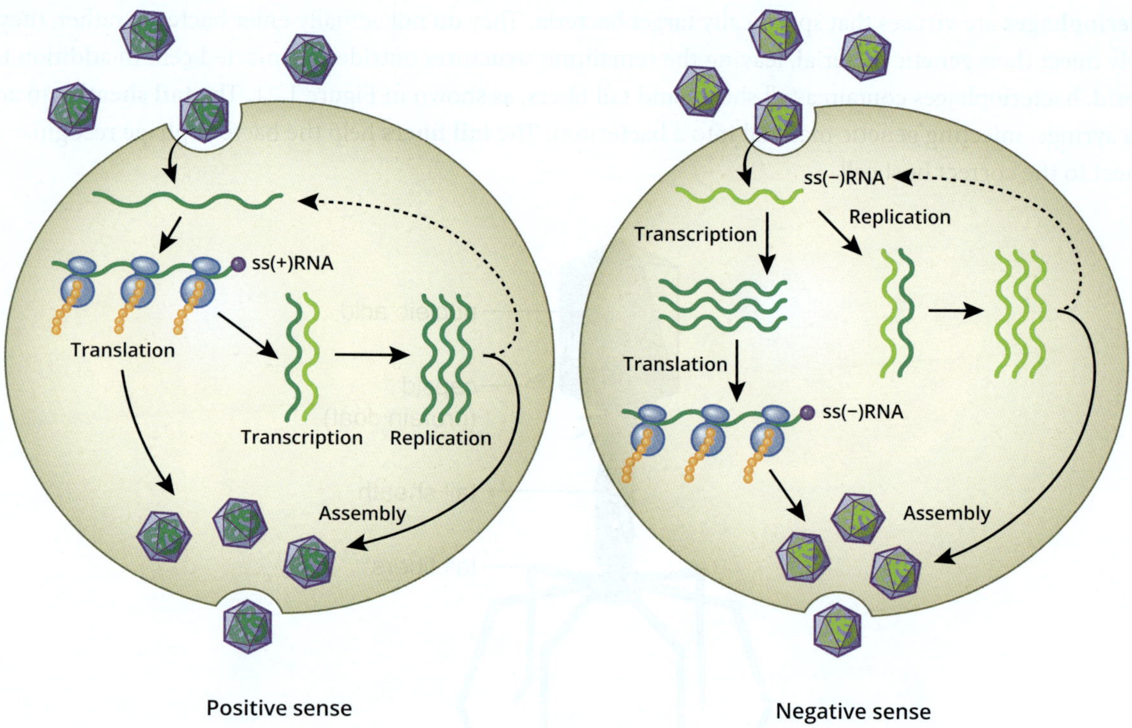

Figure 1.22 Genome of RNA Viruses: Positive-Sense and Negative-Sense

Retroviruses are enveloped, single-stranded RNA viruses in the family *Retroviridae*; usually, the virion contains two identical RNA molecules. These viruses carry an enzyme known as ***reverse transcriptase***, which synthesizes DNA from single-stranded RNA. The DNA then integrates into the host cell genome, where it is replicated and transcribed as if it were the host cell's own DNA. This is a clever mechanism because the integration of the genetic material into the host cell genome allows the cell to be infected indefinitely, so the only way to remove the infection is to kill the infected cell. The human immunodeficiency virus (HIV) is a retrovirus that utilizes this life cycle, which is one of the characteristics that make HIV so difficult to treat, as shown in Figure 1.23.

REAL WORLD

Both retroviruses and transduction are under investigation as methods of gene therapy. It is theorized that retroviral and transduction methods can deliver functional versions of missing or altered genes, so that the correct proteins can be synthesized and certain diseases can be treated. Gene therapy is discussed in Chapter 6 of *MCAT Biochemistry Review*.

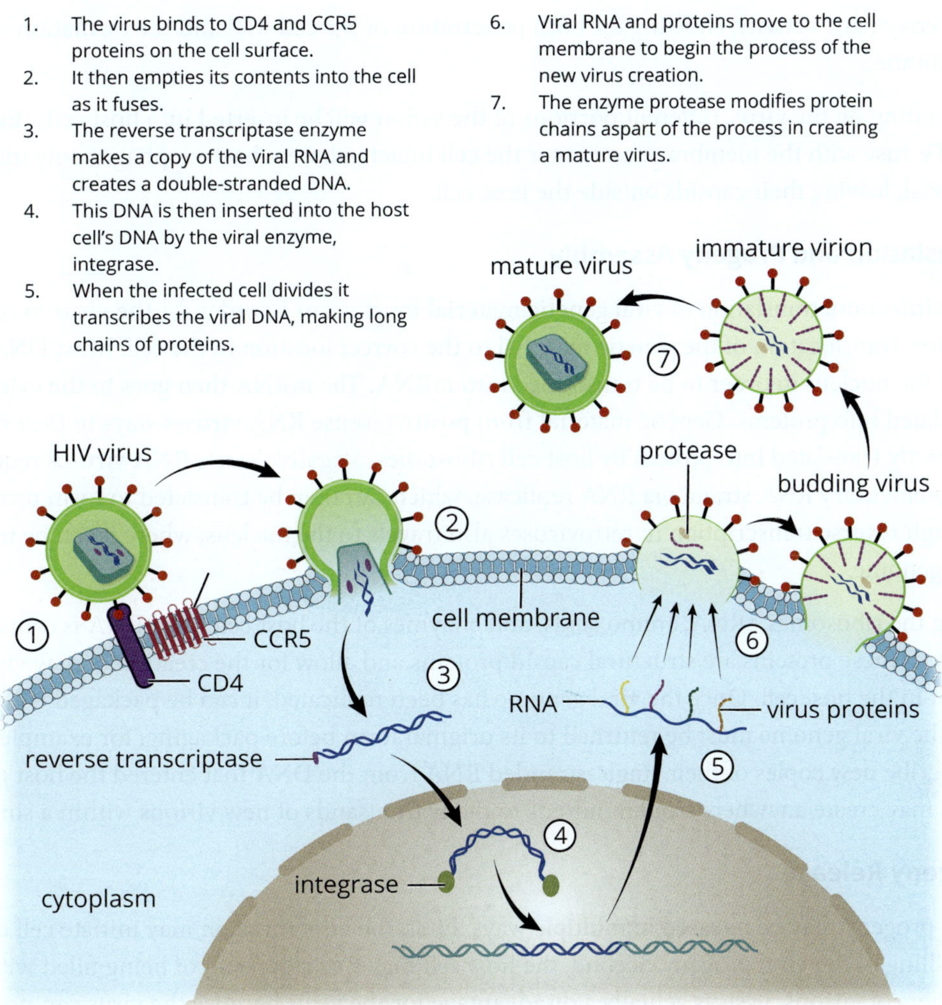

Figure 1.23 Life Cycle of the Human Immunodeficiency Virus (HIV)

Viral Life Cycle

As we have already discussed, viruses must infect a host cell and use the host cell's machinery in order to reproduce. Here, we will discuss the viral life cycle in detail.

Infection

Viruses can only infect a specific set of cells, because they must bind to specific receptors on the host cell. Without the proper receptors, a cell is essentially invisible to the virus. Once the virus binds the correct receptor, the virus and the cell are brought into close enough proximity to permit additional interactions. Enveloped viruses fuse with the plasma membrane of a cell, allowing entry of the virion into the host cell. Sometimes a host cell may mistake a virus bound to the membrane as nutrients or other useful molecules and will actually bring the virus into the cytoplasm via endocytosis. As mentioned earlier, bacteriophages use tail fibers to anchor themselves to the cell membrane and then inject their genome into the host bacterium through the tail sheath. Some tail fibers even

REAL WORLD

HIV must bind to a receptor called CCR5 on white blood cells in order to infect them. Some people lack this receptor and are thus immune to HIV. There was recently a case in which an HIV-positive individual with leukemia received a bone marrow transplant from a donor that lacked CCR5. Not only was the leukemia cured, but the patient experienced remission of the HIV infection because the white blood cells from the newly acquired bone marrow were not susceptible to HIV infection.

have enzymatic activity, allowing for both penetration of the cell wall and the formation of pores in the cell membrane.

Depending on the virus, different portions of the virion will be inserted into host cells. Enveloped viruses such as HIV fuse with the membrane and enter the cell intact, whereas bacteriophages only insert their genetic material, leaving their capsids outside the host cell.

Translation and Progeny Assembly

After infection, translation of viral genetic material must occur in order for the virus to reproduce. This requires translocation of the genetic material to the correct location in the cell. Most DNA viruses must enter the nucleus in order to be transcribed into mRNA. The mRNA then goes to the cytoplasm, where it is translated into proteins. Genetic material from positive-sense RNA viruses stays in the cytoplasm, where it is directly translated into protein by host cell ribosomes. Negative-sense RNA viruses require synthesis of a complementary RNA strand via RNA replicase, which can then be translated to form proteins. DNA formed through reverse transcription in retroviruses also travels to the nucleus, where it can be integrated into the host genome.

Using the ribosomes, tRNA, amino acids, and enzymes of the host cell, viral RNA is translated into protein. Many of these proteins are structural capsid proteins and allow for the creation of new virions in the cytoplasm in the host cell. Once the viral genome has been replicated, it can be packaged within the capsid. Note that the viral genome must be returned to its original form before packaging; for example, retroviruses must transcribe new copies of their single-stranded RNA from the DNA that entered the host genome. A single virus may create anywhere from hundreds to many thousands of new virions within a single host cell.

Progeny Release

Viral progeny may be released in multiple ways. First, the viral invasion may initiate cell death, which results in spilling of the viral progeny. Second, the host cell may lyse as a result of being filled with extremely large numbers of virions. Lysis is actually a disadvantage for the virus because the virus can no longer use the cell to carry out its life cycle. Finally, a virus can leave the cell by fusing with its plasma membrane as shown in Figure 1.24, a process known as **extrusion**. This process keeps the host cell alive, and thus allows for the continued use of the host cell by the virus. A virus in this state is said to be in a **productive cycle**.

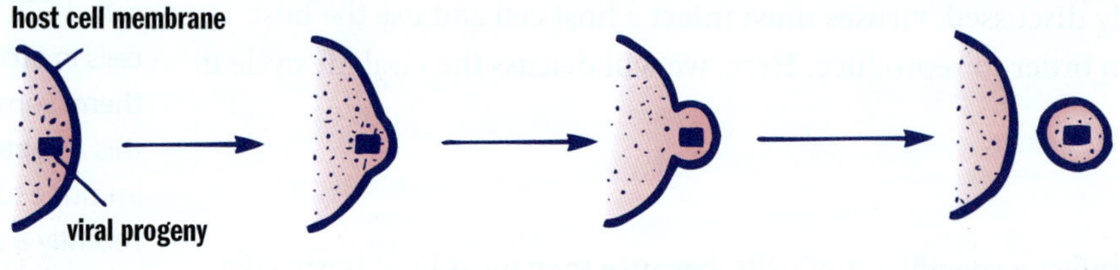

Figure 1.24 Viral Extrusion

Lytic and Lysogenic Cycles

Depending on growth conditions and the specific virus, bacteriophages may enter a lytic or lysogenic life cycle. These two phases are similar to the lysis and productive cycle methods of progeny release discussed above.

During a **lytic cycle**, the bacteriophage maximizes the use of the cell's machinery with little regard for the survival of the host cell. Once the host is swollen with new virions, the cell lyses, and other bacteria can be infected. Viruses in the lytic phase are termed **virulent**.

In the event that the virus does not lyse the bacterium, it may integrate into the host genome as a **provirus** or **prophage**, initiating the **lysogenic cycle**. In this case, the virus will be replicated as the bacterium reproduces because it is now a part of the host's genome. Although the virus may remain integrated into the host genome indefinitely, environmental factors (radiation, light, or chemicals) may cause the provirus to leave the genome and revert to a lytic cycle. As mentioned earlier, the provirus may extract bacterial genes as it leaves the genome, which allows transduction of genes from one bacterium to another. Although bacteriophages can kill their hosts, integration of the phage into the host genome may actually benefit the bacterium. Infection with one strain of phage generally makes the bacterium less susceptible to **superinfection** (simultaneous infection) with other phages. Because the provirus is relatively innocuous, this arrangement may confer an evolutionary advantage. The lytic and lysogenic cycles are contrasted in Figure 1.25.

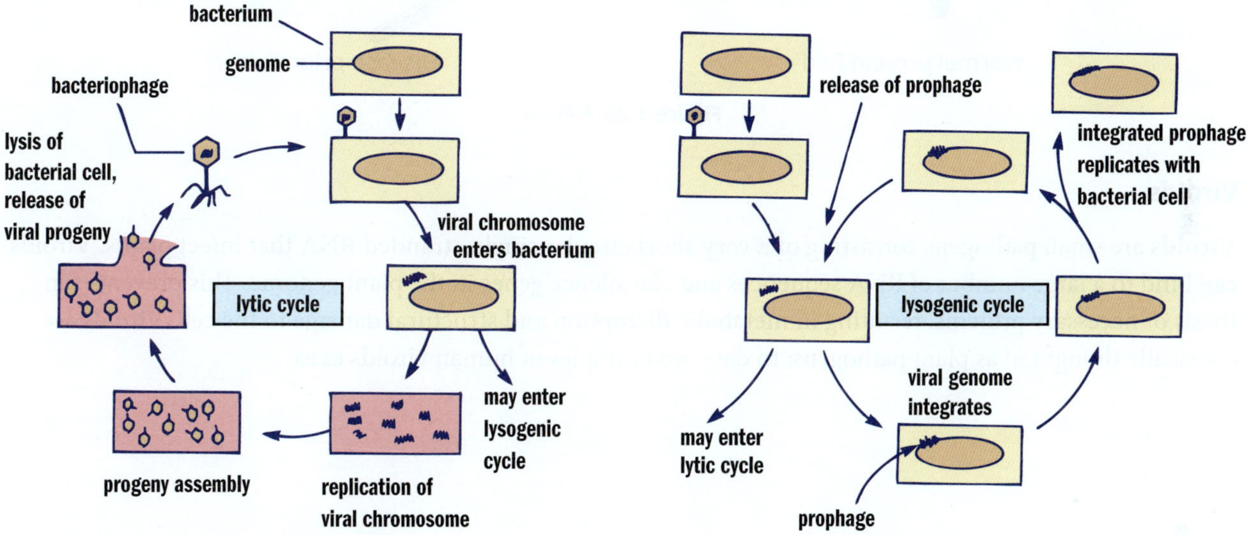

Figure 1.25 Lytic vs. Lysogenic Cycles of Bacteriophages

Prions and Viroids

Prions and viroids are very small (subviral) particles that can cause disease under certain circumstances.

Prions

Prions are infectious proteins (see Figure 1.26 for an example) and are, therefore, nonliving things. They cause disease by triggering misfolding of other proteins, usually through the conversion of a protein from an α-helical structure to a β-pleated sheet. This drastically reduces the solubility of the protein, as well as the ability of the cell to degrade the protein. Eventually, protein aggregates form, interfering with cell function. Prions are known to cause *bovine spongiform encephalopathy* (mad cow disease), *Creutzfeldt–Jakob disease*, and *familial fatal insomnia* in humans.

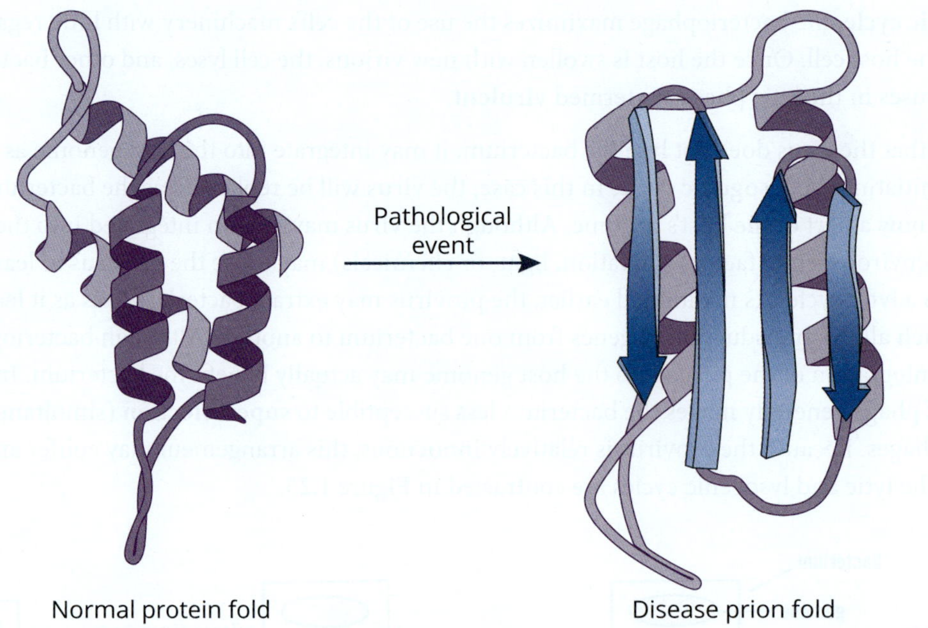

Figure 1.26 A Prion

Viroids

Viroids are small pathogens consisting of a very short circular single-stranded RNA that infect plants. Viroids can bind to a large number of RNA sequences and can silence genes in the plant genome. This prevents synthesis of necessary proteins, resulting in metabolic disruption and structural damage to the cell. Viroids are classically thought of as plant pathogens; to date, no examples of human viroids exist.

MCAT CONCEPT CHECK 1.5

Before you move on, assess your understanding of the material with these questions.

1. Why are viruses considered obligate intracellular parasites?

___

2. A coronavirus, which causes the common cold, is described as an enveloped, single-stranded positive-sense RNA virus. What does this indicate about the virus?

___

3. Briefly describe the pathway of retroviral nucleic acids from infection of a host cell to release of viral progeny:

___

4. What are the differences between the lytic and lysogenic cycles?
   - Lytic cycle:

   ___

   - Lysogenic cycle:

   ___

5. How do prions cause disease?

___

Conclusion

Our first chapter introduced the basis of all biology: cell theory. All living things are made of prokaryotic or eukaryotic cells. Prokaryotes are simpler and do not contain membrane-bound organelles. Eukaryotes contain membrane-bound organelles with highly specialized functions. While eukaryotic organisms (especially humans!) will be the primary focus on Test Day, an understanding of prokaryotic structure and physiology is necessary to understand infectious disease. Viruses are nonliving infectious particles that must invade cells in order to reproduce. Finally, we discussed the smallest infectious particles, prions and viroids.

Our discussions from here on out will focus primarily on eukaryotes, but you will spend significant time in your clinical career battling the pathogens we've presented in this chapter. Vaccines are available for a number of bacteria (*Bacillus anthracis* [anthrax], *Corynebacterium diphtheriae* [diphtheria], *Haemophilus influenzae* type B [many upper respiratory and ear infections], *Neisseria meningitidis* [some cases of bacterial meningitis], *Streptoccocus pneumoniae* [many cases of bacterial pneumonia], *Clostridium tetani* [tetanus], *Salmonella typhi* [typhoid], and *Bordetella pertussis* [whooping cough]) and viruses (varicella-zoster virus [chickenpox and shingles], hepatitis A and B viruses, human papillomavirus [HPV], influenza, measles, mumps, polio, rabies, rotavirus, rubella, and yellow fever). Those for which we do not have vaccines may be targeted with antibiotic and antiviral therapies; the appropriate pharmacotherapy usually depends on an understanding of bacterial or viral physiology and the known resistance patterns in the local area. In other words, the principles presented in this chapter will show up in your everyday life as a physician!

We've discussed one method of cellular reproduction: the division of a bacterial cell into two cells by binary fission. Eukaryotic cells also must replicate, but use a different process: mitosis. In the next chapter, we will turn our attention to mitosis, as well as meiosis and human reproduction.

GO ONLINE

You've reviewed the content, now test your knowledge and critical thinking skills by completing a test-like passage set in your online resources!

CONCEPT SUMMARY

Cell Theory

- The **cell theory** has four basic tenets:
  - All living things are composed of cells.
  - The cell is the basic functional unit of life.
  - Cells arise only from preexisting cells.
  - Cells carry genetic information in the form of DNA. This genetic material is passed on from parent to daughter cell.
- Viruses are not considered living things because they are acellular, cannot reproduce without the assistance of a host cell, and may use RNA as their genetic material.

Eukaryotic Cells

- **Eukaryotes** have membrane-bound organelles, a nucleus, and may form multicellular organisms.
- The cell membrane and membranes of organelles contain phospholipids, which organize to form hydrophilic interior and exterior surfaces with a hydrophobic core.
- The **cytosol** suspends the organelles and allows diffusion of molecules throughout the cell.
- The eukaryotic organelles each serve specific functions:
  - The **nucleus** contains DNA organized into **chromosomes**. It is surrounded by the **nuclear membrane** or **envelope**, a double membrane that contains **nuclear pores** for two-way exchange of materials between the nucleus and cytosol. DNA is organized into coding regions called **genes**.
  - The **nucleolus** is a subsection of the nucleus in which ribosomal RNA (rRNA) is synthesized.
  - **Mitochondria** contain an outer and inner membrane. The **outer membrane** forms a barrier with the cytosol; the **inner membrane** is folded into **cristae** and contains enzymes for the electron transport chain. Between the membranes is the **intermembrane space**; inside the inner mitochondrial membrane is the mitochondrial **matrix**. Mitochondria can divide independently of the nucleus via binary fission and can trigger **apoptosis** by releasing mitochondrial enzymes into the cytoplasm.
  - **Lysosomes** contain hydrolytic enzymes that can break down substances ingested by endocytosis and cellular waste products. When these enzymes are released, **autolysis** of the cell can occur.
  - The **endoplasmic reticulum** (**ER**) is a series of interconnected membranes and is continuous with the nuclear envelope. The **rough ER** (**RER**) is studded with ribosomes, which permit translation of proteins destined for secretion. The **smooth ER** (**SER**) is used for lipid synthesis and detoxification.
  - The **Golgi apparatus** consists of stacked membrane-bound sacs in which cellular products can be modified, packaged, and directed to specific cellular locations.
  - **Peroxisomes** contain hydrogen peroxide and can break down very long chain fatty acids via β-oxidation. They also participate in phospholipid synthesis and the pentose phosphate pathway.
- The **cytoskeleton** provides stability and rigidity to the overall structure of the cell, while also providing transport pathways for molecules within the cell.
  - **Microfilaments** are composed of **actin**. They provide structural protection for the cell and can cause muscle contraction through interactions with **myosin**. They also help form the **cleavage furrow** during **cytokinesis** in mitosis.

- **Microtubules** are composed of **tubulin**. They create pathways for motor proteins like **kinesin** and **dynein** to carry vesicles. They also contribute to the structure of **cilia** and **flagella**, where they are organized into nine pairs of microtubules in a ring with two microtubules at the center (**9 + 2 structure**). **Centrioles** are found in **centrosomes** and are involved in microtubule organization in the mitotic spindle.
- **Intermediate filaments** are involved in cell–cell adhesion and maintenance of the integrity of the cytoskeleton; they help anchor organelles. Common examples include keratin and desmin.

- **Epithelial tissues** cover the body and line its cavities, protecting against pathogen invasion and desiccation. Some epithelial cells absorb or secrete substances, or participate in sensation.
  - In most organs, epithelial cells form the **parenchyma**, or the functional parts of the organ.
  - Epithelial cells may be polarized, with one side facing a lumen or the outside world, and the other side facing blood vessels and structural cells.
  - Epithelia can be classified by the number of layers: **simple epithelia** have one layer, **stratified epithelia** have many layers, and **pseudostratified epithelia** appear to have multiple layers due to differences in cell heights, but actually have only one layer.
  - Epithelia can be classified by the shapes of the cells: **cuboidal cells** are cube-shaped, **columnar cells** are long and narrow, and **squamous cells** are flat and scale-like.
- **Connective tissues** support the body and provide a framework for epithelial cells.
  - In most organs, connective tissues form the **stroma** or support structure by secreting materials to form an **extracellular matrix**.
  - Bone, cartilage, tendons, ligaments, adipose tissue, and blood are all connective tissues.

Classification and Structure of Prokaryotic Cells

- **Prokaryotes** do not contain membrane-bound organelles; they contain their genetic material in a single circular molecule of DNA located in the **nucleoid region**.
- There are three overarching domains of life; prokaryotes account for two of these:
  - **Archaea** are often extremophiles, living in harsh environments (high temperature, high salinity, no light) and often use chemical sources of energy (chemosynthesis) rather than light (photosynthesis). They have similarities to both eukaryotes (start translation with methionine, similar RNA polymerases, histones) and bacteria (single circular chromosome, divide by binary fission or budding).
  - **Bacteria** have many similar structures to eukaryotes, and have complex relationships with humans, including **mutualistic symbiosis** and **pathogenesis**.
  - **Eukarya** is the only non-prokaryotic domain.
- Bacteria can be classified by shape:
  - Spherical bacteria are called **cocci**.
  - Rod-shaped bacteria are called **bacilli**.
  - Spiral-shaped bacteria are called **spirilli**.
- Bacteria can be classified based on metabolic processes:
  - **Obligate aerobes** require oxygen for metabolism.
  - **Obligate anaerobes** cannot survive in oxygen-containing environments and can only carry out anaerobic metabolism.

- **Facultative anaerobes** can survive in environments with or without oxygen and will toggle between metabolic processes based on the environment.
- **Aerotolerant anaerobes** cannot use oxygen for metabolism, but can survive in an oxygen-containing environment.

- The cell wall and cell membrane of bacteria form the **envelope**. Together, they control the movement of solutes into and out of the cell.
  - Bacteria can be classified by the color their cell walls turn during Gram staining with a crystal violet stain, followed by a counterstain with safranin. Gram-positive bacteria turn purple, while gram-negative bacteria turn pink-red.
  - Gram-positive bacteria have a thick cell wall composed of **peptidoglycan** and **lipoteichoic acid**.
  - Gram-negative bacteria have a thin cell wall composed of peptidoglycan and an outer membrane containing phospholipids and **lipopolysaccharides**.
- Bacteria may have one, two, or many flagella that generate propulsion to move the bacterium toward food or away from immune cells. Moving in response to chemical stimuli is called **chemotaxis**. Bacterial flagella contain a filament composed of flagellin, a basal body that anchors and rotates the flagellum, and a hook that connects the two.
- Prokaryotes carry out the electron transport chain using the cell membrane.
- Prokaryotic ribosomes are smaller than eukaryotic ribosomes (30S and 50S, rather than 40S and 60S).

Genetics and Growth of Prokaryotic Cells

- Prokaryotes multiply through **binary fission**, in which the chromosome replicates while the cell grows in size, until the cell wall begins to grow inward along the midline of the cell and divides it into two identical daughter cells.
- In addition to the single circular chromosome in prokaryotes, extrachromosomal material can be carried in **plasmids**. Plasmids may contain antibiotic resistance genes or **virulence factors**. Plasmids that can integrate into the genome are called **episomes**.
- Bacterial genetic recombination increases bacterial diversity.
  - **Transformation** occurs when genetic material from the surroundings is taken up by a cell, which can incorporate this material into its genome.
  - **Conjugation** is the transfer of genetic material from one bacterium to another across a **conjugation bridge**; a plasmid can be transferred from **F^+ cells** to **F^- cells**, or a portion of the genome can be transferred from an **Hfr cell** to a recipient.
  - **Transduction** is the transfer of genetic material from one bacterium to another via a bacteriophage vector.
  - **Transposons** are genetic elements that can insert into or remove themselves from the genome.
- Bacterial growth follows a predictable pattern:
  - The bacteria adapt to new local conditions during the **lag phase**.
  - Growth then increases exponentially during the **exponential (log) phase**.
  - As resources are reduced, growth levels off during the **stationary phase**.
  - As resources are depleted, bacteria undergo a **death phase**.

Viruses and Subviral Particles

- Viruses contain genetic material, a protein coat (**capsid**), and sometimes a lipid-containing envelope.
- Viruses are obligate intracellular parasites, meaning that they cannot survive and replicate outside of a **host cell**. Individual virus particles are called **virions**.
- Bacteriophages are viruses that target bacteria. In addition to the other structures, they contain a **tail sheath**, which injects the genetic material into a bacterium, and **tail fibers**, which allow the bacteriophage to attach to the host cell.
- Viral genomes may be made of various nucleic acids:
  - They may be composed of DNA or RNA and may be single- or double-stranded.
  - Single-stranded RNA viruses may be **positive sense** (that can be translated by the host cell) or **negative sense** (which requires a complementary strand to be synthesized by **RNA replicase** before translation).
  - **Retroviruses** contain a single-stranded RNA genome, from which a complementary DNA strand is made using **reverse transcriptase**. The DNA strand can then be integrated into the genome.
- Viruses infect cells by attaching to specific receptors, and can then enter the cell by fusing with the plasma membrane, being brought in by endocytosis, or injecting their genome into the cell.
- The virus reproduces by replicating and translating genetic material using the host cell's ribosomes, tRNA, amino acids, and enzymes.
- Viral progeny are released through cell death, lysis, or **extrusion**.
- Bacteriophages have two specific life cycles:
  - In the **lytic cycle**, the bacteriophage produces massive numbers of new virions until the cell lyses. Bacteria in the lytic phase are termed **virulent**.
  - In the **lysogenic cycle**, the virus integrates into the host genome as a pro-virus or prophage, which can then reproduce along with the cell. The provirus can remain in the genome indefinitely, or may leave the genome in response to a stimulus and enter the lytic cycle.
- **Prions** are infectious proteins that trigger misfolding of other proteins, usually converting an α-helical structure to a β-pleated sheet. This decreases the solubility of the protein and increases its resistance to degradation.
- **Viroids** are plant pathogens that are small circles of complementary RNA that can turn off genes, resulting in metabolic and structural changes and, potentially, cell death.

ANSWERS TO CONCEPT CHECKS

1.1

1. All living things are made of cells. The cell is the basic functional unit of life. All cells arise from other cells. Genetic information is carried in the form of deoxyribonucleic acid (DNA) and is passed from parent to daughter cell.

1.2

1. The nucleus stores genetic information and is the site of transcription. The mitochondria are involved in ATP production and apoptosis. Lysosomes break down cellular waste products and molecules ingested through endocytosis, and can also be involved in apoptosis. The rough endoplasmic reticulum synthesizes proteins destined for secretion. The smooth endoplasmic reticulum is involved in lipid synthesis and detoxification. The Golgi apparatus packages, modifies, and distributes cellular products. Peroxisomes break down very long chain fatty acids, synthesize lipids, and contribute to the pentose phosphate pathway.
2. Peroxisomes are dependent on hydrogen peroxide for their functions, so an enzyme deficiency that results in an inability to form hydrogen peroxide would likely result in an inability to digest very long chain fatty acids. These fatty acids would build up in peroxisomes until they displaced cellular contents, ultimately resulting in cell death.
3. Microfilaments are composed of actin. Microtubules are composed of tubulin. Intermediate filaments differ by cell type, but may be composed of keratin, desmin, vimentin, and lamins.
4. Centrioles consist of nine triplets of microtubules around a hollow center, while flagella consist of nine doublets on the outside, with two microtubules on the inside.
5. Endothelial cells and α-cells are epithelial cells. Fibroblasts, osteoblasts, and chondroblasts are connective tissue cells.

1.3

1. Archaea are similar to bacteria in that both are single-celled organisms that lack a nucleus or membrane-bound organelles, contain a single circular chromosome, and divide by binary fission or budding. They are similar to eukaryotes in that they start translation with methionine, contain similar RNA polymerases, and contain DNA associated with histones.
2. The three common shapes of bacteria are spherical (cocci), rod-shaped (bacilli), and spiral-shaped (spirilli).
3.

	Oxygen Present		**Oxygen Absent**	
Type of Bacteria	**Can survive**	**Can carry out aerobic metabolism**	**Can survive**	**Can carry out anaerobic metabolism**
Obligate aerobe	Yes	Yes	No	No
Facultative anaerobe	Yes	Yes	Yes	Yes
Obligate anaerobe	No	No	Yes	Yes
Aerotolerant anaerobe	Yes	No	Yes	Yes

4. The antibiotic penicillin targets the enzyme that catalyzes the cross-linking of peptidoglycan. Gram-positive bacteria have a thick layer of peptidoglycan and lipoteichoic acid, and contain no outer membrane, whereas gram-negative bacteria have only a thin layer of peptidoglycan but also have an outer membrane containing lipopolysaccharides and phospholipids. Penicillin and antibiotics with similar function can more easily reach and weaken the peptidoglycan layer of gram-positive bacteria.
5. Eukaryotic flagella contain microtubules composed of tubulin, organized in a 9 + 2 arrangement. Bacterial flagella are made of flagellin and consist of a filament, a basal body, and a hook.

1.4

1. Transformation is the acquisition of exogenous genetic material that can be integrated into the bacterial genome. Conjugation is the transfer of genetic material from one bacterium to another across a conjugation bridge; a plasmid can be transferred from F^+ cells to F^- cells, or a portion of the genome can be transferred from an Hfr cell to a recipient. Transduction is the transfer of genetic material from one bacterium to another by a bacteriophage.
2.

Phase	Features
Lag phase	Bacteria get used to environment; little growth
Exponential phase	Bacteria use available resources to multiply at an exponential rate
Stationary phase	Bacterial multiplication slows as resources are used up
Death phase	Bacteria die as resources become insufficient to support the colony

1.5

1. Viruses do not contain organelles such as ribosomes; therefore, in order to reproduce and synthesize proteins, viruses must infect cells and hijack their machinery.
2. This description indicates that the virus contains an outer layer of phospholipids with an inner capsid. Within the capsid, there is single-stranded RNA that can be immediately translated to protein by the ribosomes of the host cell.
3. The nucleic acid enters as single-stranded RNA, which undergoes reverse transcription (using reverse transcriptase) to form double-stranded DNA. This DNA enters the host genome and replicates with the host cell. The DNA is transcribed to mRNA, which can be used to make structural proteins. This mRNA doubles as the viral genome for new virions. Once new virions are assembled from the structural proteins and mRNA (single-stranded RNA) genome, the virions can be released to infect other cells.
4. In the lytic cycle, bacteriophages replicate in the host cell in extremely high numbers until the host cell lyses and releases the virions. In the lysogenic cycle, the bacteriophage genome enters the host genome and replicates with the host cell as a provirus. In response to an appropriate stimulus, the provirus may leave the host genome and can be used to synthesize new virions.
5. Prions cause disease by triggering a change in the conformation of a protein from an α-helix to a β-pleated sheet. This change reduces solubility of the protein and makes it highly resistant to degradation.

SCIENCE MASTERY ASSESSMENT EXPLANATIONS

1. **D**

Obligate anaerobes cannot survive in the presence of oxygen and would likely be killed by such a therapy, treating the infection. The other types of bacteria listed can all survive in the presence of oxygen, so infections involving these bacteria would likely not be treated using this therapy.

2. **A**

While bones and tendons are composed predominantly of connective tissue cells, muscle tissue is considered a different tissue type. Other examples of connective tissue include cartilage, ligaments, adipose tissue, and blood. Connective tissue often secretes substances to form the extracellular matrix, such as collagen and elastin, eliminating **(B)**. **(C)** and **(D)** are essentially identical and can both be eliminated: in organs, connective tissue often forms the support structure for epithelial cells, called the stroma.

3. **D**

In a virus, the nucleic acid can be either DNA or RNA and—in both cases—can be either single- or double-stranded. Therefore, all of the types of nucleic acids listed here could be used for a viral genome, making **(D)** the correct answer.

4. **C**

The process of sterilization kills all living cells. A lack of cellular growth in these conditions supports the idea that cells can only arise from preexisting cells, matching **(C)**. By contrast, since this experiment did not directly visualize the cells, nor did it analyze the genetic material, **(A)**, **(B)**, and **(D)** can be eliminated.

5. **C**

Mitochondria are thought to have evolved from an anaerobic prokaryote engulfing an aerobic prokaryote and establishing a symbiotic relationship; therefore, mitochondrial DNA, or mDNA, is likely to be similar to bacterial DNA. Both mDNA and bacterial DNA are organized into a single circular chromosome of double-stranded DNA that can replicate during binary fission. Therefore, Statements I and II are correct, while Statement III is incorrect.

6. **C**

The smooth endoplasmic reticulum is involved in the transport of materials throughout the cell, in lipid synthesis, and in the detoxification of drugs and poisons. Proteins from the rough ER can cross into the smooth ER, where they are secreted into cytoplasmic vesicles and transported to the Golgi apparatus. However, protein synthesis is not a function of the smooth ER, but rather of the free ribosomes or the ribosomes associated with the rough ER. **(C)** is therefore the correct answer.

7. **A**

The nucleolus (not to be confused with the nucleus) is a dense structure within the nucleus where ribosomal RNA (rRNA) is synthesized. **(A)** is therefore the correct answer.

8. **A**

Lysosomes are vesicular organelles that digest material using hydrolytic enzymes. They are surrounded by a single membrane. Both mitochondria and nuclei are surrounded by double membranes, eliminating **(B)** and **(C)**. Ribosomes must not be surrounded by membranes because they are found not only in eukaryotes but also in prokaryotes, which lack any membrane-bound organelles. This eliminates **(D)**.

9. **C**

Some of the main differences between prokaryotes and eukaryotes are that prokaryotes do not have a nucleus, while eukaryotes do, eliminating **(B)**; prokaryotes have ribosomal subunits of 30S and 50S, while eukaryotes have ribosomal subunits of 40S and 60S, eliminating **(A)**; and prokaryotes do not have membrane-bound organelles, whereas eukaryotes do, eliminating **(D)**. The presence of a membrane on the outer surface of the cell could not distinguish a prokaryotic cell from a eukaryotic one because both gram-negative bacteria and animal cells share this feature. Thus, **(C)** is the correct answer.

10. **C**

Tubulin is the primary protein in microtubules, which are responsible for the structure and movement of cilia and flagella, eliminating **(A)** and **(B)**. Centrioles organize microtubules into the mitotic spindle, eliminating **(D)**. Microfilaments are not composed of tubulin, but rather actin, making **(C)** the correct answer.

11. **C**

Viruses can exist in either the lytic or lysogenic cycle; they may even switch between them. During the lytic cycle, the virus's DNA takes control of the host cell's genetic machinery, manufacturing numerous progeny. In the end, the host cell bursts (lyses) and releases new virions, each capable of infecting other cells. In the lysogenic cycle, viral DNA is added to the host cell's genome, where it can remain dormant for days or years. Either spontaneously or as a result of environmental circumstances, the provirus can reactivate and enter a lytic cycle. Thus, **(A)** and **(B)** are incorrect because the terms are reversed. **(D)** describes features of bacteriophages, which are viruses that infect bacteria—not the human nervous system. **(C)** accurately describes how HSV operates during the lysogenic cycle, making it the correct answer.

12. **C**

Bacterial cells reproduce by binary fission, an asexual process in which the progeny is identical to the parent. Therefore, binary fission (Statement I) does not increase genetic variability. Conjugation can be described as sexual mating in bacteria; it is the transfer of genetic material between two bacteria that are temporarily joined. Transduction occurs when fragments of the bacterial chromosome accidentally become packaged into viral progeny produced during a viral infection and are introduced into another bacterium by the viral vector. Therefore, both conjugation and transduction (Statements II and III) increase bacterial genetic variability.

13. **A**

A bacterial cell that does not rapidly cause a phenotypic change in the rest of the colony is likely not F^+, meaning that this cell is not able to form a sex pilus for conjugation, making **(A)** correct. The expression of new phenotypic characteristics indicates that this bacterium may have acquired genetic material from the environment through transformation, **(B)**, or transduction (which occurs via bacteriophage infection), **(C)** and **(D)**.

14. **C**

Prions are infectious proteins that cause misfolding of other proteins. Prions generally cause a shift toward β-pleated sheet conformations, causing decreased solubility and increased resistance to degradation. This ultimately leads to disease. This mechanism is very similar to the one described here for Alzheimer's disease, making **(C)** the correct answer.

15. **A**

A virus that requires transport to the nucleus in order to produce viral proteins likely requires use of nuclear RNA polymerase in order to create mRNA that can be translated to protein. Therefore, only DNA viruses need to be transported to the nucleus to produce viral proteins, eliminating all answer choices but **(A)**.

GO ONLINE

Consult your online resources for additional practice.

EQUATIONS TO REMEMBER

$$(1.1)\quad \frac{\text{CFU}}{\mu\text{g of DNA}} \times \frac{\text{total volume (mL)}}{\text{volume plated (mL)}} = \text{transformation efficiency}$$

SHARED CONCEPTS

Biochemistry Chapter 3
Nonenzymatic Protein Function and Protein Analysis

Biochemistry Chapter 8
Biological Membranes

Biochemistry Chapter 10
Carbohydrate Metabolism II

Biology Chapter 2
Reproduction

Biology Chapter 8
The Immune System

Biology Chapter 12
Genetics and Evolution

CHAPTER 2

REPRODUCTION

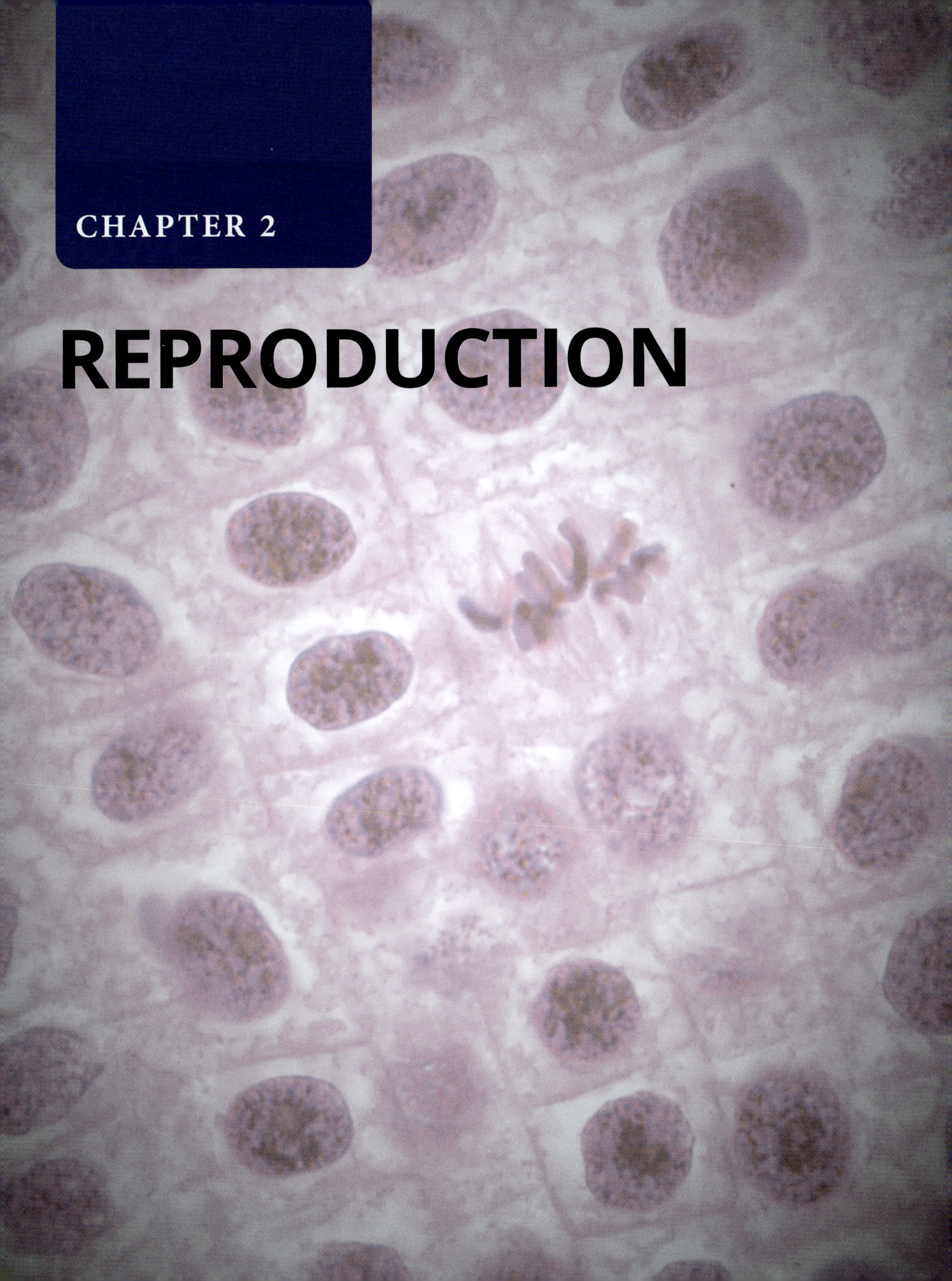

SCIENCE MASTERY ASSESSMENT

Every pre-med knows this feeling: there is so much content I have to know for the MCAT! How do I know what to do first or what's important?

While the high-yield badges throughout this book will help you identify the most important topics, this Science Mastery Assessment is another tool in your MCAT prep arsenal. This quiz (which can also be taken in your online resources) and the guidance below will help ensure that you are spending the appropriate amount of time on this chapter based on your personal strengths and weaknesses. Don't worry though—skipping something now does not mean you'll never study it. Later on in your prep, as you complete full-length tests, you'll uncover specific pieces of content that you need to review and can come back to these chapters as appropriate.

How to Use This Assessment

If you answer 0–7 questions correctly:

Spend about 1 hour to read this chapter in full and take limited notes throughout. Follow up by reviewing **all** quiz questions to ensure that you now understand how to solve each one.

If you answer 8–11 questions correctly:

Spend 20–40 minutes reviewing the quiz questions. Beginning with the questions you missed, read and take notes on the corresponding subchapters. For questions you answered correctly, ensure your thinking matches that of the explanation and you understand why each choice was correct or incorrect.

If you answer 12–15 questions correctly:

Spend less than 20 minutes reviewing all questions from the quiz. If you missed any, then include a quick read-through of the corresponding subchapters, or even just the relevant content within a subchapter, as part of your question review. For questions you answered correctly, ensure your thinking matches that of the explanation and review the Concept Summary at the end of the chapter.

1. Which of the following is the correct sequence of the development of a mature sperm cell?
   - **A.** Spermatid→1° spermatocyte→spermatogonium→2° spermatocyte→spermatozoan
   - **B.** Spermatogonium→1° spermatocyte→2° spermatocyte→spermatid→spermatozoan
   - **C.** Spermatozoan→1° spermatocyte→2° spermatocyte→spermatogonium→spermatid
   - **D.** Spermatogonium→1° spermatocyte→2° spermatocyte→spermatozoan→spermatid

2. Which of the following correctly pairs the stage of development of an egg cell with the relevant point in the life cycle?
   - **A.** From birth to menarche—prophase II
   - **B.** At ovulation—metaphase I
   - **C.** At ovulation—metaphase II
   - **D.** At fertilization—prophase II

3. Some studies suggest that, in patients who have Alzheimer's disease, there is a defect in the way the spindle apparatus attaches to the kinetochore fibers. At which stage of mitotic division would one first expect to be able to visualize this problem?
   - **A.** Prophase
   - **B.** Metaphase
   - **C.** Anaphase
   - **D.** Telophase

4. A researcher wishes to incorporate a radiolabeled deoxyadenine into the genome of one of the two daughter cells that would arise as a result of mitosis. What is the latest stage of cellular development during which the radiolabeled deoxyadenine could be added to achieve this result?
   - **A.** G_1
   - **B.** G_2
   - **C.** M
   - **D.** S

5. Certain ovarian tumors called granulosa cell tumors are known to produce excessive levels of estrogen. A physician who diagnoses a granulosa cell tumor should look for a secondary cancer in which of the following parts of the reproductive tract?
   - **A.** Fallopian tube
   - **B.** Cervix
   - **C.** Endometrium
   - **D.** Vagina

6. Upon ovulation, the oocyte is released into the:
   - **A.** fallopian tube.
   - **B.** follicle.
   - **C.** abdominal cavity.
   - **D.** uterus.

7. Cancer cells are cells in which mitosis occurs continuously, without regard to quality or quantity of the cells produced. For this reason, most chemotherapies attack rapidly dividing cells. At which point(s) in the cell cycle could chemotherapy effectively prevent cancer cell division?
   - **I.** S stage
   - **II.** Prophase
   - **III.** Metaphase
   - **A.** I only
   - **B.** I and II only
   - **C.** II and III only
   - **D.** I, II, and III

8. Which of the following INCORRECTLY pairs a structure of the male reproductive system with a feature of the structure?
   - **A.** Seminal vesicles—produce alkaline fructose-containing secretions
   - **B.** Prostate gland—surrounded by muscle to raise and lower the testes
   - **C.** Vas deferens—tube connecting the epididymis to the ejaculatory duct
   - **D.** Cowper's glands—produce a fluid to clear traces of urine in the urethra

9. What is the last point in the meiotic cycle in which the cell has a diploid number of chromosomes?
   - **A.** During interphase
   - **B.** During telophase I
   - **C.** During interkinesis
   - **D.** During telophase II

10. Which of the following does NOT likely contribute to genetic variability?
   - **A.** Random fertilization of an egg by a sperm
   - **B.** Random segregation of homologous chromosomes
   - **C.** Crossing over between homologous chromosomes during meiosis
   - **D.** Replication of the DNA during S stage

11. Which of the following statements correctly identifies a key difference between mitosis and meiosis?
   - **A.** In metaphase of mitosis, replicated chromosomes line up in single file; in metaphase II of meiosis, replicated chromosomes line up on opposite sides of the metaphase plate.
   - **B.** During anaphase of mitosis, homologous chromosomes separate; during anaphase of meiosis I, sister chromatids separate.
   - **C.** At the end of telophase of mitosis, the daughter cells are identical to each other; at the end of meiosis I, the daughter cells are identical to the parent cell.
   - **D.** During metaphase of mitosis, centromeres are present directly on the metaphase plate; during metaphase of meiosis I, there are no centromeres on the metaphase plate.

12. Which of the following is true regarding prophase?
   - **A.** The chromosomes separate and move to opposite poles of the cell.
   - **B.** The spindle apparatus disappears.
   - **C.** The chromosomes uncoil.
   - **D.** The nucleoli disappear.

13. An individual who is phenotypically female is found to have only one copy of a disease-carrying recessive allele on the X chromosome, yet demonstrates all of the classic symptoms of the disease. Geneticists determine that the individual has a genotype that likely arose from nondisjunction in one parent. What is the likely genotype of this individual?
   - **A.** 46,XX (46 chromosomes, with XX for sex chromosomes)
   - **B.** 46,XY
   - **C.** 45,X
   - **D.** 47,XXY

14. During which phase of the menstrual cycle does progesterone concentration peak?
   - **A.** Follicular phase
   - **B.** Ovulation
   - **C.** Luteal phase
   - **D.** Menses

15. Which of the following would NOT be seen during pregnancy?
   - **A.** High levels of hCG in the first trimester
   - **B.** High levels of progesterone throughout the pregnancy
   - **C.** Low levels of FSH in the first trimester
   - **D.** High levels of GnRH throughout the pregnancy

Answer Key

1. **B** (See section 2.2)
2. **C** (See section 2.2)
3. **A** (See section 2.1)
4. **D** (See section 2.1)
5. **C** (See section 2.3)
6. **C** (See section 2.3)
7. **D** (See section 2.1)
8. **B** (See section 2.3)
9. **B** (See section 2.2)
10. **D** (See section 2.2)
11. **D** (See section 2.2)
12. **D** (See section 2.1)
13. **C** (See section 2.2)
14. **C** (See section 2.3)
15. **D** (See section 2.3)

The relevant section of the chapter to review for each question is given in parentheses after the correct answer. Detailed explanations can be found at the end of the chapter.

CHAPTER 2

REPRODUCTION

In This Chapter

CHAPTER PROFILE

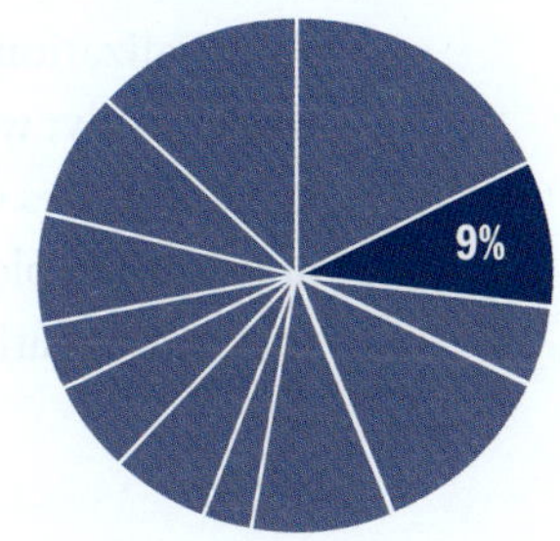

The content in this chapter should be relevant to about 9% of all questions about biology on the MCAT.

This chapter covers material from the following AAMC content categories:

1C: Transmission of heritable information from generation to generation and the processes that increase genetic diversity

2C: Processes of cell division, differentiation, and specialization

3B: Structure and integrative functions of the main organ systems

Introduction

All mammals share certain characteristics: milk-producing mammary glands, three bones in the middle ear and one in the lower jaw, fur or hair, heterodont dentition (different kinds of teeth), and both sebaceous (oil-producing) and sudoriferous (sweat) glands. What about placenta formation during embryonic development? This is a characteristic of humans, as we'll explore in Chapter 3 of *MCAT Biology Review*, but there are two groups of mammals that birth their young a bit differently: prototherians and metatherians.

Prototherians (monotremes), which include the duckbilled platypus and echidna (spiny anteater), encase their developing embryos within hard-shelled amniotic eggs and lay them to be hatched, like reptiles. This method of development is referred to as oviparity. Metatherians (marsupials) include koalas and kangaroos. A typical metatherian fetus (joey) undergoes some development in its mother's uterus and then climbs out of the birth canal and into her marsupium, or pouch. It might seem a bit strange that something as essential as reproduction can be so different between mammalian species, but there are, in fact, a wide variety of reproductive schemes in nature. Many organisms reproduce without a sexual partner. Others can reproduce sexually or asexually depending on environmental conditions. In Chapter 1 of *MCAT Biology Review*, we explored how bacteria and viruses reproduce. In this chapter, we'll explore eukaryotic reproductive systems.

2.1 The Cell Cycle and Mitosis High Yield

LEARNING OBJECTIVES

After Chapter 2.1, you will be able to:

- Describe the four phases of mitosis and the major events during each phase
- Identify the five stages of the cell cycle and the major events during each stage

In animals, autosomal cells are said to be **diploid** (**2*n***), which means that they contain two copies of each chromosome. Germ cells, on the other hand, are **haploid** (***n***), containing only one copy of each chromosome. A visualization of diploid and haploid can be seen in Figure 2.1. In humans, these numbers are 46 and 23, respectively; we inherit 23 chromosomes from each parent. Eukaryotic cells replicate through the **cell cycle**, a specific series of phases during which a cell grows, synthesizes DNA, and replicates, all while maintaining the appropriate ploidy. Derangements of the cell cycle can lead to unchecked cell division and may be responsible for the formation of cancer.

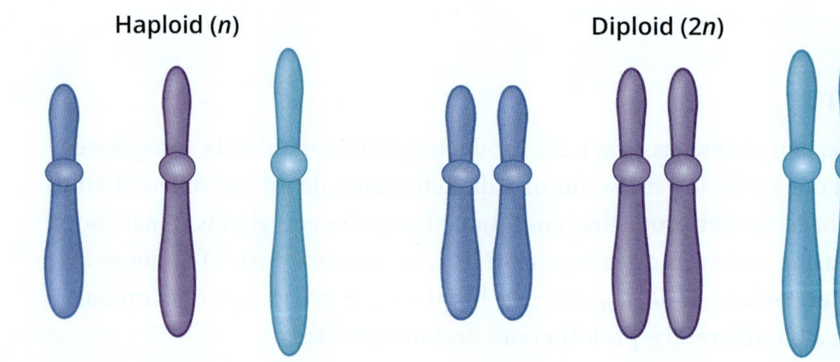

Figure 2.1 Haploid vs. Diploid

The Cell Cycle

The cell cycle, shown in Figure 2.2, is a perennial MCAT favorite. For actively dividing cells, the cell cycle consists of four stages: G_1, S, G_2, and M. There are three major checkpoints throughout these stages to ensure accurate completion of each stage. These will be discussed in more detail in their respective stage's section. The first three stages (G_1, S, and G_2) are known collectively as **interphase**. Interphase is the longest part of the cell cycle; even actively dividing cells spend about 90 percent of their time in interphase. Cells that do not divide spend all of their time in an offshoot of G_1 called G_0. During the **G_0 stage**, the cell is simply living and carrying out its functions, without any preparation for division.

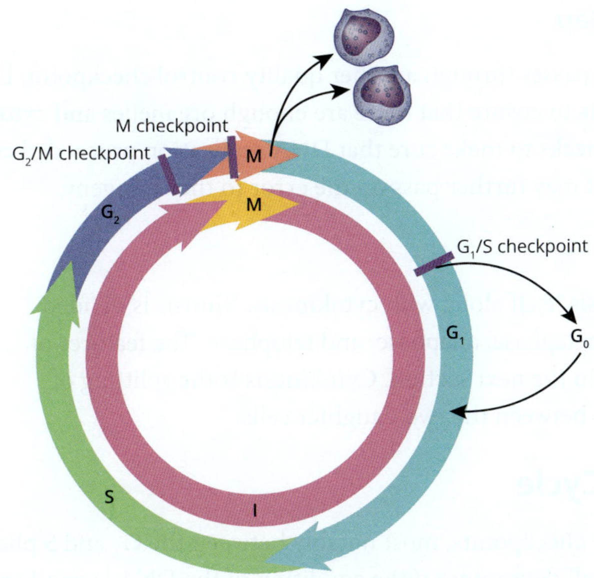

Figure 2.2 The Cell Cycle

During interphase, individual chromosomes are not visible with light microscopy because they are in a less condensed form known as **chromatin**. This is because the DNA must be available to *RNA polymerase* so that genes can be transcribed. During mitosis, however, it is preferable to condense the DNA into tightly coiled chromosomes to avoid losing any genetic material during cell division.

G_1 Stage: Presynthetic Gap

During the **G_1 stage**, cells create organelles for energy and protein production (mitochondria, ribosomes, and endoplasmic reticulum), while also increasing their size. In addition, passage into the S (synthesis) stage is governed by a **restriction point**. Certain criteria, such as containing the proper complement of DNA, must be met for the cell to pass the restriction point and enter the synthesis stage.

S Stage: Synthesis of DNA

During the **S stage**, the cell replicates its genetic material so that each daughter cell will have identical copies. After replication, each chromosome consists of two identical **chromatids** that are bound together at a specialized region known as the **centromere**, as shown in Figure 2.3. Note that the ploidy of the cell does not change even though the number of chromatids has doubled. In other words, humans in this stage still only have 46 chromosomes, even though 92 chromatids are present. Cells entering G_2 have twice as much DNA as cells in G_1.

KEY CONCEPT

Each chromatid is composed of a complete double-stranded molecule of DNA. Sister chromatids are identical copies of each other. The term *chromosome* may be used to refer to either a single chromatid before S phase or the pair of chromatids attached at the centromere after S phase.

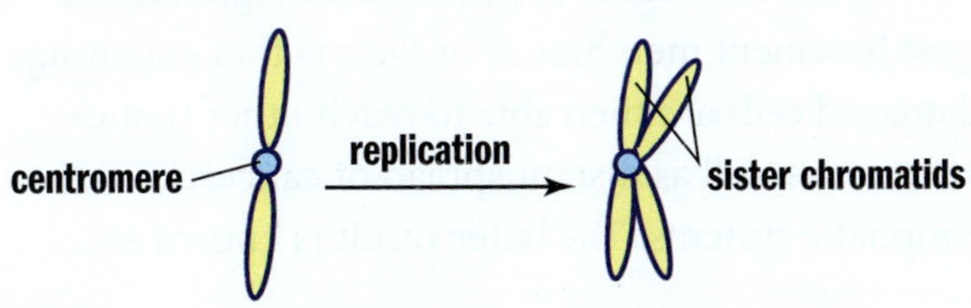

Figure 2.3 Chromosome Replication
A single chromatid replicates to form two sister chromatids.

G_2 Stage: Postsynthetic Gap

During the **G_2 stage**, the cell passes through another quality control checkpoint. DNA has already been duplicated, and the cell checks to ensure that there are enough organelles and cytoplasm for two daughter cells. Furthermore, the cell checks to make sure that DNA replication proceeded correctly to avoid passing on an error to daughter cells that may further pass on the error to their progeny.

M Stage: Mitosis

The **M stage** consists of mitosis itself along with cytokinesis. Mitosis is divided into four phases: prophase, metaphase, anaphase, and telophase. The features of each phase will be discussed in the next section. Cytokinesis is the splitting of the cytoplasm and organelles between the two daughter cells.

KEY CONCEPT

In autosomal cells, division results in two genetically identical daughter cells. In germ cells, the daughter cells are not equivalent.

Control of the Cell Cycle

The cell cycle is controlled by checkpoints, most notably between the G_1 and S phase and the G_2 and M phase. At the G_1/S checkpoint, the cell determines if the condition of the DNA is good enough for synthesis. As mentioned previously, this checkpoint is also known as the restriction point. If there has been damage to the DNA, the cell cycle goes into arrest until the DNA has been repaired. The main protein in control of this is **p53**.

At the G_2/M checkpoint, the cell is mainly concerned with ensuring that it has achieved adequate size and the organelles have been properly replicated to support two daughter cells. p53 also plays a role in the G_2/M checkpoint.

The molecules responsible for the cell cycle are known as **cyclins** and **cyclin-dependent kinases** (**CDK**). In order to be activated, CDKs require the presence of the right cyclins. During the cell cycle, concentrations of the various cyclins increase and decrease during specific stages. These cyclins bind to CDKs, creating an activated CDK–cyclin complex. This complex can then phosphorylate transcription factors. **Transcription factors** then promote transcription of genes required for the next stage of the cell cycle.

Cancer

Cell cycle control is essential to ensure that cells that are damaged or inadequately sized do not divide. When cell cycle control becomes deranged, and damaged cells are allowed to undergo mitosis, **cancer** may result. One of the most common mutations found in cancer is mutation of the gene that produces p53, called TP53. When this gene is mutated, the cell cycle is not stopped to repair damaged DNA. This allows mutations to accumulate, eventually resulting in a cancerous cell that divides continuously and without regard to the quality or quantity of the new cells produced. Often, cancer cells undergo rapid cell division, creating **tumors**. Eventually, if the cell begins to produce the right factors (such as proteases that can digest basement membranes or factors that encourage blood vessel formation), the damaged cells are then able to reach other tissues. This may include both local invasion as well as distant spread of cancerous cells through the bloodstream or lymphatic systems. The latter result is known as **metastasis**.

BRIDGE

Cancer-causing genes can often be classified into oncogenes (genes that, when mutated, actively promote cell division) and tumor suppressor genes (genes that, when mutated, lose their ability to regulate or arrest the cell cycle). Different cancer types are often associated with specific mutations in either oncogenes or tumor suppressor genes, or both. The biochemistry of these genes is discussed in Chapter 6 of *MCAT Biochemistry Review.*

Mitosis

Mitosis, shown in Figure 2.4, is the process by which two identical daughter cells are created from a single cell. Mitosis consists of four distinct phases—prophase, metaphase, anaphase, and telophase—and occurs in **somatic cells**, or cells that are not involved in sexual reproduction.

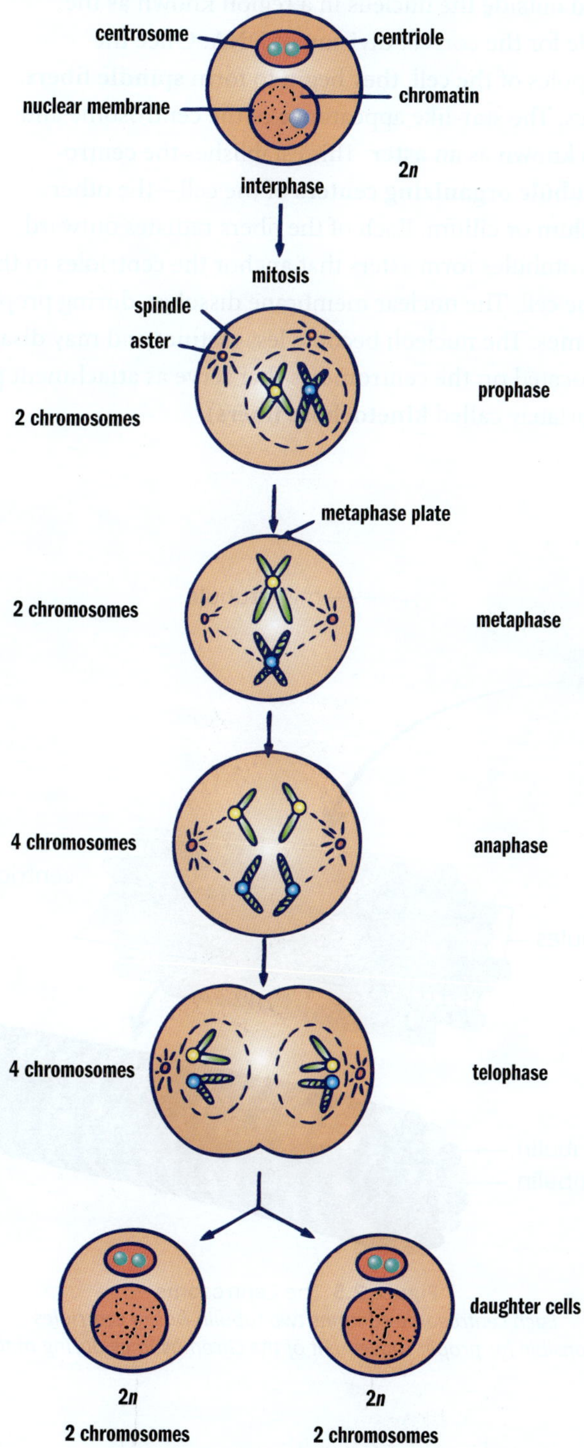

Figure 2.4 Mitosis
Mitosis results in two identical daughter cells.

Prophase

KEY CONCEPT

The phases of mitosis:

- Prophase—chromosomes condense, spindle forms
- Metaphase—chromosomes align
- Anaphase—sister chromatids separate
- Telophase—new nuclear membranes form

Prophase is the first phase in mitosis. The first step in prophase involves condensation of the chromatin into chromosomes. Also, the centriole pairs separate and move toward opposite poles of the cell. These paired cylindrical organelles, shown in Figure 2.5, are located outside the nucleus in a region known as the **centrosome** and are responsible for the correct division of DNA. Once the centrioles migrate to opposite poles of the cell, they begin to form **spindle fibers**, which are made of microtubules. The star-like appearance of the centrosome and associated microtubules is also known as an **aster**. This establishes the centrosome as one of the two **microtubule organizing centers** of the cell—the other being the basal body of a flagellum or cilium. Each of the fibers radiates outward from the centrioles. Some microtubules form asters that anchor the centrioles to the cell membrane. Others extend toward the middle of the cell. The nuclear membrane dissolves during prophase, allowing these spindle fibers to contact the chromosomes. The nucleoli become less distinct and may disappear completely. **Kinetochores** are protein structures located on the centromeres that serve as attachment points for specific fibers of the **spindle apparatus** (appropriately called **kinetochore fibers**).

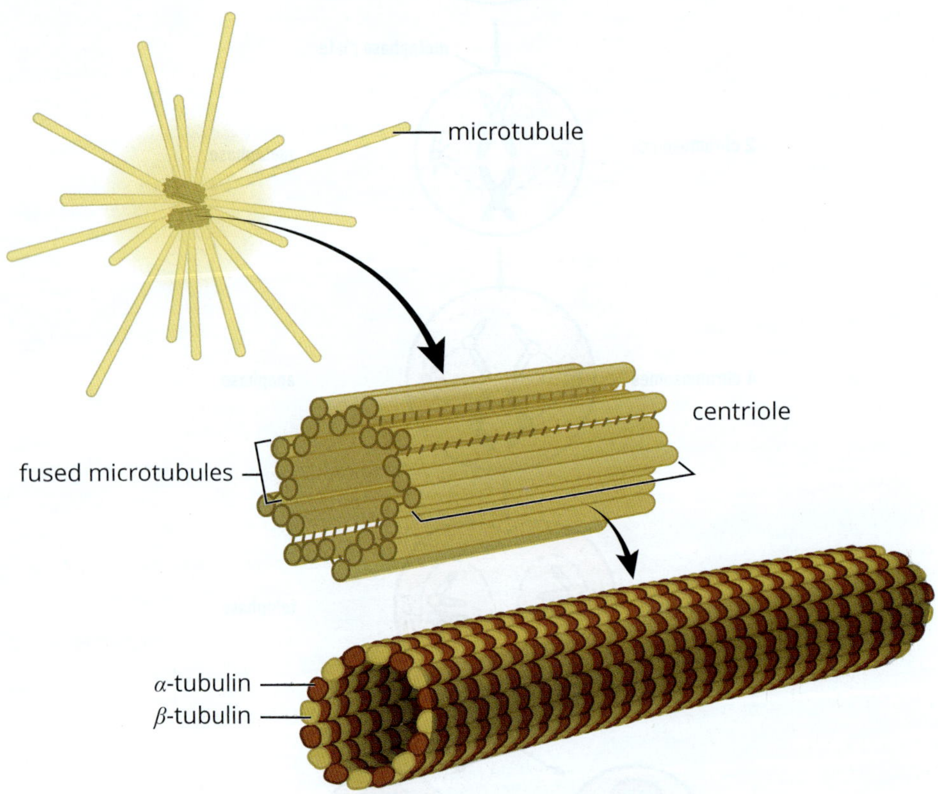

Figure 2.5 The Centrosome
Each centrosome contains two tubulin-based centrioles responsible for proper movement of the chromosomes during mitosis.

Metaphase

In **metaphase**, the centriole pairs are now at opposite ends of the cell. The kinetochore fibers interact with the fibers of the spindle apparatus to align the chromosomes at the **metaphase plate** (**equatorial plate**), which is equidistant from the two poles of the cell.

Anaphase

During **anaphase**, the centromeres split so that each chromatid has its own distinct centromere, thus allowing the sister chromatids to separate. The sister chromatids are pulled toward the opposite poles of the cell by the shortening of the kinetochore fibers.

Telophase and Cytokinesis

Telophase is essentially the reverse of prophase. The spindle apparatus disappears. A nuclear membrane reforms around each set of chromosomes, and the nucleoli reappear. The chromosomes uncoil, resuming their interphase form. Each of the two new nuclei receives a complete copy of the genome identical to the original genome and to each other.

Cytokinesis, which occurs at the end of telophase, is the separation of the cytoplasm and organelles, giving each daughter cell enough material to survive on its own. Each cell undergoes a finite number of divisions before programmed death; for human somatic cells, this is usually between 20 and 50. After that, the cell can no longer divide continuously.

BIOLOGY GUIDED EXAMPLE WITH EXPERT THINKING

The p53 tumor suppressor pathway has been heavily explored as a potential treatment for patients who have cancer. The p53 pathway induces growth arrest and apoptosis in response to cellular stress. Mutation of this pathway is thought to be nearly universal in human cancer.

Background on p53: mutation of pathway causes cancer

Researchers explored whether a retro-inverse p53C′ peptide (termed RI-TATp53C′) is a therapeutically effective means of activating the p53 tumor suppressor pathway in preclinical models of terminal metastatic cancer.

Hypothesis: Does RI-TATp53C′ activate the p53 pathway and thus treat cancer?

RI-TATp53C′ contains a protein transduction domain (PTD), which is capable of traversing the plasma membrane, and a functional sequence of the p53 C-terminus.

RI-TATp53C′ components: protein transduction domain (PTD) and functional C-terminus

A non-functional RI-TATp53C′ was developed by mutating the functional residues of the peptide.

They made a non-functional version of the treatment (RI-TATp53C′); this is going to be a negative control

Researchers exposed TA3/St mammary carcinoma cells to Wild-Type RI-TATp53C′ and the mutant peptide of RI-TATp53C′. The cells' DNA content was then analyzed to test if cell cycle arrest occurred (Figure 1).

Experiment IV: RI-TATp53C′ WT or mutant; DV: cell DNA content (determines cell cycle arrest)

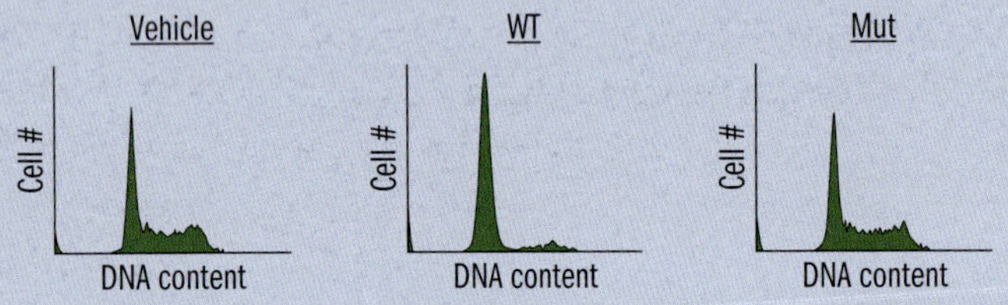

Figure 1

IV: Vehicle (no RI-TATp53C′), WT (RI-TATp53C′), or Mut (non-functional RI-TATp53C′)

DV: cell number and DNA content

Trend: Vehicle and Mut graphs have the same shape, while WT appears to make cells have less DNA

Researchers then explored the dependency of RI-TATp53C′ induction of growth arrest with endogenous p53 in cells (Figure 2). TA3/St and H1299 are both cancer cell lines.

Second experiment, asks: "Does RI-TATp53C′ depend on endogenous p53?" Probably going to manipulate endogenous p53 (IV) and measure RI-TATp53C′ effects (DV).

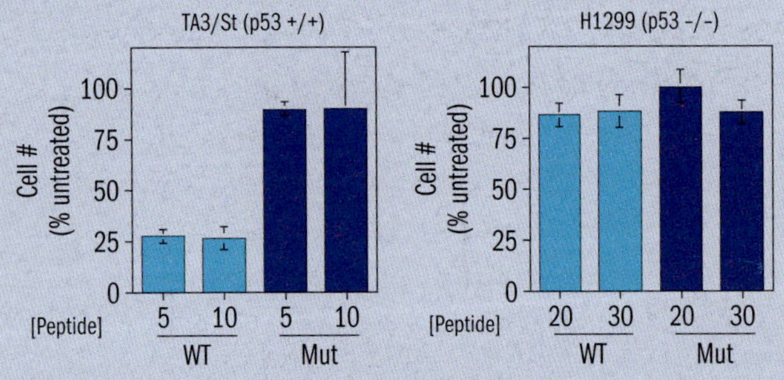

Figure 2

IV: cancer w/ endogenous p53 (TA3/St) or cancer w/ no p53 (H1299); WT or Mut; peptide concentration

DV: Cell # as % untreated

Trends: the WT peptide group produces a lower number of cells than Mut in TA3/St, but no difference in H1299; no effect with changes to peptide concentration

Adapted from: Snyder EL, Meade BR, Saenz CC, Dowdy SF (2004). Treatment of terminal peritoneal carcinomatosis by a transducible p53-activating peptide. *PLOS Biology* 2(2): e36. https://doi.org/10.1371/journal.pbio.0020036.

What stage of the cell cycle does RI-TATp53C′ arrest the cell in and does RI-TATp53C′-induced cell arrest require endogenous p53?

To answer this question we need to determine the relationship between RI-TATp53C′ and the cell cycle, as well as the relationship between RI-TATp53C′ and endogenous p53. With such an in-depth question it's worth considering the bigger picture to ensure that we understand the concepts and experiments in the passage. Start with the context: why are these experiments being done? As stated in paragraphs 1 and 2, p53 is a tumor-suppressing pathway that researchers are hoping to activate as a treatment to cancer. Both experiments, although distinct, will explore the activation of this pathway.

Keeping in mind the independent and dependent variables of the two experiments that we identified as we read, we can identify which experiment should be used to answer each question in the prompt. The first experiment has three conditions: Vehicle, WT, and Mut. The vehicle condition is something we should recognize as bio talk for "we did everything the same as the treatment condition, except the treatment," so this is a negative control. The WT condition, according to the second to last sentence in paragraph 2, is functional RI-TATp53C′. This is the treatment group! If the hypothesis at the start of the 2nd paragraph is correct we should see interesting data here. The Mut condition is described in the third to last and second to last sentences of paragraph 2 as a non-functional mutant RI-TATp53C′. In each of these conditions, the proportion of cells that have low/medium/high DNA content are measured, which, according to the last sentence of paragraph 2, determines if cell cycle arrest occurred. At this point, we know Exp 1 relates RI-TATp53C′ (IV) and the cell cycle (DV) and should, therefore, be used to answer the first question of the prompt.

Let's analyze the data from the first experiment. Looking at Figure 1, notice that the Vehicle and Mutant conditions are identical, while the WT (treatment) condition differs greatly. Specifically, the RI-TATp53C′ treatment (WT) results in a larger portion of cells having less DNA. Considering our background knowledge about the cell cycle and each phase's relative DNA content, we can deduce that G_1 has the lowest DNA content. This is because G_1 occurs after a division (decreases DNA) and before S phase (increases DNA). Thus, we can conclude RI-TATp53C′ must arrest the cell in G_1.

In order to answer the second question, the relationship between RI-TATp53C′ functionality and endogenous p53 must be determined. This aligns pretty well with paragraph 3's description of experiment 2, and is a solid indication that we need to analyze Figure 2. Looking at the titles of the graphs there are two different cancerous cell cultures, TA3/St (p53 +/+) and H1299 (p53 −/−), which differ in their expression of p53. This is the first independent variable. Analyzing the graphs further, there are two additional independent variables, WT (light blue) vs. Mut (dark blue) and peptide concentration, [Peptide]. The dependent variable in Figure 2 is the Cell # or % untreated. In other words, it's the number of cancerous cells that are unarrested and thus still cancerous after peptide exposure.

With an understanding of the variables, let's take a look at the data in Figure 2. Between the two graphs, the most striking difference is WT RI-TATp53C′ treatment in p53 +/+ cancerous cells results in a drastic drop in untreated (cancerous) cells (light blue, 1st graph), while in the p53 −/− condition WT RI-TATp53C′ cancerous cell levels remain constant (light blue, 2nd graph). This shows us that the ability of WT RI-TATp53C' to induce cell cycle arrest is dependent on endogenous p53. In addition, when both p53 +/+ and p53 −/− conditions are exposed to the mutant RI-TATp53C′ (non-functional), there is no drop in cancerous cells. This second point is to be expected, but is still worth noting, as it shows us that nothing unexpected occurred during the experiment. Thus, given the data in Figure 2, we can conclude that in order for RI-TATp53C′ to induce cell arrest, it requires endogenous p53 in the tumor.

Overall, Figure 1 shows that not only does WT RI-TATp53C′ induce cell arrest, but based on the increased proportion of cells with lower DNA content, it induces cell arrest in G_1. From Figure 2, we were able to determine that RI-TATp53C′ requires a functional p53 pathway in order to induce cell arrest due to the loss of RI-TATp53C′ functionality in the p53 −/− condition.

MCAT CONCEPT CHECK 2.1

Before you move on, assess your understanding of the material with these questions.

1. What are the five stages of the cell cycle? What happens in each stage?

Cell Cycle Stage	Features

2. What are the four phases of mitosis? What happens in each phase?

Mitotic Phase	Features

2.2 Meiosis

LEARNING OBJECTIVES

After Chapter 2.2, you will be able to:

- Predict the ploidy of daughter cells at the end of mitosis, meiosis I, and meiosis II
- Differentiate between homologous chromosomes and sister chromatids
- Compare and contrast mitosis and meiosis
- Explain the importance of crossing over events in relation to genetic diversity

Whereas mitosis occurs in somatic tissue and results in two identical daughter cells, meiosis occurs in **gametocytes** (**germ cells**) and results in up to four nonidentical sex cells (**gametes**). Meiosis shares some similarities with mitosis. In both processes, for instance, genetic material must be duplicated, chromatin is condensed to form chromosomes, and microtubules emanating from centrioles are involved in dividing genetic material. However, the MCAT tends to ask about the differences between these two processes.

In contrast to mitosis, which consists of one round each of replication and division, meiosis consists of one round of replication followed by two rounds of division, as shown in Figure 2.6. **Meiosis I** results in homologous chromosomes being separated, generating haploid daughter cells; this is known as **reductional division**. **Meiosis II** is similar to mitosis, in that it results in the separation of sister chromatids without a change in ploidy, and is therefore known as **equational division**.

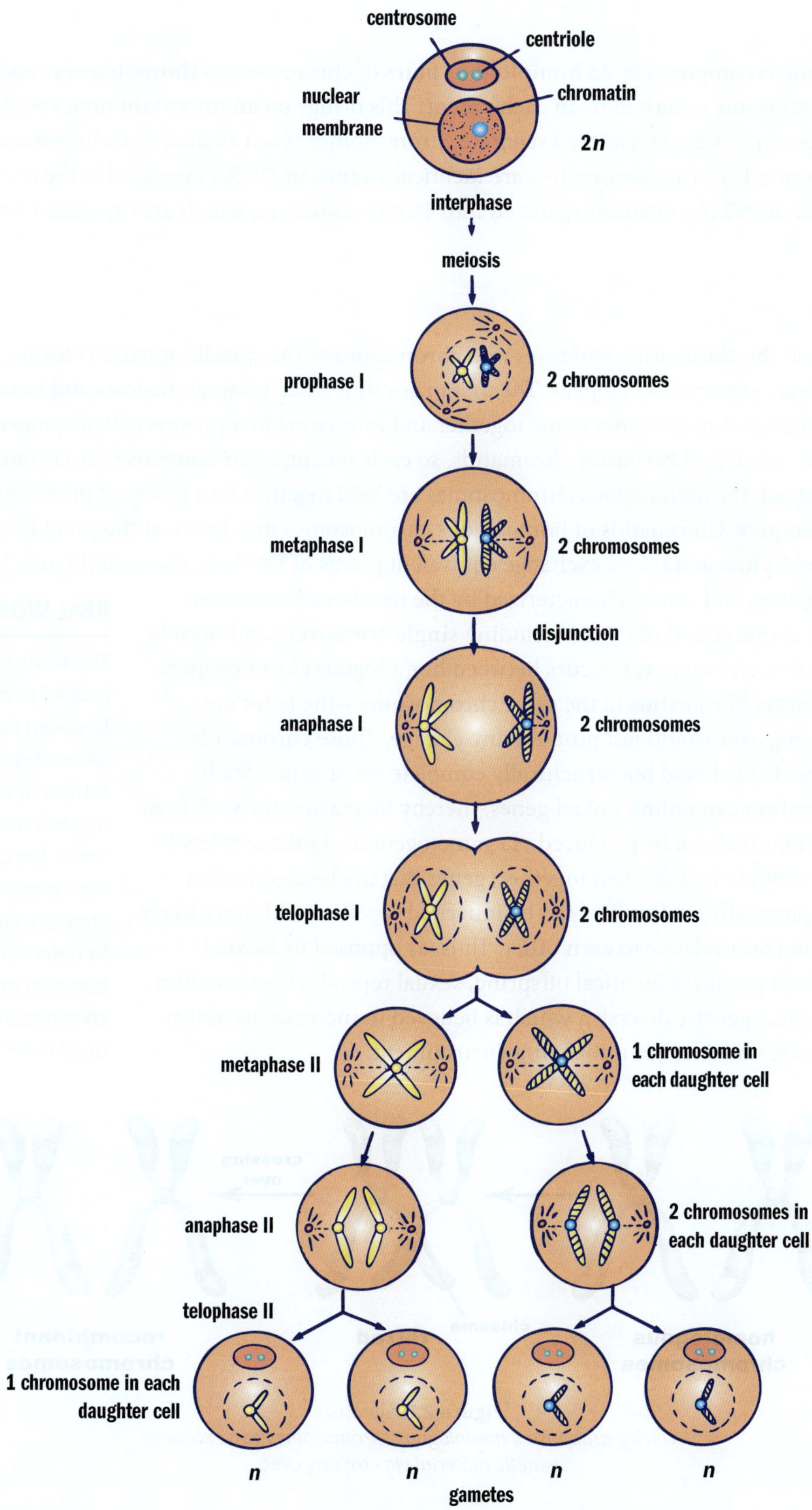

Figure 2.6 Meiosis
Meiosis results in up to four nonidentical daughter cells.

Meiosis I

The human genome is composed of 23 **homologous pairs** of chromosomes (**homologues**), each of which contains one chromosome inherited from each parent. This brings up an important note about terminology: whereas homologous pairs are considered separate chromosomes (such as maternal chromosome 15 and paternal chromosome 15), sister chromatids are identical strands of DNA connected at the centromere. Thus, after S phase, there are 92 chromatids organized into 46 chromosomes, which are organized into 23 homologous pairs.

Prophase I

During **prophase I**, the chromatin condenses into chromosomes, the spindle apparatus forms, and the nucleoli and nuclear membrane disappear. The first major difference between meiosis and mitosis occurs at this point: homologous chromosomes come together and intertwine in a process called **synapsis**. At this point, each chromosome consists of two sister chromatids, so each synaptic pair contains four chromatids and is referred to as a **tetrad**; the homologous chromosomes are held together by a group of proteins called the **synaptonemal complex**. Chromatids of homologous chromosomes may break at the point of contact, called the **chiasma** (plural: **chiasmata**) and exchange equivalent pieces of DNA, as shown in Figure 2.7. This process is called **crossing over**, and can be characterized by the number of crossover events that occur in one strand of DNA, including **single crossovers** and **double crossovers**. Note that crossing over occurs between homologous chromosomes and not between sister chromatids of the same chromosome—the latter are identical, so crossing over would not produce any change. Those chromatids involved are left with an altered but structurally complete set of genes. Such genetic **recombination** can unlink linked genes, thereby increasing the variety of genetic combinations that can be produced via gametogenesis. Linkage refers to the tendency for genes to be inherited together; genes that are located farther from each other physically are less likely to be inherited together, and more likely to undergo crossing over relative to each other. Thus, as opposed to asexual reproduction, which produces identical offspring, sexual reproduction provides the advantage of great genetic diversity, which is believed to increase the ability of a species to evolve and adapt to a changing environment.

REAL WORLD

The rate of gene unlinking is used to map differences between two genes on the same chromosome. The farther apart two genes are, the more likely they are to become unlinked during crossing over. These statistics can then be used to determine the distance between genes on the chromosome, measured in units called centimorgans.

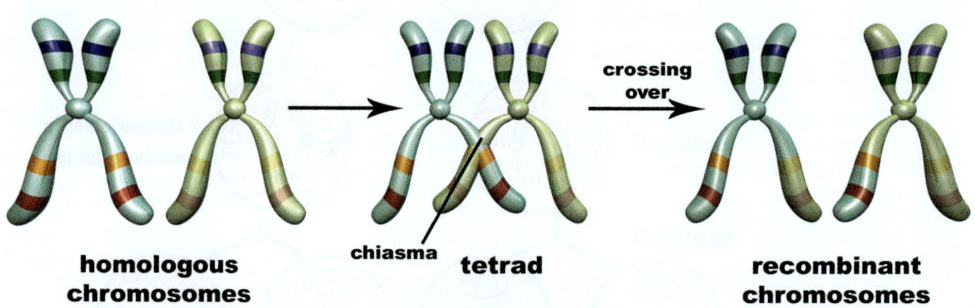

Figure 2.7 Synapsis
During prophase I, homologous chromosomes can exchange genetic material via crossing over.

Because of crossing over, each daughter cell will have a unique pool of alleles (genes coding for alternative forms of a given trait) from a random mixture of maternal and paternal origin. In classical genetics, crossing over explains **Mendel's second law (of independent assortment)**, which states that the inheritance of one allele has no effect on the likelihood of inheriting certain alleles for other genes.

Metaphase I

During **metaphase I**, homologous pairs (tetrads) align at the metaphase plate, and each pair attaches to a separate spindle fiber by its kinetochore. Note the difference from mitosis: in mitosis, each chromosome is lined up on the metaphase plate by two spindle fibers (one from each pole); in meiosis, homologous chromosomes are lined up across from each other at the metaphase plate and are held by one spindle fiber.

KEY CONCEPT

It is critical to understand how meiosis I is different from mitosis. The chromosome number is halved (reductional division) in meiosis I, and the daughter cells have the haploid number of chromosomes (23 in humans). Meiosis II is similar to mitosis in that sister chromatids are separated from one another; therefore, no change in ploidy is observed.

Anaphase I

During **anaphase I**, homologous pairs separate and are pulled to opposite poles of the cell. This process is called **disjunction**, and it accounts for **Mendel's first law (of segregation)**. During disjunction, each chromosome of paternal origin separates (or disjoins) from its homologue of maternal origin, and either chromosome can end up in either daughter cell. Thus, the distribution of homologous chromosomes to the two intermediate daughter cells is random with respect to parental origin. This separating of the two homologous chromosomes is referred to as **segregation**.

Telophase I

During **telophase I**, a nuclear membrane forms around each new nucleus. At this point, each chromosome still consists of two sister chromatids joined at the centromere. The cells are now haploid; once homologous chromosomes separate, only n chromosomes are found in each daughter cell (23 in humans). The cell divides into two daughter cells by cytokinesis. Between cell divisions, there may be a short rest period, or **interkinesis**, during which the chromosomes partially uncoil.

REAL WORLD

If, during anaphase I or II of meiosis, homologous chromosomes (anaphase I) or sister chromatids (anaphase II) fail to separate, one of the resulting gametes will have two copies of a particular chromosome and the other gamete will have none. Subsequently, during fertilization, the resulting zygote may have too many or too few copies of that chromosome. Nondisjunction can affect both autosomal chromosomes (such as trisomy 21, resulting in Down syndrome) and the sex chromosomes (such as Klinefelter and Turner syndromes).

Meiosis II

Meiosis II is very similar to mitosis in that sister chromatids—rather than homologues—are separated from each other.

Prophase II

During **prophase II**, the nuclear envelope dissolves, nucleoli disappear, the centrioles migrate to opposite poles, and the spindle apparatus begins to form.

Metaphase II

During **metaphase II**, the chromosomes line up on the metaphase plate.

Anaphase II

During **anaphase II**, the centromeres divide, separating the chromosomes into sister chromatids. These chromatids are pulled to opposite poles by spindle fibers.

Telophase II

During **telophase II**, a nuclear membrane forms around each new nucleus. Cytokinesis follows, and two daughter cells are formed. Thus, by completion of meiosis II, up to four haploid daughter cells are produced per gametocyte. We use the phrase *up to* because oogenesis, discussed later in this chapter, may result in fewer than four cells if an egg remains unfertilized after ovulation.

KEY CONCEPT

Mitosis	Meiosis
$2n \rightarrow 2n$	$2n \rightarrow n$
Occurs in all dividing cells	Occurs in sex cells only
Homologous chromosomes do not pair	Homologous chromosomes align on opposite sides of the metaphase plate
No crossing over	Crossing over can occur

MCAT CONCEPT CHECK 2.2

Before you move on, assess your understanding of the material with these questions.

1. What is the number and ploidy of the daughter cells produced from meiosis I? From meiosis II?
   - Meiosis I:

   ____

   - Meiosis II:

   ____

2. What is the difference between homologous chromosomes and sister chromatids?
   - Homologous chromosomes:

   ____

   - Sister chromatids:

   ____

3. For each phase of meiosis I listed below, what are the differences from the analogous phase of mitosis?

Meiotic Phase	Differences from Mitotic Phase
Prophase I	
Metaphase I	
Anaphase I	
Telophase I	

2.3 The Reproductive System

High Yield

LEARNING OBJECTIVES

After Chapter 2.3, you will be able to:

- Recall the functions of the interstitial cells of Leydig and Sertoli cells
- Identify the phases of meiosis in which primary and secondary oocytes are arrested
- Describe the acrosome
- Differentiate between male and female sex organs and development
- Recall the phases of the menstrual cycle, including key features and relative hormone levels for each phase:

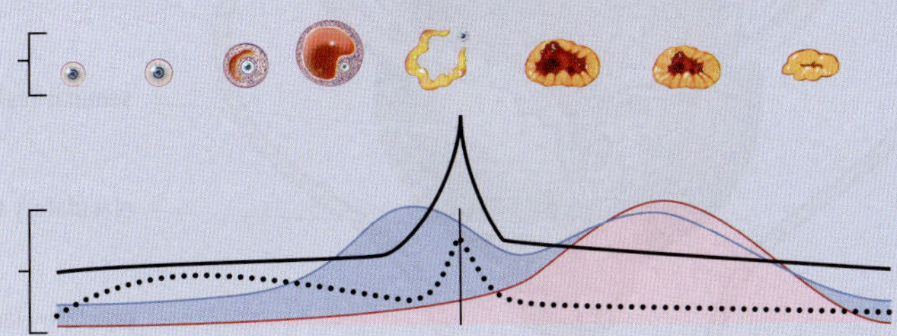

Chromosomal **sex** is determined by the 23rd pair of chromosomes, with XX being female and XY being male. Ova can only carry the X chromosome, while sperm can carry either the X or Y chromosome. The **X chromosome** carries a sizeable amount of genetic information; mutations in these genes can cause **sex-linked** (X-linked) disorders. Males are termed **hemizygous** with respect to many of the genes on the X chromosome because they only have one copy. Therefore, a male with a disease-causing allele on the unpaired part of X chromosome will necessarily express that allele. Females, on the other hand, may be homozygous or heterozygous with respect to genes on the X chromosome. Most X-linked disorders are recessively inherited; therefore, females express these disorders far less frequently than males. Females carrying a diseased allele on an X chromosome but not exhibiting the disease are said to be **carriers**.

Comparatively, the **Y chromosome** contains very little genetic information. One notable gene on the Y chromosome is ***SRY*** **(sex-determining region Y)**, which codes for a transcription factor that initiates testis differentiation and, thus, the formation of male gonads. Therefore, in the absence of the Y chromosome, all zygotes will be female. In the presence of the Y chromosome a zygote will be male.

MNEMONIC

Se**x**-linked is **X**-linked.

REAL WORLD

There are actually a handful of Y-linked diseases, most of which result in reduced fertility. A father will pass a Y-linked disease to all of his sons, assuming fertility has not been lost. These diseases are extremely rare and are not included on the official MCAT content lists.

Male Reproductive Anatomy

The male reproductive system is shown in Figure 2.8.

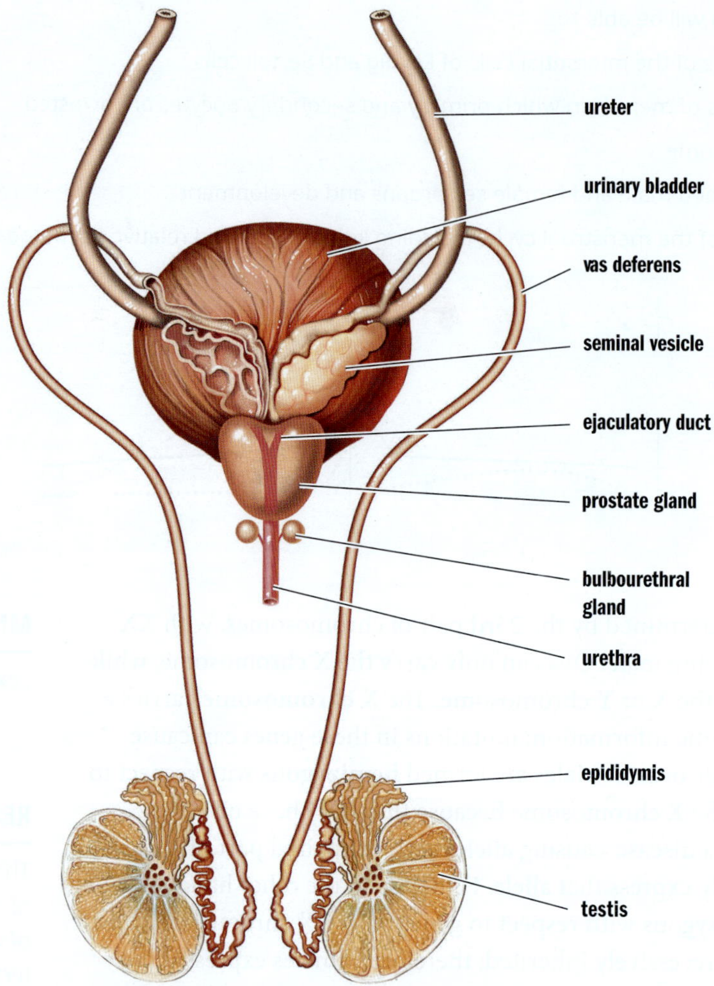

Figure 2.8 Male Reproductive System

In males, the primitive gonads develop into the **testes**. The testes have two functional components: the **seminiferous tubules** and the **interstitial cells of Leydig**. **Sperm** are produced in the highly coiled seminiferous tubules, where they are nourished by **Sertoli cells**. The cells of Leydig secrete **testosterone** and other male sex hormones (**androgens**). The testes are located in the **scrotum**, an external pouch that hangs below the **penis**, a position that allows it to maintain a temperature 2°C to 4°C lower than the body. In fact, there is a layer of muscle around the vas deferens (ductus deferens) that can raise and lower the testis to maintain the proper temperature for sperm development.

As sperm are formed they are passed to the **epididymis**, where their flagella gain motility, and they are then stored until **ejaculation**. During **ejaculation**, sperm travel through the **vas deferens** and enter the **ejaculatory duct** at the posterior edge of the prostate gland. The two ejaculatory ducts then fuse to form the

MNEMONIC

Pathway of sperm through the male reproductive system: **SEVE(N) UP**

- **S**eminiferous tubules
- **E**pididymis
- **V**as deferens (also called the ductus deferens)
- **E**jaculatory duct
- (**N**othing)
- **U**rethra
- **P**enis

urethra, which carries sperm through the penis as they exit the body. In males, the reproductive and urinary systems share a common pathway; this is not the case in females.

As sperm pass through the reproductive tract they are mixed with **seminal fluid**, which is produced through a combined effort by the seminal vesicles, prostate gland, and bulbourethral gland. The **seminal vesicles** contribute fructose to nourish sperm, and both the seminal vesicles and **prostate gland** give the fluid mildly alkaline properties so the sperm can survive in the relative acidity of the female reproductive tract. The **bulbourethral (Cowper's) glands** produce a clear viscous fluid that cleans out any remnants of urine and lubricates the urethra during sexual arousal. The combination of sperm and seminal fluid is known as **semen**.

REAL WORLD

The prostate often enlarges with age and frequently causes problems in older males, including a condition called *benign prostatic hyperplasia*. Because the prostate surrounds the urethra, classic symptoms of this condition include urinary frequency, urgency, and nighttime awakenings to use the bathroom.

Spermatogenesis

Spermatogenesis, as seen in Figure 2.9, is the formation of haploid sperm through meiosis, occurring in the seminiferous tubules. In males, the diploid stem cells are known as **spermatogonia**, which are found adjacent to the basement membrane within the seminiferous tubules. After replicating their genetic material (S stage), they develop into diploid **primary spermatocytes**, and are then found between the basement membrane and the lumen of the seminiferous tubule. The first meiotic division will result in haploid **secondary spermatocytes**, which then undergo meiosis II to generate haploid **spermatids**. Finally, the spermatids undergo maturation to become fully developed **spermatozoa** (colloquially known as sperm), which are found in the lumen of the seminiferous tubule. Spermatogenesis results in four functional sperm for each spermatogonium.

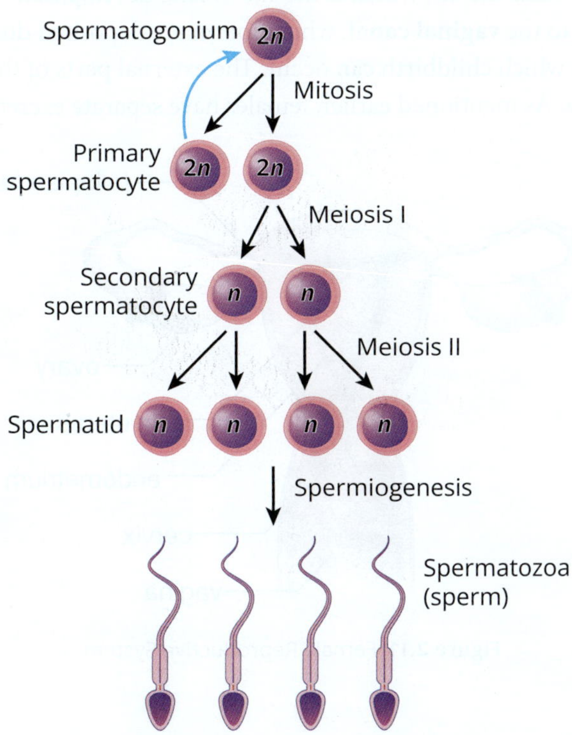

Figure 2.9 Spermatogenesis

Mature sperm are very compact. They consist of a head (containing the genetic material), a midpiece (which generates ATP from fructose), and a flagellum (for motility), as shown in Figure 2.10. The **midpiece** is filled with mitochondria, which generate the energy for swimming through the female reproductive tract to reach the ovum in the fallopian tubes. Each sperm **head** is covered by a cap known as an **acrosome**. This structure is derived from the Golgi apparatus and is necessary to penetrate the **ovum**. Once a male reaches sexual maturity during puberty, approximately 3 million sperm are produced per day, which typically continues throughout the course of that individual's lifespan.

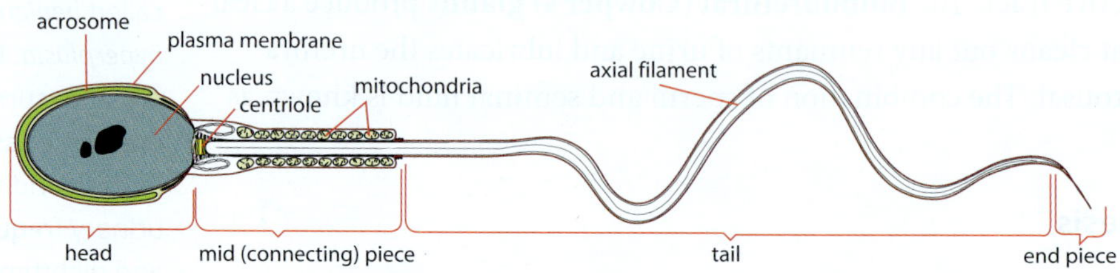

Figure 2.10 Structure of a Mature Sperm

Female Reproductive Anatomy

Female reproductive organs are primarily internal, as shown in Figure 2.11. The gonads, known as **ovaries**, produce estrogen and progesterone. The ovaries are located in the pelvic cavity; each consists of thousands of **follicles**, which are multilayered sacs that contain, nourish, and protect immature **ova** (eggs). Between puberty and menopause, one egg per month is **ovulated** into the **peritoneal sac**, which lines the abdominal cavity. It is then drawn into the **fallopian tube** or **oviduct**, which is lined with cilia to propel the egg forward. The fallopian tubes are connected to the muscular **uterus**, which is the site of fetal development. The lower end of the uterus, known as the **cervix**, connects to the **vaginal canal**, where sperm are deposited during intercourse. The vagina is also the passageway through which childbirth can occur. The external parts of the female genital organs are known collectively as the **vulva**. As mentioned earlier, females have separate excretory and reproductive tracts.

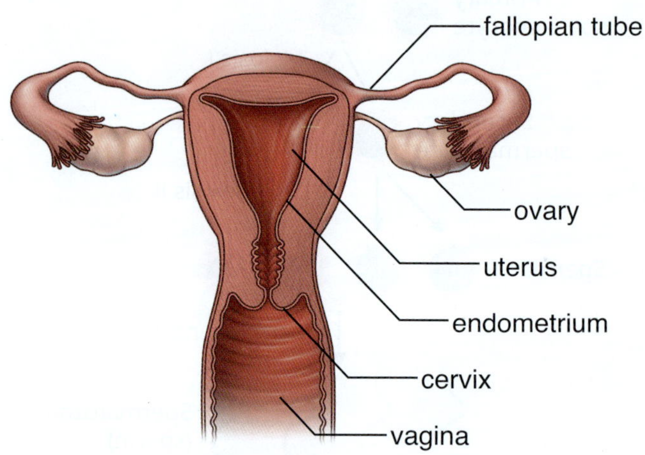

Figure 2.11 Female Reproductive System

Oogenesis

The production of female gametes is known as **oogenesis** (Figure 2.12). Although gametocytes undergo the same meiotic process in both females and males, there are some significant differences, too. First, there is no unending supply of stem cells analogous to spermatogonia in females; all of the oogonia a female will ever have are formed during fetal development. By birth, all of the oogonia have already undergone DNA replication and are considered **primary oocytes**. These cells are $2n$, like primary spermatocytes, and are actually arrested in prophase I. After **menarche** (the first menstrual cycle), one primary oocyte per month will complete meiosis I, producing a **secondary oocyte** and a polar body. The division is characterized by unequal cytokinesis, which distributes ample cytoplasm to one daughter cell (the secondary oocyte) and nearly none to the other (the polar body). The polar body generally does not divide any further and will never produce functional gametes. The secondary oocyte, on the other hand, remains arrested in metaphase II and does not complete the remainder of meiosis II unless fertilization occurs.

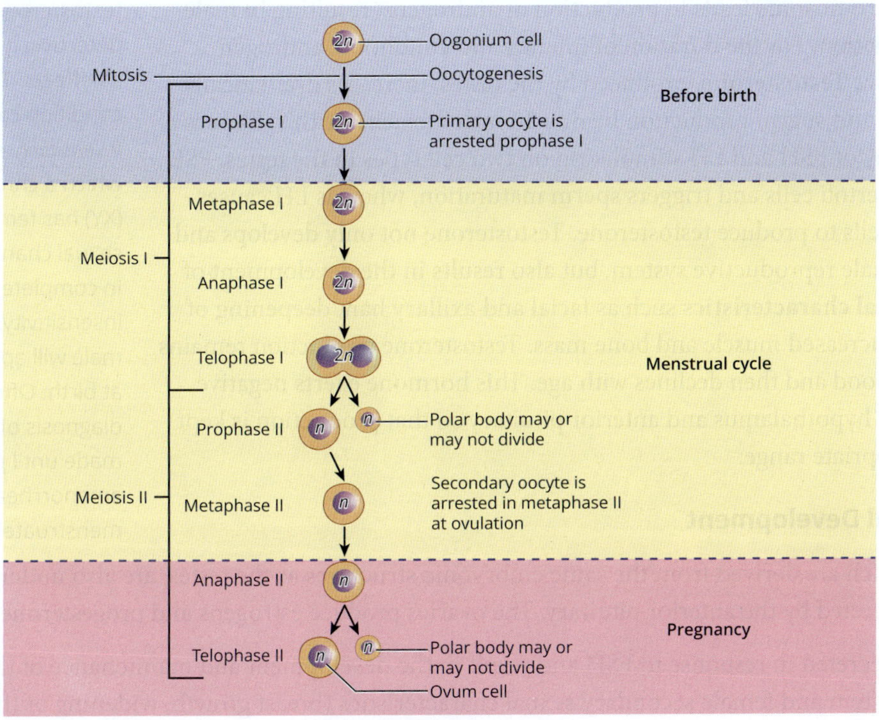

Figure 2.12 Oogenesis

Oocytes are surrounded by two layers: the zona pellucida and the corona radiata. The **zona pellucida** surrounds the oocyte itself and is an acellular mixture of glycoproteins that protects the oocyte and contains compounds necessary for sperm cell binding. The **corona radiata** lies outside the zona pellucida and is a layer of cells that adheres to the oocyte during ovulation. Meiosis II is triggered when a sperm cell penetrates these layers with the help of acrosomal enzymes. The secondary oocyte undergoes the second meiotic division to split into a mature ovum and another polar body, which will eventually be broken down.

A mature ovum is a very large cell consisting of large quantities of cytoplasm and organelles. The ovum contributes nearly everything to the zygote (half of the DNA and all of the cytoplasm, organelles [including mitochondria], and RNA for early cellular processes), and sperm contribute half of the DNA. Upon completion of meiosis II, the haploid **pronuclei** of the sperm and the ovum join, creating a diploid **zygote**.

MCAT EXPERTISE

The MCAT likes to ask about the heredity of mutations, so it is important to note that all of the zygote's mitochondria are from the mother. If someone were to inherit a mitochondrial mutation, then it almost certainly came from the mother.

Sexual Development

The ability to reproduce is under hormonal control. Prior to puberty, the **hypothalamus** restricts production of **gonadotropin-releasing hormone** (**GnRH**). At the start of puberty, this restriction is lifted as the hypothalamus releases pulses of GnRH, which then triggers the **anterior pituitary gland** to synthesize and release **follicle-stimulating hormone** (**FSH**) and **luteinizing hormone** (**LH**). These hormones trigger the production of other sex hormones that develop and maintain the reproductive system.

Male Sexual Development

During the fetal period (from nine weeks after fertilization until birth), presence of the Y chromosome leads to production of androgens, resulting in male sexual differentiation. For the duration of infancy and childhood, androgen production is low. **Testosterone**, produced by the testes, increases dramatically during puberty, and sperm production begins. In order to achieve this, there is a delicate interplay of FSH and LH stimulation on two cell types in the testes. FSH stimulates the Sertoli cells and triggers sperm maturation, whereas LH causes the interstitial cells to produce testosterone. Testosterone not only develops and maintains the male reproductive system, but also results in the development of **secondary sexual characteristics** such as facial and axillary hair, deepening of the voice, and increased muscle and bone mass. Testosterone production remains high into adulthood and then declines with age. This hormone exerts negative feedback on the hypothalamus and anterior pituitary so that production is kept within an appropriate range.

REAL WORLD

If the receptors for testosterone are absent or defective, it cannot exert its effects. The result is a condition called *androgen insensitivity syndrome* (AIS), in which a chromosomal male (XY) has female secondary sexual characteristics. In complete androgen insensitivity, a chromosomal male will appear female at birth. Oftentimes the diagnosis of AIS is not made until puberty, when amenorrhea (failure to menstruate) manifests.

Female Sexual Development

The ovaries, which are derived from the same embryonic structures as the testes, are also under the control of FSH and LH secreted by the anterior pituitary. The ovaries produce estrogens and progesterone.

Estrogens are secreted in response to FSH and result in the development and maintenance of the female reproductive system and female secondary sexual characteristics (breast growth, widening of the hips, changes in fat distribution). In the embryo, estrogens stimulate development of the reproductive tract. In adults, estrogens lead to the thickening of the lining of the uterus (**endometrium**) each month in preparation for the implantation of a zygote.

Progesterone is secreted by the **corpus luteum**—the remains of the ovarian follicle following ovulation—in response to LH. Interestingly, progesterone is involved in the development and maintenance of the endometrium, but not in the initial thickening of the endometrium—this is the role of estrogen. This means that both estrogen and progesterone are required for the generation, development, and maintenance of an endometrium capable of supporting a zygote. By the end of the first trimester of a pregnancy, progesterone is supplied by the placenta, while the corpus luteum atrophies and ceases to function.

MNEMONIC

Estrogen **est**ablishes and **pro**gesterone **pro**tects the endometrium.

The Menstrual Cycle

During the reproductive years (from menarche to menopause), estrogen and progesterone levels rise and fall in a cyclic pattern. In response, the endometrial lining will grow and be shed. This is known as the **menstrual**

cycle and can be divided into four events, as shown in Figure 2.13: the follicular phase, ovulation, the luteal phase, and menstruation.

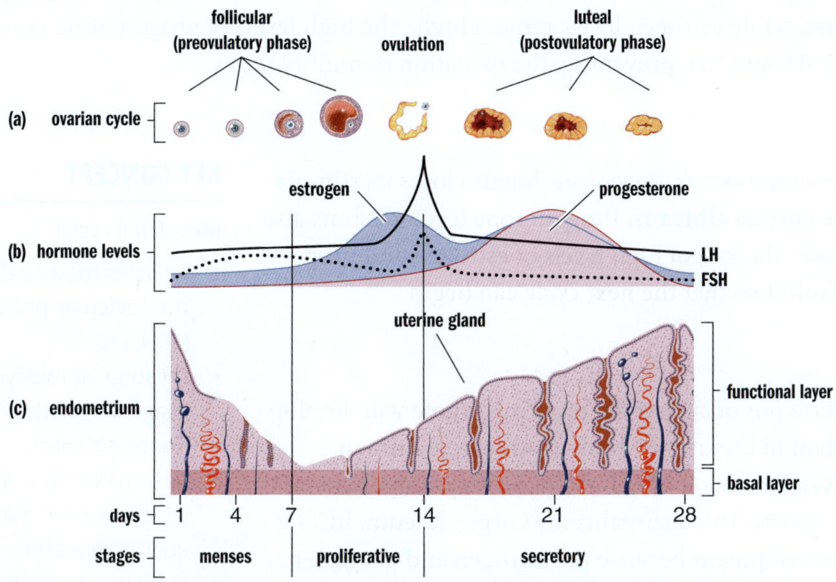

Figure 2.13 The Menstrual Cycle
(a) Follicle-stimulating hormone (FSH) facilitates the maturation of a single ovum; (b) The peak of luteinizing hormone (LH) around day 14 marks ovulation, the release of the oocyte from the follicle; (c) The endometrial lining of the uterus reaches its peak in the luteal phase and is shed at the beginning of the next cycle.

MCAT EXPERTISE

The MCAT likes to test your ability to identify graphs of the blood concentrations of FSH, LH, estrogen, and progesterone throughout the menstrual cycle. Be sure to know when each peaks by studying Figure 2.13.

Follicular Phase

The **follicular phase** begins when the **menstrual flow**, which sheds the uterine lining of the previous cycle, begins. GnRH secretion from the hypothalamus increases in response to the decreased concentrations of estrogen and progesterone, which fall off toward the end of each cycle. The higher concentrations of GnRH cause increased secretions of both FSH and LH. These two hormones work in concert to develop several ovarian follicles. The follicles begin to produce estrogen, which has negative feedback effects and causes the GnRH, LH, and FSH concentrations to level off. Estrogen stimulates regrowth of the endometrial lining, stimulating vascularization and glandularization of the **decidua**.

REAL WORLD

Oral contraceptive pills (OCPs) are simply estrogen/progesterone (or progesterone-only) preparations. These block conception by inhibiting LH and FSH release through negative feedback, thereby inhibiting ovulation. When taking the placebo pills at the end of the month, withdrawal menstruation still occurs because estrogen and progesterone levels drop, but no egg passes with the menstrual flow.

Ovulation

Estrogen is interesting in that it can have both negative and positive feedback effects. Late in the follicular phase, the developing follicles secrete higher and higher concentrations of estrogen. Eventually, estrogen concentrations reach a threshold that paradoxically results in positive feedback, and GnRH, LH, and FSH levels spike. The surge in LH is important; it induces **ovulation**, the release of the ovum from the ovary into the abdominal (peritoneal) cavity.

Luteal Phase

After ovulation, LH causes the ruptured follicle to form the corpus luteum, which secretes progesterone. Remember that estrogen helps regenerate the uterine lining, but progesterone maintains it for implantation. Progesterone levels begin to rise, while estrogen levels remain high. The high levels of progesterone cause negative feedback on GnRH, FSH, and LH, preventing the ovulation of multiple eggs.

Menstruation

Assuming that implantation does not occur, the corpus luteum loses its stimulation from LH, turning into the **corpus albicans**. Progesterone levels decline, and the uterine lining is sloughed off. The loss of high levels of estrogen and progesterone removes the block on GnRH so that the next cycle can begin.

Pregnancy

On the other hand, if fertilization *has* occurred the resulting zygote will develop into a blastocyst that will implant in the uterine lining and secrete **human chorionic gonadotropin (hCG)**, an analog of LH—it looks very similar chemically and can stimulate LH receptors. This maintains the corpus luteum. hCG is critical during first trimester development because the estrogen and progesterone secreted by the corpus luteum keep the uterine lining in place. By the second trimester, hCG levels decline because the placenta has grown to a sufficient size to secrete enough progesterone and estrogen by itself. The high levels of estrogen and progesterone continue to serve as negative feedback on GnRH secretion.

Menopause

With aging, the ovaries become less sensitive to FSH and LH, resulting in ovarian atrophy. As estrogen and progesterone levels drop, the endometrium also atrophies, and menstruation stops. Also, because the negative feedback on FSH and LH is removed, the blood levels of these two hormones rise. This is called **menopause**. Profound physical and physiological changes usually accompany this process, including flushing, hot flashes, bloating, and headaches. Menopause usually occurs between the ages of 45 and 55.

KEY CONCEPT

Menstrual cycle:

- Follicles mature during the follicular phase (FSH, LH)
- LH surge at midcycle triggers ovulation
- Ruptured follicle becomes corpus luteum, which secretes estrogen and progesterone to build up uterine lining in preparation for implantation; LH and FSH are inhibited
- If fertilization does not occur, corpus luteum atrophies, progesterone and estrogen levels decrease, menses occurs, and LH and FSH levels begin to rise again

MCAT CONCEPT CHECK 2.3

Before you move on, assess your understanding of the material with these questions.

1. What are the functions of interstitial cells of Leydig and Sertoli cells?
   - Interstitial cells of Leydig:

   - Sertoli cells:

2. During which phase of meiosis is a primary oocyte arrested? During which phase of meiosis is a secondary oocyte arrested?
   - Primary oocyte:

   - Secondary oocyte:

3. What is the acrosome? What organelle forms the acrosome?

4. Which hormones are key to sexual differentiation in a fetus with XY genotype? Describe the expected phenotype if receptors to these hormones are absent.

5. What are the four phases of the menstrual cycle? What are the features and relative hormone concentrations of each phase? (Note: Draw in symbols to signify the levels of each hormone, such as ↑, =, and ↓.)

Phase	Key Features	FSH	LH	Estrogen	Progesterone

Conclusion

In this chapter, we explored one of the key tenets of the cell theory—how cells produce more copies of themselves. We first examined mitosis, which results in genetically identical diploid daughter cells. We then moved on to meiosis, which results in genetically nonidentical haploid daughter cells, or gametes. We then looked at the male and female reproductive systems, which form these gametes, each of which contains half of the normal complement of genetic information. Finally, we explored basic reproductive endocrinology and saw how testosterone and estrogen are key in the development of the reproductive systems and the secondary sex characteristics that develop at puberty.

Formation of gametes is only half the story, of course. It serves us no good as a species to form sex cells if the cells cannot interact to form another human. Ultimately, gametes must accomplish their purpose: passing on the genes, the instructions for life, from one generation to another. Thus, we turn our attention in the next chapter to the next steps of fertilization, embryogenesis, and birth. Indeed, it is through the union of one egg and one sperm that every human being on the planet today—and since the beginning of the human race—came into existence.

GO ONLINE

You've reviewed the content, now test your knowledge and critical thinking skills by completing a test-like passage set in your online resources!

CONCEPT SUMMARY

The Cell Cycle and Mitosis

- **Diploid** ($2n$) cells have two copies of each chromosome; **haploid** (n) cells have one copy.
- The cell cycle contains five stages. The G_1, S, and G_2 stages are collectively called **interphase**, during which the DNA is uncoiled in the form of **chromatin**.
  - In the G_1 stage (**presynthetic gap**), cells create organelles for energy and protein production, and increase their size. The **restriction point**, during which the DNA is checked for quality, must be passed for the cell to move into the S stage.
  - In the **S** stage (**synthesis**), DNA is replicated. The strands of DNA, called **chromatids**, are held together at the centromere.
  - In the G_2 stage (**postsynthetic gap**), there is further cell growth and replication of organelles in preparation for mitosis. Another quality checkpoint must be passed for the cell to enter into mitosis.
  - In the **M** stage (**mitosis**), mitosis and cytokinesis occur.
  - In the G_0 stage, the cell performs its functions without preparing for division.
- **p53** plays a role in the two major checkpoints of the cell cycle (G_1 to S, and G_2 to M).
- **Cyclins** and **cyclin-dependent kinases** (**CDK**) rise and fall during the cell cycle. Cyclins bind to CDKs, phosphorylating and activating **transcription factors** for the next stage of the cell cycle.
- **Cancer** occurs when cell cycle control becomes deranged, allowing damaged cells to undergo mitosis without regard to quality or quantity of the new cells produced. Cancerous cells may begin to produce factors that allow them to delocalize and invade adjacent tissues or **metastasize** elsewhere.
- Mitosis produces two genetically identical diploid daughter cells from a single cell and occurs in **somatic cells**.
- Mitosis has four phases:
  - In **prophase**, the chromosomes condense, the nuclear membrane dissolves, nucleoli disappear, centrioles migrate to opposite sides of the cell, and the **spindle apparatus** begins to form. The **kinetochore** of each chromosome is contacted by a spindle fiber.
  - In **metaphase**, chromosomes line up along the **metaphase plate** (**equatorial plate**).
  - In **anaphase**, sister chromatids are separated and pulled to opposite poles.
  - In **telophase**, the nuclear membrane reforms, spindle apparatus disappears, and cytosol and organelles are split between the two daughter cells through **cytokinesis**.

Meiosis

- **Meiosis** occurs in **gametocytes** (**germ cells**) and produces up to four nonidentical haploid sex cells (**gametes**).
- Meiosis has one round of replication and two rounds of division (the **reductional** and **equational** divisions).
- In **meiosis I**, homologous pairs of chromosomes (homologues) are separated from each other. **Homologues** are chromosomes that are given the same number, but are of opposite parental origin.
  - In **prophase I**, the same events occur as in prophase of mitosis, except that homologues come together and intertwine in a process called **synapsis**. The four chromatids are referred to as a **tetrad**, and **crossing over** exchanges genetic material between one chromatid and material from a chromatid in the homologous chromosome. This accounts for **Mendel's second law (of independent assortment)**.

    - In **metaphase I**, homologous chromosomes line up on opposite sides of the metaphase plate.
    - In **anaphase I**, homologous chromosomes are pulled to opposite poles of the cell. This accounts for **Mendel's first law (of segregation)**.
    - In **telophase I**, the chromosomes may or may not fully decondense, and the cell may enter **interkinesis** after cytokinesis.
- In **meiosis II**, sister chromatids are separated from each other in a process that is functionally identical to mitosis. **Sister chromatids** are copies of the same DNA held together at the centromere.

The Reproductive System

- Chromosomal sex is determined by the 23rd pair of chromosomes in humans, with XX being female and XY being male.
    - The **X chromosome** carries a sizeable amount of genetic information; mutations of X-linked genes can cause sex-linked disorders. Males are **hemizygous** with respect to the unpaired genes on the X chromosome, so they will express sex-linked disorders, even if they only have one recessive disease-carrying allele. Females with only one copy of the affected allele are called **carriers**.
    - The **Y chromosome** carries little genetic information, but does contain the ***SRY*** **(sex-determining region Y)** gene, which causes the gonads to differentiate into testes.
- The male reproductive system contains both internal and external structures.
    - **Sperm** develop in the **seminiferous tubules** in the **testes**. They are nourished by **Sertoli cells**.
    - **Interstitial cells of Leydig**, in the testes, secrete **testosterone** and other male sex hormones (**androgens**).
    - The testes are located in the **scrotum**, which hangs outside of the abdominal cavity and has a temperature 2°C to 4°C lower than the rest of the body.
    - Once formed, sperm gain motility in the **epididymis** and are stored there until ejaculation.
    - During **ejaculation**, sperm travel through the **vas deferens** to the **ejaculatory duct**, and then to the **urethra** and out through the **penis**.
    - The **seminal vesicles** contribute fructose to nourish sperm and produce alkaline fluid.
    - The **prostate gland** also produces alkaline fluid.
    - The **bulbourethral glands** produce a clear viscous fluid that cleans out any remnants of urine and lubricates the urethra during sexual arousal.
    - **Semen** is composed of sperm and **seminal fluid** from the glands above.
- In **spermatogenesis**, four haploid sperm are produced from a **spermatogonium**.
    - After S stage, the germ cells are called **primary spermatocytes**.
    - After meiosis I, the germ cells are called **secondary spermatocytes**.
    - After meiosis II, the germ cells are called **spermatids**.
    - After maturation, the germ cells are called **spermatozoa**.
- Sperm contain a head, midpiece, and flagellum.
    - The **head** contains the genetic material and is covered with an **acrosome**—a modified Golgi apparatus that contains enzymes that help the sperm fuse with and penetrate the ovum.
    - The **midpiece** generates ATP from fructose and contains many mitochondria.
    - The **flagellum** promotes motility.

- The female reproductive system primarily contains internal structures.
  - **Ova** (eggs) are produced in **follicles** in the **ovaries**.
  - Once each month, an egg is **ovulated** into the **peritoneal sac** and is drawn into the **fallopian tube** or **oviduct**.
  - The fallopian tubes are connected to the **uterus**, the lower end of which is the **cervix**.
  - The **vaginal canal** lies below the cervix and is the site where sperm are deposited during intercourse.
  - The vaginal canal also can be the site of childbirth.
  - The external parts of the female genital organs are collectively known as the **vulva**.
- In **oogenesis**, one haploid ovum and a variable number of polar bodies are formed from an **oogonium**.
  - At birth, all oogonia have already undergone replication and are considered **primary oocytes**. They are arrested in prophase I.
  - The ovulated egg each month is a **secondary oocyte**, which is arrested in metaphase II.
  - If the oocyte is fertilized, it will complete meiosis II to become a true ovum.
  - Cytokinesis is uneven in oogenesis. The cell receiving very little cytoplasm and organelles is called a **polar body**.
  - Oocytes are surrounded by the **zona pellucida**, an acellular mixture of glycoproteins that protects the oocyte and contains the compounds necessary for sperm binding; and the **corona radiata**, which is a layer of cells that adheres to the oocyte during ovulation.
- **Gonadotropin-releasing hormone** (**GnRH**) from the **hypothalamus** causes the release of **follicle-stimulating hormone** (**FSH**) and **luteinizing hormone** (**LH**), the functions of which depend on the sex of the individual.
  - In males, FSH stimulates the Sertoli cells and triggers spermatogenesis, while LH causes the interstitial cells to produce testosterone. **Testosterone** is responsible for the maintenance and development of the male reproductive system and male secondary sex characteristics (facial and axillary hair, deepening of the voice, and increased bone and muscle mass).
  - In females, FSH stimulates development of the ovarian follicles, while LH causes ovulation. These hormones also stimulate production of estrogens and progesterone.
- The menstrual cycle is a periodic growth and shedding of the endometrial lining.
  - In the **follicular phase**, GnRH secretion stimulates FSH and LH secretion, which promotes follicle development. Estrogen is released, stimulating vascularization and glandularization of the **decidua**.
  - **Ovulation** is stimulated by a sudden surge in LH. This surge is triggered when estrogen levels reach a threshold and switch from negative to positive feedback effects.
  - In the **luteal phase**, LH causes the ruptured follicle to become the corpus luteum, which secretes progesterone that maintains the uterine lining. High estrogen and progesterone levels cause negative feedback on GnRH, LH, and FSH.
  - **Menstruation** occurs if there is no fertilization. As the estrogen and progesterone levels drop, the endometrial lining is sloughed off, and the block on GnRH production is removed.
  - If fertilization does occur, the blastula produces **human chorionic gonadotropin** (**hCG**) which, as an LH analog, can maintain the corpus luteum. Near the end of the first trimester, hCG levels drop as the placenta takes over progesterone production.
- **Menopause** occurs when the ovaries stop producing estrogen and progesterone, usually between ages 45 and 55. Menstruation stops and FSH and LH levels rise. Physical and physiological changes accompanying menopause include flushing, hot flashes, bloating, and headaches.

ANSWERS TO CONCEPT CHECKS

2.1

1.

Cell Cycle Stage	Features
G_1	Cell grows and performs its normal functions. DNA is examined and repaired.
S	DNA is replicated.
G_2	Cell continues to grow and replicates organelles in preparation for mitosis. Cell continues to perform its normal functions.
M	Mitosis (cell division) occurs.
G_0	The cell performs its normal functions and is not preparing to divide.

2.

Mitotic Phase	Features
Prophase	Chromosomes condense, nuclear membrane dissolves, nucleoli disappear, centrioles migrate to opposite poles and begin forming the spindle apparatus
Metaphase	Chromosomes gather along the metaphase plate in the center of the cell under the guidance of the spindle apparatus
Anaphase	Sister chromatids separate, and a copy of each chromosome migrates to opposite poles
Telophase and Cytokinesis	Chromosomes decondense, nuclear membrane reforms, nucleoli reappear, spindle apparatus breaks down, cell divides into two identical daughter cells

2.2

1. After meiosis I, there are two haploid daughter cells. After meiosis II, there are up to four haploid gametes.
2. Homologous chromosomes are related chromosomes of opposite parental origin (such as maternal chromosome 15 and paternal chromosome 15, or—in males—the X and Y chromosomes). Sister chromatids are identical copies of the same DNA that are held together at the centromere. After S phase, a cell contains 92 chromatids, 46 chromosomes, and 23 homologous pairs.

3.

Meiotic Phase	Differences from Mitotic Phase
Prophase I	Homologous chromosomes come together as tetrads during synapsis; crossing over
Metaphase I	Homologous chromosomes line up on opposite sides of the metaphase plate, rather than individual chromosomes lining up on the metaphase plate
Anaphase I	Homologous chromosomes separate from each other; centromeres do not break
Telophase I	Chromatin may or may not decondense; interkinesis occurs as the cell prepares for meiosis II

2.3

1. The interstitial cells of Leydig secrete testosterone and other male sex hormones (androgens). Sertoli cells nourish sperm during their development.
2. A primary oocyte is arrested in prophase I, while a secondary oocyte is arrested in metaphase II.
3. The acrosome contains enzymes that are capable of penetrating the corona radiata and zona pellucida of the ovum, permitting fertilization to occur. It is a modified Golgi apparatus.
4. Androgens, such as testosterone, lead to male sexual differentiation. Absence of androgen receptors, a condition known as androgen insensitivity syndrome, leads to an XY genotype with phenotypically female characteristics.

5.

Phase	Key Features	FSH	LH	Estrogen	Progesterone
Follicular	Egg develops, endometrial lining becomes vascularized and glandularized	↑	=	↓, then ↑	↓
Ovulation	Egg is released from follicle into peritoneal cavity	↑	↑↑	↑	↓
Luteal	Corpus luteum produces progesterone to maintain endometrium	↓	=	↑	↑
Menses	Shedding of endometrial lining	↓	↓	↓	↓

SCIENCE MASTERY ASSESSMENT EXPLANATIONS

1. **B**

Diploid cells called spermatogonia differentiate into primary spermatocytes, which undergo the first meiotic division to yield two haploid secondary spermatocytes. These undergo a second meiotic division to become immature spermatids. The spermatids then undergo a series of changes leading to the production of mature sperm, or spermatozoa.

2. **C**

From the time of birth until shortly before ovulation, all egg cells are arrested at the prophase stage of meiosis I. These cells are referred to as primary oocytes. At ovulation, the egg cell has completed meiosis I and is now arrested in metaphase II as a haploid cell called a secondary oocyte. When a sperm penetrates the outer layers of the secondary oocyte, it completes meiosis II to become a mature ovum.

3. **A**

The spindle apparatus first interacts with the kinetochore fibers near the end of prophase. While the spindle apparatus aligns the chromosomes at the equatorial plate during metaphase, **(B)**, the initial connection of the microtubule to the kinetochore occurs in prophase.

4. **D**

To ensure that the labeled deoxyadenine will be incorporated into the DNA of one of the daughter cells, we have to insert the nucleotide before DNA replication has been completed. Because replication occurs during S stage, we could introduce the deoxyadenine during G_1 or S stage. Because G_1 precedes S, the latest point at which the deoxyadenine could be added is the S stage.

5. **C**

Estrogen is known to cause growth of the endometrial lining during the follicular phase of the menstrual cycle, and its levels stay high during the luteal phase to promote vascularization and glandularization of this tissue. Excessive levels of estrogen may provide a strong enough signal for cell growth to promote tumor formation or even cancer. The other tissues listed in this question require estrogen for development, but are not strongly dependent on estrogen for growth.

6. **C**

This subtle point about ovulation is missed by most students and remains hard to believe until the organs are examined in anatomy class in medical school. The ruptured ovarian follicle releases an oocyte into the abdominal cavity, close to the entrance of the fallopian tube. With the aid of beating cilia, the oocyte is drawn into the fallopian tube, through which it travels until it reaches the uterus. If it is fertilized in the fallopian tube, it will implant in the uterine wall. If fertilization does not occur, it will be expelled along with the uterine lining during menstruation.

7. **D**

The question is asking us to determine at which points in the cell cycle we can prevent or at least lower the number of cells undergoing mitosis. One idea would be to prevent DNA synthesis during the S stage of the cell cycle. Without the DNA being replicated, two viable daughter cells could not be formed. Other ideas would be preventing the mitotic cycle from forming altogether in prophase by preventing spindle apparatus formation, preventing the nuclear membrane from dissolving, or interfering with other processes during this phase. Similarly, a treatment that would act on cells in the metaphase stage of the cell cycle would also interfere with the mitotic cycle. Therefore, any of the three solutions presented would be a viable option.

8. **B**

The prostate gland, along with the seminal vesicles and the bulbourethral gland, secretes seminal fluid that combines with sperm to produce semen. It is the cremaster muscle which surrounds the testes that raises and lowers the testes in response to changes in temperature.

9. **B**

The first meiotic division (reductional division) pulls homologous chromosomes to opposite poles of the cell during anaphase I. Near the end of telophase I, cytokinesis occurs, resulting in two haploid (n) daughter cells. Thus, during interkinesis and anaphase II, the daughter cells are already haploid, eliminating **(C)** and **(D)**. The cell is diploid during interphase, **(A)**, but remains diploid up until the end of telophase I.

10. **D**

The safest way to answer this question correctly is to go through each answer choice and eliminate the ones that contribute to genetic variability. The random fertilization of an egg by a sperm, the random segregation of homologous chromosomes during anaphase I, and crossing over between homologous chromosomes during prophase I all contribute to genetic variability during sexual reproduction because they result in novel combinations of genetic material, eliminating **(A)**, **(B)**, and **(C)**. S stage, **(D)**, should *not* cause increased genetic variability; the DNA should be copied precisely, without error, meaning that both strands of DNA should be identical.

11. **D**

The key differences between mitosis and meiosis primarily appear during meiosis I. Of note, synapsis and crossing over occur during prophase I, and homologous chromosomes are separated during meiosis I (rather than sister chromatids, as in mitosis). While the location of the centromeres relative to the metaphase plate may seem trivial, it is representative of the fact that homologous chromosomes line up on opposite sides of the equatorial plate in meiosis, in contrast to the positioning of each chromosome directly upon the metaphase plate in mitosis.

12. **D**

In prophase, the chromatin condenses into chromosomes, the spindle apparatus forms, and the nucleoli and nuclear membrane disappear. **(A)** describes anaphase, whereas **(B)** and **(C)** describe telophase.

13. **C**

Nondisjunction refers to the incorrect segregation of homologous chromosomes during anaphase I, or of sister chromatids during anaphase II. In either case, one daughter cell ends up with two copies of related genetic material, while the other receives zero. Immediately, this should eliminate **(A)** and **(B)**, which show a normal complement of chromosomes (46). An individual who has only one recessive disease-carrying allele, and yet still expresses the disease, likely does not have a dominant allele for the given trait. This is seen in males, who are hemizygous for many X-linked genes, and can also be seen in females who have Turner syndrome (45,X) and only one X chromosome. Thus, **(C)** is the answer.

14. **C**

Progesterone peaks during the luteal phase, as it supports the endometrium for potential implantation of a blastula. Progesterone levels are relatively low during the follicular phase and ovulation, eliminating **(A)** and **(B)**. Withdrawal of progesterone actually causes menses, eliminating **(D)**.

15. **D**

During the first trimester of pregnancy, the corpus luteum is preserved by human chorionic gonadotropin (hCG); hence, progesterone secretion by the corpus luteum is maintained during the first trimester. This eliminates **(A)**. During the second trimester, hCG levels decline, but progesterone levels rise because the hormone is now secreted by the placenta itself, eliminating **(B)**. High levels of progesterone and estrogen inhibit GnRH secretion, thus preventing FSH and LH secretion and the onset of a new menstrual cycle. This eliminates **(C)** and validates **(D)**.

GO ONLINE

Consult your online resources for additional practice.

SHARED CONCEPTS

Behavioral Sciences Chapter 1
Biology and Behavior

Biochemistry Chapter 6
DNA and Biotechnology

Biology Chapter 1
The Cell

Biology Chapter 3
Embryogenesis and Development

Biology Chapter 5
The Endocrine System

Biology Chapter 12
Genetics and Evolution

CHAPTER 3

EMBRYOGENESIS AND DEVELOPMENT

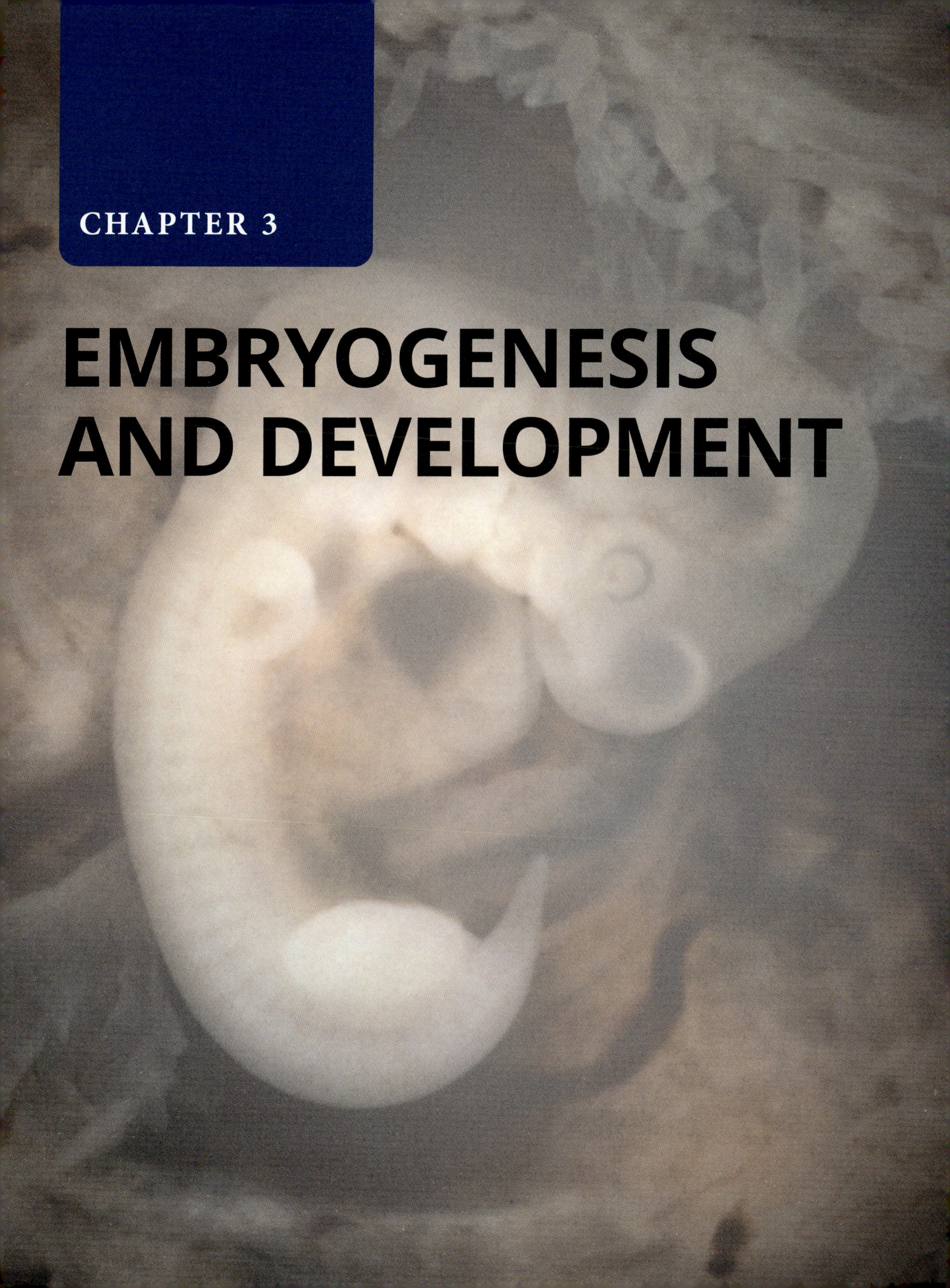

SCIENCE MASTERY ASSESSMENT

Every pre-med knows this feeling: there is so much content I have to know for the MCAT! How do I know what to do first or what's important?

While the high-yield badges throughout this book will help you identify the most important topics, this Science Mastery Assessment is another tool in your MCAT prep arsenal. This quiz (which can also be taken in your online resources) and the guidance below will help ensure that you are spending the appropriate amount of time on this chapter based on your personal strengths and weaknesses. Don't worry though—skipping something now does not mean you'll never study it. Later on in your prep, as you complete full-length tests, you'll uncover specific pieces of content that you need to review and can come back to these chapters as appropriate.

How to Use This Assessment

If you answer 0–7 questions correctly:

Spend about 1 hour to read this chapter in full and take limited notes throughout. Follow up by reviewing **all** quiz questions to ensure that you now understand how to solve each one.

If you answer 8–11 questions correctly:

Spend 20–40 minutes reviewing the quiz questions. Beginning with the questions you missed, read and take notes on the corresponding subchapters. For questions you answered correctly, ensure your thinking matches that of the explanation and you understand why each choice was correct or incorrect.

If you answer 12–15 questions correctly:

Spend less than 20 minutes reviewing all questions from the quiz. If you missed any, then include a quick read-through of the corresponding subchapters, or even just the relevant content within a subchapter, as part of your question review. For questions you answered correctly, ensure your thinking matches that of the explanation and review the Concept Summary at the end of the chapter.

1. Which of the following signaling molecules coordinate uterine contractions during childbirth?
   - **A.** Oxytocin and prolactin
   - **B.** Progesterone and prostaglandins
   - **C.** Oxytocin and progesterone
   - **D.** Oxytocin and prostaglandins

2. Which of the following associations of a primary germ layer and an adult organ is correct?
   - **A.** Endoderm—cardiac muscle
   - **B.** Endoderm—lens of the eye
   - **C.** Ectoderm—fingernails
   - **D.** Mesoderm—lining of digestive tract

3. From which of the following layers does the notochord form?
   - **A.** Ectoderm
   - **B.** Mesoderm
   - **C.** Endoderm
   - **D.** Archenteron

4. The influence of a specific group of cells on the differentiation of another group of cells is called:
   - **A.** competence.
   - **B.** senescence.
   - **C.** determination.
   - **D.** induction.

5. Which of the following is likely to be found in the blood of a person who is pregnant?
   - **A.** Immunoglobulins produced by the fetus
   - **B.** Fetal hemoglobin released from fetal red blood cells
   - **C.** Progesterone produced by placental cells
   - **D.** Carbon dioxide exhaled from fetal lungs

6. A cell releases a substance that diffuses through the environment, resulting in differentiation of a nearby cell. This is an example of what type of cell–cell communication?
   - **A.** Autocrine
   - **B.** Juxtacrine
   - **C.** Paracrine
   - **D.** Endocrine

7. A cancer cell is removed from a patient and cultured. The cells in this culture seem to be able to divide indefinitely with no cellular senescence. Which protein is likely activated in these cells that accounts for this characteristic?
   - **A.** Epidermal growth factor
   - **B.** Sonic hedgehog
   - **C.** Transforming growth factor beta
   - **D.** Telomerase

8. Anencephaly is a rare physiological abnormality in which the cerebrum fails to develop. During which trimester of pregnancy would this disorder manifest?
   - **A.** First trimester
   - **B.** Second trimester
   - **C.** Third trimester
   - **D.** Any trimester

9. Which of the following is FALSE with regard to adult stem cells?
   - **A.** They retain inherent pluripotency if harvested from selected organs.
   - **B.** They are less controversial than embryonic stem cells.
   - **C.** They require treatment with various transcription factors.
   - **D.** There is a reduced risk of rejection if the patient's own stem cells are used.

10. A child is born with an imperforate anus, in which the anal canal fails to form correctly and the rectum is not connected to the outside world. This pathology is most likely accounted for by a failure of:
    - **A.** cell differentiation.
    - **B.** cell determination.
    - **C.** apoptosis.
    - **D.** neurulation.

11. Following a myocardial infarction, the heart often heals by the creation of a scar by fibroblasts. This is an example of:

A. complete regeneration.
B. incomplete regeneration.
C. competency.
D. multipotency.

12. Neurofibromatosis type I, or von Recklinghausen's disease, is a disorder that causes formation of tumors in multiple nervous system structures as well as the skin. While all cells carry the same mutation on chromosome 17, selective transcription of the genome appears to cause the most significant tumorigenesis in which of the following primary germ tissue layers?

A. Ectoderm
B. Mesoderm
C. Endoderm
D. Notochord

13. Which of the following shows the correct order of early developmental milestones during embryogenesis?

A. Blastula → gastrula → morula
B. Morula → gastrula → blastula
C. Morula → blastula → gastrula
D. Gastrula → blastula → morula

14. A woman who is pregnant is accidentally given a single dose of a teratogenic drug late in the third trimester. The baby is born three days later. Which of the following is the most likely outcome?

A. Complete failure of organ development and death of the fetus
B. Partial failure of organ development with survival of the fetus
C. Serious disfigurement of the fetus
D. Respiratory distress at birth, but no long-term effects

15. Which of the following statements regarding fetal circulation is FALSE?

A. In the umbilical cord, there are more arteries than veins.
B. The foramen ovale is the only shunt that connects two chambers of the heart.
C. Blood flow in the ductus arteriosus is from the aorta to the pulmonary artery.
D. The ductus venosus is the only shunt that bypasses the liver.

Answer Key

1. **D** (See section 3.4)
2. **C** (See section 3.1)
3. **B** (See section 3.1)
4. **D** (See section 3.1)
5. **C** (See section 3.3)
6. **C** (See section 3.2)
7. **D** (See section 3.2)
8. **A** (See section 3.4)
9. **A** (See section 3.2)
10. **C** (See section 3.2)
11. **B** (See section 3.2)
12. **A** (See section 3.1)
13. **C** (See section 3.1)
14. **D** (See section 3.1)
15. **C** (See section 3.3)

The relevant section of the chapter to review for each question is given in parentheses after the correct answer. Detailed explanations can be found at the end of the chapter.

CHAPTER 3

EMBRYOGENESIS AND DEVELOPMENT

In This Chapter

CHAPTER PROFILE

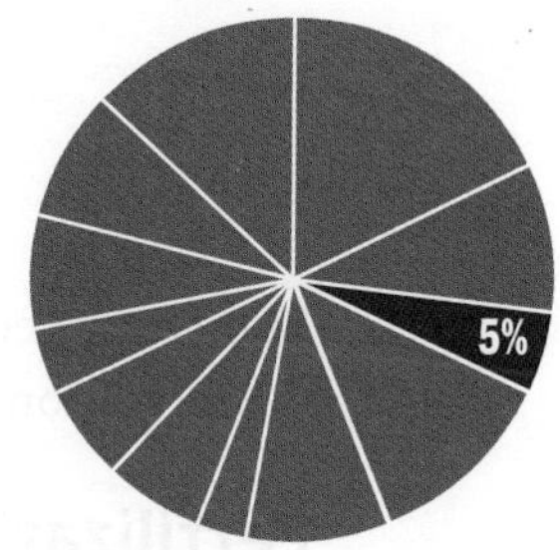

The content in this chapter should be relevant to about 5% of all questions about biology on the MCAT.

This chapter covers material from the following AAMC content categories:

1B: Transmission of genetic information from the gene to the protein

2C: Processes of cell division, differentiation, and specialization

3B: Structure and integrative functions of the main organ systems

7A: Individual influences on behavior

Introduction

Ultrasonography is a radiographic technique performed by placing a probe that emits high-frequency sound waves near the tissue to be examined. When used during pregnancy, the probe transduces an image onto a computer screen to determine gestational age, screen for multiple pregnancies or anomalies, and identify the baby's phenotypical sex. The latter typically cannot be determined before 16 to 17 weeks without a blood test, because ultrasonography equipment does not have high enough resolution.

In this chapter, we'll continue the discussion from Chapter 2 by beginning with fertilization, the formation of a diploid zygote from the union of a sperm and an ovum. We'll then follow development from this point until the birth of an autonomously breathing baby. We'll examine how the cells of a developing human divide and differentiate. We'll also explore some specific system differences that exist between developing fetuses and adults as we present an overview of the stages of pregnancy and childbirth.

3.1 Early Developmental Stages

LEARNING OBJECTIVES

After Chapter 3.1, you will be able to:

- Distinguish between determinate and indeterminate cleavage of a zygote
- Describe the process of implantation and the stage of development at which it occurs
- Connect the ectoderm, mesoderm, neural crest, and endoderm to the organs they will form
- Describe how induction influences development
- Recall the stages of embryonic development up to the gastrula:

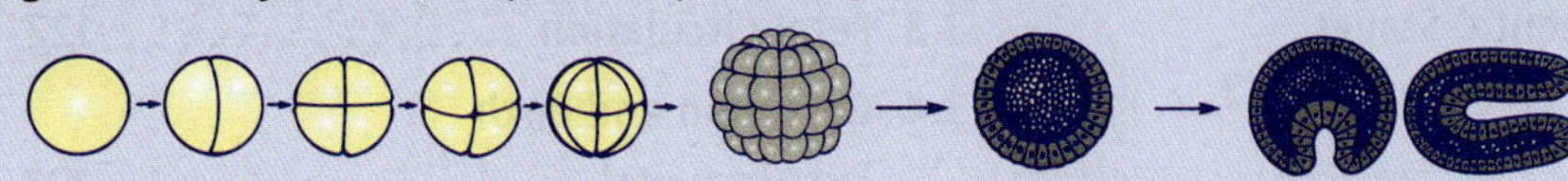

In this first section, we will explore development from the formation of a diploid zygote until neurulation, or the formation of the neural tube that will differentiate into the nervous system.

Fertilization

As discussed in Chapter 2 of *MCAT Biology Review*, a secondary oocyte is ovulated from the follicle on approximately day 14 of the menstrual cycle. The secondary oocyte travels into the fallopian tube, where it can be fertilized up to 24 hours after ovulation. Fertilization, shown in Figure 3.1, usually occurs in the widest part of the fallopian tube, called the **ampulla**. When the sperm meets the secondary oocyte in the fallopian tube, it binds to the oocyte and releases acrosomal enzymes that enable the head of the sperm to penetrate the corona radiata and zona pellucida. The first sperm to come into direct contact with the secondary oocyte's cell membrane forms a tube-like structure known as the **acrosomal apparatus**, which extends to and penetrates the cell membrane. Its pronucleus may then freely enter once the oocyte completes meiosis II.

After penetration of the sperm through the cell membrane, the **cortical reaction**, a release of calcium ions, occurs. These calcium ions depolarize the membrane of the ovum, which serves two purposes: depolarization prevents fertilization of the ovum by multiple sperm cells, and the increased calcium concentration increases the metabolic rate of the newly formed diploid **zygote**. The now depolarized and impenetrable membrane is called the **fertilization membrane**.

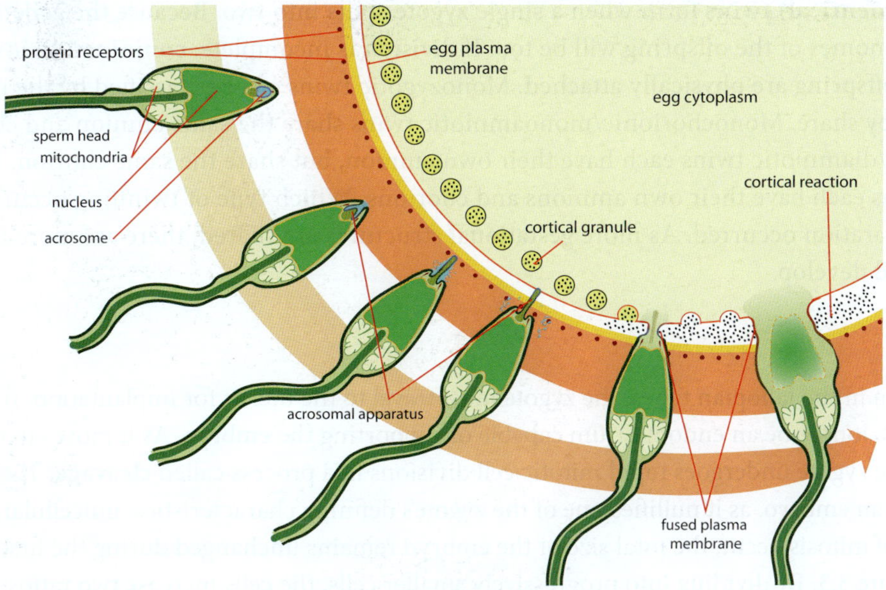

Figure 3.1 Fertilization

Twins

As seen in Figure 3.2, twinning can occur by two different mechanisms. **Dizygotic (fraternal) twins** form from fertilization of two different eggs released during one ovulatory cycle by two different sperm. Each zygote will implant in the uterine wall, and each develops its own placenta, chorion, and amnion—these structures are discussed later in the chapter. If the zygotes implant close together, the placentas may grow onto each other. Fraternal twins are no more genetically similar than any other pair of siblings.

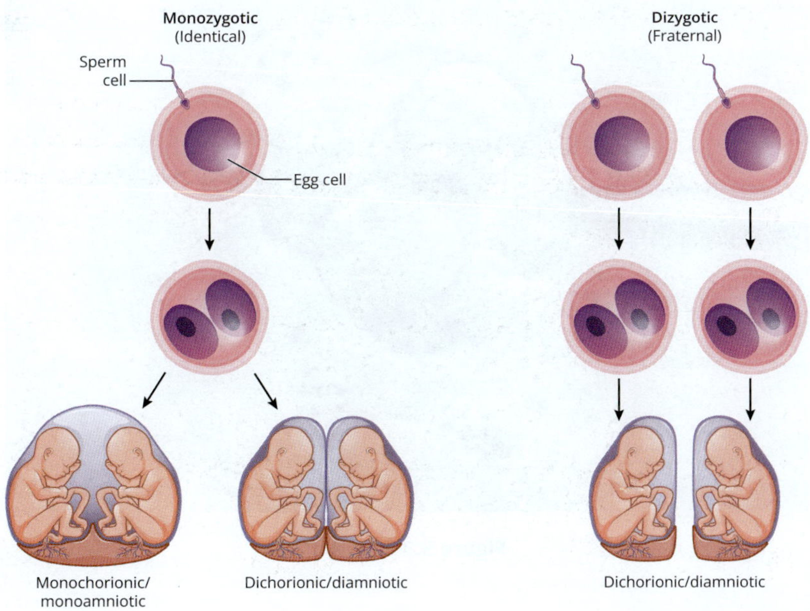

Figure 3.2 Monozygotic (Identical) Twins vs. Dizygotic (Fraternal) Twins

Monozygotic (identical) twins form when a single zygote splits into two. Because the genetic material is identical, the genomes of the offspring will be too. If division is incomplete, **conjoined twins** may result, where the two offspring are physically attached. Monozygotic twins can be classified by the number of structures they share. Monochorionic/monoamniotic twins share the same amnion and chorion. Monochorionic/diamniotic twins each have their own amnion, but share the same chorion. Dichorionic/diamniotic twins each have their own amnions and chorions. Which type of twinning occurs is a result of when the separation occurred. As more gestational structures are shared, there are more risks as the fetuses grow and develop.

Cleavage

After fertilization in the fallopian tubes, the zygote must travel to the uterus for implantation. If it arrives too late, there will no longer be an endometrium capable of supporting the embryo. As it moves to the uterus for implantation, the zygote undergoes rapid mitotic cell divisions in a process called **cleavage**. The first cleavage officially creates an embryo, as it nullifies one of the zygote's defining characteristics: unicellularity. Although several rounds of mitosis occur, the total size of the embryo remains unchanged during the first few divisions, as shown in Figure 3.3. By dividing into progressively smaller cells, the cells increase two ratios: the nuclear-to-cytoplasmic (N:C) ratio and the surface area-to-volume ratio. Thus, the cells achieve increased area for gas and nutrient exchange relative to overall volume.

There are two types of cleavage: indeterminate and determinate. **Indeterminate cleavage** results in cells that can still develop into complete organisms. In fact, monozygotic twins have identical genomes because they both originate from indeterminately cleaved cells of the same embryo. **Determinate cleavage** results in cells with fates that are, as the term implies, already determined. In other words, these cells are committed to **differentiating** into a certain type of cell.

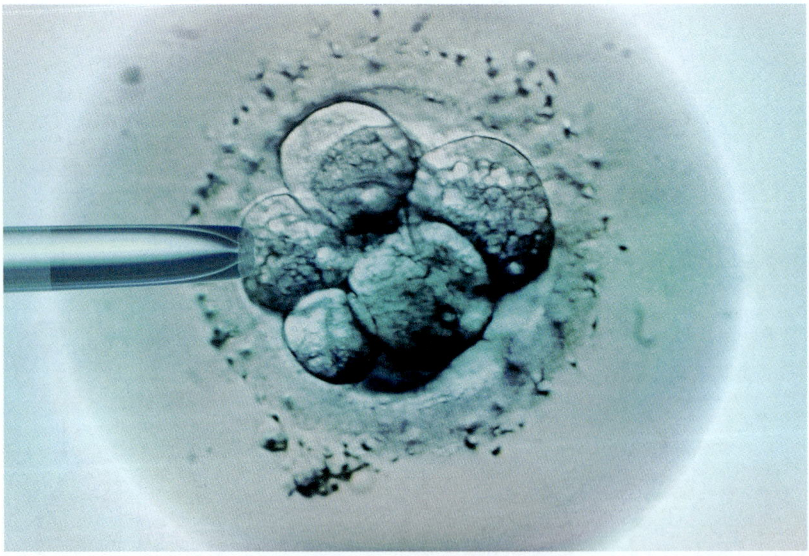

Figure 3.3 Embryo

Blastulation

Several divisions later, the embryo becomes a solid mass of cells known as a **morula**, as shown in Figure 3.4. This term comes from the Latin word for mulberry, which might help us grasp what an embryo at this stage looks like.

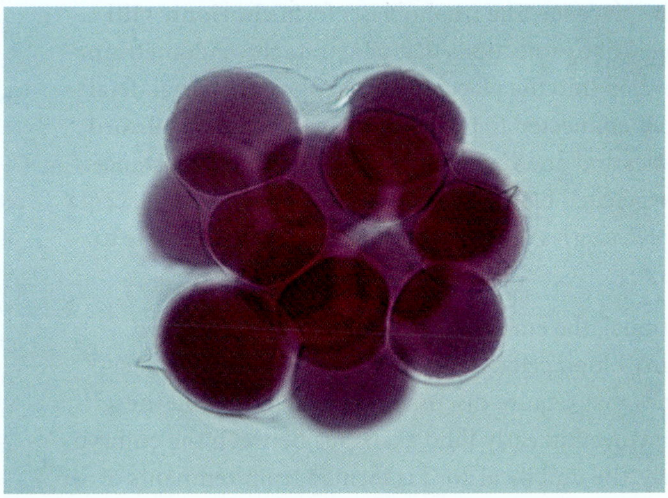

Figure 3.4 Morula
The morula is a solid ball of cells.

Once the morula is formed, it undergoes **blastulation**, which forms the **blastula**, a hollow ball of cells with a fluid-filled inner cavity known as a **blastocoel**. The mammalian blastula is known as a **blastocyst** and consists of two noteworthy cell groups, the trophoblast and inner cell mass. The **trophoblast cells** surround the blastocoel and give rise to the chorion and later the placenta, whereas the **inner cell mass** protrudes into the blastocoel and gives rise to the organism itself. The development of the blastocyst occurs in roughly the first week of pregnancy (see Figure 3.5).

MNEMONIC

Remember that a **blast**ula is an embryo with a **blast**ed-out cavity.

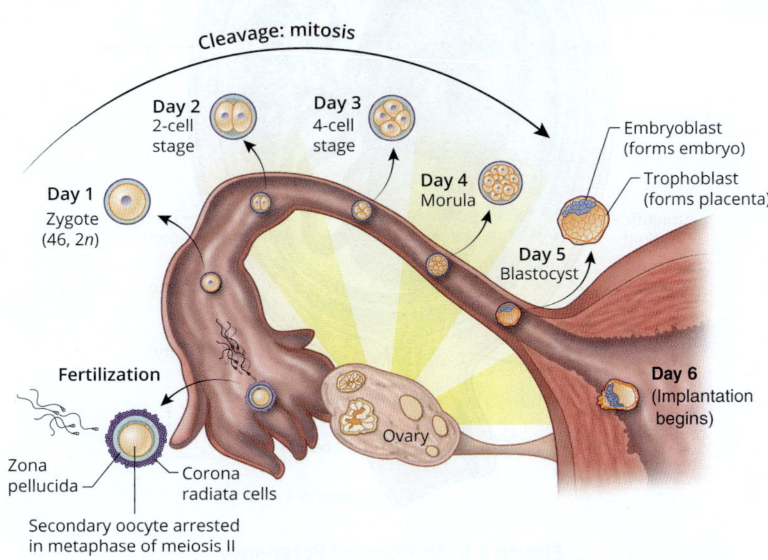

Figure 3.5 Week One Development

Implantation

The blastula moves through the fallopian tube to the uterus, where it burrows into the endometrium. The trophoblast cells are specialized to create an interface between the maternal blood supply and the developing embryo. These trophoblastic cells give rise to the **chorion**, an extraembryonic membrane that develops into the placenta. The trophoblasts form **chorionic villi**, which are microscopic finger-like projections that penetrate the endometrium. As these chorionic villi develop into the placenta they support maternal–fetal gas exchange. The embryo is connected to the placenta by the **umbilical cord**, which consists of two arteries and one vein encased in a gelatinous substance. The vein carries freshly oxygenated blood rich with nutrients from the placenta to the embryo. The umbilical arteries carry deoxygenated blood and waste to the placenta for exchange.

Until the placenta is functional, the embryo is supported by the **yolk sac**, which is also the site of early blood cell development. There are two other extraembryonic membranes that require discussion: the allantois and the amnion. The **allantois** is involved in early fluid exchange between the embryo and the yolk sac. Ultimately, the umbilical cord is formed from remnants of the yolk sac and the allantois. The allantois is surrounded by the **amnion**, a thin, tough membrane filled with amniotic fluid. This fluid serves as a shock absorber during pregnancy, lessening the impact of maternal motion on the developing embryo. In addition to forming the placenta, the chorion also forms an outer membrane around the amnion, adding an additional level of protection. The anatomy of these structures is shown in Figure 3.6.

REAL WORLD

Sometimes the blastula implants itself outside the uterus, a situation known as an ectopic pregnancy. Over 95% of ectopic pregnancies occur in the fallopian tube. Ectopic pregnancies are generally not viable because the narrow fallopian tube is not an environment in which an embryo can properly grow. If the embryo does not spontaneously abort, the tube may rupture and a considerable amount of hemorrhaging may result. In fact, a suspected ectopic pregnancy is often a surgical emergency.

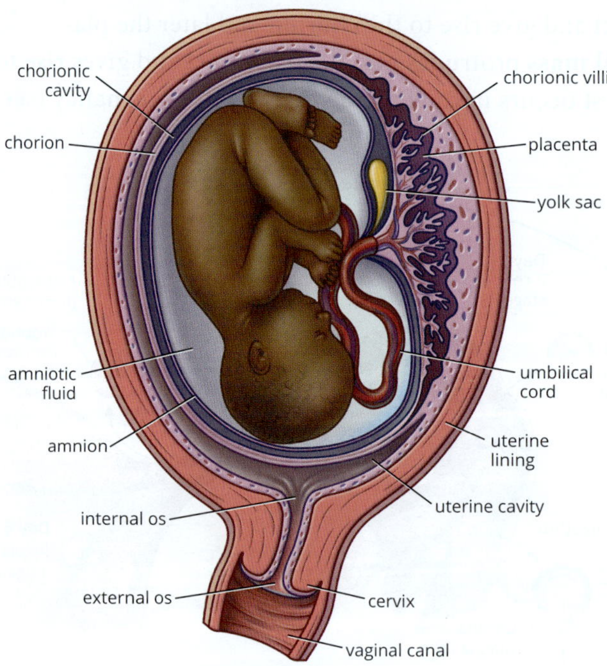

Figure 3.6 Anatomy of Pregnancy

Gastrulation

Once the cell mass implants it can begin further developmental processes such as **gastrulation**, the generation of three distinct cell layers. The early developmental processes up to this point are shown in Figure 3.7. Much of today's understanding of development comes from the study of other organisms with varying degrees of similarity to human development. In sea urchins, gastrulation begins with a small invagination in the blastula. Cells continue moving toward the invagination, resulting in elimination of the blastocoel. To visualize this, imagine inflating a balloon and poking it with your finger. If you kept pushing, eventually the rubber from that side of the balloon would come into contact with the other side. If the two membranes could merge, as occurs in development, this would create a tube through the middle of the balloon. In living things, the result of this process is called a **gastrula**. The membrane invagination into the blastocoel is called the **archenteron**, which later develops into the gut. The opening of the archenteron is called the **blastopore**. In **deuterostomes**, such as humans, the blastopore develops into the anus. In **protostomes**, such as snails and spiders, it develops into the mouth. Figure 3.8 depicts the difference in initial development of deuterostomes and protostomes.

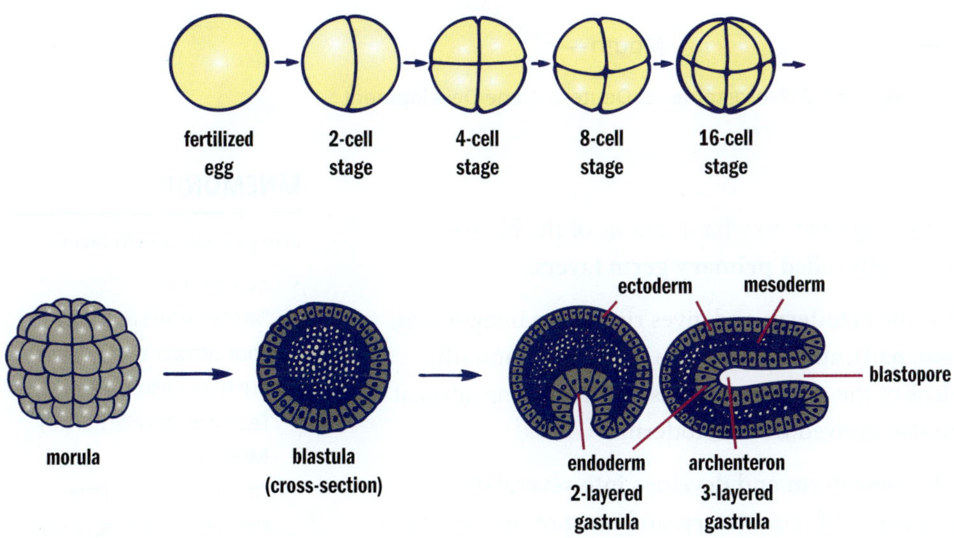

Figure 3.7 Early Stages of Embryonic Development

REAL WORLD

Amniocentesis is the process of aspirating amniotic fluid by inserting a thin needle into the amniotic sac. The amniotic fluid contains fetal cells that can be examined for chromosomal abnormalities as well as sex determination. Amniocentesis is recommended for people who are over 35 and pregnant if earlier screening tests (blood tests and ultrasound) indicate a high chance of chromosomal abnormalities in the fetus. Individuals in this age group have a higher rate of meiotic nondisjunction, which can result in genetic deviations such as Down syndrome.

MNEMONIC

How can we remember the blastopore's fate in protostomes vs. deuterostomes? Think about how some adults talk to toddlers—*deuterostome* starts with *deu*, which looks like *duo*, meaning *two*. Thus, **deu**terostomes develop the anus—the orifice associated with "**number two**"—from the blastopore. Protostomes must start at the other end (the mouth).

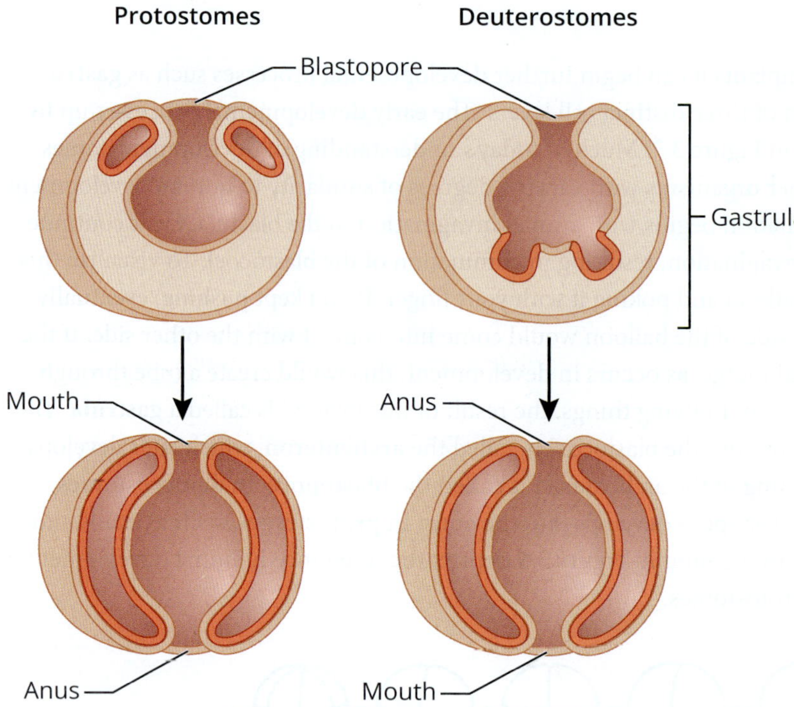

Figure 3.8 Protostome vs. Deuterostome Development

Primary Germ Layers

Eventually, some cells will also migrate into what remains of the blastocoel. This establishes three layers of cells called **primary germ layers**.

The outermost layer is called the **ectoderm** and gives rise to the integument, including the epidermis, hair, nails, and the epithelia of the nose, mouth, and lower anal canal. The lens of the eye, nervous system (including adrenal medulla), and inner ear are also derived from ectoderm.

The middle layer is called the **mesoderm** and develops into several different systems including the musculoskeletal, circulatory, and most of the excretory systems. Mesoderm also gives rise to the gonads as well as the muscular and connective tissue layers of the digestive and respiratory systems and the adrenal cortex.

The innermost layer is called the **endoderm** and forms the epithelial linings of the digestive and respiratory tracts, including the lungs. The pancreas, thyroid, bladder, and distal urinary tracts, as well as parts of the liver, are derived from endoderm.

MNEMONIC

The primary germ layers:

- Ectoderm—"attracto"derm (things that attract us to others, such as cosmetic features and "smarts")
- Mesoderm—"means"oderm (the means of getting around as an organism, such as bones and muscle; the means of getting around in the body, such as the circulatory system; the means of *getting around*, such as the gonads)
- Endoderm—linings of "endernal" (internal) organs (the digestive and respiratory tract, and accessory organs attached to these systems)

Differentiation

So how is it that cells with the same genes are able to develop into such distinctly different cell types with highly specialized functions? Primarily, it is by **selective transcription** of the genome. In other words, only the genes needed for that particular cell type are transcribed. Thus, in pancreatic islet cells the genes to produce specific hormones (insulin, glucagon, or somatostatin) are turned on, while these same genes are turned off in other cell types. Selective transcription is often related to the concept of **induction**, which is the ability of one group of cells to influence the fate of nearby cells. This process is mediated by chemical substances called **inducers** which diffuse from the **organizing cells** to the **responsive cells**. These chemicals are responsible for processes such as the guidance of neuronal axons. Induction also ensures the proximity of different cell types that work together within an organ.

MCAT EXPERTISE

The MCAT likes to test on the dual embryonic origin of the adrenal glands. The adrenal cortex is derived from the mesoderm, but the adrenal medulla is derived from the ectoderm (because the adrenal medulla contains some nervous tissue).

Neurulation

Once the three germ layers are formed, **neurulation**, or development of the nervous system, can begin. Remember that the nervous system is derived from the ectoderm. How, then, do cells originating on the surface of the embryo (ectoderm) end up inside the final organism? First, a rod of mesodermal cells known as the **notochord** forms along the long axis of the organism like a primitive spine (in fact, remnants of notochord persist in the intervertebral discs between vertebrae). The notochord induces a group of overlying ectodermal cells to slide inward to form **neural folds**, which surround a **neural groove**, as shown in Figure 3.9. The neural folds grow toward one another until they fuse into a **neural tube**, which gives rise to the central nervous system. At the tip of each neural fold are **neural crest cells**. These cells migrate outward to form the peripheral nervous system (including the sensory ganglia, autonomic ganglia, adrenal medulla, and Schwann cells) as well as specific cell types in other tissues (such as calcitonin-producing cells of the thyroid, melanocytes in the skin, and others). Finally, ectodermal cells will migrate over the neural tube and crest to cover the rudimentary nervous system.

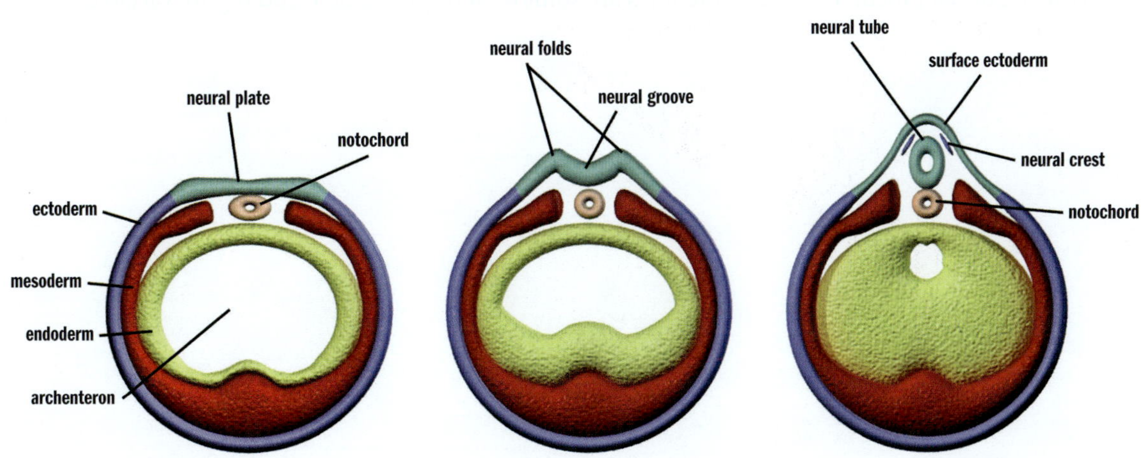

Figure 3.9 Formation of the Neural Tube

Problems in Early Development

Early development is a highly sensitive time. During this stage, as the germ layers are forming and as organogenesis (the production of organs) begins, teratogens may have far-reaching and highly detrimental effects. **Teratogens** are substances that interfere with development, causing defects or even death of the developing embryo. However, each teratogen will not have the same effect on every embryo. It is believed that the unique genetics of the embryo influences the effects of the teratogen. In addition to genetics, the route of exposure, length of exposure, rate of placental transmission of the teratogen, and the exact identity of the teratogen will also affect the outcome. Some common teratogens include alcohol, prescription drugs, viruses, bacteria, and environmental chemicals including polycyclic aromatic hydrocarbons.

In addition to teratogens, maternal health can also influence development. Certain conditions may cause changes in the overall physiology of the person who is pregnant, resulting in overexposure or underexposure of the embryo or fetus to certain chemicals. For example, pregnant individuals who have diabetes and hyperglycemia (high blood glucose) can have poor birth outcomes. Overexposure to sugar *in utero* can lead to a fetus that is too large to be delivered and that could become hypoglycemic soon after birth (due to synthesizing very high levels of insulin to compensate). Maternal folic acid deficiency may prevent complete closure of the neural tube, resulting in spina bifida, in which parts of the nervous system are exposed to the outside world or covered with a thin membrane, or anencephaly, in which the brain fails to develop. However, like teratogens, maternal health issues can have variable effects on the developing embryo or fetus. Spina bifida may be so severe as to result in profound disability, or may be completely asymptomatic and only detected by a tuft of hair overlying the area. Overall, trends and associations can certainly be found between various environmental conditions and genes during development; however, outcomes are somewhat unpredictable and highly variable.

REAL WORLD

Failure of the neural tube to close results in either spina bifida (in which some or all of the spinal cord may be exposed to the outside world) or anencephaly (in which the brain fails to develop and the skull is left open). The severity of spina bifida's effects range from no significant distress to death, whereas anencephaly is universally fatal. Individuals who are likely to get pregnant are encouraged to take folate (folic acid) to prevent this complication; furthermore, it is recommended that all individuals who could become pregnant supplement their diets with folate because neurulation often occurs before pregnancy is detected.

MCAT CONCEPT CHECK 3.1

Before you move on, assess your understanding of the material with these questions.

1. What is the difference between determinate and indeterminate cleavage?
   - Determinate cleavage:
   - Indeterminate cleavage:
2. From zygote to gastrula, what are the various stages of development?
3. During which stage of development does implantation occur?
4. What are the primary germ layers, and what organs are formed from each?

Germ Layer	Organs

5. What is induction and how does it influence development?
6. What tissues do neural crest cells develop into?

3.2 Mechanisms of Development High Yield

LEARNING OBJECTIVES

After Chapter 3.2, you will be able to:

- Explain the difference between determination and differentiation
- Connect totipotency, pluripotency, and multipotency to their respective levels of differentiation
- Recall the four types of cell–cell communication
- Distinguish between apoptosis and necrosis

As described earlier, cells undergo determinate cleavage to commit to a particular cell line, and inducers can be used for communication between one group of differentiating cells and another. In this section, we take a more specific look at the biochemical properties of these developmental mechanisms, as well as a few others.

Cell Specialization

An adult human being is composed of approximately 37 trillion cells. These cells are organized into tissues that form organs within organ systems. In order to create an organism as complex as a human being, each cell must perform a specialized function. In addition, the cells in an organ must be organized such that the organ can function properly. For example, the pancreas must create both digestive enzymes (*trypsin*, *carboxypeptidases A* and *B*, *pancreatic lipase*, and others) and endocrine hormones (*insulin*, *glucagon*, and *somatostatin*). The cells that synthesize digestive enzymes must be located where cell products can enter ducts to ultimately empty into the duodenum. Likewise, the cells that synthesize endocrine hormones must be located near a blood vessel to put their products into systemic circulation. In order to accomplish this the cell must go through three stages: specification, determination, and differentiation.

Specification/Determination

The initial stage of cell specialization is **specification**, in which the cell is reversibly designated as a specific cell type. This is followed by **determination**, which was previously defined as the commitment of a cell to a particular function in the future. Prior to determination the cell can become any cell type, even if it has already gone through specification. After determination the cell is irreversibly committed to a specific lineage. There are multiple pathways by which determination may occur. During cleavage, where the existing mRNA and protein in the parent cell has been asymmetrically distributed between the daughter cells, the presence of specific mRNA and protein molecules may result in determination. Determination may also occur due to secretion of specific molecules from nearby cells. These molecules, also called **morphogens**, may cause neighboring cells to follow a particular developmental pathway. Determination is a commitment to a particular cell type, but note that the cell has not yet actually produced what it needs to carry out the functions of that cell type—that is the goal of differentiation.

Differentiation

After a cell's fate has been determined, the cell must begin to undertake changes that cause the cell to develop into the determined cell type. This includes changing the structure, function, and biochemistry of the cell to match the cell type, a process called **differentiation**.

Cells that have not yet differentiated or that give rise to *other* cells that will differentiate are known as **stem cells**. Stem cells exist in embryonic tissues as well as adult tissues. The tissues a particular stem cell can differentiate into are determined by its **potency** (see Figure 3.10). Cells with the greatest potency are called **totipotent** and include embryonic stem cells; totipotent cells can differentiate into any cell type, either in the fetus or in placental structures. After the 16-cell stage, the cells of the morula begin to differentiate into two groups: the inner cell mass and the trophoblast. After a few more cycles of cell division these totipotent cells start to differentiate into the three germ cell layers. At this stage, the cells are said to be **pluripotent**; these cells can differentiate into any cell type except for those found in the placental structures. Finally, as the cells continue to become more specialized they are said to be **multipotent** stem cells, which can differentiate into multiple types of cells within a particular group. For example, hematopoietic stem cells are capable of differentiating into all of the cells found in blood, including the various types of white blood cells, red blood cells, and platelets—but not into skin cells, neurons, or muscle cells.

While we use all of these different terms to describe potency, it is important to recognize that potency is a spectrum—not a series of strict definitions. Also, note that stem cells exist not only in embryos, but also in adults, who have stem cells that give rise to skin, blood, and the epithelial lining of the digestive tract, among others. Adults still need stem cells because cells die and need to be replaced. Human life would not be sustainable with only one batch of skin cells or blood cells.

KEY CONCEPT

When a cell is determined, it is committed to a particular cell lineage. When the cell differentiates, it assumes the structure, function, and biochemistry of that cell type.

KEY CONCEPT

Stem cells are able to differentiate into different cell types. The potency of the stem cell determines how many different cell types a stem cell can become. As cells become more differentiated, the potency of the cell decreases (from totipotent to pluripotent to multipotent).

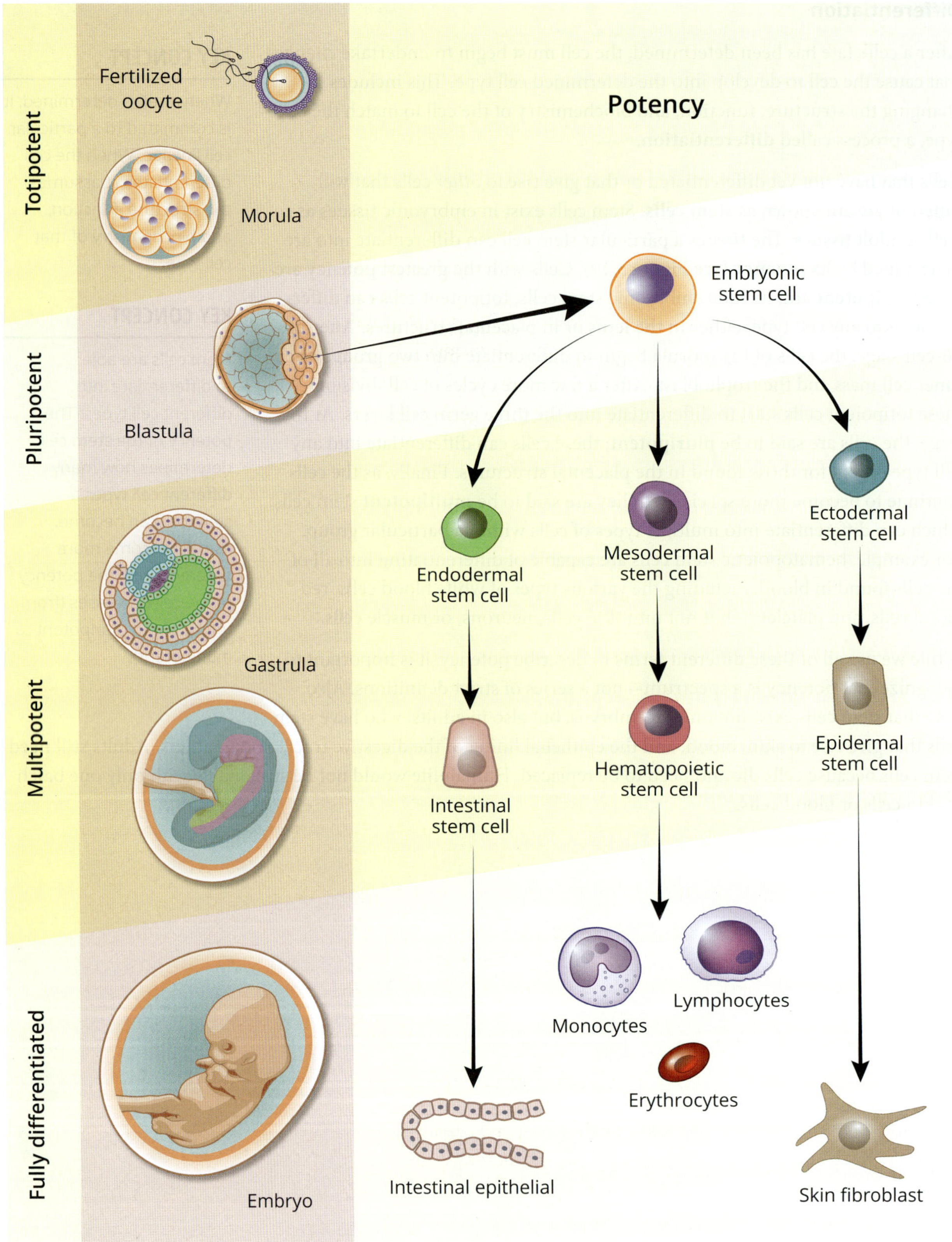

Figure 3.10 Levels of Cell Potency

Over the last few decades, stem cell research has been a hotly contested issue. While harvesting of embryonic stem cells, as seen in Figure 3.11, ultimately results in termination of the embryo, it is thought that these cells could be used to regenerate human tissues, including the spinal cord (following injury) and the heart (following a heart attack). There are also immunologic concerns, as transplantation of stem cells of a different genetic makeup could evoke an immune response, resulting in rejection. In addition, once implanted, pluripotent cells may not necessarily differentiate into the desired tissue and may even become cancerous.

BRIDGE

Stem cells are a cornerstone of biotechnology. Gene studies can be performed by introducing altered embryonic stem cells that contain transgenes into mice. Stem cells lacking a particular gene can be used to create knockout mice. These processes are discussed in Chapter 6 of *MCAT Biochemistry Review*.

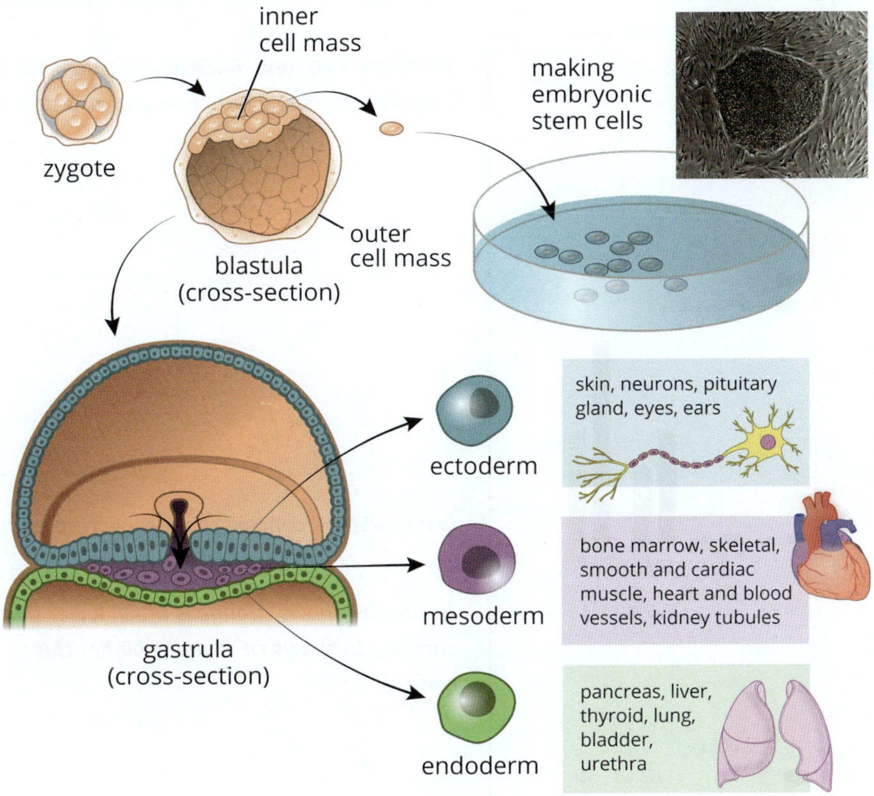

Figure 3.11 Embryonic Stem Cells

In order to address this controversy, many researchers have begun investigating adult stem cells. At best, these cells are multipotent, able to differentiate into only a few different cell types. Researchers may take adult stem cells and use various transcription factors to increase potency in these cells. One of the potential advantages of this approach is that a stem cell can be taken from a patient (usually from blood, bone marrow, or adipose tissue), induced to become a different tissue type, and then implanted into that same patient. This offers reduced risk of rejection of foreign tissue. However, it is challenging to induce differentiation into the correct cell type, and most organs have a complex structure that depends on a number of different cell types, each of which requires different signals. Research is ongoing and holds promise, despite limited success.

BIOLOGY GUIDED EXAMPLE WITH EXPERT THINKING

The role of microRNA-29b in controlling the differentiation of neuroectoderm cells into neural tube epithelial cells (NTE) and neural crest cells (NCC) remains unclear. To study the impact of microRNA-29b, researchers engineered microRNA sponges to contain multiple tandem binding sites for the target microRNA to competitively bind with microRNA-29b. In addition to the sponge, researchers also engineered microRNA-29b-overexpressed cells by inserting a microRNA-29b sequence into the embryonic stem cell genome. Both are driven by a CAG promoter and inserted into the ROSA26 site.

Study goal: clarify the role of microRNA-29b

It sounds like these sponges will "pick up" the microRNA-29b that is present

They made cells that overexpress microRNA-29b

The terms "CAG" and "ROSA26" are unfamiliar, but both have the same promoter and insertion site

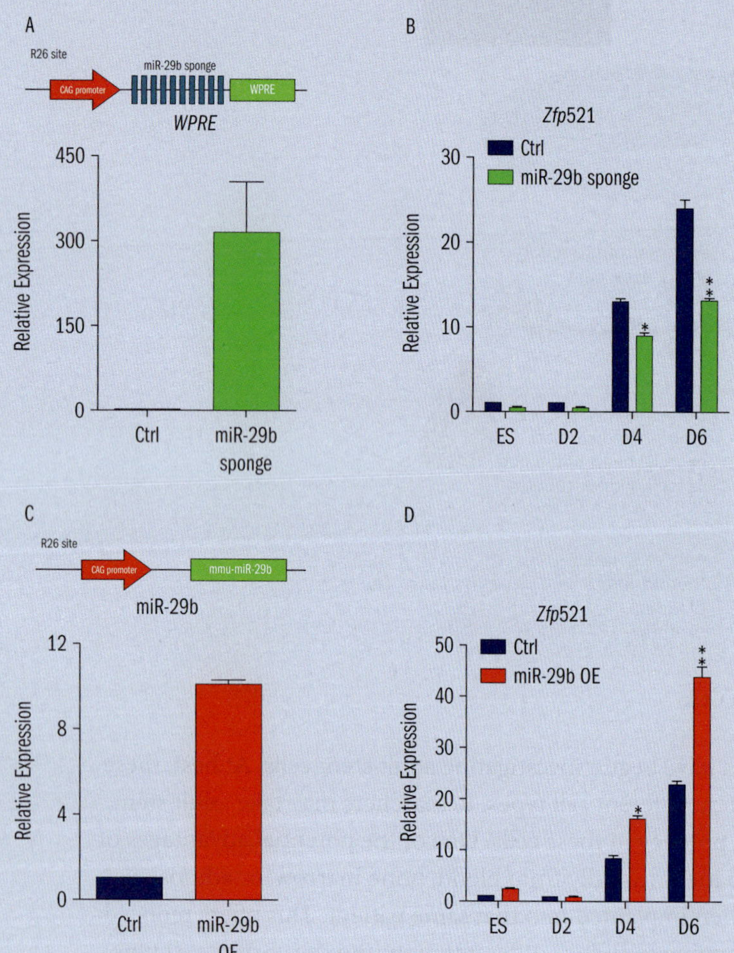

IVs: condition (control, sponge, overexpression)

DV: relative expression

Trends: (B) shows sponge is much lower than control, (D) shows OE is much higher than control

Figure 1 Neural tube epithelial cells differentiation experiment results. (A) The expression level of microRNA-29b sponge verified by qPCR. (B) qPCR results of NTE marker genes Zfp521 expression levels in microRNA-29b sponge condition. (C) The expression level of microRNA-29b verified by qPCR. (D) qPCR results of NTE marker genes Zfp521 in microRNA-29b overexpression condition.

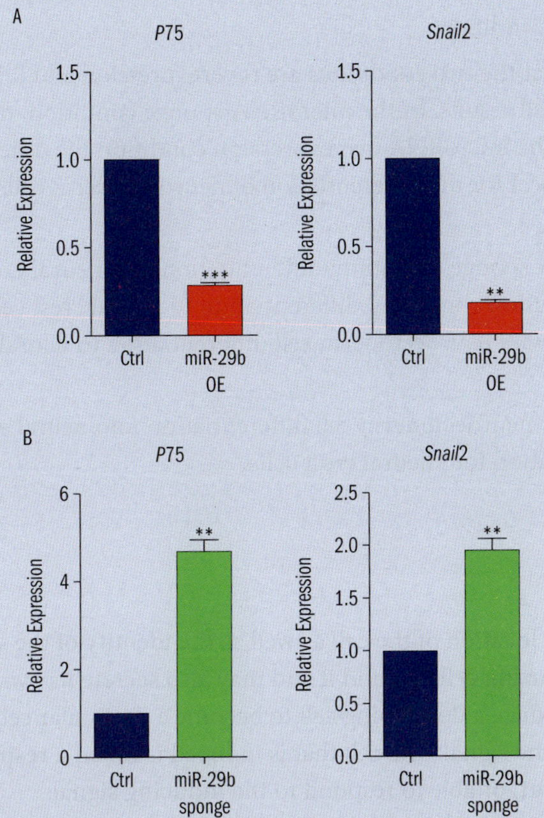

IVs: condition (control, sponge, OE)

DV: relative expression

Trends: (A) shows OE is much lower than control; (B) shows sponge is much higher than control

Figure 2 Neural crest cells differentiation experiment results. (A) qPCR results of NCC markers P75 and Snail2 expression in microRNA-29b overexpression condition. (B) qPCR results of NCC markers P75 and Snail2 expression in microRNA-29b sponge condition.

Adapted from Xi, J., Wu, Y., Li, G., Ma, L., Feng, K., Guo, X., ... Kang, J. (2017). Mir-29b mediates the neural tube versus neural crest fate decision during embryonic stem cell neural differentiation. *Stem Cell Reports*, 9(2), 571–586.

How does microRNA-29b influence the differentiation of neuroectoderm cells into neural epithelial cells and neural crest cells, respectively?

This question asks us to draw conclusions based on the data provided. To start, we'll want to define the terms in the question stem and make sure we're clear on exactly what we're being asked for. We are told in the first paragraph that the neuroectoderm cells will differentiate into two types of cells, the neural epithelial cells and the neural crest cells. We are also told that microRNA-29b influences this process, but we do not know how it impacts differentiation.

Now we must parse out how the target microRNA are being manipulated to see how those changes alter the neuroectoderm cells' differentiation. The researchers created two experimental conditions, the microRNA sponge and the microRNA overexpression. Recall that microRNA works by binding to complementary sites on mRNA, which blocks translation mechanisms and prevents the synthesis of the gene product. As stated in the passage, the microRNA sponge has several sites that are complementary to the microRNA, which will act like a sponge by grabbing all the microRNA in the cell. As a result, the microRNA will bind to the sponge instead of just binding to local RNA, meaning that there is functionally less microRNA-29b binding to the RNA as compared to normal. In other words, it is the opposite of the overexpressed condition.

Now that we know what our action is (differentiation) and what the two conditions are (overexpression and inhibition), we can analyze the data. Figure 1 shows the neural epithelial cell results. In the microRNA sponge condition, the differentiation level is reduced compared to control, while in the microRNA overexpression condition the differentiation level is increased. This implies that microRNA-29b is critical for the differentiation of neuroectoderm cells to neural epithelial cells.

Looking at Figure 2, we see opposing effects. In the microRNA sponge condition, differentiation into neural crest cells is increased compared to control. In the microRNA overexpression condition, differentiation to neural crest cells is reduced. From these data, we can infer that microRNA suppresses neuroectoderm cell differentiation to neural crest cells.

In conclusion, the presence of microRNA-29b is important for neuroectoderm cell differentiation into neural epithelial cells, but the presence of microRNA-29b suppresses differentiation into neural crest cells.

Cell–Cell Communication

The determination and differentiation of a cell depends on the location of the cell as well as the identity of the surrounding cells. The developing cell receives signals from organizing cells around it and may also secrete its own signaling molecules. As discussed previously, surrounding tissues induce a developing cell to become a particular cell type via inducers; the term *inducer* may also refer to the cell secreting the signal. The cell that is induced is called a **responder** (responsive cell); to be induced, a responder must be **competent**, or able to respond to the inducing signal.

As depicted in Figure 3.12, cell–cell communication can occur via autocrine, paracrine, juxtacrine, or endocrine signals. **Autocrine** signals act on the same cell that secreted the signal in the first place. An example of autocrine signaling is a T-cell releasing a molecule (IL-2) in order to bind to itself and proliferate T-cell replication. **Paracrine** signals act on cells in the local area, as seen in neurotransmission between neurons. **Juxtacrine** signals do not usually involve diffusion, but involve a cell directly stimulating receptors of an adjacent cell. For example, helper T-cells interact with antigen-presenting cells (APCs) that contain major histocompatibility complex II (MHC-2). This complex physically binds to and initiates the activation of the ready T-cell. Finally, **endocrine** signals involve secreted hormones that travel through the bloodstream to a distant target tissue. The hormone insulin is a commonly tested example of an endocrine signal.

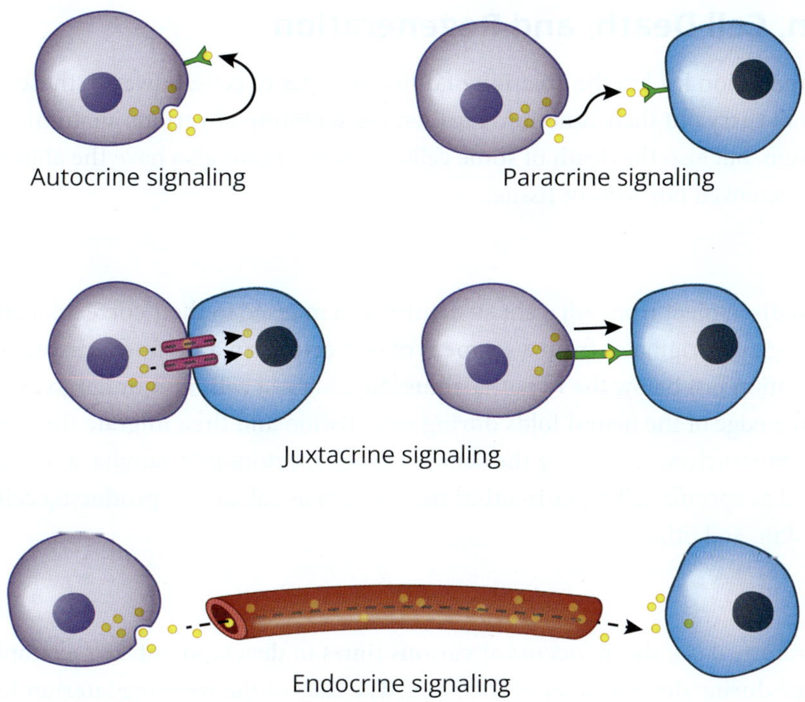

Figure 3.12 Types of Cell Signaling

Inducers

Inducers are often **growth factors**, which are peptides that promote differentiation and mitosis in certain tissues. Most growth factors only function on specific cell types or in certain areas, as determined by the competence of these cells. In this way, certain growth factors can code for particular tissues. For example, *PAX6* is expressed in the ectoderm of the head, but in no other location. Therefore, as the optic vesicle approaches the overlying ectoderm producing this factor, development of the lens of the eye is induced. Interestingly, induction is not always a one-way pathway. To that end, differentiation of the lens then triggers the optic vesicle to form the optic cup, which ultimately becomes the retina. This is known as **reciprocal development**. Most tissues will be exposed to multiple inducers during the course of development.

One of the main methods of signaling occurs via the use of gradients. Morphogens, or molecules that cause determination of cells, diffuse throughout the organism. Locations closer to the origin of the morphogen will be exposed to higher concentrations, while areas further away will have less exposure. Multiple morphogens are secreted simultaneously, resulting in unique combinations of morphogen exposure throughout the organism, which can thereby induce the differentiation of specific cell types. Some common morphogens include transforming growth factor beta (TGF-β), sonic hedgehog (Shh), and epidermal growth factor (EGF).

REAL WORLD

In development of the eyes, lateral outpocketings from the brain (optic vesicles) grow out and touch the overlying ectoderm. The optic vesicle induces the ectoderm to form the lens placode. The lens placode in turn induces the optic vesicle to create the optic cup. The optic cup then induces the lens placode to develop into the cornea and lens. Experiments with frog embryos show that if this ectoderm is subsequently transplanted to the trunk (after the optic vesicles have grown out), a lens will develop in the trunk. If, however, the ectoderm is transplanted before the outgrowth of the optic vesicles, it will not.

Cell Migration, Cell Death, and Regeneration

Induction and differentiation lead to the creation of different types of cells; however, these cells are not always in the right location to carry out their function. Further, the sculpting of various anatomic structures requires not only differentiation, but also the death of some cells. Certain organs also have the ability to recreate injured or surgically removed portions of tissue.

Cell Migration

Cells must be able to disconnect from adjacent structures and migrate to their correct location. For example, the anterior pituitary gland originates from a segment of oral ectoderm and must migrate from the top of the mouth to its final location just below the hypothalamus. Neural crest cells also undergo extensive migration. These cells form at the edge of the neural folds during neurulation and then migrate throughout the body to form many different structures including the sensory ganglia, autonomic ganglia, adrenal medulla, and Schwann cells, as well as specific cell types in other tissues such as calcitonin-producing cells of the thyroid, melanocytes in the skin, and others.

Cell Death

Apoptosis, or programmed cell death, occurs at various times in development. For example, the fingers are originally webbed during development of the hand. The cells of the webbing later undergo apoptosis, resulting in separation of each individual finger and toe. Apoptosis may occur via apoptotic signals or preprogramming.

During the process of apoptosis the cell undergoes changes in morphology and divides into many self-contained protrusions called **apoptotic blebs**, which can then be broken apart into **apoptotic bodies** and digested by other cells, as shown in Figure 3.13. This allows recycling of materials. Because the blebs are contained by a membrane, this also prevents the release of potentially harmful substances into the extracellular environment. This is different from **necrosis**, which is a process of cell death in which a cell dies as a result of injury. In necrosis, internal substances can be leaked, causing irritation of nearby tissues or even an immune response.

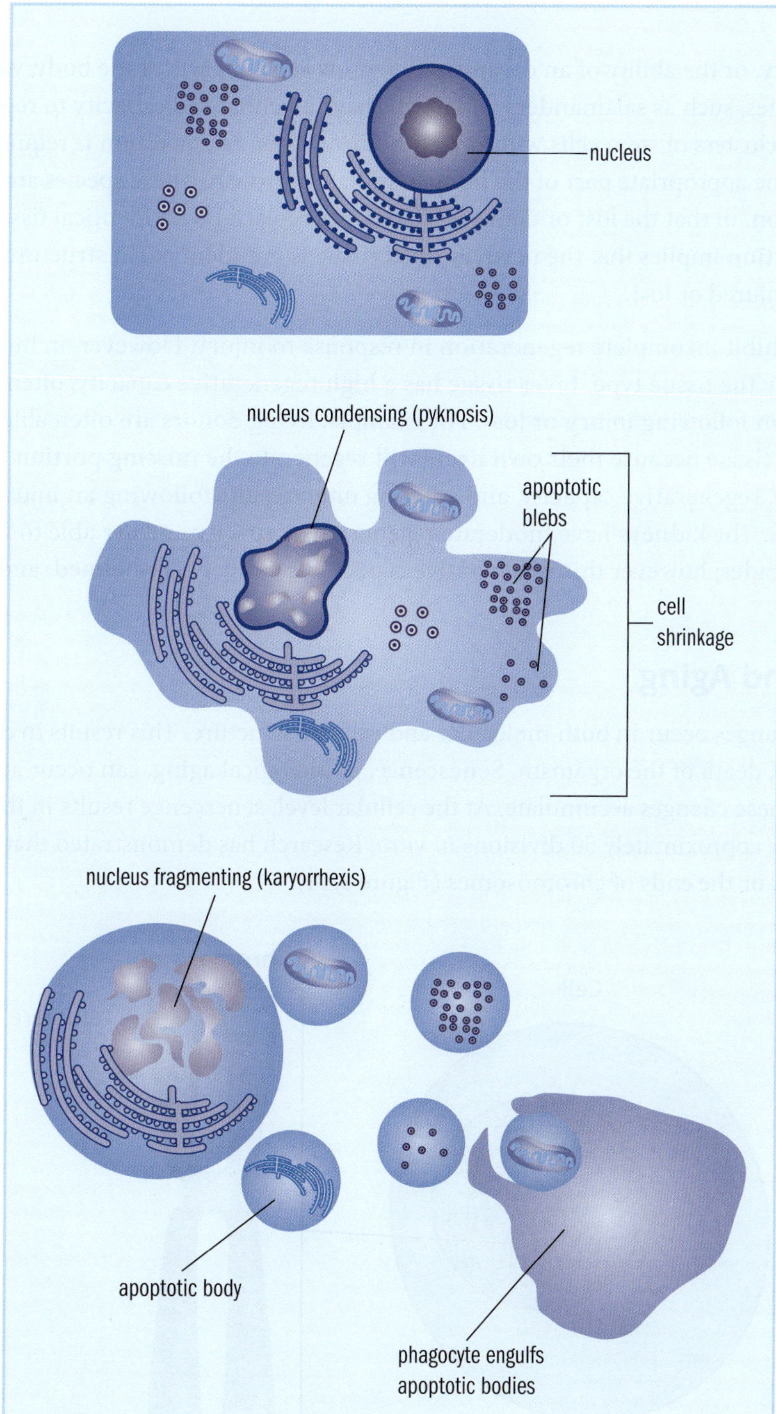

Figure 3.13 Apoptosis
An apoptotic cell disintegrates so that it can be absorbed and digested by other cells.

Regeneration

Regenerative capacity, or the ability of an organism to regrow certain parts of the body, varies from species to species. Some species, such as salamanders and newts, have an enhanced capacity to regenerate because they retain extensive clusters of stem cells within their bodies. When regeneration is required, these stem cells can then migrate to the appropriate part of the body to initiate regrowth. These species are said to undergo **complete regeneration**, in that the lost or damaged tissues are replaced with identical tissues. In contrast, **incomplete regeneration** implies that the newly formed tissue is not identical in structure or function to the tissue that has been injured or lost.

Humans typically exhibit incomplete regeneration in response to injury. However, in humans regenerative capacity varies by the tissue type. Liver tissue has a high regenerative capacity, often able to undergo extensive regeneration following injury or loss. For example, living donors are often able to donate up to 50 percent of their liver tissue because their own livers will regenerate the missing portion. Unfortunately, the heart has little, if any, regenerative capacity, and scarring often results following an injury due to an event such as a heart attack. The kidneys have moderate regenerative capacity and are able to repair nephrons after injury to the tubules; however this regenerative capacity is easily overwhelmed, and kidney failure may result.

Senescence and Aging

As organisms age, changes occur in both molecular and cellular structure. This results in disruption of metabolism and, eventually, death of the organism. **Senescence**, or biological aging, can occur at the cellular and organismal level as these changes accumulate. At the cellular level, senescence results in the failure of cells to divide, normally after approximately 50 divisions *in vitro*. Research has demonstrated that this may be due to shortened **telomeres**, or the ends of chromosomes (Figure 3.14).

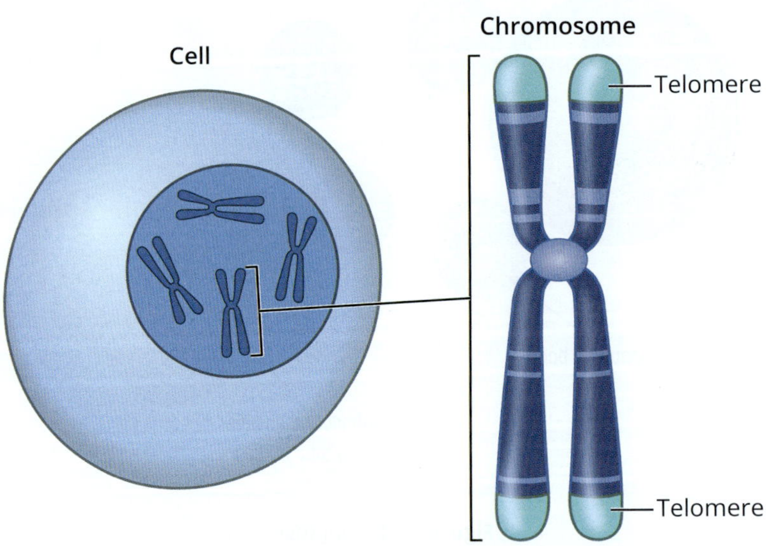

Figure 3.14 Telomeres

Telomeres reduce the loss of genetic information from the ends of chromosomes and help prevent the DNA from unraveling—their high concentration of guanine and cytosine enables telomeres to "knot off" the end of the chromosome. Telomeres are difficult to replicate due to a lack of *telomerase* activity in most human cells, however, so they shorten during each round of DNA synthesis. Eventually, the telomeres become too short, and the cell is no longer able to replicate. Some cells, including germ cells, fetal cells, and tumor cells, express telomerase, a reverse transcriptase that is able to synthesize the ends of chromosomes, preventing senescence. Telomerase allows cells to divide indefinitely and may play a role in the survival of cancer cells.

At the organismal level, senescence represents changes in the body's ability to respond to a changing environment. Aging is complex and often involves not only cellular senescence but also the accumulation of chemical and environmental damage over time.

MCAT CONCEPT CHECK 3.2

Before you move on, assess your understanding of the material with these questions.

1. What is the difference between determination and differentiation?
   - Determination:
   - Differentiation:

2. What are the three types of potency? What lineages can a cell of each type differentiate into?

Type of Potency	Cell Lineages

3. What are the four types of cell–cell communication?
   -
   -
   -
   -

4. What is the difference between apoptosis and necrosis?
   - Apoptosis:

   ____

   - Necrosis:

   ____

3.3 Fetal Circulation

LEARNING OBJECTIVES

After Chapter 3.3, you will be able to:

- Recall the oxygenation status of blood in umbilical arteries and umbilical veins
- Identify the three fetal shunts, their locations, and the organs they bypass

Recall that the placenta, shown in Figure 3.15, is the organ where nutrient, gas, and waste exchange occurs. It is crucial that maternal and fetal blood do not mix because they may be different blood types. The simplest method to move nutrients and waste products is by diffusion, the preferred method for water, glucose, amino acids, and inorganic salts. Diffusion requires a gradient, which implies there is a higher partial pressure of oxygen in maternal blood than in fetal blood. To further enhance the transfer of oxygen from maternal to fetal circulation, fetal blood cells contain **fetal hemoglobin** (**HbF**), which has a greater affinity for oxygen than adult hemoglobin (primarily HbA). This also assists with the transfer (and retention) of oxygen into the fetal circulatory system. Waste material and carbon dioxide move in the opposite direction.

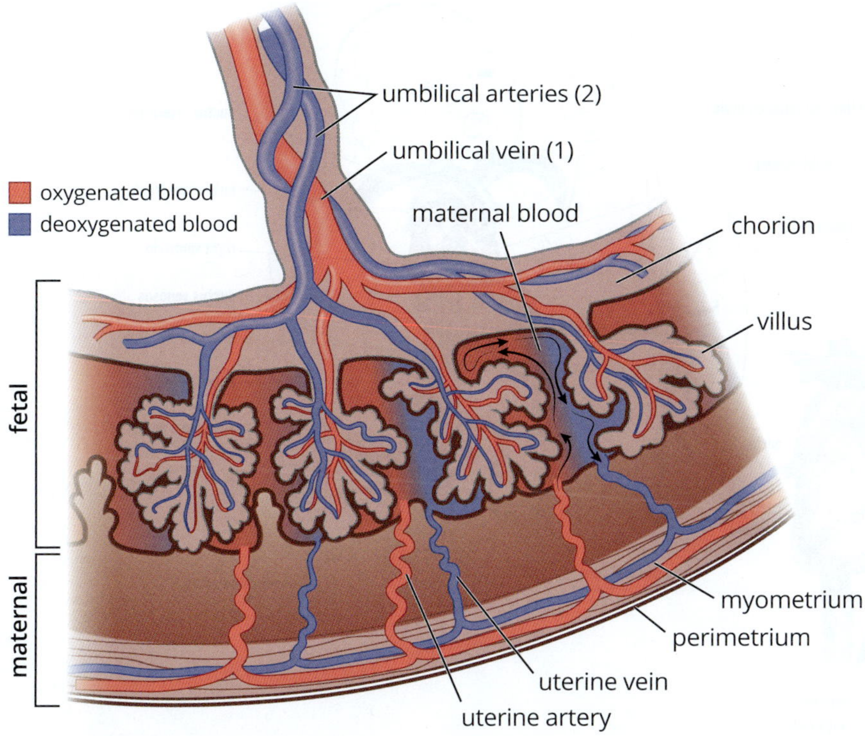

Figure 3.15 Placental Structure

The placental barrier also serves another function: immunity. The fetus is immunologically naïve because it has not yet been exposed to any pathogens; however, accidental exposure can happen *in utero*. Thus, the crossing of antibodies across the placental membrane serves a protective function. The placenta also qualifies as an endocrine organ because it produces progesterone, estrogen, and human chorionic gonadotropin (hCG), all which are essential for maintaining pregnancy.

The umbilical vessels are commonly tested on the MCAT because they demonstrate the need to understand the proper biological definitions of artery and vein. Like all other arteries that carry blood away from the heart, the **umbilical arteries** carry blood away from the fetus toward the placenta. And, like all of the other veins that carry blood toward the heart, the **umbilical vein** carries blood toward the fetus from the placenta. Remember that oxygenation occurs at the placenta, rather than in the fetal lungs. Therefore, the umbilical arteries carry deoxygenated blood and the umbilical vein carries oxygenated blood.

There are several key differences between fetal and adult circulation that demonstrate important characteristics of the developing organism. The lungs and liver both do not serve significant functions prior to birth. Gas exchange does not occur at the lungs, but rather at the placenta. Detoxification and metabolism are primarily controlled by the mother's liver, and nutrient and waste exchange occurs at the placenta as well. Thus, the fetus does not depend on its own lungs and liver. Notably, these two organs are both underdeveloped and sensitive to the high blood pressures they will receive in postnatal life; thus, the fetus constructs three **shunts** to actively direct blood away from these organs while they develop, as shown in Figure 3.16.

KEY CONCEPT

Although the embryo obtains its nutrients and oxygen from the person who is pregnant, there is no actual mixing of the blood. Instead, the placenta depends on the close proximity of the embryonic and maternal bloodstreams, facilitating diffusion between them.

KEY CONCEPT

Remember, gas exchange in the fetus occurs across the placenta. Fetal lungs do not function until birth.

REAL WORLD

Many pathogens are too large to cross the placental barrier by diffusion, but a set of pathogens called TORCHES infections can cross this barrier and cause significant birth defects. Therefore, screening for (and sometimes immunization against) these infections is recommended in pregnancy. TORCHES stands for ***TO****xoplasma gondii*, **R**ubella, **C**ytomegalovirus, **HE**rpes or **H**IV, and **S**yphilis.

KEY CONCEPT

Unlike most other arteries, the umbilical arteries carry deoxygenated blood with waste products. Unlike most other veins, the umbilical vein carries oxygenated blood with nutrients.

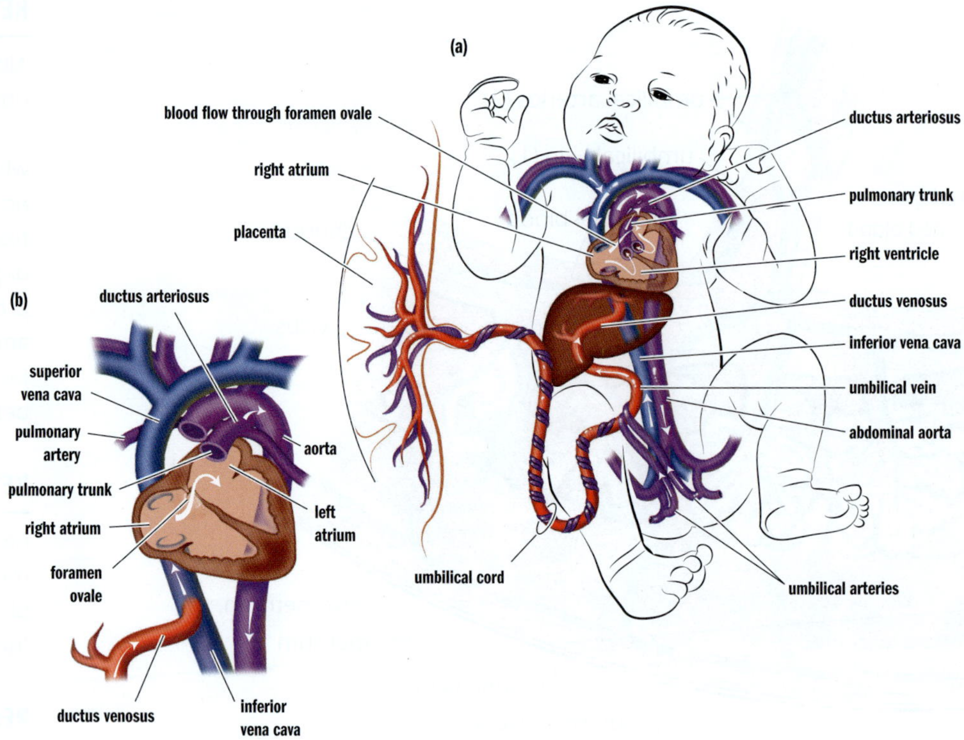

Figure 3.16 Fetal Circulation
(a) Systemic fetal circulation; (b) Enlarged view of fetal circulation highlighting the three fetal shunts

Two different shunts are used to reroute blood from the lungs. The first, called the **foramen ovale**, is a one-way valve that connects the right atrium to the left atrium. This allows blood entering the right atrium from the inferior vena cava to flow into the left atrium instead of the right ventricle, and thereby be pumped through the aorta into systemic circulation directly. Unlike in adult circulation, the right side of the heart is at a higher pressure in the developing fetus than the left side, which pushes blood through the opening. After birth, this pressure differential reverses, shutting the foramen ovale. Second, the **ductus arteriosus** shunts leftover blood from the pulmonary artery to the aorta. Again, the pressure differential between the right and left sides of the heart pushes blood through this opening and into systemic circulation.

The liver is bypassed via the **ductus venosus**, which shunts blood returning from the placenta via the umbilical vein directly into the inferior vena cava. The liver still receives some blood supply from smaller hepatic arteries in the systemic circulation.

MCAT CONCEPT CHECK 3.3

Before you move on, assess your understanding of the material with these questions.

1. What is the oxygenation status of the blood in the umbilical arteries? In the umbilical vein?
   - Umbilical arteries:
   - Umbilical vein:

2. What are the three fetal shunts? What vessels or heart chambers do they connect? What organ does each shunt bypass?

Shunt	Connected Vessels or Chambers	Organ Bypassed

3.4 Gestation and Birth

LEARNING OBJECTIVES

After Chapter 3.4, you will be able to:

- Identify the major developmental features of each trimester
- Describe the three stages of birth
- Recall key concepts and terms used for the birth process, including parturition, prostaglandins, oxytocin, and afterbirth

Human gestation lasts an estimated 280 days, which are divided into three trimesters (see Figure 3.17). As a general rule, the larger the animal, the longer the gestational period and the fewer the offspring per pregnancy. For example, elephants usually have one calf and gestate for 22 months. In contrast, mice have 10 to 12 offspring per litter and gestate for only 20 days. Although you don't need to know every detail of gestation for the MCAT, there are key developmental events in each trimester with which you should be familiar.

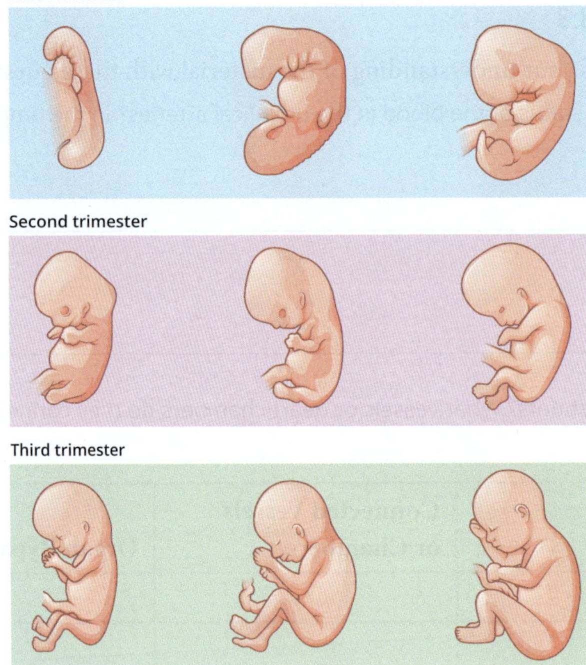

Figure 3.17 Fetal Development by Trimester

First Trimester

The major organs begin to develop during the first few weeks. The heart begins to beat at approximately 22 days, and soon afterward the eyes, gonads, limbs, and liver start to form. By five weeks the embryo is 10 mm in length, and by week six it has grown to 15 mm. The cartilaginous skeleton begins to harden into bone by the seventh week. By the end of eight weeks most of the organs have formed, the brain is fairly developed, and the embryo becomes known as a **fetus**. At the end of the third month the fetus is about 9 cm long.

Second Trimester

During the second trimester the fetus undergoes a tremendous amount of growth. It begins to move within the amniotic fluid, its face takes on a human appearance, and its toes and fingers elongate. By the end of the sixth month the fetus measures 30 to 36 cm long.

Third Trimester

The seventh and eighth months are characterized by continued rapid growth and further brain development. Antibodies are transported by highly selective active transport from the pregnant individual to the fetus for protection against foreign agents in preparation for life outside the womb; this transfer begins earlier in pregnancy, but is highest in the ninth month just before birth. The growth rate slows and the fetus becomes less active, as it has less room to move about.

REAL WORLD

Advances in medicine have allowed premature babies born as early as 24 weeks to survive—far short of the normal 40 weeks. While these neonates may survive, there are often severe complications because fetal development is not complete at 24 weeks. These problems are most apparent in the respiratory, gastrointestinal, and nervous systems.

Birth

Vaginal childbirth, or **parturition**, is accomplished by rhythmic contractions of uterine smooth muscle, coordinated by **prostaglandins** and the peptide hormone **oxytocin**. Birth consists of three basic phases. First, the cervix thins out and the amniotic sac ruptures, which is commonly called *water breaking*. Next, strong uterine contractions result in the birth of the fetus. Finally, the placenta and umbilical cord are expelled; these are often referred to as the **afterbirth**.

MCAT CONCEPT CHECK 3.4

Before you move on, assess your understanding of the material with these questions.

1. What are some of the key developmental features of each trimester?
   - First trimester:

     ____

     ____

   - Second trimester:

     ____

     ____

   - Third trimester:

     ____

     ____

2. What occurs in each of the three phases of birth?
   - ______________________________
   - ______________________________
   - ______________________________

Conclusion

In this chapter, we have seen how a just-fertilized ovum (zygote) becomes an embryo. As organs develop and the body organizes into complex organ systems, that embryo will turn into a newborn baby. Development certainly does not stop there, however—humans nurture their young for years (sometimes decades!) as they undergo physical, cognitive, and sexual development. Embryonic development is extremely important because it lays the foundation for further development to proceed correctly. Most of the time, the process goes exactly as planned; however, this is not always the case. In medical school, you will study the wide spectrum of teratology—the study of birth defects.

Adult structures that arise from embryonic germ layers are of special importance to us because they are commonly tested on the MCAT. For the remainder of embryology—from the first cleavage event to the last uterine contraction—focus on the main terminology and highlights of each stage, in addition to the differences between fetal and adult physiology. Now that we have seen from where the organ systems derive, we will begin our survey of anatomy and physiology. For the next eight chapters (Chapters 4 to 11 of *MCAT Biology Review*), we will explore the cells, tissues, organs, and interactions of each of the major organ systems. Our discussion begins with the nervous system.

GO ONLINE

You've reviewed the content, now test your knowledge and critical thinking skills by completing a test-like passage set in your online resources!

CONCEPT SUMMARY

Early Developmental Stages

- **Fertilization** is the joining of a sperm and an ovum.
  - It usually occurs in the **ampulla** of the fallopian tube.
  - The sperm uses acrosomal enzymes to penetrate the corona radiata and zona pellucida.
  - Once it contacts the oocyte's plasma membrane, the sperm establishes the **acrosomal apparatus** and injects its pronucleus.
  - When the first sperm penetrates it causes a release of calcium ions, which prevents additional sperm from fertilizing the egg and increases the metabolic rate of the resulting diploid **zygote**. This is called the **cortical reaction**.
- **Fraternal (dizygotic) twins** result from the fertilization of two eggs by two different sperm. **Identical (monozygotic) twins** result from the splitting of a zygote in two. Monozygotic twins can be classified by the placental structures they share (mono- vs. diamniotic, mono- vs. dichorionic).
- **Cleavage** refers to the early divisions of cells in the embryo. These mitotic divisions result in a larger number of smaller cells, as the overall volume does not change.
  - The zygote becomes an embryo after the first cleavage because it is no longer unicellular.
  - **Indeterminate cleavage** results in cells that are capable of becoming any cell in the organism, while **determinate cleavage** results in cells that are committed to differentiating into a specific cell type.
- The **morula** is a solid mass of cells seen in early development.
- The **blastula (blastocyst)** has a fluid-filled center called a **blastocoel** and has two different structures: the **trophoblast** (which becomes placental structures) and the **inner cell mass** (which becomes the developing organism).
  - The blastula implants in the endometrial lining and forms the **placenta**.
  - The **chorion** contains **chorionic villi**, which penetrate the endometrium and create the interface between maternal and fetal blood.
  - Before the placenta is established, the embryo is supported by the **yolk sac**.
  - The **allantois** is involved in early fluid exchange between the embryo and the yolk sac.
  - The **amnion** lies just inside the chorion and produces amniotic fluid.
  - The developing organism is connected to the placenta via the **umbilical cord**.
- During **gastrulation**, the **archenteron** is formed with a **blastopore** at the end. As the archenteron grows through the blastocoel it contacts the opposite side, establishing three primary germ layers.
  - The **ectoderm** becomes epidermis, hair, nails, and the epithelia of the nose, mouth, and anal canal, as well as the nervous system (including adrenal medulla) and lens of the eye.
  - The **mesoderm** becomes much of the musculoskeletal, circulatory, and excretory systems. Mesoderm also gives rise to the gonads and the muscular and connective tissue layers of the digestive and respiratory systems, as well as the adrenal cortex.
  - The **endoderm** becomes much of the epithelial linings of the respiratory and digestive tracts and parts of the pancreas, thyroid, bladder, and distal urinary tracts.

- **Neurulation**, or development of the nervous system, begins after the formation of the three germ layers.
  - The **notochord** induces a group of overlying ectodermal cells to form **neural folds** surrounding a **neural groove**.
  - The neural folds fuse to form the **neural tube**, which becomes the central nervous system.
  - The tip of each neural fold contains **neural crest cells**, which become the peripheral nervous system (sensory ganglia, autonomic ganglia, adrenal medulla, and Schwann cells), as well as specific cell types in other tissues (calcitonin-producing cells of the thyroid, melanocytes in the skin, and others).
- Teratogens are substances that interfere with development, causing defects or even death of the developing embryo. Teratogens include alcohol, certain prescription drugs, viruses, bacteria, and environmental chemicals.
- Maternal conditions can affect development, including diabetes (increased fetal size and hypoglycemia after birth) and folic acid deficiency (neural tube defects).

Mechanisms of Development

- Cell specialization occurs as a result of determination and differentiation.
  - **Determination** is the commitment to a specific cell lineage, which may be accomplished by uneven segregation of cellular material during mitosis or with **morphogens**, which promote development down a specific cell line. To respond to a specific morphogen, a cell must have **competency**.
  - **Differentiation** refers to the changes a cell undergoes due to **selective transcription** to take on characteristics appropriate to its cell line.
- Stem cells are cells that are capable of developing into various cell types. They can be classified by potency.
  - **Totipotent cells** are able to differentiate into all cell types, including the three germ layers and placental structures.
  - **Pluripotent cells** are able to differentiate into all three of the germ layers and their derivatives.
  - **Multipotent cells** are able to differentiate only into a specific subset of cell types.
- Cells communicate through a number of different signaling methods. An **inducer** releases factors to promote the differentiation of a competent **responder**.
  - **Autocrine** signals act on the same cell that released the signal.
  - **Paracrine** signals act on local cells.
  - **Juxtacrine** signals act through direct stimulation of adjacent cells.
  - **Endocrine** signals act on distant tissues after traveling through the bloodstream.
  - These are often **growth factors**, which are peptides that promote differentiation and mitosis in certain tissues.
  - If two tissues both induce further differentiation in each other, this is **reciprocal induction**.
  - Signaling often occurs via gradients.
- Cells may need to migrate to arrive at their correct location.
- **Apoptosis** is programmed cell death via the formation of **apoptotic blebs** that can subsequently be absorbed and digested by other cells. Apoptosis can be used for sculpting certain anatomical structures, such as removing the webbing between digits.

- **Regenerative capacity** is the ability of an organism to regrow certain parts of the body. The liver has high regenerative capacity, while the heart has low regenerative capacity.
- **Senescence** is the result of multiple molecular and metabolic processes, most notably, the shortening of telomeres during cell division.

Fetal Circulation

- Nutrient, gas, and waste exchange occurs at the placenta.
- Oxygen and carbon dioxide are passively exchanged due to concentration gradients.
- **Fetal hemoglobin** (**HbF**) has a higher affinity for oxygen than adult hemoglobin (primarily HbA); this affinity assists in the transfer (and retention) of oxygen into the fetal circulatory system.
- The placental barrier also serves as immune protection against many pathogens, and antibodies are transferred from the pregnant individual to child.
- The placenta serves endocrine functions, secreting estrogen, progesterone, and human chorionic gonadotropin (hCG).
- The **umbilical arteries** carry deoxygenated blood from the fetus to the placenta; the **umbilical vein** carries oxygenated blood from the placenta back to the fetus.
- The fetal circulatory system differs from its adult version by having three shunts:
  - The **foramen ovale** connects the right atrium to the left atrium, bypassing the lungs.
  - The **ductus arteriosus** connects the pulmonary artery to the aorta, bypassing the lungs.
  - The **ductus venosus** connects the umbilical vein to the inferior vena cava, bypassing the liver.

Gestation and Birth

- In the first trimester, organogenesis occurs (development of heart, eyes, gonads, limbs, liver, brain).
- In the second trimester, tremendous growth occurs, movement begins, the face becomes distinctly human, and the digits elongate.
- In the third trimester, rapid growth and brain development continue, and there is transfer of antibodies to the fetus.
- During birth the cervix thins out and the amniotic sac ruptures. Then, uterine contractions, coordinated by prostaglandins and oxytocin, result in birth of the fetus. Finally, the placenta and umbilical cord are expelled.

ANSWERS TO CONCEPT CHECKS

3.1

1. Determinate cleavage refers to cell division that results in cells having definitive lineages; that is, at least one daughter cell is programmed to differentiate into a particular cell type. Indeterminate cleavage refers to cell division that results in cells that can differentiate into any cell type (or a whole organism).
2. Zygote → 2-, 4-, 8-, and 16-cell embryo → morula → blastula (blastocyst) → gastrula
3. Implantation occurs during the blastula (blastocyst) stage.
4.

Germ Layer	Organs
Ectoderm	Integument (including the epidermis, hair, nails, and epithelia of the nose, mouth, and anal canal), lens of the eye, nervous system (including adrenal medulla), inner ear
Mesoderm	Musculoskeletal system, circulatory system, excretory system, gonads, muscular and connective tissue layers of the digestive and respiratory systems, adrenal cortex
Endoderm	Epithelial linings of digestive and respiratory tracts, and parts of the liver, pancreas, thyroid, bladder, and distal urinary and reproductive tracts

5. Induction is the process by which nearby cells influence the differentiation of adjacent cells. This ensures proper spatial location and orientation of cells that share a function or have complementary functions.
6. Neural crest cells become the peripheral nervous system (including the sensory ganglia, autonomic ganglia, adrenal medulla, and Schwann cells) as well as specific cell types in other tissues (such as calcitonin-producing cells of the thyroid, melanocytes in the skin, and others).

3.2

1. Determination is the commitment of a cell to a particular lineage. Differentiation refers to the actual changes that occur in order for the cell to assume the structure and function of the determined cell type.
2.

Type of Potency	Cell Lineages
Totipotency	Any cell type in the developing embryo (primary germ layers) or in extraembryonic tissues (amnion, chorion, placenta)
Pluripotency	Any cell type in the developing embryo (primary germ layers)
Multipotency	Any cell type within a particular lineage (for example, hematopoietic stem cells)

3. Autocrine (the signal acts on the same cell that secreted it), paracrine (the signal acts on local cells), juxtacrine (a cell triggers adjacent cells through direct receptor stimulation), endocrine (the signal travels via the bloodstream to act on cells at distant sites)
4. Apoptosis is programmed cell death and results in contained blebs of the dead cell that can be picked up and digested by other cells. Necrosis is cell death due to injury and results in spilling of cytoplasmic contents.

3.3

1. The umbilical arteries carry deoxygenated blood. The umbilical vein carries oxygenated blood.
2.

Shunt	Connected Vessels or Chambers	Organ Bypassed
Foramen ovale	Right atrium to left atrium	Lungs
Ductus arteriosus	Pulmonary artery to aorta	Lungs
Ductus venosus	Umbilical vein to inferior vena cava	Liver

3.4

1. In the first trimester, organogenesis occurs (development of heart, eyes, gonads, limbs, liver, brain). In the second trimester, tremendous growth occurs, movement begins, the face becomes distinctly human, and the digits elongate. In the third trimester, rapid growth and brain development continue, and there is transfer of antibodies to the fetus.
2. In the first phase of birth, the cervix thins out and the amniotic sac ruptures. In the second phase, uterine contractions, coordinated by prostaglandins and oxytocin, result in birth of the fetus. In the third phase, the placenta and umbilical cord are expelled.

SCIENCE MASTERY ASSESSMENT EXPLANATIONS

1. **D**

Prostaglandins promote cervical dilation and the onset of contractions, and oxytocin promotes uterine contractions in a positive feedback loop. Oxytocin is also involved in milk letdown and helps the uterus to contract (shrink) following delivery. These factors together lead to **(D)** as the right answer. By contrast, prolactin, which promotes milk production, is produced following childbirth, which eliminates **(A)**, and progesterone maintains the pregnancy and actually inhibits uterine contractions, eliminating **(B)** and **(C)**.

2. **C**

To answer this question, it could be useful to review quickly the embryonic layers. The ectoderm gives rise to the integument (the epidermis, hair, nails, and the epithelia of the nose, mouth, and anal canal), the lens of the eye, and the nervous system (including the adrenal medulla). The endoderm gives rise to the epithelial linings of the digestive and respiratory tracts and parts of the liver, pancreas, thyroid, and bladder. Finally, the mesoderm gives rise to the musculoskeletal system, the circulatory system, the excretory system, the gonads, and the adrenal cortex. Therefore, the only correct association can be found in **(C)** because the fingernails are derived from ectoderm.

3. **B**

A rod of mesodermal cells called the notochord develops along the longitudinal axis just under the dorsal layer of ectoderm. Through inductive effects from the notochord, the overlying ectoderm starts bending inward and forms a groove on the dorsal surface of the embryo. The dorsal ectoderm will eventually pinch off and develop into the spinal cord and brain. While the neural tube forms from ectoderm, the notochord itself is mesodermal.

4. **D**

The influence of a specific group of cells on the differentiation of another group of cells is termed induction. For example, the eyes are formed through reciprocal induction between the brain and the ectoderm. Competence refers to the ability of a cell to respond to a given inducer, but not the influence of the group of organizing cells, eliminating **(A)**. Senescence is a term for biological aging, eliminating **(B)**. Determination may be the result of induction, but this term does not refer to the general concept of the effect of one group of cells on the differentiation of another group of cells, eliminating **(C)**.

5. **C**

During pregnancy, the placenta produces estrogen and progesterone to maintain the endometrium. These hormones are necessary for proper gestation of the fetus and should be measurable in maternal blood because they act on maternal organs. Prior to birth, the fetus is immunologically naïve and does not yet produce immunoglobulins, eliminating **(A)**. It is worth noting, though, that maternal immunoglobulins cross the placenta to enter fetal blood. Fetal hemoglobin is a large protein and, thus, cannot easily cross the placenta. Further, red blood cells are much too large to cross the barrier themselves, eliminating **(B)**. Carbon dioxide from fetal metabolism can be found in maternal blood, but the fetal lungs are nonfunctional prior to birth as the fetus is suspended in amniotic fluid. Carbon dioxide is transferred across the placenta directly from the fetal bloodstream, eliminating **(D)**.

6. **C**

The question stem states that a cell releases a substance that diffuses through the environment and causes differentiation of a nearby cell. Because the cell is acting on a nearby cell and the molecule spreads by diffusion, this is an example of paracrine signaling. Autocrine signaling, **(A)**, occurs when a molecule secreted by a cell acts on the same cell. Juxtacrine signaling, **(B)**, occurs between adjacent cells, but the signal does not spread by diffusion. In endocrine signaling, **(D)**, a molecule is secreted that travels via the bloodstream to a distant target.

7. **D**

Cells that are able to divide indefinitely with no senescence are not exhibiting normal cell behavior. Normally, somatic cells divide a limited number of times until the telomeres become too short to be effective protectors of genomic material. When this occurs, the cells stop dividing. However, in this case, the cells have continued to divide indefinitely. It is likely that the enzyme telomerase has been activated, which allows for synthesis of telomeres to counteract shortening during DNA replication.

8. **A**

Organogenesis primarily occurs during the first trimester of pregnancy; after 8 weeks of gestation, the brain is fairly developed and most of the organs have formed. The severity of anencephaly suggests a defect very early in fetal development, leading to **(A)** as the correct answer. The second and third trimesters are marked by significant growth and further development. Defects in these stages may cause structural abnormalities, but the absence of an organ is unlikely.

9. **A**

Embryonic stem cells are controversial because they require termination of an embryo to harvest, eliminating **(B)**. Adult stem cells are significantly less controversial, but require treatment with various transcription factors in order to increase the level of potency, eliminating **(C)**. Rejection is a concern when foreign cells are introduced into an individual; using one's own stem cells should remove this risk, eliminating **(D)**. Adult stem cells are not naturally pluripotent, unless pluripotency has been induced by strategic use of transcription factors. Therefore, **(A)** is the correct answer.

10. **C**

During development, programmed cell death occurs in multiple locations in order to ensure development of the correct adult structures. One of the places in which this occurs is between fingers and toes; another is the digestive tract, where a central lumen is formed. If apoptosis does not occur correctly in the digestive tract, an imperforate anus could result. Failure of determination or differentiation would likely result in the absence of anorectal structures altogether, eliminating **(A)** and **(B)**. Failure of neurulation would lead to the absence of a nervous system and would not be compatible with life, eliminating **(D)**.

11. **B**

After an injury, healing occurs by some sort of regenerative process. In humans, some tissues, such as the liver, are capable of regenerating tissue with much the same function and structure as the original tissue. However, the heart is not capable of this sort of regeneration, often forming a fibrous scar in an area of injury. This is an example of incomplete regeneration, in which newly formed tissues are not identical in structure or function to the tissues that have been injured or lost.

12. **A**

Here, the mutation affects the skin and the nervous system, both of which are derived from ectoderm. The other germ tissue layers do not lead to skin or nervous system formation, eliminating **(B)** and **(C)**. The notochord is not actually a primary germ tissue layer, and thus cannot be an answer to the question, eliminating **(D)**.

13. **C**

After the first cell divisions occur, the embryo consists of a solid ball of cells known as a morula. Then a hollow center forms, creating the blastula. Finally, as the cells begin to differentiate into the three germ layers, the embryo is considered a gastrula. **(C)** is therefore the correct answer.

14. **D**

The question stem states that the woman was given the drug three days before the baby was born. It is important to remember that organogenesis occurs during the first trimester. The last structure to become fully functional is the lungs. Because the organs were already largely formed prior to the administration of the teratogenic drug, it is likely that there was no major effect on the development of most organs as a result of exposure to the teratogen, eliminating **(A)**, **(B)**, and **(C)**. However, because lung tissues are so sensitive and because they mature so late, it is likely that the infant may have some respiratory distress at birth.

15. **C**

Blood flow in the ductus arteriosus is from the pulmonary artery to the aorta. The direction of flow is determined by the pressure differential between the right side of the heart (and pulmonary circulation) and the left side of the heart (and systemic circulation). Unlike in adults, the right side of the heart is at a higher pressure during prenatal life than the left side, so blood will shunt from the pulmonary circulation to the systemic circulation through both the foramen ovale and ductus arteriosus.

GO ONLINE

Consult your online resources for additional practice.

SHARED CONCEPTS

Behavioral Sciences Chapter 1
Biology and Behavior

Biochemistry Chapter 3
Nonenzymatic Protein Function and Protein Analysis

Biochemistry Chapter 6
DNA and Biotechnology

Biology Chapter 1
The Cell

Biology Chapter 2
Reproduction

Biology Chapter 5
The Endocrine System

CHAPTER 4

THE NERVOUS SYSTEM

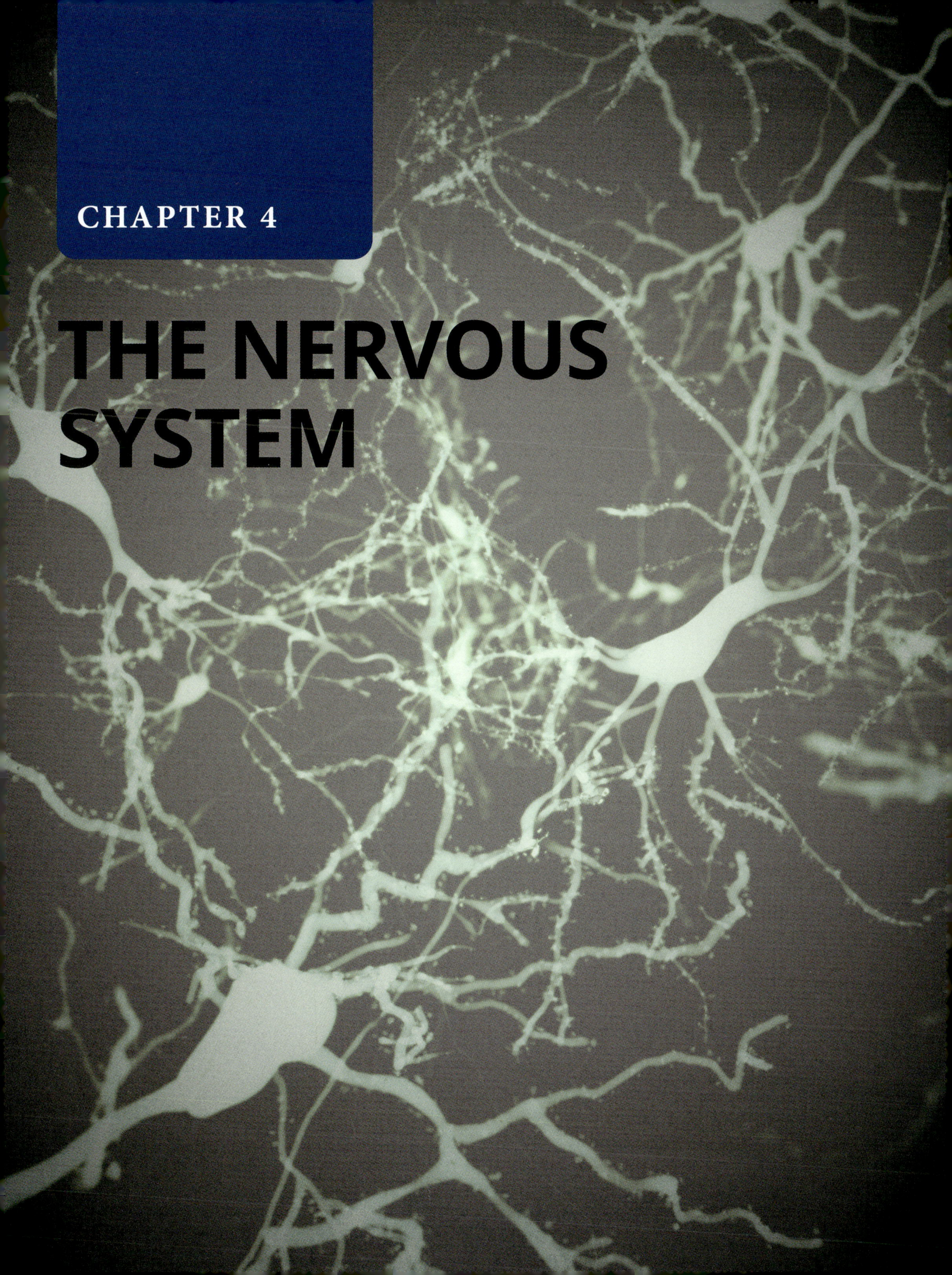

SCIENCE MASTERY ASSESSMENT

Every pre-med knows this feeling: there is so much content I have to know for the MCAT! How do I know what to do first or what's important?

While the high-yield badges throughout this book will help you identify the most important topics, this Science Mastery Assessment is another tool in your MCAT prep arsenal. This quiz (which can also be taken in your online resources) and the guidance below will help ensure that you are spending the appropriate amount of time on this chapter based on your personal strengths and weaknesses. Don't worry though—skipping something now does not mean you'll never study it. Later on in your prep, as you complete full-length tests, you'll uncover specific pieces of content that you need to review and can come back to these chapters as appropriate.

How to Use This Assessment

If you answer 0–7 questions correctly:

Spend about 1 hour to read this chapter in full and take limited notes throughout. Follow up by reviewing **all** quiz questions to ensure that you now understand how to solve each one.

If you answer 8–11 questions correctly:

Spend 20–40 minutes reviewing the quiz questions. Beginning with the questions you missed, read and take notes on the corresponding subchapters. For questions you answered correctly, ensure your thinking matches that of the explanation and you understand why each choice was correct or incorrect.

If you answer 12–15 questions correctly:

Spend less than 20 minutes reviewing all questions from the quiz. If you missed any, then include a quick read-through of the corresponding subchapters, or even just the relevant content within a subchapter, as part of your question review. For questions you answered correctly, ensure your thinking matches that of the explanation and review the Concept Summary at the end of the chapter.

1. Resting membrane potential depends on:
   - **I.** differential distribution of ions across the axon membrane.
   - **II.** the opening of voltage-gated calcium channels.
   - **III.** active transport of ions across the membrane.

   A. I only
   B. I and II only
   C. I and III only
   D. II and III only

2. All of the following are associated with the myelin sheath EXCEPT:
   A. faster conduction of nerve impulses.
   B. nodes of Ranvier forming gaps along the axon.
   C. increased magnitude of the potential difference during an action potential.
   D. saltatory conduction of action potentials.

3. Which of the following is true with regard to the action potential?
   A. All hyperpolarized stimuli will be carried to the axon terminal without a decrease in size.
   B. The size of the action potential is proportional to the size of the stimulus that produced it.
   C. Increasing the intensity of the depolarization increases the size of the impulse.
   D. Once an action potential is triggered, an impulse of a given magnitude and speed is produced.

4. Which of the following correctly describes a difference between nerves and tracts?
   A. Nerves are seen in the central nervous system; tracts are seen in the peripheral nervous system.
   B. Nerves have cell bodies in nuclei; tracts have cell bodies in ganglia.
   C. Nerves may carry more than one type of information; tracts can only carry one type of information.
   D. Nerves contain only one neuron; tracts contain many neurons.

5. Which of the following accurately describes sensory neurons?
   A. Sensory neurons are afferent and enter the spinal cord on the dorsal side.
   B. Sensory neurons are efferent and enter the spinal cord on the dorsal side.
   C. Sensory neurons are afferent and enter the spinal cord on the ventral side.
   D. Sensory neurons are efferent and enter the spinal cord on the ventral side.

6. When a sensory neuron receives a stimulus that brings it to threshold, it will do all of the following EXCEPT:
   A. become depolarized.
   B. transduce the stimulus to an action potential.
   C. inhibit the spread of the action potential to other sensory neurons.
   D. cause the release of neurotransmitters onto cells in the central nervous system.

7. When the potential across the axon membrane is more negative than the normal resting potential, the neuron is said to be in a state of:
   A. depolarization.
   B. hyperpolarization.
   C. repolarization.
   D. polarization.

8. Which of the following statements concerning the somatic division of the peripheral nervous system is INCORRECT?
   A. Its pathways innervate skeletal muscle.
   B. Its pathways are usually voluntary.
   C. Some of its pathways are referred to as reflex arcs.
   D. Its pathways always involve more than two neurons.

9. Which of the following is a function of the parasympathetic nervous system?
   A. Increasing blood sugar during periods of stress
   B. Dilating the pupils to enhance vision
   C. Increasing oxygen delivery to muscles
   D. Decreasing heart rate and blood pressure

10. Which of the following neurotransmitters is used in the ganglia of both the sympathetic and parasympathetic nervous systems?

A. Acetylcholine
B. Dopamine
C. Norepinephrine
D. Serotonin

11. In which neural structure are ribosomes primarily located?

A. Dendrites
B. Soma
C. Axon hillock
D. Axon

12. An autoimmune disease attacks the voltage-gated calcium channels in the synaptic terminal of an excitatory neuron. What is a likely symptom of this condition?

A. Spastic paralysis (inability to relax the muscles)
B. Flaccid paralysis (inability to contract the muscles)
C. Inability to reuptake neurotransmitters once released
D. Retrograde flow of action potentials

13. A neuron only fires an action potential if multiple presynaptic cells release neurotransmitters onto the dendrites of the neuron. This is an example of:

A. saltatory conduction.
B. summation.
C. a feedback loop.
D. inhibitory transmission.

14. A disease results in the death of Schwann cells. Which portion of the nervous system is NOT likely to be affected?

A. Central nervous system
B. Somatic nervous system
C. Autonomic nervous system
D. Parasympathetic nervous system

15. A surgeon accidentally clips a dorsal root ganglion during a spinal surgery. What is a likely consequence of this error?

I. Loss of reflexes at that level
II. Loss of sensation at that level
III. Loss of cognitive function

A. I only
B. II only
C. I and II only
D. I, II, and III

Answer Key

1. **C** (See section 4.2)
2. **C** (See section 4.2)
3. **D** (See section 4.2)
4. **C** (See section 4.1)
5. **A** (See section 4.2)
6. **C** (See section 4.2)
7. **B** (See section 4.2)
8. **D** (See section 4.2)
9. **D** (See section 4.2)
10. **A** (See section 4.2)
11. **B** (See section 4.1)
12. **B** (See section 4.2)
13. **B** (See section 4.2)
14. **A** (See section 4.1)
15. **C** (See section 4.2)

The relevant section of the chapter to review for each question is given in parentheses after the correct answer. Detailed explanations can be found at the end of the chapter.

CHAPTER 4

THE NERVOUS SYSTEM

In This Chapter

CHAPTER PROFILE

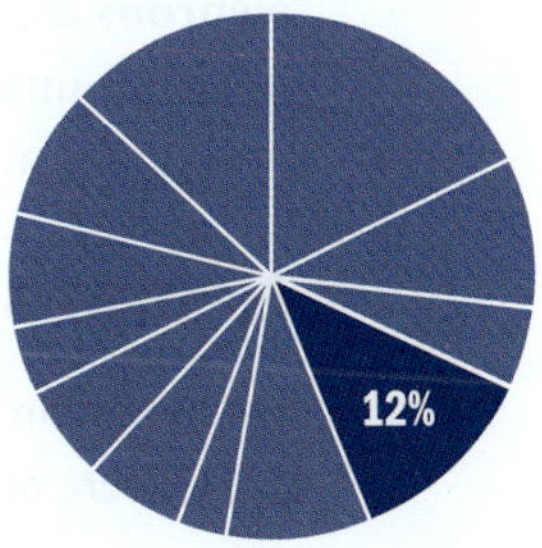

The content in this chapter should be relevant to about 12% of all questions about biology on the MCAT.

This chapter covers material from the following AAMC content categories:

2A: Assemblies of molecules, cells, and groups of cells within single cellular and multicellular organisms

3A: Structure and functions of the nervous and endocrine systems and ways in which these systems coordinate the organ systems

4C: Electrochemistry and electrical circuits and their elements

6A: Sensing the environment

Introduction

For generations, some indigenous peoples of South America used blow darts laced with a paralytic plant extract to hunt their prey. In the 1800s, English physicians who interacted with these indigenous South Americans recognized the possible uses of this paralytic agent, now known as *tubocurarine*, as an anesthetic agent for surgeries. Physicians noticed that animals under the influence of *tubocurarine* would become temporarily immobilized, but would recover after a period of paralysis. According to these physicians, this anesthetic agent would revolutionize surgery. To test the effectiveness of the new drug, one of the physicians volunteered to demonstrate its effectiveness by being tested for pain perception while under the influence of *tubocurarine*. While the drug was an effective paralyzing agent, it did not have any effect on the sensory receptors of the body—he felt every test without being able to move or express his discomfort.

Organisms sense pain, temperature, and all aspects of their environment through the nervous system, which also coordinates this sensory information and responds to stimuli. Specifically, the nervous system is responsible for the control of muscular movement, neuromuscular reflexes, and glandular secretions (such as salivation and lacrimation). In addition, the nervous system is responsible for higher-level thinking and mental function.

Despite all of its complex functions, the nervous system operates through basic electrical and chemical signals. Biomedical scientists have discovered much about the nervous system: its anatomical and functional divisions, the nature of the action potential, and its histological features under the microscope. However, there is so much more that we do not know. It is an inspirational challenge for future physicians to realize that the brain continues to be a vast frontier for human exploration and discovery.

4.1 Cells of the Nervous System High Yield

LEARNING OBJECTIVES

After Chapter 4.1, you will be able to:

- Recall the different terms used for myelin-producing cells in the peripheral and the central nervous systems
- Identify the functions of the five main categories of glial cells
- Describe the purpose of each major structure of the neuron

Neurons are specialized cells capable of transmitting electrical impulses and then translating those electrical impulses into chemical signals. In this section, we will consider the structure of the neuron as well as how neurons communicate with other parts of the nervous system.

Neurons

Each neuron has a shape that matches its function, as dictated by the other cells with which that neuron interacts. There are a variety of different types of neurons in the body, but they all share some specific features.

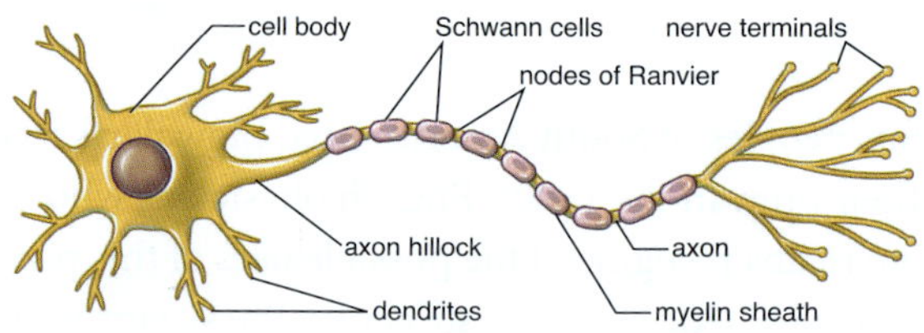

Figure 4.1 Structure of a Neuron

MNEMONIC

Axons carry neural signals **a**way from the soma; dendrites carry signals toward the soma.

The anatomy of a neuron is shown in Figure 4.1. Like all other cells (besides mature red blood cells), neurons have nuclei. The nucleus is located in the **cell body**, also called the **soma**. The soma is also the location of the endoplasmic reticulum and ribosomes. The cell has many appendages emanating directly from the soma called **dendrites**, which receive incoming messages from other cells. The information received from the dendrites is transmitted through the cell body before it reaches the **axon hillock**, which integrates the incoming signals. The axon hillock plays an important role in **action potentials**, or the transmission of electrical impulses down the axon. Signals arriving from the dendrites can be either excitatory or inhibitory; the axon hillock sums up these signals, and if the result is excitatory enough (reaching threshold, as discussed later in this chapter), it will initiate an action potential. The **axon** is a long appendage that terminates in close proximity to a target structure (a muscle, a gland, or another neuron). Most mammalian nerve fibers are insulated by **myelin**, a fatty membrane, to prevent signal loss or crossing of signals. Just like insulation prevents wires next to each other from accidentally discharging each other, the **myelin sheath** maintains the electrical signal within one neuron. In addition, myelin increases the speed of conduction in the axon. Myelin is produced by **oligodendrocytes** in the central nervous system and **Schwann cells** in the peripheral nervous system. At certain intervals along the axon, there are small breaks in the myelin sheath with exposed areas of axon membrane called **nodes of Ranvier**. As will be explored in the discussion of action potentials to follow, nodes of Ranvier are critical for rapid signal conduction. Finally, at the end of the axon is the **nerve terminal** or **synaptic bouton (knob)**. This structure is enlarged and flattened to maximize transmission of the signal to the next neuron and ensure proper release of **neurotransmitters**, the chemicals that transmit information between neurons.

Neurons are not physically connected to each other. Between the neurons, there is a small space into which the terminal portion of the axon releases neurotransmitters, which bind to the dendrites of the adjacent neuron (the postsynaptic neuron). This space is known as the **synaptic cleft**; together, the nerve terminal, synaptic cleft, and postsynaptic membrane are known as a **synapse**. Neurotransmitters released from the axon terminal traverse the synaptic cleft and bind to receptors on the postsynaptic neuron.

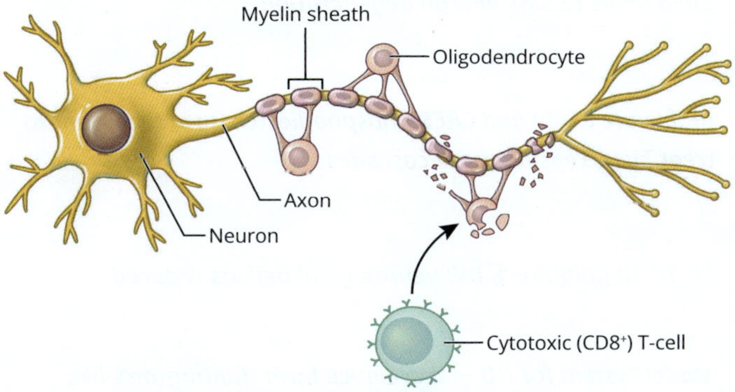

Figure 4.2 Destruction of Myelin as a Result of Multiple Sclerosis

Multiple neurons may be bundled together to form a **nerve** in the peripheral nervous system. These nerves may be **sensory**, **motor**, or **mixed**, which refers to the type(s) of information they carry; mixed nerves carry both sensory and motor information. The cell bodies of neurons of the same type are clustered together into ganglia.

In the central nervous system, axons may be bundled together to form **tracts**. Unlike nerves, tracts only carry one type of information. The cell bodies of neurons in the same tract are grouped into **nuclei**. Figure 4.3 illustrates the differences between peripheral and central nervous system organization.

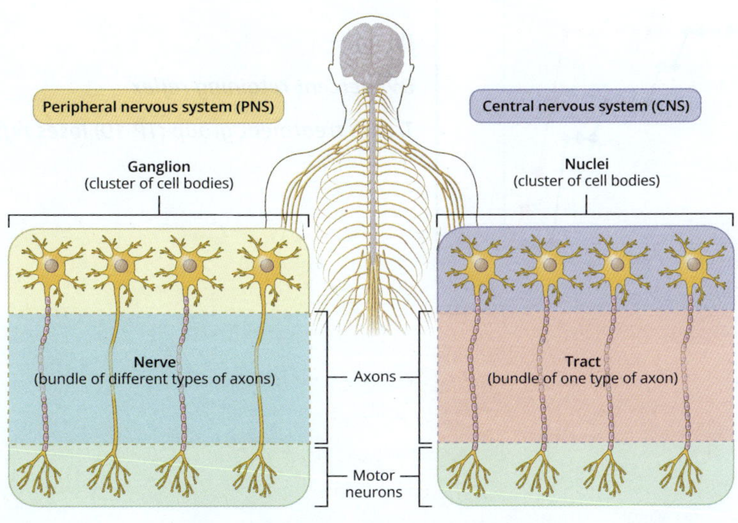

Figure 4.3 PNS vs. CNS Neural Paths

REAL WORLD

Sometimes the body mounts an immune response against its own myelin, leading to the destruction of this insulating substance (demyelination). Because myelin speeds the conduction of impulses along a neuron, the absence of myelin slows down or dissipates the transferring signal. A common demyelinating disorder is multiple sclerosis (MS). In MS, oligodendrocytes (the myelin-producing cells of the brain and spinal cord) are selectively targeted by immune cells (see Figure 4.2). Because there is demyelination across different tracts responsible for a range of tasks, patients who have MS experience a wide variety of symptoms including weakness, lack of balance, vision problems, and incontinence.

BIOLOGY GUIDED EXAMPLE WITH EXPERT THINKING

Huntington's disease (HD) is a devastating neurodegenerative condition caused by expansion of a CAG repeat in exon 1 of *IT15*, which encodes for the protein huntingtin.

Background: Huntington's disease

Although huntingtin is widely expressed, HD is associated with the neurodegeneration of the striatal medium spiny neurons. This particular vulnerability is hypothesized to result from transcriptional dysregulation within the cAMP and CREB signaling cascades in these neurons.

Hypothesis: dysregulation of transcription within cAMP and CREB leads to SMS neuron degeneration

Thus, a potential treatment would be to target phosphodiesterases (PDE) that inactivate cAMP and CREB cascades.

Inactivate cAMP and CREB phosphodiesterase = they want to treat by increasing these cascades

To test this hypothesis, and the potential therapeutic approach, researchers investigated whether administration of TP-10, a highly specific phosphodiesterase inhibitor would alleviate neurological deficits

IV: TP-10 (inhibitor), DV: neurological deficits reduced

in a highly utilized HD model system, the R6/2 mouse.

Model system for HD = these mice have Huntington's-like symptoms

Loss of reflexes, loss of body weight, and increased instances of clasping behavior in the mice were monitored in the TP-10 intervention group and the vehicle control group. Righting reflex is assessed by laying the mice on their side and monitoring their ability to get back to the upright position. Clasping is a behavior correlated to neurodegeneration.

Behavior on these tests must correlate to symptom relief from HD

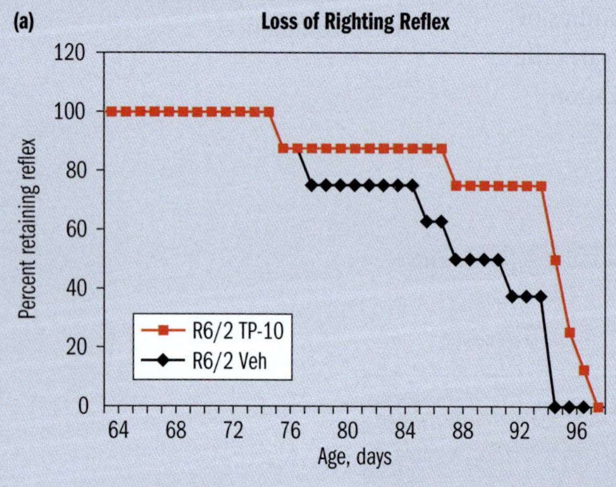

IV: age

DV: percent retaining reflex

Trend: treatment group (TP-10) loses reflex at a later age

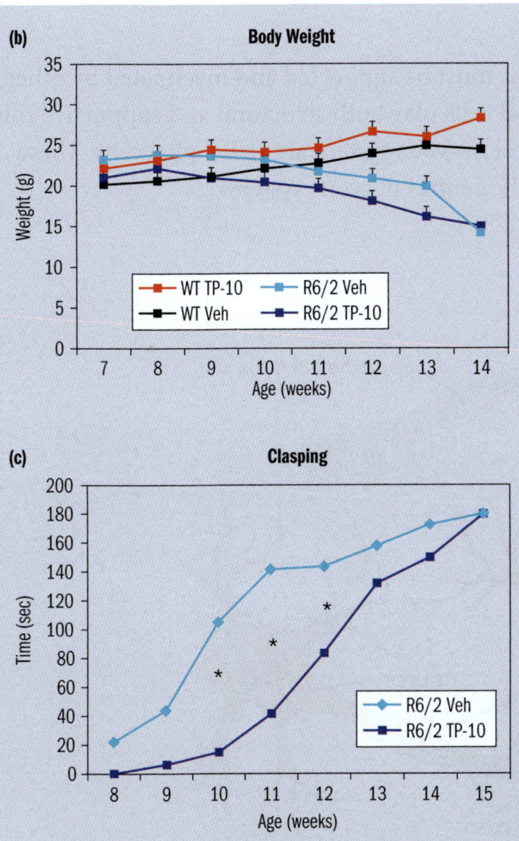

IV: age

DV: weight

Trend: wild-type (WT) gain weight toward the end of the experiment; R6/2 lose weight

IV: age

DV: time

Trend: vehicle group develops "clasping" before treatment (TP-10) group

Figure 1

Adapted from: Giampà, C., Laurenti, D., Anzilotti, S., Bernardi, G., Menniti, F. S., & Fusco, F. R. (2010). Inhibition of the striatal specific phosphodiesterase PDE10a ameliorates striatal and cortical pathology in R6/2 mouse model of Huntingtons disease. *PLoS One*, 5(10). doi:10.1371/journal.pone.0013417.

Does TP-10 treatment alleviate neurological deficits associated with Huntington's disease?

This question asks about the results of the associated study, so we are going to have to use the information in the article and the results in the figures in order to answer. The article says that TP-10 is a possible treatment for Huntington's disease (HD), and the second paragraph describes the dependent variables used to measure success in this experiment. There appears to be a figure associated with each dependent variable, so we will need to evaluate the results in each figure to reach a conclusion.

Based on the label and axes of the graph, Figure 1(a) shows the age at which mice lose their righting reflex. Specifically, we can see that that R6/2 TP-10 (red) retains their righting reflex longer than R6/2 Vehicle (black). According to the passage, the loss of the righting reflex indicates neurodegeneration; therefore, TP-10 appears to be alleviating this particular symptom. However, Figure 1(b) shows that mice who had the HD genetic condition lost weight in both treatment and vehicle conditions, meaning TP-10 doesn't appear to have helped with weight maintenance. Finally, Figure 1(c) shows that clasping occurs more readily in R6/2 Vehicle than R6/2 TP-10. The term clasping alone doesn't imply positive or negative effects on the brain, but the article tells us that clasping is a sign of neurodegeneration. Thus, the data showing that R6/2 TP-10-treated mice have later onset of clasping demonstrates that neurological deficits are being alleviated.

Overall, Figures 1(a) and 1(c) indicate that TP-10 may have potential to treat neurological deficits associated with Huntington's disease. Figure 1(b), however, indicates that this treatment may not be addressing all aspects of the disease.

Other Cells in the Nervous System

Neurons are not the only cells in the nervous system. Neurons must be supported and myelinated by other cells. These cells are often called **glial cells**, or **neuroglia**. Glial cells play both structural and supportive roles, as shown in Figure 4.4. The progenitor stem cells of the central nervous system are radial glial cells. These cells divide and differentiate into all the different kinds of glia in the central nervous system.

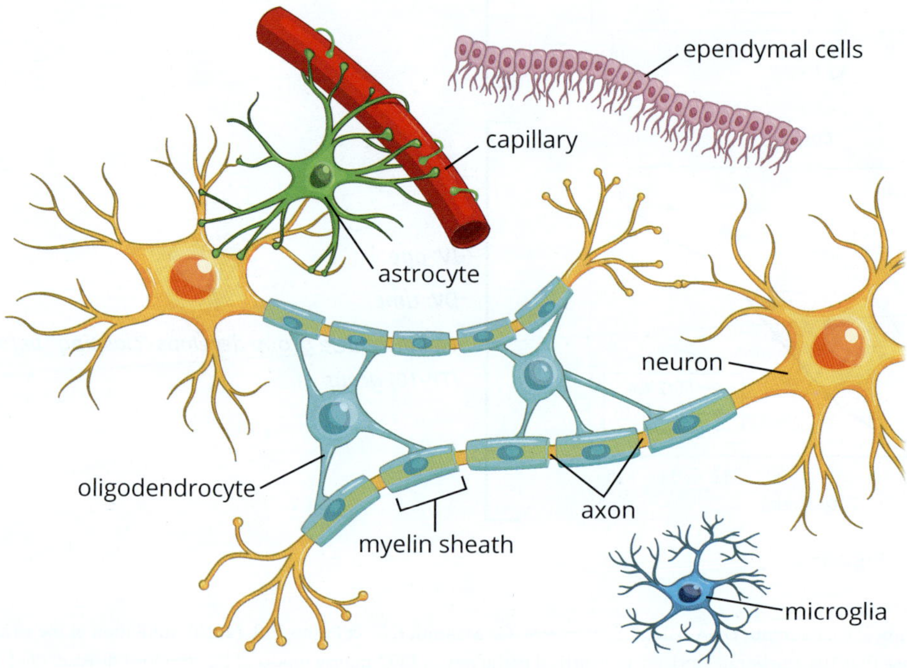

Figure 4.4 Glial Cells: Astrocytes and Oligodendrocytes

A detailed knowledge of these cell types is not necessary for the MCAT, so a familiarity with their basic functions will suffice:

- **Astrocytes** nourish neurons and form the blood–brain barrier, which controls the transmission of solutes from the bloodstream into nervous tissue.
- **Ependymal cells** line the ventricles of the brain and produce cerebrospinal fluid, which physically supports the brain and serves as a shock absorber.
- **Microglia** are phagocytic cells that ingest and break down waste products and pathogens in the central nervous system.
- **Oligodendrocytes** (CNS) and **Schwann cells** (PNS) produce myelin around axons.

MCAT CONCEPT CHECK 4.1

Before you move on, assess your understanding of the material with these questions.

1. For each of the following neuron structures, provide a brief description of its purpose:
    - Axon:

    - Axon hillock:

    - Dendrite:

    - Myelin sheath:

    - Soma:

    - Synaptic bouton:

    ---

2. What is a collection of cell bodies called in the CNS? In the PNS?
    - CNS:

    - PNS:

    ---

3. Which two types of glial cells, if not properly functioning, will make an individual most susceptible to a CNS infection?

    ---

4. Guillain-Barré syndrome (GBS) is an autoimmune disease that causes demyelination in the peripheral nervous system. What type of glial cell is being targeted in GBS?

4.2 Transmission of Neural Impulses

High Yield

LEARNING OBJECTIVES

After Chapter 4.2, you will be able to:

- Explain the ion channels and regulatory steps involved in the process of initiating, propagating, and terminating an action potential
- Describe the resting membrane potential and how it is maintained
- Differentiate between temporal and spatial summation
- Identify the ion responsible for the fusion of neurotransmitter-containing vesicles at the nerve terminal membrane
- Recall the three main methods to block the action of a neurotransmitter
- Identify the ion channel changes that occur during the shifts in voltage associated with an action potential:

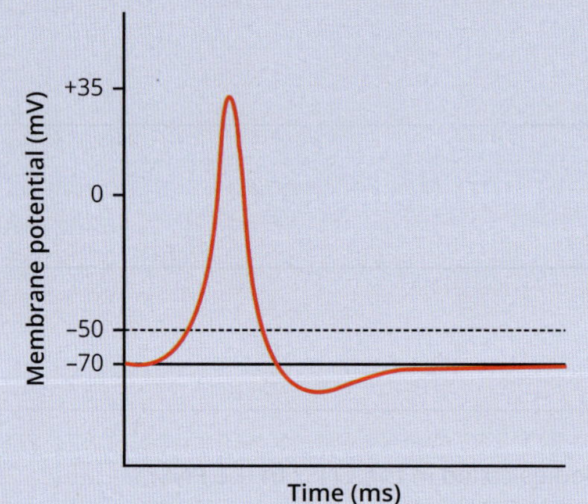

Now that we have discussed the basic anatomy of the neuron, we can turn to the physiology that underlies neuronal signaling.

The Action Potential

Neurons use all-or-nothing messages called **action potentials** to relay electrical impulses down the axon to the synaptic bouton. As we will explore in the following section, action potentials ultimately cause the release of neurotransmitters into the synaptic cleft.

Resting Potential

A cell's **resting membrane potential** is the net electric potential difference that exists across the cell membrane, created by movement of charged molecules across that membrane. For neurons, this potential is about −70 mV, with the inside of the neuron being negative relative to the outside. The two most important ions involved in generating and maintaining the resting potential are potassium (K^+) and sodium (Na^+).

The potassium concentration inside the cell averages about 140 mM, as compared to 4 mM outside of the cell. This concentration difference makes it favorable for potassium to move to the outside of the cell. To facilitate the outward movement of potassium, the cell membrane has transmembrane **potassium leak channels**, which allow the slow leak of potassium out of the cell. As potassium continually leaks out of the cell, the cell loses a small amount of positive charge, leaving behind a small amount of negative charge and making the outside of the cell slightly positively charged.

However, as negative charge builds up inside the cell, some potassium will be drawn back into the cell due to the attraction between the positive potassium ions and the negative potential building inside the cell. As the potential difference continues to grow, potassium will also be more strongly drawn back into the cell. And at a certain potential, each potassium cation that is pushed out due to the concentration gradient will be matched by another potassium cation pulled back in due to the electric potential. At this point, there is no more net movement of the ion, as the cell is in equilibrium with respect to potassium. The potential difference that represents this potassium equilibrium is called the **equilibrium potential of potassium**. Potassium's equilibrium potential is around −90 mV. The negative sign is assigned due to convention, and because a positive ion (potassium) is leaving the cell.

Next, let's consider in isolation the other important ion, sodium. Sodium's concentration gradient is the reverse of potassium's, with a concentration of about 12 mM inside and 145 mM outside of the cell, meaning there is a driving force pushing sodium into the cell. This movement is facilitated by **sodium leak channels**. The slow leak of sodium into the cell causes a buildup of electric potential. The **equilibrium potential of sodium** is around 60 mV, and is positive because sodium is moving into the cell.

REAL WORLD

Even though we may think of these influxes and effluxes as big events, only a very small amount of potassium needs to exit the cell before the resulting electrostatic force equals the force of the concentration gradient. In fact, during an action potential the change to potassium's intracellular concentration is so small that it cannot even be accurately measured using current devices! The action potential is reliant only on local voltage changes at the membrane itself, so this overall lack of change in intracellular ion concentration does not impact transmission. This is the reason why you see membrane potentials reported in units of voltage, which are easily measurable, instead of concentration change, which is almost negligible. Because so little potassium needs to exit, the equilibrium potential with respect to potassium is established almost instantly.

In a living system, sodium and potassium are flowing across the cell's membrane at the same time. Potassium's concentration gradient causes potassium to leak out of the cell through potassium leak channels. At the same time, sodium is moving in the opposite direction, with the opposite effect. In a certain sense, sodium undoes the effect of potassium's movement. The resting potential is thus a tug-of-war: Potassium's movement pulls the cell potential toward −90 mV, while sodium's movement pulls the cell potential the opposite way, toward +60 mV. But neither ion ever "wins" the tug-of-war. Instead, a balance of these two effects is reached at around −70 mV for the average nerve cell, as can be seen in Figure 4.5. This balance, the net effect of sodium's and potassium's equilibrium potentials, is the **resting membrane potential**. The resting potential is significantly closer to potassium's equilibrium potential because the cell is much more permeable to potassium. Neither ion is ever able to establish its own equilibrium, so both ions continue leaking across the cell membrane.

BRIDGE

The resting membrane potential is dependent on the intra- and extracellular ion concentrations, relative permeability of the membrane to these different ions, and charges of these ions. The Goldman–Hodgkin–Katz voltage equation brings together these different factors into one equation that predicts the resting membrane potential. This equation is discussed in Chapter 8 of *MCAT Biochemistry Review*.

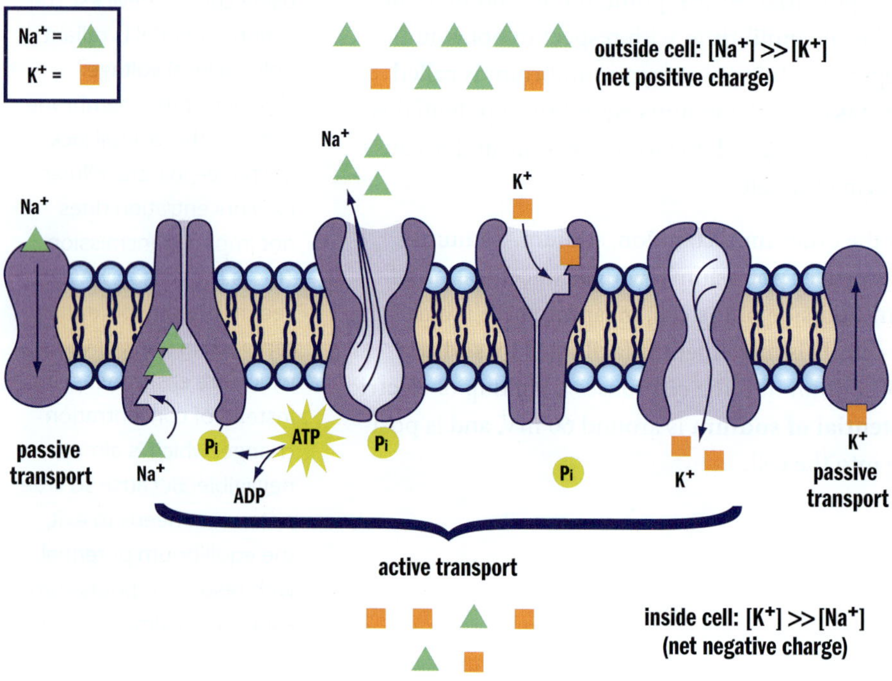

Figure 4.5 Maintenance of Resting Membrane Potential
The action of Na^+/K^+ ATPase, Na^+ leak channels, and K^+ leak channels creates and maintains a resting membrane potential of −70 mV.

Given the continual ion leaking at the membrane, there must be a means of moving both sodium and potassium ions back against their gradients if a resting potential is to be maintained. **Na^+/K^+ ATPase** continually pumps sodium and potassium back to where they started: potassium into the cell and sodium out of the cell, to maintain their respective gradients. In fact, in a person's body more ATP is spent by the Na^+/K^+ ATPase to maintain these gradients than for any other single purpose.

MNEMONIC

To remember the direction of ion movement by Na^+/K^+ ATPase, think *pumpKin*.

The Axon Hillock

Neurons can receive both excitatory and inhibitory input. Excitatory input causes **depolarization** (raising the membrane potential, V_m, from its resting potential) and thus makes the neuron more likely to fire an action potential. Inhibitory input causes **hyperpolarization** (lowering the membrane potential from its resting potential) and thus makes the neuron less likely to fire an action potential. If the axon hillock receives enough excitatory input to be depolarized to the **threshold** value (usually in the range of −55 mV to −40 mV), an action potential will be triggered.

This implies that not every stimulus necessarily generates a response. A small excitatory signal may not be sufficient to bring the axon hillock to threshold. Further, a postsynaptic neuron may receive information from several different presynaptic neurons, some of which are excitatory and some of which are inhibitory. The additive effect of multiple signals is known as **summation**.

There are two types of summation: temporal and spatial (Figure 4.6). In **temporal summation**, multiple signals are integrated during a relatively short period of time. A number of small excitatory signals firing at nearly the same moment could bring a postsynaptic cell to threshold, enabling an action potential. In **spatial summation**, the additive effects are based on the number and location of the incoming signals. A large number of inhibitory signals firing directly on the soma will cause more profound hyperpolarization of the axon hillock than the depolarization caused by a few excitatory signals firing on the dendrites of a neuron.

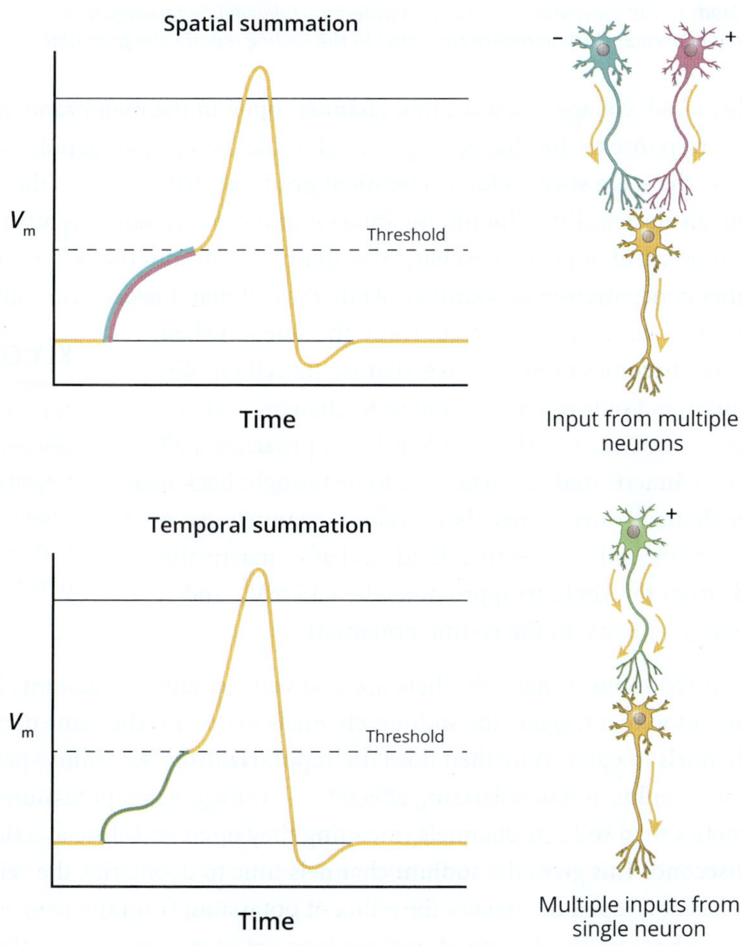

Figure 4.6 Spatial vs. Temporal Summation

Ion Channels and Membrane Potential

A graph of membrane potential vs. time during an action potential is shown in Figure 4.7.

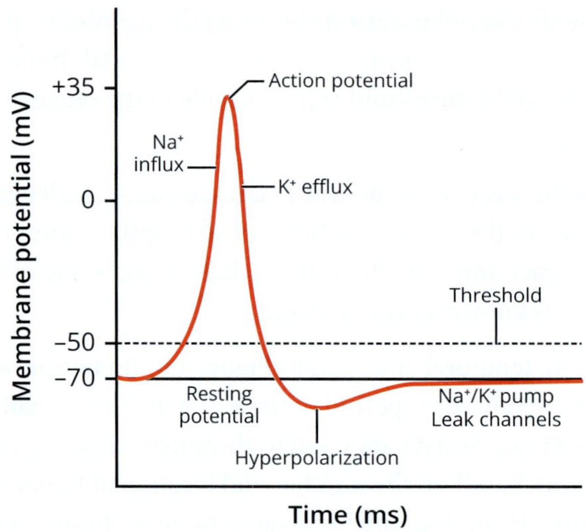

Figure 4.7 Action Potential Generation
Sufficient depolarization across the cell membrane to threshold leads to the generation of an action potential, followed by repolarization and hyperpolarization before returning to the resting membrane potential.

If the cell is brought to threshold, voltage-gated sodium channels open in the membrane. As the name implies, these ion channels open in response to the change in potential of the membrane (depolarization) and permit the passage of sodium ions. There is a strong **electrochemical gradient** that promotes the migration of sodium into the cell. From an electrical standpoint, the interior of the cell is more negative than the exterior of the cell, which favors the movement of positively charged sodium cations into the cell. From a chemical standpoint, there is a higher concentration of sodium outside the cell than inside, which also favors the movement of sodium into the cell. As sodium passes through these ion channels, the membrane potential becomes more positive; that is, the cell rapidly depolarizes. Sodium channels not only open in response to changes in membrane potential, but are also inactivated by them. When V_m approaches +35 mV, the sodium channels are **inactivated** and will have to be brought back near the resting potential to be **deinactivated**. Thus, these sodium channels can exist in three states: **closed** (before the cell reaches threshold, and after inactivation has been reversed), **open** (from threshold to approximately +35 mV), and **inactive** (from approximately +35 mV to the resting potential).

KEY CONCEPT

Na^+ wants to go into the cell because the cell is more negative inside (electrical gradient) and has a lower concentration of Na^+ inside (chemical gradient).

In addition to the voltage-gated sodium channels, there are also voltage-gated potassium channels. Interestingly enough, the depolarization that triggers the sodium channels to open is the same depolarization that triggers the potassium channels to open. Why then does the **repolarization** (K^+ efflux) part of the action potential occur after sodium's influx and depolarizing effects? The voltage-gated potassium channels are slower in their conformation kinetics than sodium-channels (meaning they open and close at a slower rate). This delay is roughly one millisecond. This gives the sodium channels time to depolarize the cell. At this point, an electrochemical gradient has developed that favors the efflux of potassium from the neuron. The potassium efflux is called repolarization because the driving of positive ions out of the cell restores the negative membrane potential. However, due to the slower closing of the voltage-gated potassium channels, more potassium than needed to reach resting membrane potential is released. This results in an overshoot of the resting membrane potential, hyperpolarizing the neuron. This hyperpolarization serves an important function: it makes the neuron refractory to further action potentials. There are two types of **refractory periods**. During the **absolute refractory period**, no amount of stimulation can cause another action potential to occur. During the **relative refractory period**, there must be *greater than normal* stimulation to cause an action potential because the membrane is starting from a potential that is more negative than its resting value.

The Na^+/K^+ ATPase acts to restore the concentration gradients of Na^+ (outside the cell) and K^+ (inside the cell). These concentration gradients, as discussed earlier, result in the formation of an electrochemical gradient. This electrochemical gradient stabilizes the cell's potential at -70 mV. At that point, the resting membrane potential is restored, all thanks to the hard work of Na^+/K^+ ATPase.

Impulse Propagation

So far, we have discussed the movements of ions at one small segment of the axon. For a signal to be conveyed to another neuron, the action potential must travel down the axon and initiate neurotransmitter release. This movement is called **impulse propagation** and is shown in Figure 4.8. As sodium rushes into one segment of the axon, it will cause depolarization in the surrounding regions of the axon. This depolarization will bring subsequent segments of the axon to threshold, opening the sodium channels in those segments. Each of these segments then continues through the rest of the action potential in a wave-like fashion until the action potential reaches the nerve terminal. After the action potential has fired in one segment of the axon, that segment becomes momentarily refractory, as described previously. The functional consequence of this is that information can only flow in one direction.

KEY CONCEPT

Action potentials rely on both electrical and chemical gradients. The neuron starts at the resting potential, around -70 mV. At the resting potential, potassium is high inside the cell and low outside the cell, while sodium is high outside the cell and low inside the cell. Once the cell reaches threshold, sodium channels open and sodium floods the cell, making it more positive inside (depolarization). Then, sodium channels are inactivated and the potassium channels open. This allows potassium to flow out of the cell, bringing the potential into the negative range (repolarization), and actually overshooting the resting potential (hyperpolarization). Na^+/K^+ ATPase then works to restore the resting potential.

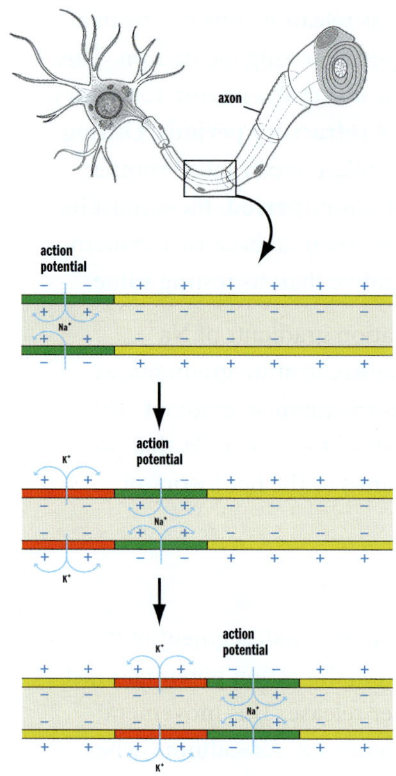

Figure 4.8 Action Potential Propagation
Action potentials are propagated down the axon when proximal sodium channels open and depolarize the membrane, inducing distal sodium channels to open as well; because of the refractory character of these channels, the action potential can move in only one direction.

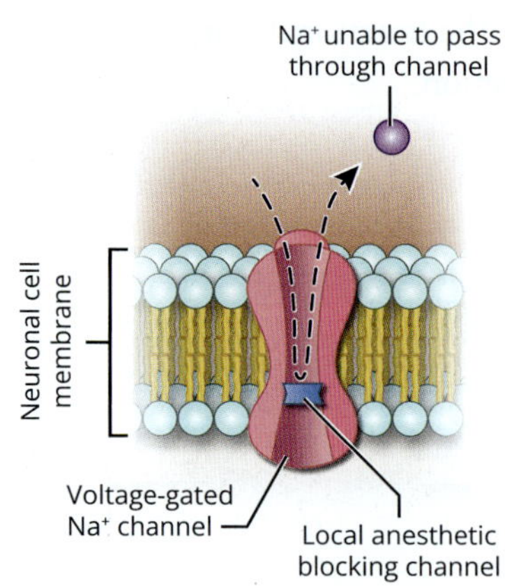

Figure 4.9 Local Anesthetic Function

REAL WORLD

A toxin called *tetrodotoxin* (TTX) is found in the pufferfish, a delicacy in some parts of the world. TTX blocks voltage-gated Na^+ channels, blocking neuronal transmission. This can rapidly cause death because the phrenic nerves innervating the diaphragm can no longer depolarize, leading to paralysis of the muscle and cessation of breathing. For this reason, chefs who prepare pufferfish must be specially trained and licensed.

REAL WORLD

As seen in Figure 4.9, local anesthetics work by blocking voltage-gated Na^+ channels. They favor blocking pain neurons because these neurons have small axonal diameters and little or no myelin, allowing easy access to the sodium channels. Anesthetic concentrations are kept sufficiently low to block pain neurons without significant effects on neurons performing other functions.

The speed at which action potentials move depends on the length and cross-sectional area of the axon. Increased length of the axon results in higher resistance and slower conduction. Greater cross-sectional areas allow for faster propagation due to decreased resistance. The effect of cross-sectional area is more significant than the effect of length. In order to maximize the speed of transmission, mammals have myelin. Myelin is an extraordinarily good insulator, preventing the dissipation of the electric signal. The insulation is so effective that the membrane is only permeable to ion movement at the nodes of Ranvier. Thus, the signal "hops" from node to node—what is called **saltatory conduction**.

It is important to note that all action potentials within the same type of neuron have the same potential difference during depolarization. Increased intensity of a stimulus does not result in an increased potential difference of the action potential, but rather an increased frequency of firing.

MNEMONIC

Saltatory conduction can be recalled by thinking of the Spanish verb *saltar*, to jump.

REAL WORLD

Insulation by myelin is extremely effective. A human spinal cord is about the thickness of a finger. Without this insulation, the cord would have to be almost as wide as a telephone pole to prevent signal loss.

The Synapse

As discussed previously, neurons are not actually in direct physical contact. There is a small space between neurons called the synaptic cleft into which neurotransmitters are secreted, as shown in Figure 4.10. To clarify the terminology, the neuron preceding the synaptic cleft is called the **presynaptic neuron**; the neuron after the synaptic cleft is called the **postsynaptic neuron**. If a neuron signals to a gland or muscle, rather than another neuron, the postsynaptic cell is termed an **effector**. Most synapses are **chemical** in nature; they use small molecules referred to as **neurotransmitters** to send messages from one cell to the next.

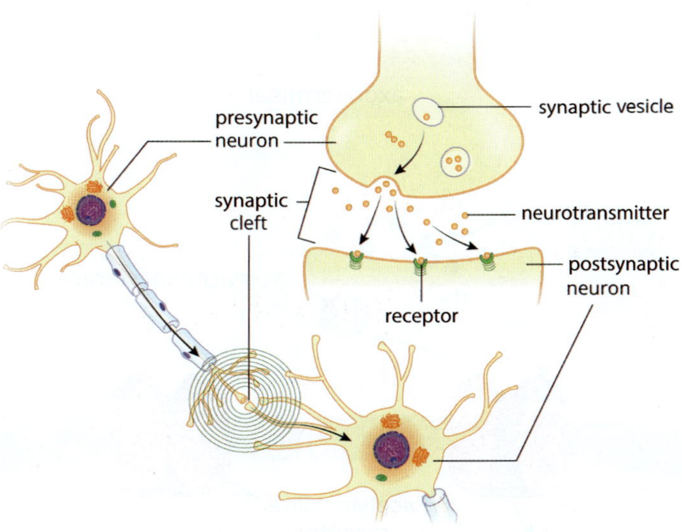

Figure 4.10 The Synapse
Synaptic vesicles are released from the presynaptic neuron and diffuse across the synaptic cleft to activate receptors on the postsynaptic neuron (or gland or muscle).

Neurotransmitters

Prior to release, neurotransmitter molecules are stored in membrane-bound vesicles in the nerve terminal. When the action potential reaches the nerve terminal, voltage-gated calcium channels open, allowing calcium to flow into the cell. This sudden increase in intracellular calcium triggers fusion of the membrane-bound vesicles with the cell membrane at the synapse, causing exocytosis of the neurotransmitter.

Once released into the synapse, the neurotransmitter molecules diffuse across the cleft and bind to receptors on the postsynaptic membrane. This allows the message to be passed from one neuron to the next. As stated earlier, neurons may be either excitatory or inhibitory; this distinction truly comes at the level of the neurotransmitter receptors. If the receptor is a ligand-gated ion channel, the postsynaptic cell will either be depolarized or hyperpolarized. If it is a G protein–coupled receptor, it will cause either changes in the levels of cyclic AMP (cAMP) or an influx of calcium. Note that the physiology of receptors is further discussed in Chapter 3 of *MCAT Biochemistry Review*.

KEY CONCEPT

It is critical to understand the difference between electrical and chemical transmission. Within a neuron, electricity is used to pass signals down the length of the axon. Between neurons, chemicals (neurotransmitters) are used to pass signals to the subsequent neuron (or gland or muscle).

Neurotransmission must be regulated—there are almost no circumstances under which constant signaling to the postsynaptic cell would be desirable. Therefore, the neurotransmitter must be removed from the synaptic cleft. There are three main mechanisms to accomplish this goal. First, neurotransmitters can be broken down by enzymatic reactions. The breakdown of **acetylcholine** (**ACh**) by *acetylcholinesterase* (AChE), shown in Figure 4.11, is a classic example.

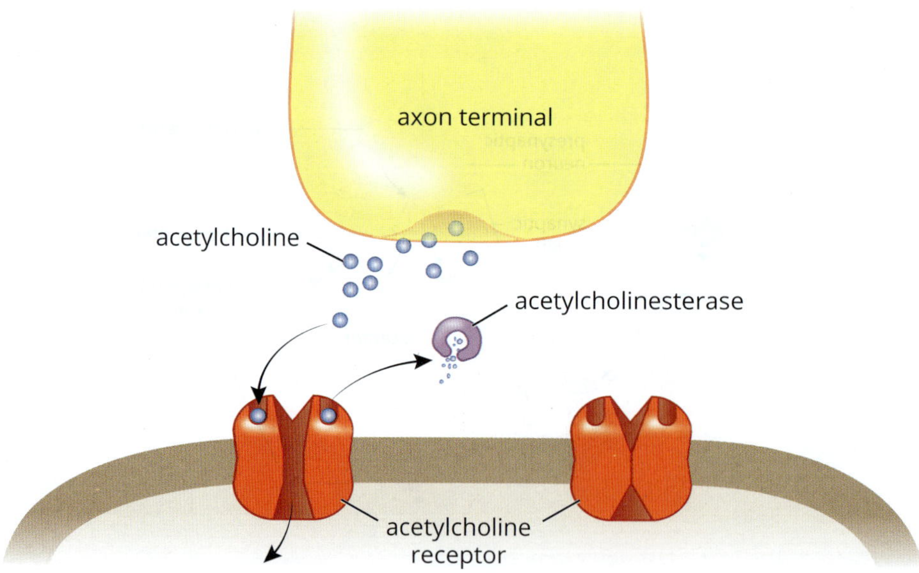

Figure 4.11 Breakdown of a Neurotransmitter by an Enzyme
Acetylcholine (ACh) can be broken down by acetylcholinesterase (AChE).

Second, neurotransmitters can be brought back into the presynaptic neuron using **reuptake transporters**. The reuptake of **serotonin** (**5-HT**), shown in Figure 4.12, is a classic example of this mechanism. **Dopamine** (**DA**) and **norepinephrine** (**NE**) also use reuptake transporters.

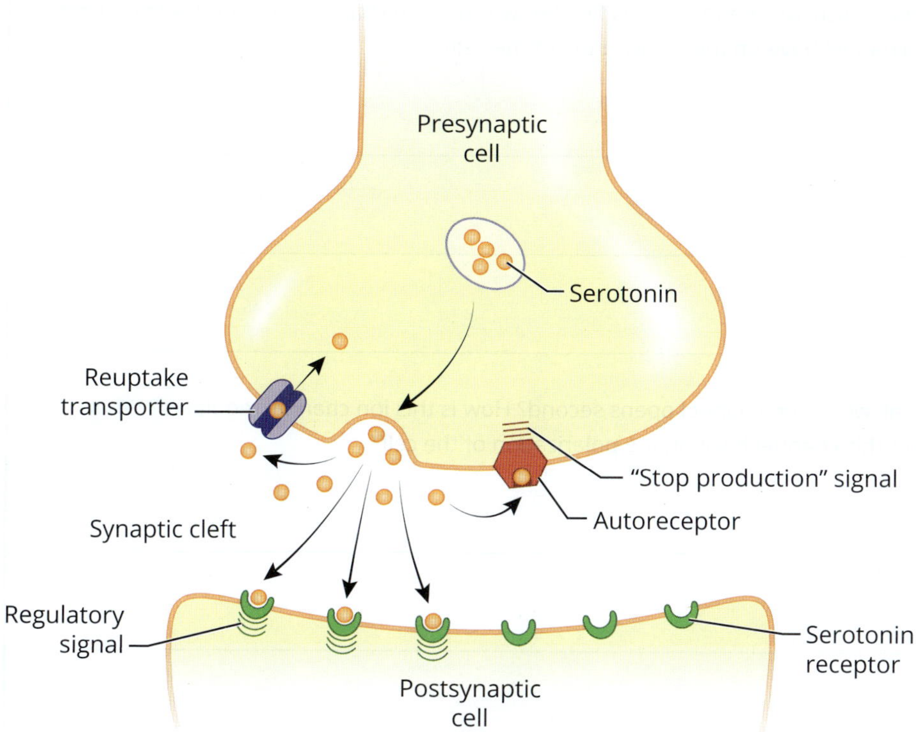

Figure 4.12 Reuptake of a Neurotransmitter
Serotonin (5-HT) can be taken back up by the presynaptic cell; an autoreceptor will signal the presynaptic cell to stop releasing serotonin and start the reuptake process.

REAL WORLD

Many common drugs modify processes that occur in the synapse. For instance, cocaine acts by blocking neuronal reuptake carriers, thus prolonging the action of neurotransmitters in the synapse. There are clinically useful drugs (some of which are used to treat Alzheimer's disease, glaucoma, and myasthenia gravis) that inhibit acetylcholinesterase, thereby elevating synaptic levels of acetylcholine. Nerve gases, which have been used in warfare and terrorism, are extremely potent acetylcholinesterase inhibitors. Nerve gas causes rapid death by preventing the relaxation of skeletal muscle (most importantly, the diaphragm), leading to respiratory arrest.

Third, neurotransmitters may simply diffuse out of the synaptic cleft. **Nitric oxide** (**NO**), a gaseous signaling molecule, fits into this category.

MCAT CONCEPT CHECK 4.2

Before you move on, assess your understanding of the material with these questions.

1. What neural structure initiates the action potential?

____

2. What entity maintains the resting membrane potential? What is the approximate voltage of the resting membrane potential?

____

3. What is the difference between temporal and spatial summation?
   - Temporal summation:

   ____

   - Spatial summation:

   ____

4. During the action potential, which ion channel opens first? How is this ion channel regulated? What effect does the opening of this channel have on the polarization of the cell?
   - Ion channel:
   - Regulation:
   - Effect on polarization:

5. During the action potential, which ion channel opens second? How is this ion channel regulated? What effect does the opening of this channel have on the polarization of the cell?
   - Ion channel:
   - Regulation:
   - Effect on polarization:

6. What is the difference between the absolute and relative refractory period?
   - Absolute refractory period:
   - Relative refractory period:

7. What ion is primarily responsible for the fusion of neurotransmitter-containing vesicles with the nerve terminal membrane?

8. What are the three main methods by which a neurotransmitter's action can be stopped?
   -
   -
   -

4.3 Organization of the Human Nervous System High Yield

LEARNING OBJECTIVES

After Chapter 4.3, you will be able to:

- Classify elements of the nervous system as components of either the central nervous system or the peripheral nervous system
- Differentiate between afferent and efferent neurons
- Describe the functions of the somatic and autonomic nervous systems
- Recall the physiological effects of activating the sympathetic nervous system and the parasympathetic nervous system
- Distinguish between the neural pathways for a monosynaptic and a polysynaptic reflex

The nervous system is a remarkable collection of cells that governs both involuntary and voluntary behavior, while also maintaining **homeostasis**. Functions of the nervous system include:

- Sensation and perception
- Motor function
- Cognition (thinking) and problem solving
- Executive function and planning
- Language comprehension and creation
- Memory
- Emotion and emotional expression
- Balance and coordination
- Regulation of endocrine organs
- Regulation of heart rate, breathing rate, vascular resistance, temperature, and exocrine glands

The human nervous system is a complex web of over 100 billion cells that communicate, coordinate, and regulate signals for the rest of the body. Action occurs when the body can react to external stimuli using the nervous system. In this section, we will look at the nervous system and its basic organization.

Note: Much of the information contained in this section is also discussed in Chapter 1 of MCAT Behavioral Sciences Review.

Central and Peripheral Nervous Systems

Generally speaking, there are three kinds of nerve cells in the nervous system: sensory neurons, motor neurons, and interneurons. **Sensory neurons** (also known as **afferent neurons**) transmit sensory information from sensory receptors to the spinal cord and brain. **Motor neurons** (also known as **efferent neurons**) transmit motor information from the brain and spinal cord to muscles and glands. **Interneurons** are found between other neurons and are the most numerous of the three types. Interneurons are located predominantly in the brain and spinal cord and are often linked to reflexive behavior.

MNEMONIC

Afferent neurons **a**scend in the spinal cord toward the brain; **e**fferent neurons **e**xit the spinal cord on their way to the rest of the body.

Different types of information require different types of processing. Processing of stimuli and response generation may happen at the level of the spinal cord, or may require input from the brainstem or cerebral cortex. Reflexes, discussed later in this section, only require processing at the level of the spinal cord. For example, when a reflex hammer hits the patellar tendon, the sensory information goes to the spinal cord, where a motor signal is sent to the quadriceps muscles, causing the leg to jerk forward at the knee. No input from the brain is required. However, some scenarios require input from the brain or brainstem. When this happens, **supraspinal** circuits are used.

Let's turn to the overall structure of the human nervous system, which is diagrammed in Figure 4.13.

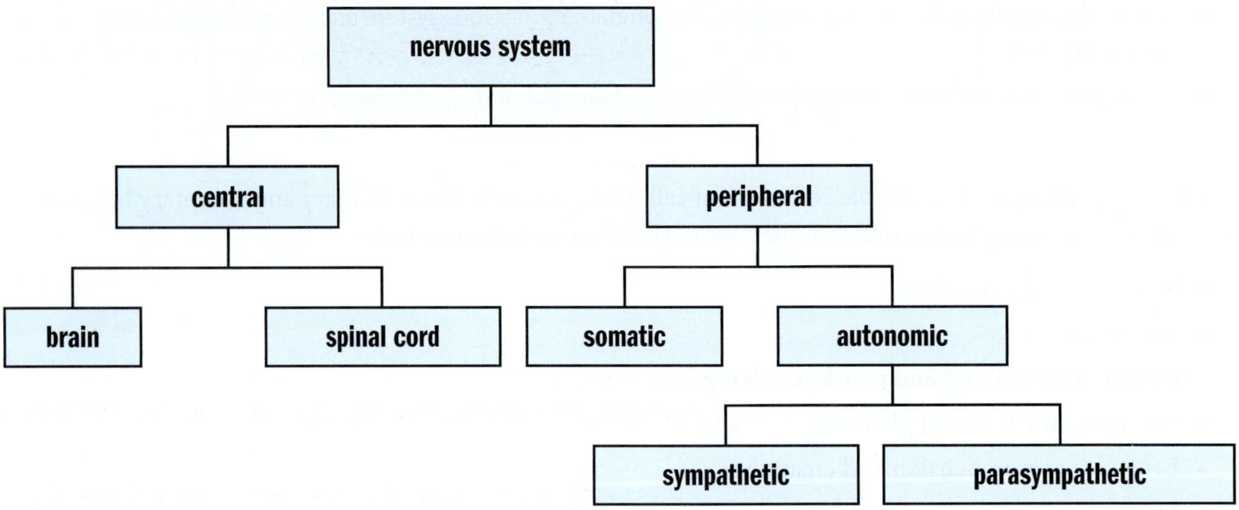

Figure 4.13 Major Divisions of the Nervous System

The nervous system can be broadly divided into two primary components: the central and peripheral nervous systems. The **central nervous system (CNS)** is composed of the brain and spinal cord. The brain consists of white matter and grey matter. The **white matter** consists of axons encased in myelin sheaths. The **grey matter** consists of unmyelinated cell bodies and dendrites. In the brain, the white matter lies deeper than the grey matter. At the base of the brain is the brainstem, which is largely responsible for basic life functions such as breathing. Note that the lobes of the brain and major brain structures are discussed in Chapter 1 of *MCAT Behavioral Sciences Review*.

The spinal cord extends downward from the brainstem and can be divided into four regions: **cervical**, **thoracic**, **lumbar**, and **sacral**. Almost all of the structures below the neck receive sensory and motor innervation from the spinal cord. The spinal cord is protected by the **vertebral column**, which transmits nerves at the space between adjacent vertebrae. Like the brain, the spinal cord also consists of white and grey matter. The white matter lies on the outside of the cord, and the grey matter is deep within it. The axons of motor and sensory neurons are in the spinal cord. The sensory neurons bring information in from the periphery and enter on the dorsal (back) side of the spinal cord. The cell bodies of these sensory neurons are found in the **dorsal root ganglia**. Motor neurons exit the spinal cord ventrally, or on the side closest to the front of the body. The structure of the spinal cord can be seen in Figure 4.14.

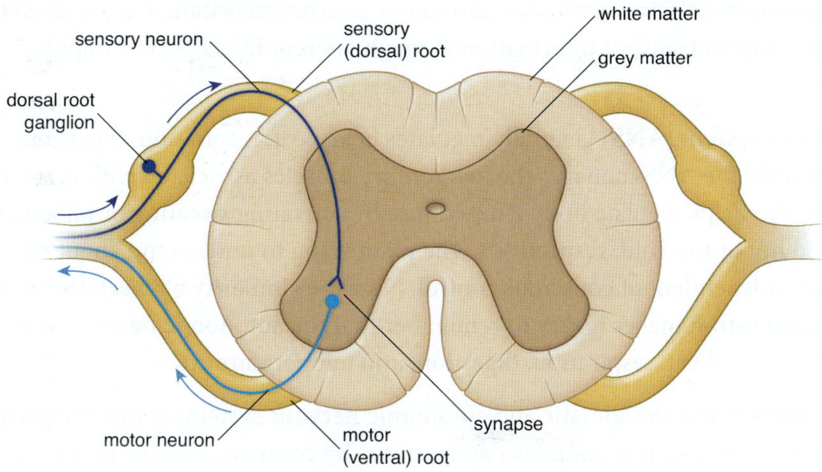

Figure 4.14 The Spinal Cord
Sensory neurons transmit information about pain, temperature, and vibration up to the brain and have cell bodies in the dorsal root ganglia toward the back of the spinal cord; the motor neurons run from the brain along the opposite side of the spinal cord and in the ventral root to control movements of skeletal muscle and glandular secretions.

The **peripheral nervous system** (**PNS**), in contrast, is made up of nerve tissue and fibers outside the brain and spinal cord, including all 31 pairs of spinal nerves and 10 of the 12 pairs of cranial nerves (the olfactory and optic nerves are technically outgrowths of the central nervous system). The PNS thus connects the CNS to the rest of the body and can itself be subdivided into the somatic and autonomic nervous systems, as shown in Figure 4.15.

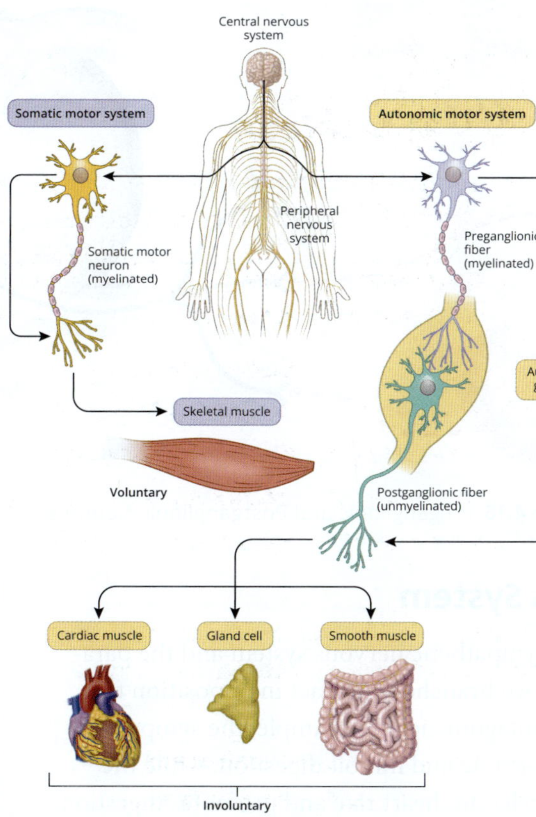

Figure 4.15 The Somatic Nervous System and the Autonomic Nervous System

The **somatic nervous system** consists of sensory and motor neurons distributed throughout the skin, joints, and muscles. Sensory neurons transmit information through afferent fibers. Motor impulses, in contrast, travel along efferent fibers.

The **autonomic nervous system** (**ANS**) generally regulates heartbeat, respiration, digestion, and glandular secretions. In other words, the ANS manages the involuntary muscles associated with many internal organs and glands. The ANS also helps regulate body temperature by activating sweating or piloerection, depending on whether we are too hot or too cold, respectively. The main thing to understand about these functions is that they are automatic, or independent of conscious control. Note the similarity between the words autonomic and automatic. This association makes it easy to remember that the autonomic nervous system manages automatic functions such as heartbeat, respiration, digestion, and temperature control.

One primary difference between the somatic and autonomic nervous systems is that the peripheral component of the autonomic nervous system contains two neurons. By contrast, a motor neuron in the somatic nervous system goes directly from the spinal cord to the muscle without synapsing. In the autonomic nervous system, two neurons work in series to transmit messages from the spinal cord. As demonstrated in Figure 4.16, the first neuron is known as the **preganglionic neuron**, whereas the second is the **postganglionic neuron**. The soma of the preganglionic neuron is in the CNS, and its axon travels to a ganglion in the PNS. Here it synapses on the cell body of the postganglionic neuron, which then stimulates the target tissue.

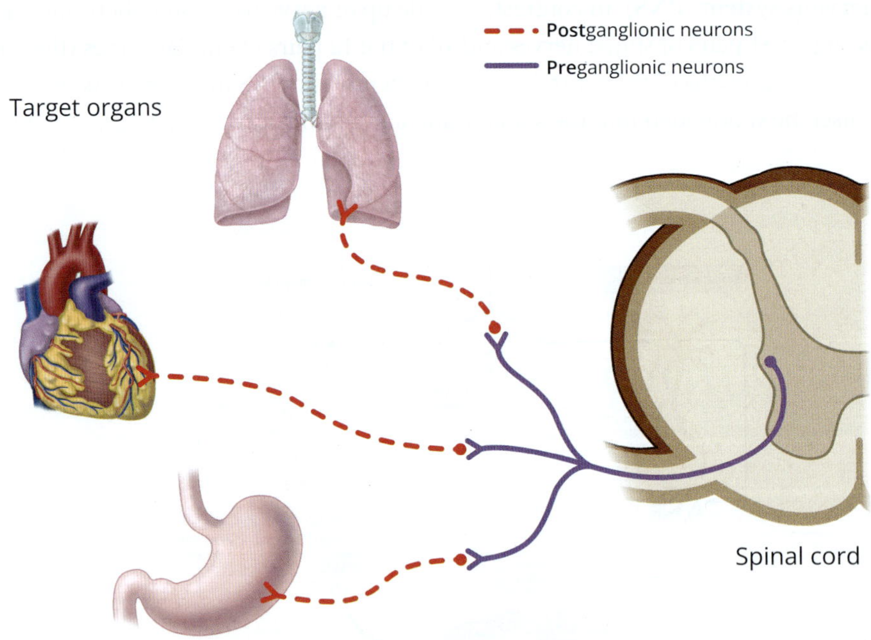

Figure 4.16 Preganglionic and Postganglionic Neurons

The Autonomic Nervous System

The ANS has two subdivisions: the sympathetic nervous system and the parasympathetic nervous system. These two branches often act in opposition to one another, meaning that they are antagonistic. For example, the sympathetic nervous system acts to accelerate heart rate and inhibit digestion, while the parasympathetic nervous system decelerates heart rate and promotes digestion.

KEY CONCEPT

The first neuron in the autonomic nervous system is called the preganglionic neuron. The second neuron is the postganglionic neuron.

The main role of the **parasympathetic nervous system** is to conserve energy. It is associated with resting and sleeping states and acts to reduce heart rate and constrict the bronchi. The parasympathetic nervous system is also responsible for managing digestion by increasing peristalsis and exocrine secretions. Acetylcholine is the neurotransmitter responsible for parasympathetic responses in the body and is released by both preganglionic and postganglionic neurons. The vagus nerve (cranial nerve X) is responsible for much of the parasympathetic innervation of the thoracic and abdominal cavity. The functions of the parasympathetic nervous system are summarized in Figure 4.17.

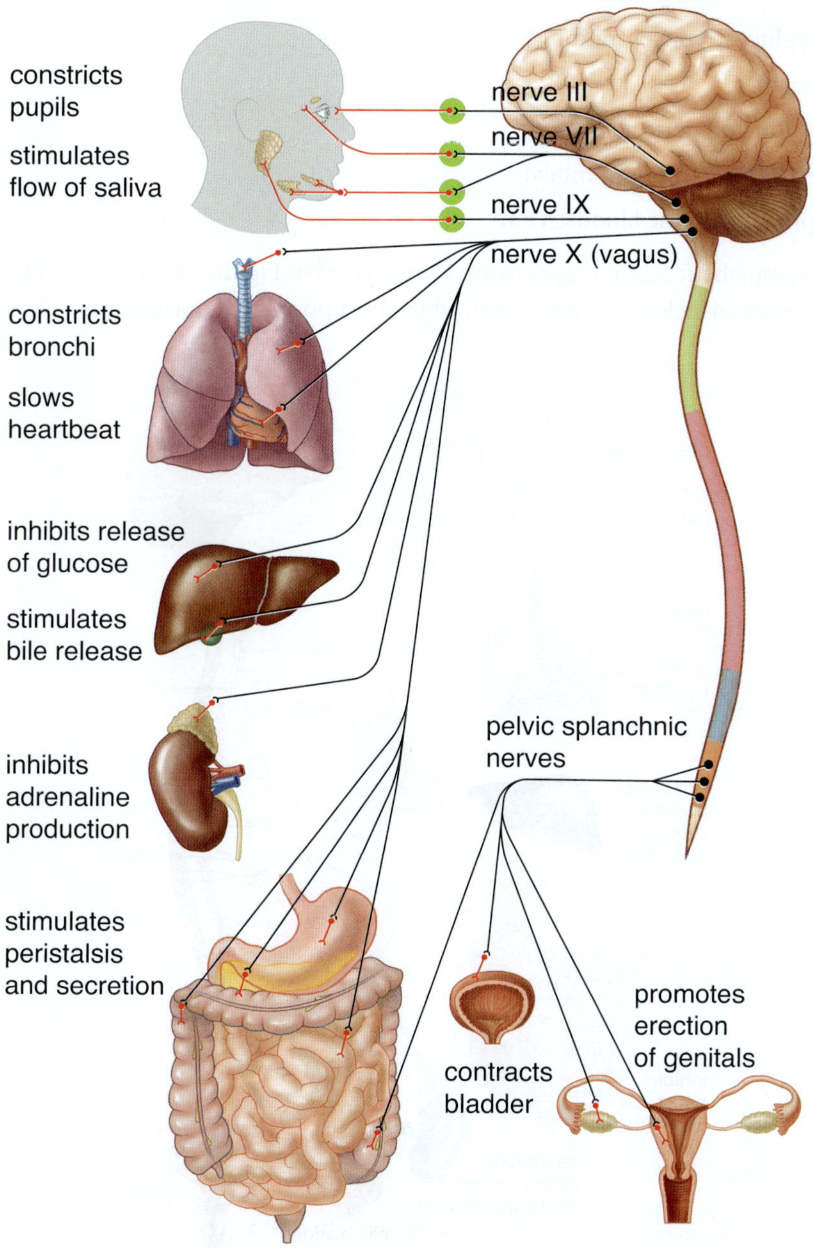

Figure 4.17 Functions of the Parasympathetic Nervous System

In contrast, the **sympathetic nervous system** is activated by stress. This can include everything from a mild stressor, such as keeping up with school or work deadlines, to emergencies that mean the difference between life and death. The sympathetic nervous system is closely associated with rage and fear reactions, also known as "fight-or-flight" reactions. When activated, the sympathetic nervous system:

- Increases heart rate
- Redistributes blood to muscles of locomotion
- Increases blood glucose concentration
- Relaxes the bronchi
- Decreases digestion and peristalsis
- Dilates the eyes to maximize light intake
- Releases epinephrine into the bloodstream

MNEMONIC

Sympathetic and parasympathetic nervous systems:

- Sympathetic: "**fight**-or-**flight**"
- Parasympathetic: "**rest**-and-**digest**"

The functions of the sympathetic nervous system are summarized in Figure 4.18. In the sympathetic nervous system, preganglionic neurons release acetylcholine, while most postganglionic neurons release norepinephrine.

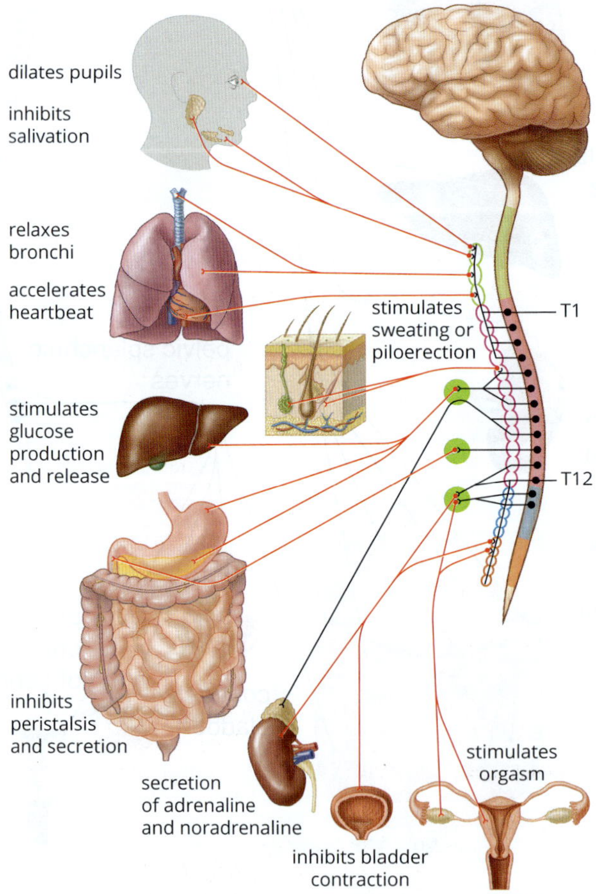

Figure 4.18 Functions of the Sympathetic Nervous System

Reflexes

Neural circuits called **reflex arcs** control reflexive behavior. For example, consider what occurs when someone steps on a nail. Receptors in the foot detect pain, and the pain signal is transmitted by sensory neurons up to the spinal cord. At that point, the sensory neurons connect with interneurons, which can then relay pain impulses up to the brain. Rather than wait for the brain to send out a signal, interneurons in the spinal cord can also send signals to the muscles of both legs directly, causing the individual to withdraw the foot with pain while supporting with the other foot. The original sensory information still makes its way up to the brain; however, by the time it arrives there, the muscles have already responded to the pain, thanks to the reflex arc. There are two types of reflex arcs: monosynaptic and polysynaptic.

KEY CONCEPT

Consider the purpose of reflexes. Although it may be amusing to watch your leg jump when a doctor tests your knee-jerk reflex, there is a more functional reason why this response occurs. The stretch on the patellar tendon makes the body think that the muscle may be getting overstretched. In response, the muscle contracts in order to prevent injury.

Monosynaptic

In a **monosynaptic reflex arc**, there is a single synapse between the sensory neuron that receives the stimulus and the motor neuron that responds to it. A classic example is the **knee-jerk reflex**, shown in Figure 4.19. When the patellar tendon is stretched, information travels up the sensory (afferent, presynaptic) neuron to the spinal cord, where it interfaces with the motor (efferent, postsynaptic) neuron that causes contraction of the quadriceps muscles. The net result is extension of the leg, which lessens the tension on the patellar tendon. Note that the reflex is simply a feedback loop and a response to potential injury. If the patellar tendon or quadriceps muscles are stretched too far, they may tear, damaging the knee joint. Thus, the reflex serves to protect the muscles.

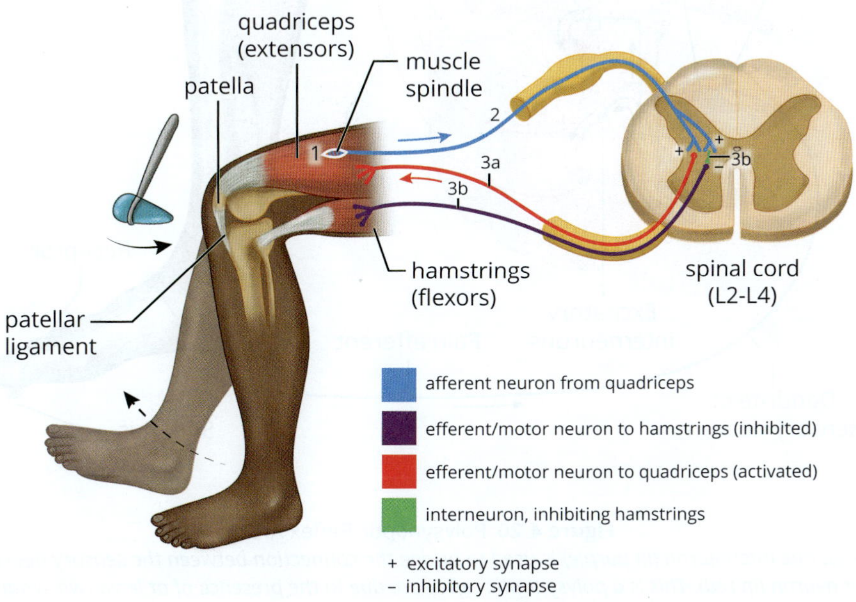

Figure 4.19 The Knee-Jerk Reflex
The knee-jerk or knee extension reflex may be elicited by swiftly stretching the patellar tendon with a reflex hammer.

Polysynaptic

In a **polysynaptic reflex arc**, there is at least one interneuron between the sensory and motor neurons. A real-life example is the reaction to stepping on a nail described earlier, which involves the **withdrawal reflex**. The extremity with which one steps on the nail will be stimulated to flex, using the hip muscles and hamstring muscles, pulling the foot away from the nail. This is a monosynaptic reflex, similar to the knee-jerk reflex described previously. However, if the person is to maintain balance, the other foot must be planted firmly on the ground. For this to occur, the motor neuron that controls the quadriceps muscles in the opposite limb must be stimulated, extending it. Interneurons in the spinal cord provide the connections from the incoming sensory information to the motor neurons in the supporting limb. This pathway is illustrated in Figure 4.20. Note the color-coding of the different sets of neurons: sensory neurons in blue, interneurons in purple, and motor neurons in red.

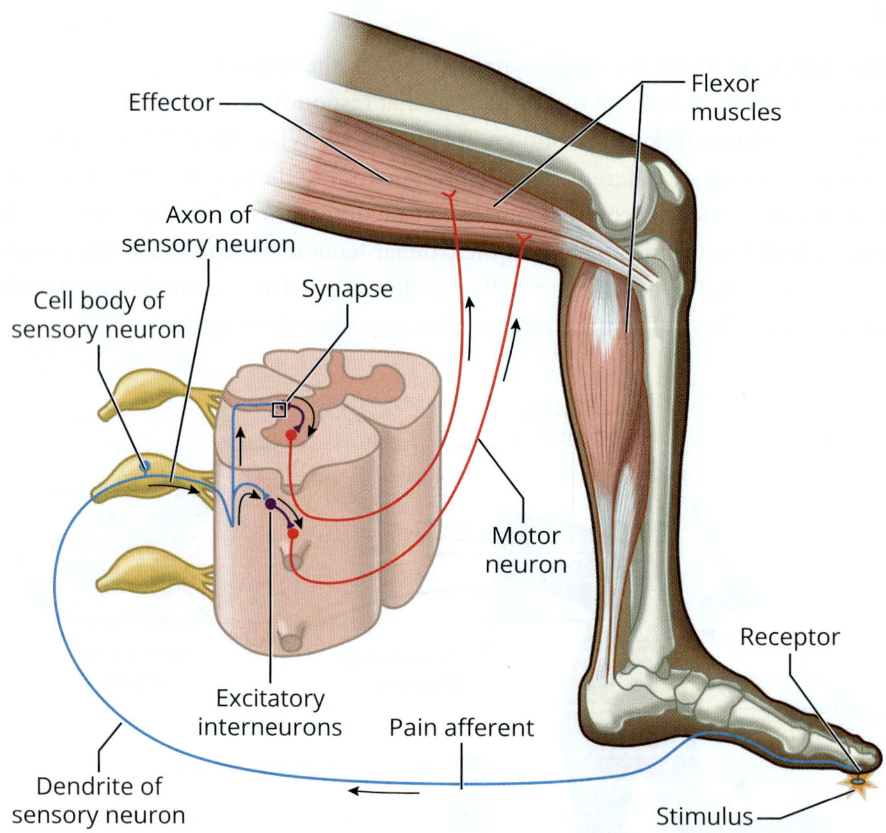

Figure 4.20 Polysynaptic Reflex Arc
The presence of at least one interneuron (in purple) is used to bridge the connection between the sensory neuron (in blue) and the motor neuron (in red). This is a polysynaptic reflex arc due to the presence of at least two synapses.

MCAT CONCEPT CHECK 4.3

Before you move on, assess your understanding of the material with these questions.

1. What parts of the nervous system are in the central nervous system (CNS)? Peripheral nervous system (PNS)?
   - CNS:

   - PNS:

   ---

2. What do afferent neurons do? Efferent neurons?
   - Afferent:

   - Efferent:

   ---

3. What functions are accomplished by the somatic nervous system? The autonomic nervous system?
   - Somatic:

   - Autonomic:

   ---

4. What are the effects of the sympathetic nervous system? The parasympathetic nervous system?
   - Sympathetic:

   - Parasympathetic:

   ---

5. What is the pathway of neural impulses in a monosynaptic reflex? In a polysynaptic reflex?
   - Monosynaptic reflex:

   - Polysynaptic reflex:

Conclusion

The nervous system is one of the most fascinating and complex systems of the human body; millions upon millions of cells allow for appropriate interactions in the everyday world. It is the seat of personality and, ultimately, the system that makes you *you*. In medical school, your courses on neuroscience will go into astounding detail about the nervous system, including the circuits that govern sensations such as pain and temperature, and circuits that allow your body to move and function.

In this chapter, we explored the nervous system at both the cellular and organizational level. Neurons are the primary cells of the nervous system, propagating impulses through both electrical and chemical means—action potentials and synaptic transmission, respectively. Neurons can be grouped together to form nerves, which are the primary organizational structures in one major branch of the nervous system, the peripheral nervous system. The central nervous system consists of the brain and spinal cord. The peripheral nervous system can be subdivided into the somatic and autonomic nervous systems, the latter of which can be further subdivided into the sympathetic and parasympathetic nervous systems.

The nervous system is heavily tested on the MCAT because it plays a role in the function of almost every other major organ system. Neurons cause muscles to move and digestive structures to carry food along through peristalsis, and they regulate breathing rate, heart rate, and glandular secretions. The nervous system is not the only system that has such a profound effect throughout the body, however. The endocrine system, which we will explore in the next chapter, serves a similar role—but through chemical messengers carried in the blood called hormones.

GO ONLINE

You've reviewed the content, now test your knowledge and critical thinking skills by completing a test-like passage set in your online resources!

CONCEPT SUMMARY

Cells of the Nervous System

- **Neurons** are highly specialized cells responsible for the conduction of impulses.
- Neurons communicate using both electrical and chemical forms of communication.
  - Electrical communication occurs via ion exchange and the generation of membrane potentials down the length of the axon.
  - Chemical communication occurs via neurotransmitter release from the presynaptic cell and the binding of these neurotransmitters to the postsynaptic cell.
- Neurons consist of many different parts.
  - **Dendrites** are appendages that receive signals from other cells.
  - The cell body or **soma** is the location of the nucleus as well as organelles such as the endoplasmic reticulum and ribosomes.
  - The **axon hillock** is where the cell body transitions to the axon, and where action potentials are initiated.
  - The **axon** is a long appendage down which an action potential travels.
  - The **nerve terminal** or **synaptic bouton** is the end of the axon from which neurotransmitters are released.
  - **Nodes of Ranvier** are exposed areas of myelinated axons that permit saltatory conduction.
  - The **synapse** consists of the nerve terminal of the presynaptic neuron, the membrane of the postsynaptic cell, and the space between the two, called the **synaptic cleft**.
- Many axons are coated in **myelin**, an insulating substance that prevents signal loss.
  - Myelin is created by **oligodendrocytes** in the central nervous system and **Schwann cells** in the peripheral nervous system.
  - Myelin prevents dissipation of the neural impulse and crossing of neural impulses from adjacent neurons.
- Individual axons are bundled into **nerves** or **tracts**.
  - A single nerve may carry multiple types of information, including sensory, motor, or both. Tracts contain only one type of information.
  - Cell bodies of neurons of the same type within a nerve cluster together in **ganglia** in the peripheral nervous system.
  - Cell bodies of the individual neurons within a tract cluster together in **nuclei** in the central nervous system.
- **Neuroglia** or **glial cells** are other cells within the nervous system in addition to neurons.
  - **Astrocytes** nourish neurons and form the blood–brain barrier, which controls the transmission of solutes from the bloodstream into nervous tissue.
  - **Ependymal cells** line the ventricles of the brain and produce cerebrospinal fluid, which physically supports the brain and serves as a shock absorber.
  - **Microglia** are phagocytic cells that ingest and break down waste products and pathogens in the central nervous system.
  - Oligodendrocytes (CNS) and Schwann cells (PNS) produce myelin around axons.

Transmission of Neural Impulses

- All neurons exhibit a **resting membrane potential** of approximately −70 mV.
  - Resting potential is maintained using selective permeability of ions as well as the Na^+/K^+ ATPase.
  - The **Na^+/K^+ ATPase** pumps three sodium ions out of the cell for every two potassium ions pumped in.
- Incoming signals can be either excitatory or inhibitory.
  - Excitatory signals cause depolarization of the neuron.
  - Inhibitory signals cause hyperpolarization of the neuron.
  - **Temporal summation** refers to the integration of multiple signals near each other in time.
  - **Spatial summation** refers to the addition of multiple signals near each other in space.
- An **action potential** is used to propagate signals down the axon.
  - When enough excitatory stimulation occurs, the cell is **depolarized** to the **threshold voltage** and voltage-gated sodium channels open.
  - Sodium flows into the neuron due to its strong **electrochemical gradient**. This continues depolarizing the neuron.
  - At the peak of the action potential (approximately +35 mV), sodium channels are inactivated and potassium channels open.
  - Potassium flows out of the neuron due to its strong electrochemical gradient, **repolarizing** the cell. Potassium channels stay open long enough to overshoot the resting potential, resulting in a **hyperpolarized** neuron; then, the potassium channels close.
  - The Na^+/K^+ ATPase brings the neuron back to the resting potential and restores the sodium and potassium gradients.
  - While the axon is hyperpolarized, it is in its **refractory period**. During the **absolute refractory period**, the cell is unable to fire another action potential. During the **relative refractory period**, the cell requires a larger than normal stimulus to fire an action potential.
  - The impulse propagates down the length of the axon because the influx of sodium in one segment of the axon brings the subsequent segment of the axon to threshold. The fact that the preceding segment of the axon is in its refractory period means that the action potential can only travel in one direction.
- At the nerve terminal, neurotransmitters are released into the synapse.
  - When the action potential arrives at the nerve terminal, voltage-gated calcium channels open.
  - The influx of calcium causes fusion of vesicles filled with neurotransmitters with the presynaptic membrane, resulting in exocytosis of neurotransmitters into the synaptic cleft.
  - The neurotransmitters bind to receptors on the postsynaptic cell, which may be ligand-gated ion channels or G protein–coupled receptors.
- Neurotransmitters must be cleared from the postsynaptic receptors to stop the propagation of the signal. There are three ways this can happen:
  - The neurotransmitter can be enzymatically broken down.
  - The neurotransmitter can be absorbed back into the presynaptic cell by **reuptake channels**.
  - The neurotransmitter can diffuse out of the synaptic cleft.

Organization of the Human Nervous System

- There are three types of neurons in the nervous system: **motor** (**efferent**) neurons, **interneurons**, and **sensory** (**afferent**) neurons.
- The nervous system is made up of the **central nervous system** (**CNS**: brain and spinal cord) and **peripheral nervous system** (**PNS**: cranial and spinal nerves).
  - In the CNS, **white matter** consists of myelinated axons, and **grey matter** consists of unmyelinated cell bodies and dendrites. In the brain, white matter is deeper than grey matter. In the spinal cord, grey matter is deeper than white matter.
  - The PNS is divided into the **somatic** (voluntary) and **autonomic** (automatic) nervous systems.
  - The autonomic nervous system is further divided into the **parasympathetic** (rest-and-digest) and **sympathetic** (fight-or-flight) branches.
- **Reflex arcs** use the ability of interneurons in the spinal cord to relay information to the source of a stimulus while simultaneously routing it to the brain.
  - In a **monosynaptic reflex arc**, the sensory (afferent, presynaptic) neuron fires directly onto the motor (efferent, postsynaptic) neuron.
  - In a **polysynaptic reflex arc**, the sensory neuron may fire onto a motor neuron as well as interneurons that fire onto other motor neurons.

ANSWERS TO CONCEPT CHECKS

4.1

1. The axon transmits an electrical signal (the action potential) from the soma to the synaptic knob. The axon hillock integrates excitatory and inhibitory signals from the dendrites and fires an action potential if the excitatory signals are strong enough to reach threshold. Dendrites receive incoming signals and carry them to the soma. The myelin sheath acts as insulation around the axon and speeds conduction. The soma is the cell body and contains the nucleus, endoplasmic reticulum, and ribosomes. The synaptic bouton lies at the end of the axon and releases neurotransmitters.
2. A collection of cell bodies in the central nervous system is called a nucleus. In the peripheral nervous system, it is called a ganglion.
3. Astrocytes nourish neurons and form the blood–brain barrier, which helps protect the brain from foreign pathogens gaining entrance. Microglia ingest and break down waste products and pathogens. Disruption of either of these mechanisms would increase susceptibility to a CNS infection.
4. Oligodendrocytes produce myelin in the central nervous system while Schwann cells produce myelin in the peripheral nervous system. Since GBS causes demyelination in the PNS, it can be inferred that Schwann cells are targeted for immune destruction.

4.2

1. The action potential is initiated at the axon hillock.
2. The resting membrane potential is maintained by the Na^+/K^+ATPase at approximately -70 mV.
3. Temporal summation is the integration of multiple signals close to each other in time. Spatial summation is the integration of multiple signals close to each other in space.
4. The sodium channel opens first at threshold (around -50 mV). It is regulated by inactivation, which occurs around $+35$ mV. Inactivation can only be reversed by repolarizing the cell. The opening of the sodium channel causes depolarization.
5. The potassium channel opens second at approximately $+35$ mV. It is regulated by closing at low potentials (slightly below -70 mV). The opening of the potassium channel causes repolarization and, eventually, hyperpolarization.
6. During the absolute refractory period, the cell is unable to fire an action potential regardless of the intensity of a stimulus. During the relative refractory period, the cell can fire an action potential only with a stimulus that is stronger than normal.
7. Calcium is responsible for fusion of neurotransmitter vesicles with the nerve terminal membrane.
8. A neurotransmitter's action can be stopped by enzymatic degradation, reuptake, or diffusion.

4.3

1. The central nervous system includes the brain and spinal cord. The peripheral nervous system includes cranial and spinal nerves and sensory nerves.
2. Afferent (sensory) neurons bring signals from a sensor to the central nervous system. Efferent (motor) neurons bring signals from the central nervous system to an effector.

3. The somatic nervous system is responsible for voluntary actions—most notably, moving muscles. The autonomic nervous system is responsible for involuntary processes like heart rate, bronchial dilation, dilation of the pupils, exocrine gland function, and peristalsis.
4. The sympathetic nervous system promotes a "fight-or-flight" response, with increased heart rate and bronchial dilation, redistribution of blood to locomotor muscles, dilation of the pupils, and slowing of digestive and urinary function. The parasympathetic nervous system promotes "rest-and-digest" functions, slowing heart rate and constricting the bronchi, redistributing blood to the gut, promoting exocrine secretions, constricting the pupils, and promoting peristalsis and urinary function.
5. In a monosynaptic reflex, a sensory (afferent, presynaptic) neuron fires directly onto a motor (efferent, postsynaptic) neuron. In a polysynaptic reflex, a sensory neuron may fire directly onto a motor neuron, but interneurons are used as well. These interneurons fire onto other motor neurons.

SCIENCE MASTERY ASSESSMENT EXPLANATIONS

1. **C**

The polarization of the neuron at rest is the result of an uneven distribution of ions between the inside and outside of the cell. This difference is achieved through the active pumping of ions into and out of the neuron (using the Na^+/K^+ ATPase). Voltage-gated calcium channels are important in the nerve terminal, where the influx of calcium triggers the fusion of vesicles containing neurotransmitters with the membrane, but not in maintaining resting membrane potential.

2. **C**

Myelin is a white lipid-containing material surrounding the axons of many neurons in the central and peripheral nervous systems. It is arranged on the axon discontinuously; the gaps between the segments of myelin are called nodes of Ranvier, eliminating **(B)**. Myelin increases the conduction velocity by insulating segments of the axon so that the membrane is permeable to ions only at the nodes of Ranvier, eliminating **(A)**. The action potential jumps from node to node, a process known as saltatory conduction, eliminating **(D)**. Action potentials are often described as being "all-or-nothing"; the magnitude of the potential difference of an action potential is fixed, regardless of the intensity of the stimulus. Thus, myelin does not affect the magnitude of the potential difference in an action potential, making **(C)** the correct answer.

3. **D**

As in the previous question, the action potential is often described as an all-or-nothing response. This means that, whenever the threshold membrane potential is reached, an action potential with a consistent size and duration is produced. Neuronal information is coded by the frequency and number of action potentials, not the size of the action potential, eliminating **(B)** and **(C)** and making **(D)** the correct answer. Hyperpolarizing (inhibitory) signals are not transmitted to the nerve terminal, eliminating **(A)**.

4. **C**

Nerves are collections of neurons in the peripheral nervous system and may contain multiple types of information (sensory or motor); they contain cell bodies in ganglia. Tracts are collections of neurons in the central nervous system and contain only one type of information; they contain cell bodies in nuclei.

5. **A**

Sensory neurons are considered afferent (carrying signals from the periphery to the central nervous system) and enter the spinal cord on the dorsal side. Motor neurons are considered efferent (carrying signals from the central nervous system to the periphery) and exit the spinal cord on the ventral side.

6. **C**

When a sensory neuron receives a signal that is strong enough to bring it to threshold, one can assume that the receptor becomes depolarized, allowing it to transduce the stimulus to an action potential. The action potential will then be carried by sensory neurons to the central nervous system, where the cell will release neurotransmitters. Therefore, among the given choices, the only incorrect statement is found in **(C)**. If a receptor is stimulated, it will promote the spread of the action potential to postsynaptic sensory neurons in the spinal cord, which can send the signal toward the brain.

7. **B**

When the potential across the axon membrane is more negative than the normal resting potential, the neuron is referred to as hyperpolarized. Hyperpolarization occurs right after an action potential and is caused by excess potassium exiting the neuron.

8. **D**

The somatic division of the peripheral nervous system innervates skeletal muscles and is responsible for voluntary movement. Some of the pathways in this part of the nervous system are reflex arcs, which are reflexive responses to certain stimuli that involve only a sensory and a motor neuron. These neurons synapse in the spinal cord and do not require signaling from the brain. The pathways of the somatic division can involve two, three, or more neurons, depending on the type of signal. The correct answer therefore is **(D)**.

9. **D**

The parasympathetic nervous system governs the "rest-and-digest" response. The parasympathetic nervous system slows the heart rate, decreases blood pressure, promotes bloodflow to the GI tract, and constricts the pupils, among other functions. The sympathetic nervous system governs the fight-or-flight response, including increased heart rate and blood pressure, decreased bloodflow to the digestive tract, and increased bloodflow to the muscles. **(D)** is the only answer choice that represents a function of the parasympathetic nervous system.

10. **A**

Acetylcholine is the neurotransmitter released by the preganglionic neuron in both the sympathetic and parasympathetic nervous systems. The postganglionic neuron in the sympathetic nervous system usually releases norepinephrine, while the postganglionic neuron in the parasympathetic nervous system releases acetylcholine.

11. **B**

Neurons contain very specialized structures, including dendrites, axons, and the axon hillock. However, neurons are still cells and must carry out cellular functions including protein synthesis. The cell body or soma contains the nucleus, endoplasmic reticulum, and ribosomes.

12. **B**

First, consider the function of voltage-gated calcium channels. When the nerve terminal depolarizes, voltage-gated calcium channels open, allowing for influx of calcium. This influx of calcium triggers fusion of the synaptic vesicles containing neurotransmitters with the membrane of the neuron at the nerve terminal. This allows for exocytosis of the neurotransmitters into the synapse. If a disease blocked the influx of calcium, there would be no release of neurotransmitters. A lack of neurotransmitters means that the neuron cannot send excitatory signals. Thus, any symptoms resulting from this disease would be due to an inability of neurons to transmit excitatory signals to the muscle. If neurons cannot communicate, flaccid paralysis may be one of the results.

13. **B**

Some neurons require multiple instances of excitatory transmission to be brought to threshold. These excitatory signals may be close to each other in time (temporal) or in space (spatial); either way, this pattern of excitation is termed summation.

14. **A**

Schwann cells are responsible for myelination of cells in the peripheral nervous system. Thus, the central nervous system is unlikely to be affected. The peripheral nervous system includes the somatic nervous system and the autonomic nervous system. The autonomic nervous system is composed of both the parasympathetic and sympathetic nervous systems. Thus, **(A)** is the right answer.

15. **C**

The dorsal root ganglion contains cell bodies of sensory neurons only. If a dorsal root ganglion is disrupted at a certain level, there will be a loss of sensation at that level. Furthermore, reflexes rely on sensory afferents that are part of the dorsal root ganglion. As a result, reflex arcs will also be affected.

GO ONLINE
Consult your online resources for additional practice.

SHARED CONCEPTS

Behavioral Sciences Chapter 1
Biology and Behavior

Behavioral Sciences Chapter 2
Sensation and Perception

Biochemistry Chapter 3
Nonenzymatic Protein Function and Protein Analysis

Biochemistry Chapter 8
Biological Membranes

Biology Chapter 11
The Musculoskeletal System

General Chemistry Chapter 12
Electrochemistry

CHAPTER 5

THE ENDOCRINE SYSTEM

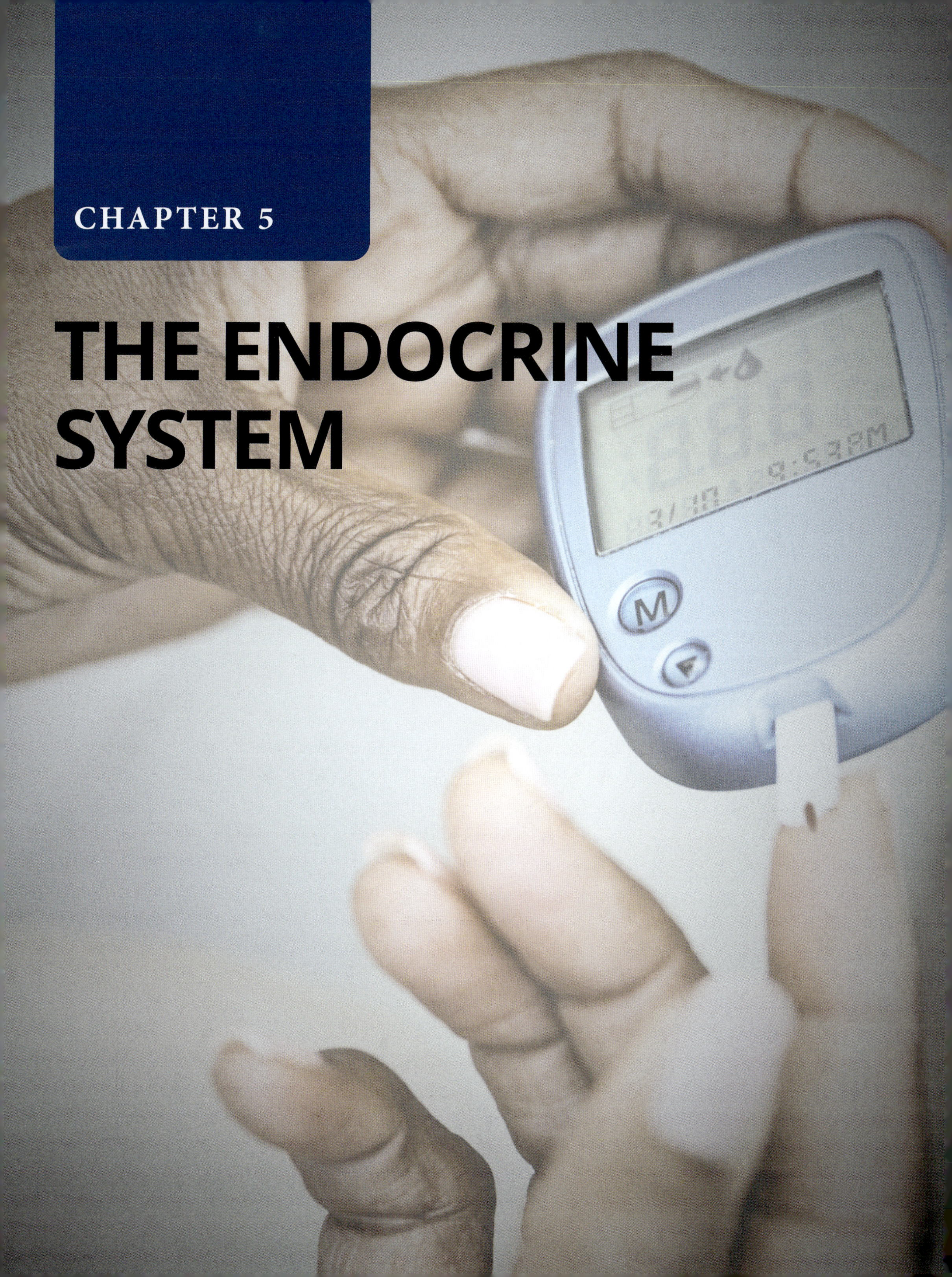

SCIENCE MASTERY ASSESSMENT

Every pre-med knows this feeling: there is so much content I have to know for the MCAT! How do I know what to do first or what's important?

While the high-yield badges throughout this book will help you identify the most important topics, this Science Mastery Assessment is another tool in your MCAT prep arsenal. This quiz (which can also be taken in your online resources) and the guidance below will help ensure that you are spending the appropriate amount of time on this chapter based on your personal strengths and weaknesses. Don't worry though—skipping something now does not mean you'll never study it. Later on in your prep, as you complete full-length tests, you'll uncover specific pieces of content that you need to review and can come back to these chapters as appropriate.

How to Use This Assessment

If you answer 0–7 questions correctly:

Spend about 1 hour to read this chapter in full and take limited notes throughout. Follow up by reviewing **all** quiz questions to ensure that you now understand how to solve each one.

If you answer 8–11 questions correctly:

Spend 20–40 minutes reviewing the quiz questions. Beginning with the questions you missed, read and take notes on the corresponding subchapters. For questions you answered correctly, ensure your thinking matches that of the explanation and you understand why each choice was correct or incorrect.

If you answer 12–15 questions correctly:

Spend less than 20 minutes reviewing all questions from the quiz. If you missed any, then include a quick read-through of the corresponding subchapters, or even just the relevant content within a subchapter, as part of your question review. For questions you answered correctly, ensure your thinking matches that of the explanation and review the Concept Summary at the end of the chapter.

1. Which of the following associations between a hormone and its category is INCORRECT?
   - **A.** Aldosterone—mineralocorticoid
   - **B.** Testosterone—cortical sex hormone
   - **C.** ADH—mineralocorticoid
   - **D.** Cortisone—glucocorticoid

2. Which of the following hormones directly stimulates a target tissue that is NOT an endocrine organ?
   - **A.** ACTH
   - **B.** TSH
   - **C.** LH
   - **D.** GH

3. Increased synthetic activity of the parathyroid glands would lead to:
   - **A.** an increase in renal calcium reabsorption.
   - **B.** a decrease in the rate of bone resorption.
   - **C.** a decrease in basal metabolic rate.
   - **D.** a decrease in blood glucose concentration.

4. Which of the following best describes the structure and mechanism of action of a peptide hormone?
   - **A.** Cholesterol derivative that binds to a receptor on the cell surface
   - **B.** Chain of amino acids that signals through a second messenger
   - **C.** Chain of amino acids that directly binds to DNA to alter gene expression
   - **D.** Cholesterol derivative that binds to an intracellular receptor and alters gene expression

5. Iodine deficiency may result in:
   - **A.** galactorrhea.
   - **B.** cretinism.
   - **C.** gigantism.
   - **D.** hyperthyroidism.

6. A patient has a very high TSH level. Which of the following would NOT cause a high TSH level?
   - **A.** Autoimmune destruction of thyroid cells that produce T_3 and T_4
   - **B.** A tumor in the hypothalamus that secretes high levels of TRH
   - **C.** High levels of T_4 from thyroid replacement medications
   - **D.** Cancerous growth of parafollicular cells in the thyroid, destroying other cell types in the organ

7. Testing of a novel hormone indicates nuclear localization and a composition of carbon, hydrogen, and oxygen. Based on these findings, how would this hormone most likely be classified?
   - **A.** Peptide hormone
   - **B.** Steroid hormone
   - **C.** Amino acid derivative
   - **D.** Direct hormone

8. Which of the following is true regarding pancreatic somatostatin?
   - **A.** Its secretion is increased by low blood glucose.
   - **B.** It is always inhibitory.
   - **C.** It is regulated by cortisol levels.
   - **D.** It stimulates insulin and glucagon secretion.

9. Destruction of all β-cells in the pancreas would cause:
   - **A.** glucagon secretion to stop and an increase in blood glucose concentration.
   - **B.** glucagon secretion to stop and a decrease in blood glucose concentration.
   - **C.** insulin secretion to stop and an increase in blood glucose concentration.
   - **D.** insulin secretion to stop and a decrease in blood glucose concentration.

10. Which of the following is FALSE regarding aldosterone regulation?

- **A.** Renin converts the plasma protein angiotensinogen to angiotensin I.
- **B.** Angiotensin II stimulates the adrenal cortex to secrete aldosterone.
- **C.** Angiotensin I is converted to angiotensin II by angiotensin-converting enzyme.
- **D.** A decrease in blood oxygen concentrations stimulates renin production.

11. A scientist discovers a new hormone that is relatively large in size and triggers the conversion of ATP to cAMP. Which of the following best describes the type of hormone that was discovered?

- **A.** Amino acid–derivative hormone
- **B.** Peptide hormone
- **C.** Steroid hormone
- **D.** Tropic hormone

12. A patient presents with muscle weakness, slow movement, and calcium deposits in some tissues. A blood test reveals very low calcium levels in the blood. Administration of which of the following would be an appropriate treatment for the blood test findings?

- **A.** Calcitonin
- **B.** Parathyroid hormone
- **C.** Aldosterone
- **D.** Thymosin

13. Oxytocin and antidiuretic hormone are:

- **A.** peptide hormones produced and released by the pituitary.
- **B.** steroid hormones produced and released by the pituitary.
- **C.** peptide hormones produced by the hypothalamus and released by the pituitary.
- **D.** steroid hormones produced by the hypothalamus and released by the pituitary.

14. Excessive levels of dopamine in the brain are associated with psychosis. Accordingly, many antipsychotic medications block dopamine receptors. Which of the following effects may be seen in an individual taking antipsychotics?

- **A.** Increased secretion of growth hormone
- **B.** Decreased secretion of growth hormone
- **C.** Increased secretion of prolactin
- **D.** Decreased secretion of prolactin

15. A genotypically female infant is born with ambiguous genitalia. Soon after birth, the infant suffers from hyponatremia, or low blood concentrations of sodium. Which endocrine organ is most likely to be affected?

- **A.** Hypothalamus
- **B.** Pituitary
- **C.** Kidneys
- **D.** Adrenal cortex

Answer Key

1. **C** (See section 5.2)
2. **D** (See section 5.2)
3. **A** (See section 5.2)
4. **B** (See section 5.1)
5. **B** (See section 5.2)
6. **C** (See section 5.2)
7. **B** (See section 5.1)
8. **B** (See section 5.2)
9. **C** (See section 5.2)
10. **D** (See section 5.2)
11. **B** (See section 5.1)
12. **B** (See section 5.2)
13. **C** (See section 5.2)
14. **C** (See section 5.2)
15. **D** (See section 5.2)

The relevant section of the chapter to review for each question is given in parentheses after the correct answer. Detailed explanations can be found at the end of the chapter.

CHAPTER 5

THE ENDOCRINE SYSTEM

In This Chapter

CHAPTER PROFILE

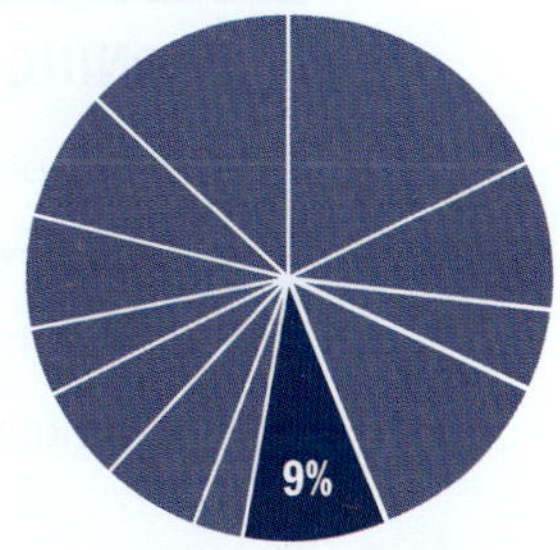

The content in this chapter should be relevant to about 9% of all questions about biology on the MCAT.

This chapter covers material from the following AAMC content categories:

3A: Structure and functions of the nervous and endocrine systems and ways in which these systems coordinate the organ systems

3B: Structure and integrative functions of the main organ systems

Introduction

The human body consists of many trillions of cells that must work together to sustain life. In order to work effectively, fuel resources must be conserved or used appropriately, such as when responding to stressful situations. In addition, organs must be able to communicate with the brain to cause changes in behavior and physiology to maintain homeostasis. As the messengers in the endocrine system, hormones play an essential role in this communication. For example, the pancreas produces insulin and glucagon. Insulin induces the transport of glucose into organs and the storage of excess glucose when blood glucose concentrations are high. Conversely, glucagon triggers the release of sugar stores which raises blood glucose concentration. Working together, these hormones ensure that there are adequate levels of glucose for organ function, but that glucose levels are not so high as to cause damage to organ systems.

Diabetes mellitus is one of the most common diseases in the United States and a major cause of morbidity and mortality. Type 1 diabetes mellitus is an autoimmune disease in which insulin-producing cells in the islets of Langerhans are destroyed. Type 2 diabetes mellitus is caused by end-organ insensitivity to insulin. In both cases, blood glucose concentrations rise to dangerous levels (sometimes up to ten times the normal concentration), which can cause significant damage to organs, including the retina of the eye, the glomeruli of the kidneys, the coronary vessels of the heart and cerebral vessels of the brain, and peripheral nerves. Left untreated (or, to be frank, even if treated in many cases), diabetes can lead to blindness, kidney failure, heart attacks, strokes, and limb amputations.

Regardless of the field you enter, you will spend a significant amount of time working with diabetic patients and will have to think about the effects of this disease on other conditions and their treatment.

In this chapter, we will explore the different types of hormones and how they work. We'll survey the various endocrine organs and discuss the hormones each one produces. This is an extremely high-yield chapter: the MCAT frequently tests not only the makeup of the endocrine system (hormones and their functions), but also the processes of the endocrine system (feedback loops and their regulation). Return to this chapter frequently; a thorough knowledge of this system will definitely pay off on Test Day.

5.1 Mechanisms of Hormone Action High Yield

LEARNING OBJECTIVES

After Chapter 5.1, you will be able to:

- Compare and contrast the traits and actions of peptide vs. steroid hormones
- Recall the process for synthesizing amino acid–derivative hormones
- Distinguish between direct and tropic hormones

The endocrine system consists of organs, known as **glands**, that secrete hormones. **Hormones** are signaling molecules that are secreted directly into the bloodstream to distant target tissues. At target tissues, hormones bind to receptors, inducing a change in gene expression or cellular functioning. Not all hormones share the same structure and function. In order to understand how each hormone functions, it is first important to understand basic hormone structure.

Classification of Hormones by Chemical Structure

Hormones can be subdivided into categories based on different criteria. First, hormones can be classified by their chemical identities. Hormones can be **peptides**, **steroids**, or **amino acid derivatives**.

Peptide Hormones

Peptide hormones are made up of amino acids, ranging in size from quite small (such as anti-diuretic hormone, ADH, which is 9 amino acids long) to relatively large (such as calcitonin in Figure 5.1, which is 32 amino acids long). Peptide hormones are all derived from larger precursor polypeptides that are cleaved during posttranslational modification. These smaller units are transported to the Golgi apparatus for further modifications that activate the hormones and direct them to the correct locations in the cell. Such hormones are released by exocytosis after being packaged into vesicles.

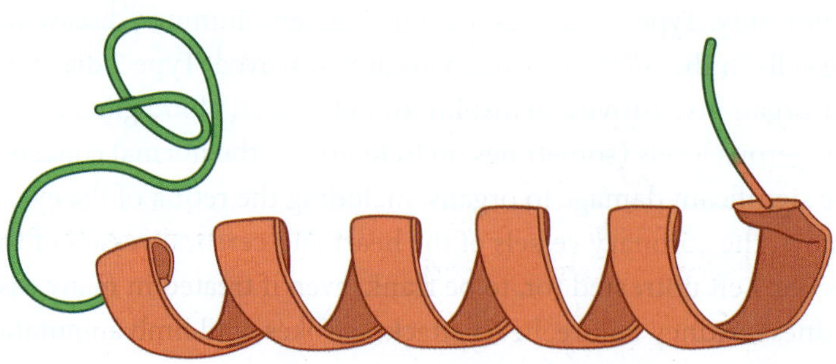

Figure 5.1 A Peptide Hormone: Calcitonin

Because peptide hormones are charged and cannot pass through the plasma membrane, they must bind to an extracellular receptor. The peptide hormone is considered the **first messenger**; it binds to the receptor and triggers the transmission of a second signal, known as the **second messenger**. There are many different receptor subtypes, and the type of receptor determines what happens once the hormone has stimulated the receptor.

The connection between the hormone at the surface and the effect brought about by second messengers within the cell is known as a **signaling cascade**. At each step, there is the possibility of **amplification**. For example, one hormone molecule may bind to multiple receptors before it is degraded. Also, each receptor may activate multiple enzymes, each of which will trigger the production of large quantities of second messengers. Thus, each step can result in an increase in signal intensity. Some common second messengers are **cyclic adenosine monophosphate** (**cAMP**), **inositol triphosphate** (**IP_3**), and calcium. The activation of a G protein–coupled receptor is shown in Figure 5.2. In this system, the binding of a peptide hormone triggers the receptor to either activate or inhibit an enzyme called ***adenylate cyclase***, raising or lowering the levels of cAMP accordingly. cAMP can bind to intracellular targets, such as *protein kinase A*, which phosphorylates transcription factors like cAMP response element-binding protein (CREB) to exert the hormone's ultimate effect. Keep in mind that protein kinase A can modify other enzymes as well as transcription factors, and therefore it can have a rapid or slow effect on the cell.

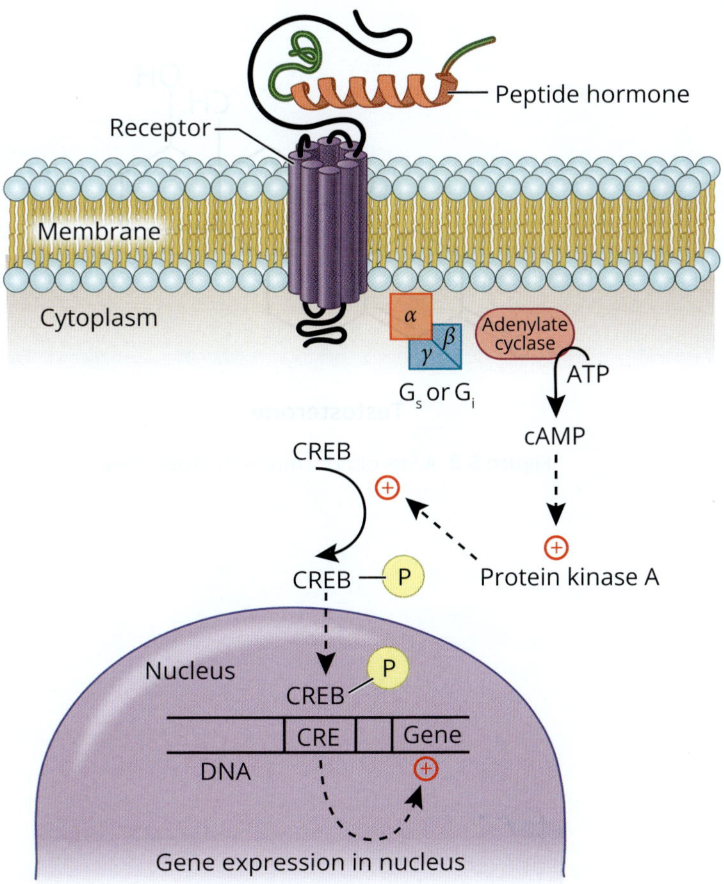

Figure 5.2 Mechanism of Action of a Peptide Hormone
Peptide hormones bind to membrane-bound receptors to intiate a signal cascade, using second messengers like cAMP.

The effects of peptide hormones are usually rapid but short lived because these hormones act through second messenger cascades, which are transient. It is quicker to turn them on and off, compared with steroid hormones, but their effects do not last without relatively constant stimulation.

Because peptides are generally water-soluble, peptide hormones can travel freely in the bloodstream and usually do not require carriers. This is in stark contrast to steroid hormones, which are lipid-soluble.

Steroid Hormones

Steroid hormones (as seen in testosterone in Figure 5.3) are derived from cholesterol and are produced primarily by the gonads and adrenal cortex. Because steroid hormones are derived from nonpolar molecules, they can easily cross the cell membrane. Hence, their receptors are usually intracellular (in the cytosol) or intranuclear (in the nucleus). Upon binding to the receptor, steroid hormone–receptor complexes undergo conformational changes. The receptor can then bind directly to DNA, resulting in either increased or decreased transcription of particular genes, depending on the identity of the hormone, as shown in Figure 5.4. One common form of conformational change is **dimerization**, or pairing of two receptor–hormone complexes. The effects of steroid hormones are slower but longer lived than peptide hormones because steroid hormones participate in gene regulation, causing alterations in the amount of mRNA and protein present in a cell by direct action on DNA.

KEY CONCEPT

Peptide hormones have surface receptors and act via second messenger systems. Steroid hormones bind to intracellular receptors and function by binding to DNA to alter gene transcription.

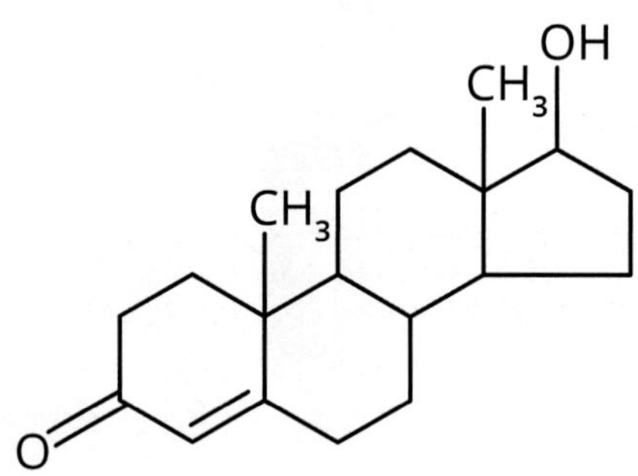

Testosterone

Figure 5.3 A Steroid Hormone: Testosterone

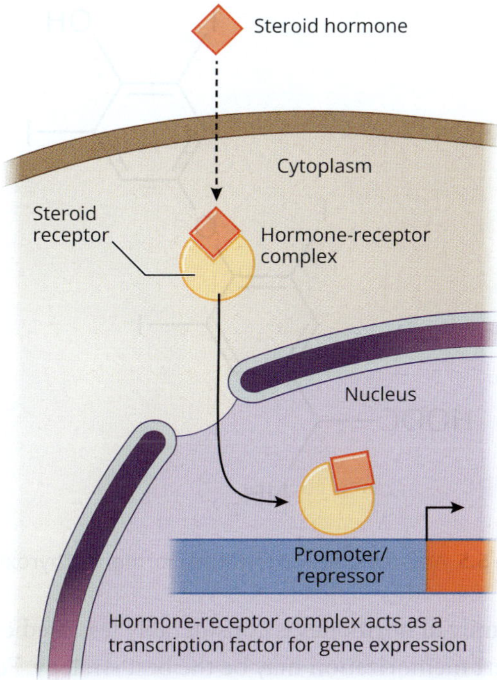

Figure 5.4 Mechanism of Action of a Steroid Hormone
Steroid hormones influence cell behavior by modifying transcription.

Steroid hormones are not water-soluble, so they must be carried by proteins in the bloodstream to travel around the body. Some of these proteins are very specific and carry only one hormone (such as *sex hormone-binding globulin*), while other proteins are nonspecific (such as ***albumin***). Note that hormones are generally inactive while attached to a carrier protein and must dissociate from the carrier to function. Therefore, levels of carrier proteins can change the levels of *active* hormone. For example, some conditions increase the quantity of a protein that carries thyroid hormones, *thyroxine-binding globulin* (TBG). This causes the body to perceive a lower level of thyroid hormone because the increased quantity of TBG binds a larger proportion of the hormone, meaning there is less free hormone available.

Amino Acid–Derivative Hormones

Finally, **amino acid–derivative hormones** are less common than peptide and steroid hormones, but include some of the most important hormones discussed in this chapter, including epinephrine, norepinephrine, triiodothyronine (T_3), and thyroxine (T_4). Figure 5.5 presents the structure of T_4. These hormones are derived from one or two amino acids, usually with a few additional modifications. For example, thyroid hormones are made from tyrosine modified by the addition of several iodine atoms.

MNEMONIC

Insulin is a peptide hormone, and it has to be released at every meal in order to be active. Thus, it has fast onset but is short-acting (like most peptide hormones). Estrogen and testosterone are steroid hormones that promote sexual maturation. This is a slower, but longer-lasting change (as is true for most steroid hormones).

REAL WORLD

During pregnancy, high levels of estrogen and progesterone cause increased production of TBG, thyroxine-binding globulin. In order to compensate, people who are pregnant secrete much higher levels of the thyroid hormones. Thus, in order to diagnose thyroid disease during pregnancy, different reference values must be used.

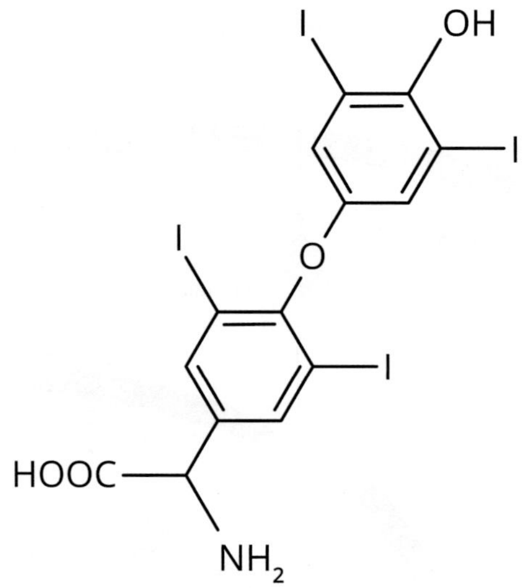

Figure 5.5 An Amino Acid-Derivative Hormone: Thyroxine (T_4)

The chemistry of this family of hormones is considerably less predictable and is one of the few instances where overt memorization may be the best strategy. For instance, the **catecholamines** (epinephrine and norepinephrine) bind to G protein–coupled receptors, while thyroid hormones bind intracellularly.

Classification of Hormones by Target Tissue

Some hormones, known as **direct hormones**, are secreted and then act directly on a target tissue. For example, insulin released by the pancreas causes increased uptake of glucose by muscles. Other hormones, known as **tropic hormones**, require an intermediary to act. For example, as discussed in Chapter 2 of *MCAT Biology Review*, gonadotropin-releasing hormone (GnRH) from the hypothalamus stimulates the release of luteinizing hormone (LH) and follicle-stimulating hormone (FSH). LH then acts on the gonads to stimulate testosterone production in males and estrogen production in females. GnRH and LH do not cause direct changes in the physiology of muscle, bone, and hair follicles; rather, they stimulate the production of another hormone by another endocrine gland that acts on these target tissues. Tropic hormones usually originate in the brain and anterior pituitary gland, allowing for the coordination of multiple processes within the body.

MCAT EXPERTISE

The mechanism of action of the amino acid–derivative hormones should be memorized because it is so unpredictable. Epinephrine and norepinephrine have extremely fast onset but are short-lived, like peptide hormones—think of an *adrenaline rush*. Thyroxine and triiodothyronine, on the other hand, have slower onset but a longer duration, like steroid hormones—they regulate metabolic rate over a long period of time.

MNEMONIC

Most peptide and amino acid–derivative hormones have names that end in ***–in*** or ***–ine*** (insul***in***, vasopress***in***, thyrox***ine***, triiodothyron***ine***, and so on). Most steroid hormones have names that end in ***–one***, ***–ol***, or ***–oid*** (testoster***one***, aldoster***one*** and other mineralocortic***oid***s, cortis***ol*** and other glucocortic***oid***s, and so on). This is not exhaustive, but may help you identify the chemistry of a hormone on Test Day.

MCAT CONCEPT CHECK 5.1

Before you move on, assess your understanding of the material with these questions.

1. Compare and contrast peptide and steroid hormones based on the following criteria:

Criterion	Peptide Hormones	Steroid Hormones
Chemical precursor		
Location of receptor		
Mechanism of action		
Method of travel in the bloodstream		
Speed of onset		
Duration of action		

2. How are amino acid–derivative hormones synthesized?

____

3. What is the difference between a direct and a tropic hormone?

   - Direct hormone:

____

   - Tropic hormone:

____

5.2 Endocrine Organs and Hormones High Yield

LEARNING OBJECTIVES

After Chapter 5.2, you will be able to:

- Recall the hormones involved in calcium homeostasis and their impact on blood calcium
- Identify the tissue that synthesizes catecholamines and the major catecholamines it produces
- List the pancreatic hormones, their regulators, and their impact on blood glucose concentration
- Recall details about the hormones involved in water homeostasis, including their production, action, and ultimate impact on blood volume and osmolarity
- Recall the releasing hormones produced by the hypothalamus, their pituitary targets, and the end result of each signaling pathway on the final target organ:

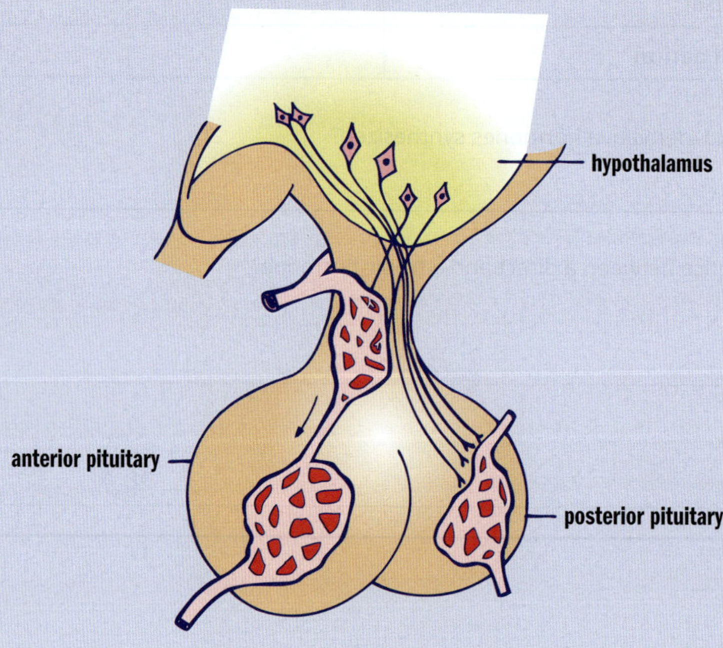

The hypothalamus, the pituitary, the thyroid, the parathyroid glands, the adrenal glands, the pancreas, the gonads (testes and ovaries), and the pineal gland are all endocrine glands, as shown in Figure 5.6. Each of these organs is capable of synthesizing and secreting one or more hormones. Furthermore, there are collections of cells within organs, such as the kidneys, gastrointestinal glands, heart, and thymus, that serve important endocrine roles. The organs in this second group are traditionally not called endocrine organs because hormone production is not their main function.

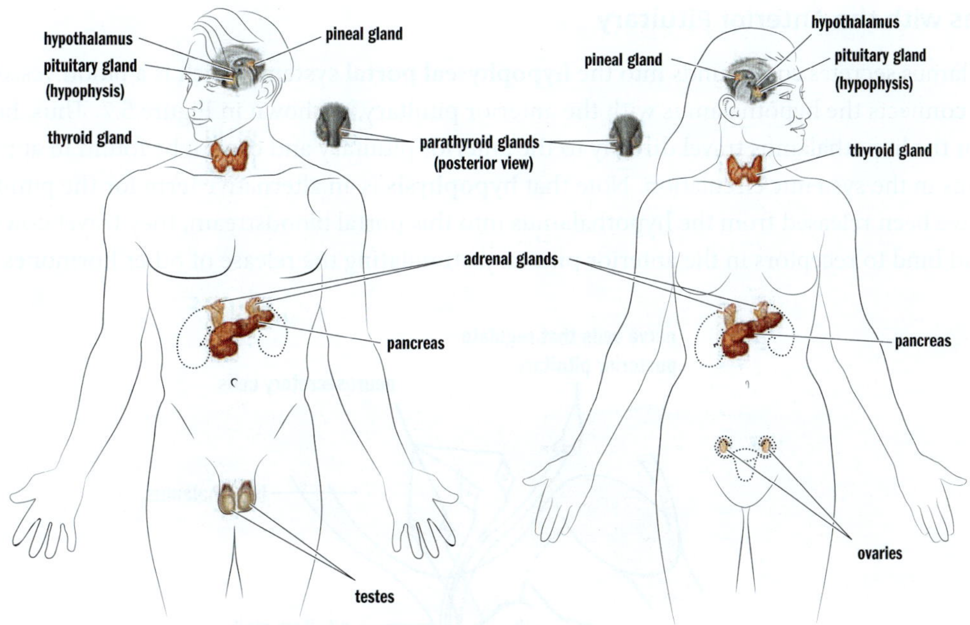

Figure 5.6 Organs of the Endocrine System
Endocrine organs produce hormones that are secreted into the bloodstream to act on distant target tissues.

Now that we have discussed the mechanisms through which hormones act and their classification, we can discuss the individual endocrine organs and the hormones secreted by each.

Hypothalamus

Let's begin with the **hypothalamus**, the bridge between the nervous and endocrine systems. By regulating the pituitary gland through tropic hormones, the hypothalamus is capable of having organism-wide effects. The hypothalamus is located in the forebrain, directly above the pituitary gland and below the thalamus (hence the name *hypo*thalamus). Because the hypothalamus and the pituitary are close to each other, the hypothalamus controls the pituitary through paracrine release of hormones into a portal system that directly connects the two organs. The hypothalamus receives input from a wide variety of sources. For example, a part of the hypothalamus called the *suprachiasmatic nucleus* receives some of the light input from the retinae and helps to control sleep–wake cycles. Other parts of the hypothalamus respond to increases in blood osmolarity. Still other parts of the hypothalamus regulate appetite and satiety.

BRIDGE

The hypothalamus contains a number of nuclei in its three sections, called the lateral, ventromedial, and anterior hypothalamus. These nuclei play roles in emotional experience, aggressive behavior, sexual behavior, metabolism, temperature regulation, and water balance. The parts of the hypothalamus are discussed in Chapter 1 of *MCAT Behavioral Sciences Review.*

The release of hormones by the hypothalamus is regulated by negative feedback. **Negative feedback** occurs when a hormone (or product) later in the pathway inhibits hormones (or enzymes) earlier in the pathway. This type of feedback maintains homeostasis and conserves energy by restricting production of substances that are already present in sufficient quantities. The hypothalamus and pituitary gland are inextricably linked. The pituitary gland has an anterior and posterior component, each with a unique interaction with the hypothalamus. We will discuss each in turn.

Interactions with the Anterior Pituitary

The hypothalamus secretes compounds into the **hypophyseal portal system**, which is a blood vessel system that directly connects the hypothalamus with the anterior pituitary, as shown in Figure 5.7. Thus, hormones released from the hypothalamus travel directly to the anterior pituitary and cannot be found in appreciable concentrations in the systemic circulation. Note that **hypophysis** is an alternative term for the pituitary. Once hormones have been released from the hypothalamus into this portal bloodstream, they travel down the pituitary stalk and bind to receptors in the anterior pituitary, stimulating the release of other hormones.

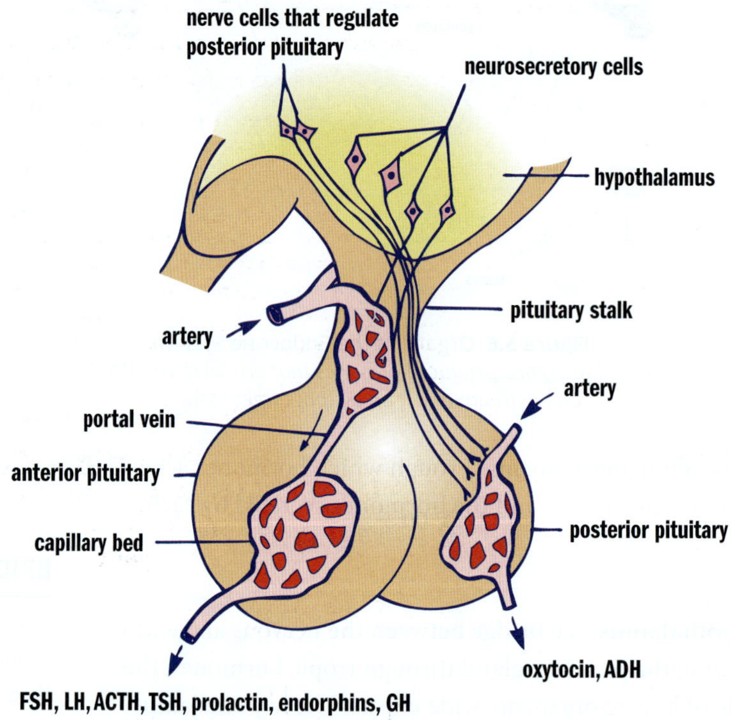

Figure 5.7 The Hypophyseal Portal System
A system of blood vessels connects the hypothalamus to the pituitary.

The hypothalamus secretes several different tropic hormones. The following indicates each hormone released by the hypothalamus and the hormone(s) released by the anterior pituitary in response:

- Gonadotropin-releasing hormone (GnRH) → follicle-stimulating hormone (FSH) and luteinizing hormone (LH)
- Growth hormone–releasing hormone (GHRH) → growth hormone (GH)
- Thyroid-releasing hormone (TRH) → thyroid-stimulating hormone (TSH)
- Corticotropin-releasing factor (CRF) → adrenocorticotropic hormone (ACTH)

There is one exception to this pattern—prolactin-inhibiting factor (PIF), which is actually dopamine, is released by the hypothalamus and causes a *decrease* in prolactin secretion.

KEY CONCEPT

Although it seems as if the anterior pituitary has all the power in the endocrine system, it is controlled by the hypothalamus, which is located directly above it.

Each of the tropic hormones then causes the release of another hormone from an endocrine gland that has negative feedback effects. For example, release of CRF from the hypothalamus will stimulate the anterior pituitary to secrete ACTH. ACTH will then cause the adrenal cortex to increase the level of **cortisol** being secreted into the blood. However, cortisol is detrimental when levels become too high. To prevent excess cortisol secretion, cortisol inhibits the hypothalamus and anterior pituitary from releasing CRF and ACTH, respectively, as shown in Figure 5.8. This makes sense because CRF and ACTH have already accomplished their desired effect: getting more cortisol into the blood. What does this mean in terms of receptors in the hypothalamus and pituitary? Cortisol receptors must be present in these organs; otherwise, they wouldn't be able to recognize that cortisol levels had increased. Three-organ s ystems like these are commonly referred to as **axes**; for example, the hypothalamic–pituitary–adrenal (HPA) axis, the hypothalamic–pituitary–ovarian (HPO) axis, and so on.

KEY CONCEPT

Whereas most of the hormones in the anterior pituitary require a factor from the hypothalamus to be released, prolactin is the exception. As long as the hypothalamus releases PIF (which is actually dopamine), no prolactin will be released. It is the *absence* of PIF that allows prolactin to be released.

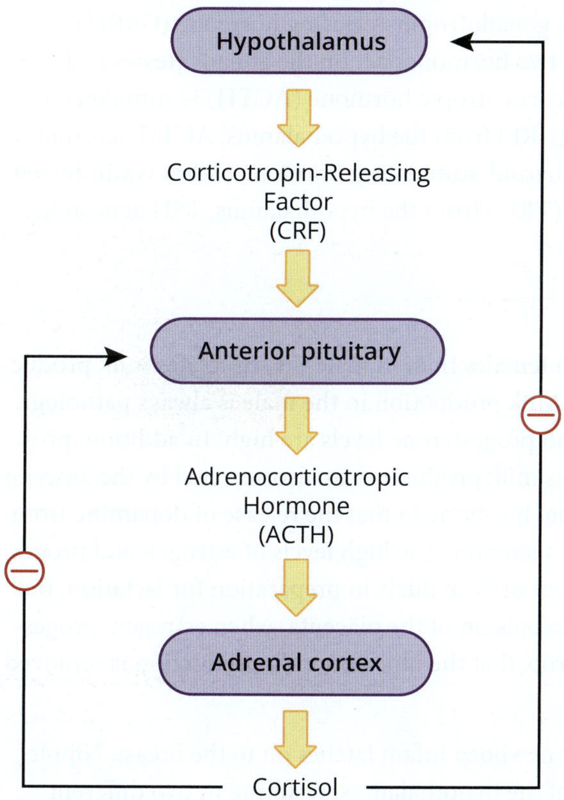

Figure 5.8 Hypothalamic Negative Feedback Mechanism

Interactions with the Posterior Pituitary

The posterior pituitary does not receive tropic hormones through the hypophyseal portal system. Rather, neurons in the hypothalamus send their axons down the pituitary stalk directly into the posterior pituitary, which can then release oxytocin and antidiuretic hormone. **Oxytocin** stimulates uterine contractions during labor, as well as milk letdown during lactation. There is evidence that oxytocin is also involved in bonding behavior. **Antidiuretic hormone** (**ADH**, also called **vasopressin**) increases reabsorption of water in the collecting ducts of the kidneys. ADH is secreted in response to increased plasma osmolarity, or increased concentration of solutes within the blood.

Anterior Pituitary

As described earlier, the pituitary gland is divided into anterior and posterior sections. Because this distinction has already been covered, our discussion of the pituitary gland here will focus on the hormones released by each section.

The **anterior pituitary** synthesizes and secretes seven different products. Four of these are tropic hormones, while the other three are direct hormones.

Tropic Hormones

We are going to mention the tropic hormones only briefly here. These hormones work by causing the release of another hormone at the organ level. Thus, we will discuss the tropic hormones in tandem with the endocrine organ on which they act. The release of both follicle-stimulating hormone (FSH) and luteinizing hormone (LH) is stimulated by gonadotropin-releasing hormone (GnRH) from the hypothalamus. These two hormones act on the gonads (testes and ovaries). The release of adrenocorticotropic hormone (ACTH) is stimulated by corticotropin-releasing factor (CRF) from the hypothalamus; ACTH acts on the adrenal cortex. The release of thyroid-stimulating hormone (TSH) is stimulated by thyroid-releasing hormone (TRH) from the hypothalamus; TSH acts on the thyroid.

Direct Hormones

Prolactin is more important in females than in males; it stimulates milk production in the **mammary glands**. Milk production in the male is always pathologic. During pregnancy, estrogen and progesterone levels are high. In addition, prolactin, a hormone that increases milk production, is also secreted by the anterior pituitary. Prolactin is an unusual hormone in that the release of dopamine from the hypothalamus *decreases* its secretion. The high levels of estrogen and progesterone allow for the development of milk ducts in preparation for lactation, but it is not until shortly after the expulsion of the placenta, when estrogen, progesterone, and dopamine levels drop, that the block on milk production is removed and lactation actually begins.

Milk ejection occurs when the newborn infant latches on to the breast. Nipple stimulation causes activation of the hypothalamus, resulting in two different reactions. First, oxytocin is released from the posterior pituitary, resulting in contraction of the smooth muscle of the breast and ejection of milk through the nipple. Second, the hypothalamus stops releasing dopamine onto the anterior pituitary, which allows prolactin release, causing production of milk and regulation of the milk supply.

REAL WORLD

A tumor of the pituitary gland may result in compression of the portal system that connects the pituitary to the hypothalamus. This will block the ability of PIF to reach the pituitary and exert its effect. Thus, more prolactin will be released. This may result in lactation (galactorrhea), even in males. Thus, milk production in a male or nonpregnant female should lead a physician to suspect the presence of a pituitary tumor.

MNEMONIC

Products of the anterior pituitary:

FLAT PEG

- **F**ollicle-stimulating hormone (FSH)
- **L**uteinizing hormone (LH)
- **A**drenocorticotropic hormone (ACTH)
- **T**hyroid-stimulating hormone (TSH)
- **P**rolactin
- **E**ndorphins
- **G**rowth hormone (GH)

Additionally, the four hormones in **FLAT** are all tropic hormones, while the three hormones in **PEG** are all direct hormones.

Endorphins decrease the perception of pain. For example, after completing a marathon, many people will say they are on an endorphin "high" or "rush." Endorphins mask the pain from having run 26.2 miles and can even induce a sense of euphoria. Many pharmaceutical agents, such as morphine, mimic the effect of these naturally occurring painkillers.

Growth hormone (**GH**) is named for exactly what it does: it promotes the growth of bone and muscle. This sort of growth is energetically expensive and requires large quantities of glucose. Growth hormone prevents glucose uptake in certain tissues (those that are not growing) and stimulates the breakdown of fatty acids. This increases the availability of glucose overall, allowing muscle and bone to use it. GH release is stimulated by growth hormone–releasing hormone (GHRH) from the hypothalamus.

Bone growth originates in special regions of the bone known as epiphyseal plates, which seal shut during puberty. An excess of GH released in childhood (before this closure) can cause **gigantism**, and a deficit results in **dwarfism**. In adults, the situation is slightly different. Because the long bones are sealed, GH still has an effect, but it is primarily in the smaller bones. The resulting medical condition is known as **acromegaly**. The bones most commonly affected are those in the hands, feet, and head. Patients with acromegaly tend to seek medical help because they have had to buy larger shoes, cannot wear their rings, and can no longer fit into their hats.

Posterior Pituitary

The **posterior pituitary** contains the nerve terminals of neurons with cell bodies in the hypothalamus. As mentioned earlier, the posterior pituitary receives and stores two hormones produced by the hypothalamus: ADH and oxytocin.

ADH is secreted in response to low blood volume (as sensed by baroreceptors) or increased blood osmolarity (as sensed by osmoreceptors), shown in Figure 5.9. Its action is at the level of the collecting duct, where it increases the permeability of the duct to water. This increases the reabsorption of water from the filtrate in the nephron. This results in greater retention of water, which results in increased blood volume and higher blood pressure.

Oxytocin is secreted during childbirth and allows for coordinated contraction of uterine smooth muscle. Its secretion may also be stimulated by suckling, as it promotes milk ejection through contraction of smooth muscle in the breast. Finally, oxytocin may be involved in bonding behavior. Oxytocin is unusual in that it has a **positive feedback** loop: the release of oxytocin promotes uterine contraction, which promotes more oxytocin release, which promotes stronger uterine contractions, and so on. Positive feedback loops can usually be identified by a "spiraling forward" scheme and usually have a definitive endpoint—in this case, delivery.

KEY CONCEPT

The two hormones released from the posterior pituitary are actually synthesized in the hypothalamus and simply released from the posterior pituitary gland. The posterior pituitary does not synthesize any hormones itself.

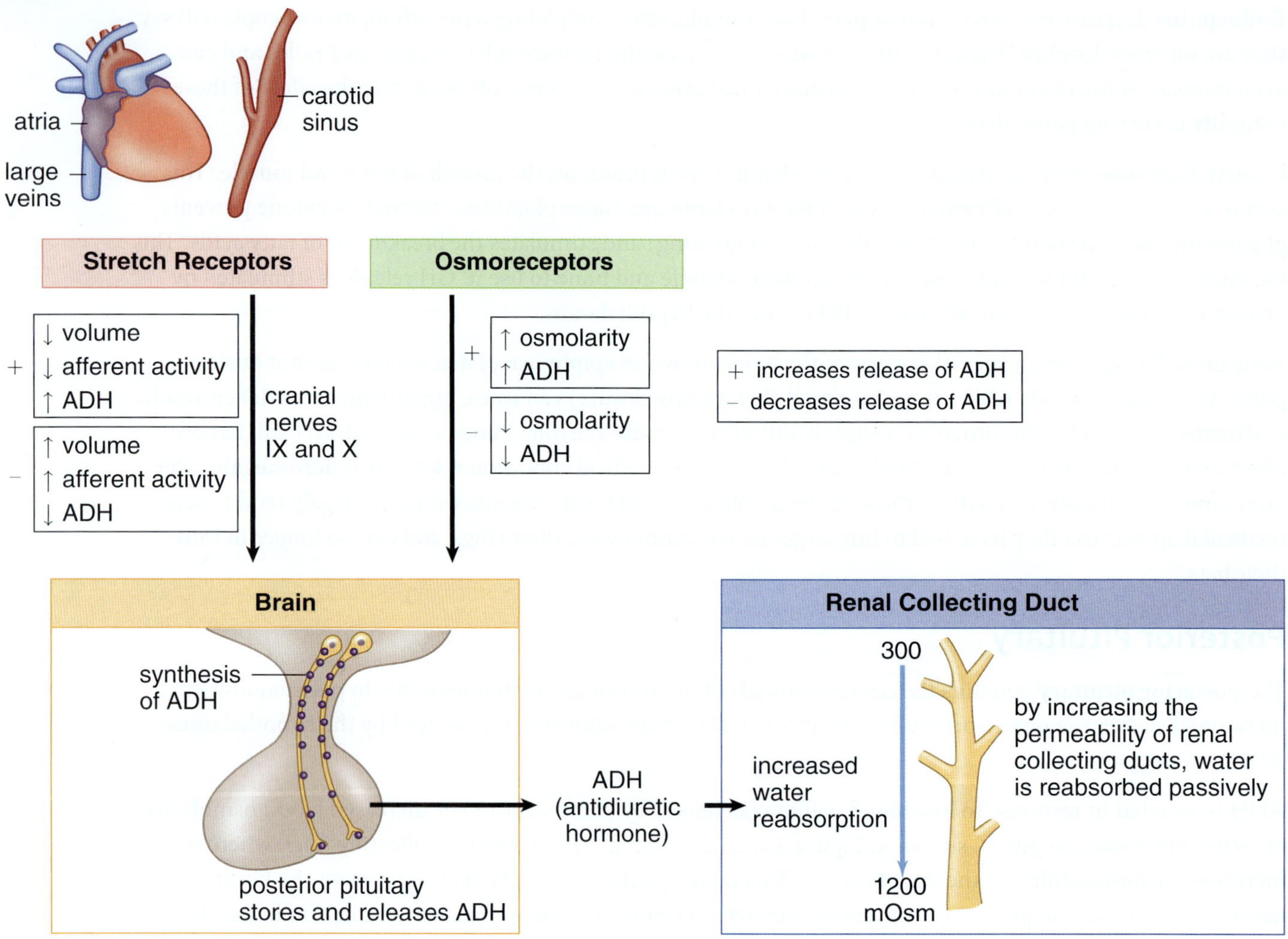

Figure 5.9 Antidiuretic Hormone (ADH)

Thyroid

The **thyroid** is controlled by **thyroid-stimulating hormone** from the anterior pituitary. The thyroid is on the front surface of the trachea; it can be palpated (felt) as an organ near the base of the neck that moves up and down with swallowing. The thyroid has two major functions: setting basal metabolic rate and promoting calcium homeostasis. It mediates the first effect by releasing triiodothyronine (T_3) and thyroxine (T_4), while it carries out the second effect through the release of calcitonin.

Triiodothyronine and Thyroxine

Triiodothyronine (T_3) and **thyroxine** (T_4) are both produced by the iodination of the amino acid tyrosine in the **follicular cells** of the thyroid (see Figure 5.10). The numbers 3 and 4 refer to the number of iodine atoms attached to the tyrosine. T_4 is actually the less active version that will be converted to T_3 for a stronger effect. Thyroid hormones are capable of resetting the basal metabolic rate of the body by making energy production more or less efficient, as well as altering the utilization of glucose and fatty acids. Increased amounts of T_3 and T_4 will lead to increased cellular respiration. This leads to increased protein and fatty acid turnover by speeding up both synthesis and degradation of these compounds. High plasma levels of thyroid hormones will lead to decreased TSH and TRH synthesis; negative feedback prevents excessive secretion of T_3 and T_4, as shown in Figure 5.11.

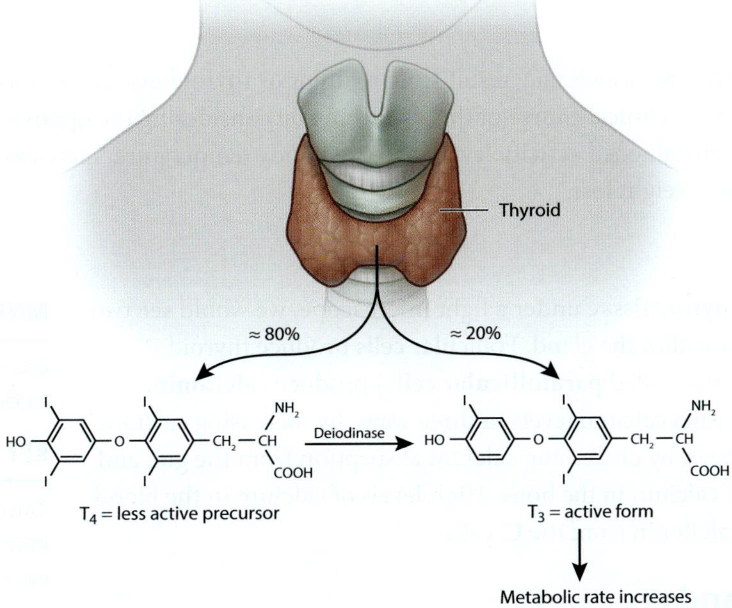

Figure 5.10 The Pathway of Thyroid Hormones: T_4 and T_3

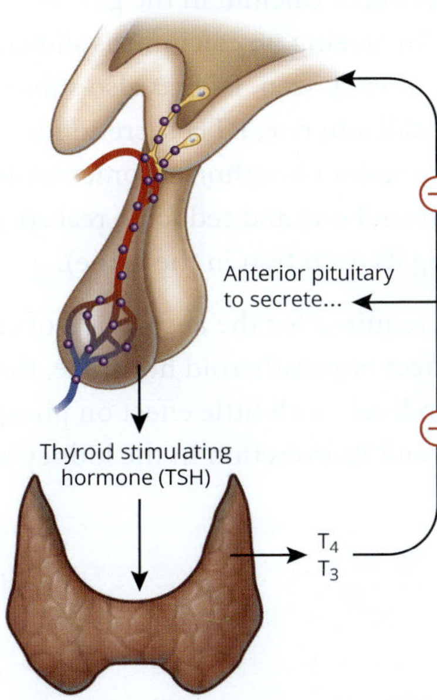

Figure 5.11 Thyroid Hormone Negative Feedback Mechanism

A deficiency of iodine or inflammation of the thyroid may result in **hypothyroidism**, in which thyroid hormones are secreted in insufficient amounts or not at all. The condition is characterized by lethargy, decreased body temperature, slowed respiratory and heart rate, cold intolerance, and weight gain. Thyroid hormones are required for appropriate neurological and physical development in children. Most children are tested at birth for appropriate levels because a deficiency will result in intellectual disability and developmental delay (**cretinism**).

An excess of thyroid hormone, which may result from a tumor or thyroid overstimulation, is called **hyperthyroidism**. We can predict the clinical course of this syndrome by considering the opposite of each of the effects seen in hypothyroidism: heightened activity level, increased body temperature, increased respiratory and heart rate, heat intolerance, and weight loss.

Calcitonin

If we were to examine thyroid tissue under a light microscope, we would see two distinct cell populations within the gland. Follicular cells produce thyroid hormones and **C-cells** (also called **parafollicular cells**) produce **calcitonin**. Calcitonin decreases plasma calcium levels in three ways: by increasing calcium excretion from the kidneys, by decreasing calcium absorption from the gut, and by increasing storage of calcium in the bone. High levels of calcium in the blood stimulate secretion of calcitonin from the C-cells.

MNEMONIC

Calci**ton**in **ton**es down calcium levels in the blood.

KEY CONCEPT

Calcium is an exceptionally important ion. The critically important functions of calcium include:

- Bone structure and strength
- Release of neurotransmitters from neurons
- Regulation of muscle contraction
- Clotting of blood (calcium is a cofactor)

In addition, calcium also plays a role in cell movement and exocytosis of cellular materials.

Parathyroid Glands

The parathyroids are four small pea-sized structures that sit on the posterior surface of the thyroid. The hormone produced by the parathyroid glands is aptly named **parathyroid hormone** (**PTH**). PTH serves as an antagonistic hormone to calcitonin, raising blood calcium levels; specifically, it decreases excretion of calcium by the kidneys, increases absorption of calcium in the gut (via vitamin D), and increases bone resorption, thereby freeing up calcium, as shown in Figure 5.12. Like the hormones we have already seen, PTH is also subject to feedback inhibition. As levels of plasma calcium rise, PTH secretion is decreased. Parathyroid hormone also promotes phosphorus homeostasis by increasing the resorption of phosphate from bone and reducing reabsorption of phosphate in the kidney (thus promoting its excretion in the urine).

PTH also activates **vitamin D**, which is required for the absorption of calcium and phosphate in the gut. The overall effect of parathyroid hormone, therefore, is a significant increase in blood calcium levels with little effect on phosphate (the absorption of phosphate in the gut and its excretion in the kidney somewhat cancel each other).

KEY CONCEPT

Just like glucagon and insulin, PTH and calcitonin are antagonistic to each other. We should think of these hormones as a pair with the primary function of regulating calcium levels in the blood. PTH increases serum calcium levels, whereas calcitonin decreases calcium levels.

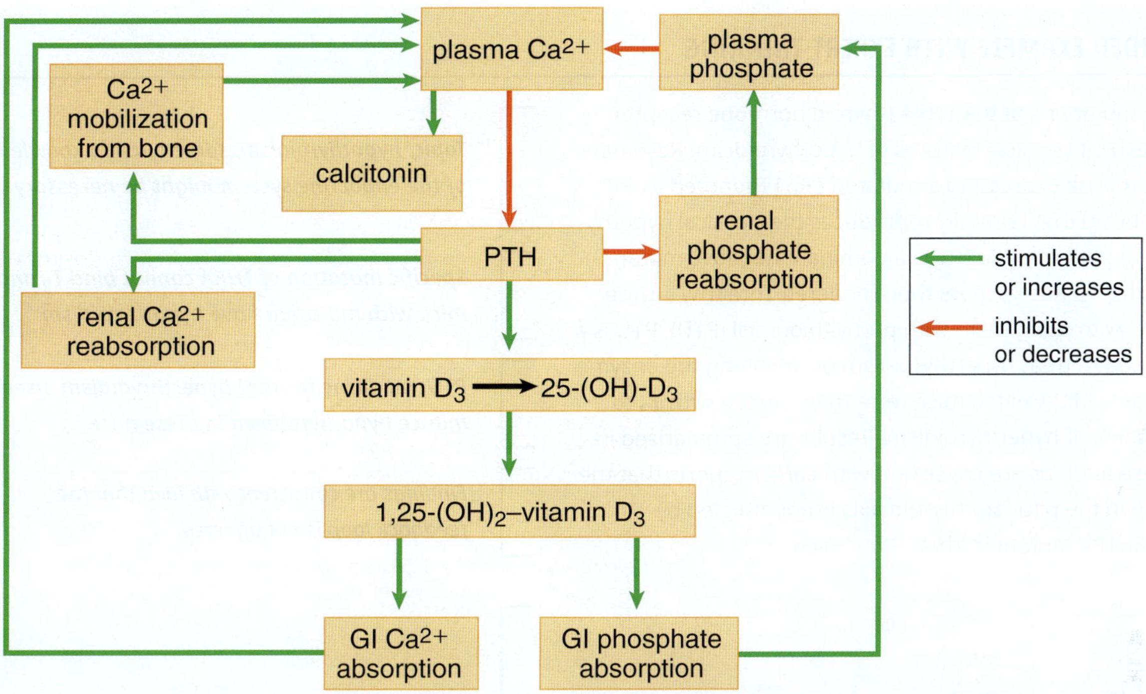

Figure 5.12 Calcium and Phosphorus Homeostasis

BIOLOGY GUIDED EXAMPLE WITH EXPERT THINKING

Patients with mutations of the THRA (thyroid hormone receptor alpha) gene exhibit classical features of hypothyroidism. Researchers created a mouse expressing a mutated TRα1 (denoted as PV; Thra1PV/+ mouse) that faithfully reproduces the classical hypothyroidism seen in patients. TRα1PV is a dominant negative mutant and cannot bind T_3. Researchers then rendered Thra1PV/+ mice hypothyroidic by treating them with propylthiouracil (PTU). PTU is a medication used to treat hyperthyroidism by inhibiting the enzyme thyroperoxidase. PTU-treated mice were then treated with T_3 to induce symptoms of hyperthyroidism. Results are summarized in Figure 1. These findings are consistent with earlier reports that the feedback loop in the pituitary-thyroid axis is not affected by expressing TRα1PV mutant in Thra1PV/+ mice.

Topic: hypothyroidism; some outside knowledge of the endocrine system might be necessary

Specific mutation of THRA cannot bind T_3 and mice with mutation have hypothyroidism

PTU: medicine to treat hyperthryoidism, used to induce hypothyroidism in these mice

Findings are consistent with idea that the feedback loop is not affected

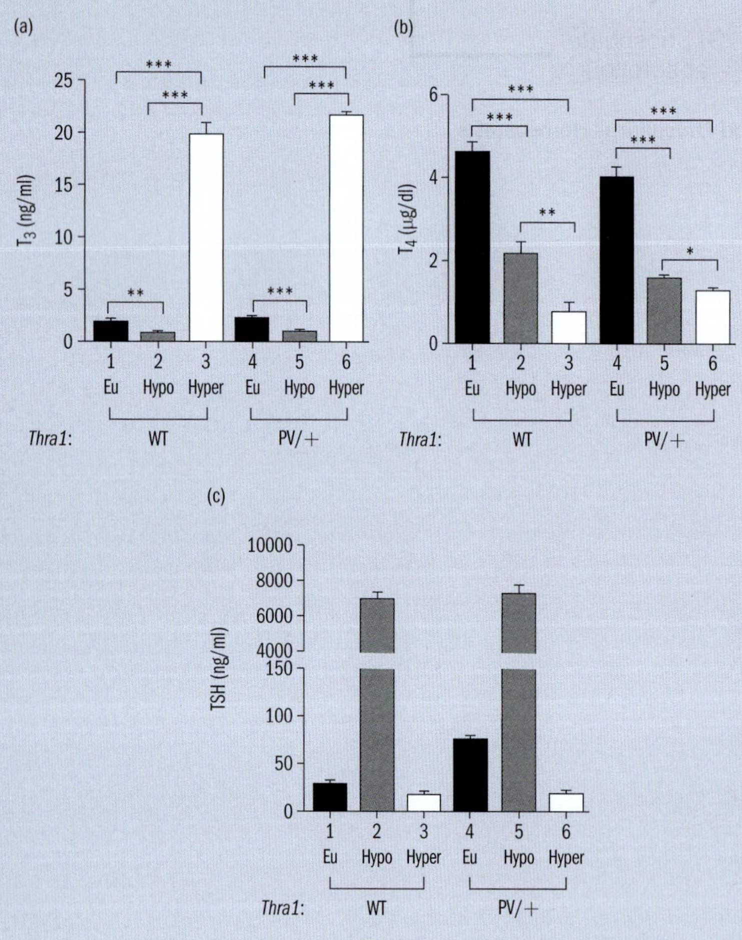

Figure 1 Thyroid experiment results. Eu = euthyroid condition.

IVs: Eu, Hypo, Hyper

DVs: T_3, T_4, TSH

Trends: Euthryoid means the thyroid is kept normal, so this is the control. The changes in T_3, T_4, and TSH are pretty consistent for each condition (Eu, Hypo, Hyper) between WT and PV/+ mice.

Adapted from Park, S., Han, C. R., Park, J. W., Zhao, L., Zhu, X., Willingham, M., … Cheng, S. Y. (2017). Defective erythropoiesis caused by mutations of the thyroid hormone receptor α gene. *PLoS Genetics*, 13(9), e1006991. doi:10.1371/journal.pgen.1006991.

Why are TSH levels elevated in mice given propylthiouracil (PTU)?

A question like this is asking us to explain the underlying biological cause for an observed phenomenon. The MCAT often tests our ability to reason with a concept or mechanism that we are already familiar with. For this question, the stated change to the system is "propylthiouracil" and the effect observed is "elevated TSH levels". It is now our job to determine how the two are related.

First, we'll want to identify what information we'll need, both from the passage and from our science background. MCAT questions will often intentionally include terms that we aren't familiar with. The key to answering these questions, even if we're not familiar with the phenomenon described, is finding the relevant information from the passage and using that information in conjunction with our scientific understanding to solve the problem. We already identified the change to the system in this question as the application of PTU. According to the passage, PTU is a medication that inhibits thyroperoxidase and it is used to treat hyperthyroidism. In the experiment, they used PTU to "render[ed] Thra1PV/+ mice hypothyroidic". If we look to Figure 1(a), we can see that in the T_3 and T_4 graphs, the hypothyroid (gray) bar is significantly smaller than the euthyroid (black) bar. If we weren't sure what euthyroid referred to, we could infer that, given that the other two categories in each graph are hypothyroid and hyperthyroid, this must be wild-type or normal function. Based on these data and the context from the passage, it is reasonable to infer that PTU is a drug that functions by lowering the production of thyroid hormone (T_3 and T_4).

Now we must consider how having low thyroid hormones would be related to elevated TSH levels. TSH is a tropic hormone released from the anterior pituitary, and it is regulated by a negative feedback mechanism involving thyroid hormone. Specifically, we should know that the hypothalamus releases thyroid-releasing hormone (TRH), which causes the anterior pituitary to release thyroid-stimulating hormone (TSH). TSH acts upon the thyroid to stimulate the release of thyroid hormone triiodothyronine (T_3) and thyroxine (T_4). T_3 and T_4 then act as negative feedback on the hypothalamus and the pituitary gland, lowering TRH and TSH levels. We can reason that, if T_3 and T_4 levels were low, TRH and TSH would be continuously produced, as they would not be inhibited by the presence of T3 and T_4.

The mice in the experiment have normally functioning endocrine glands prior to treatment. We can always assume this to be the case unless the passage explicitly states otherwise: subjects should be assumed to be healthy individuals with normal hormone levels. When PTU is administered, the thyroid hormone levels in the mice decreased. As a result, there is now less thyroid hormone in circulation. As we predicted, there is now little to no negative feedback on the hypothalamus and the anterior pituitary gland. TRH and TSH levels in the mice would be elevated as a result of this lack of feedback. Normally, that would work to create more T_3 and T_4, but in this case, the mice are under the influence of PTU, and despite TSH stimulation, the thyroid will not be able to produce more T_3 and T_4. The cycle will continue, and more TRH and TSH will be secreted.

In short, the reason why TSH level is elevated in mice administered with PTU is that there is no T_3 or T_4 to activate the negative feedback mechanism on TSH and TRH, which "tricks" the brain into secreting more TSH (and TRH).

Adrenal Cortex

As seen in Figure 5.13, the **adrenal glands** are located on top of the kidneys. Adrenal actually translates to *near* or *next to the kidney*. Each adrenal gland consists of a cortex and a medulla. This distinction is more than anatomical. Each part of the gland is responsible for the secretion of different hormones. The **adrenal cortex** secretes **corticosteroids**. These are steroid hormones that can be divided into three functional classes: **glucocorticoids**, **mineralocorticoids**, and **cortical sex hormones**.

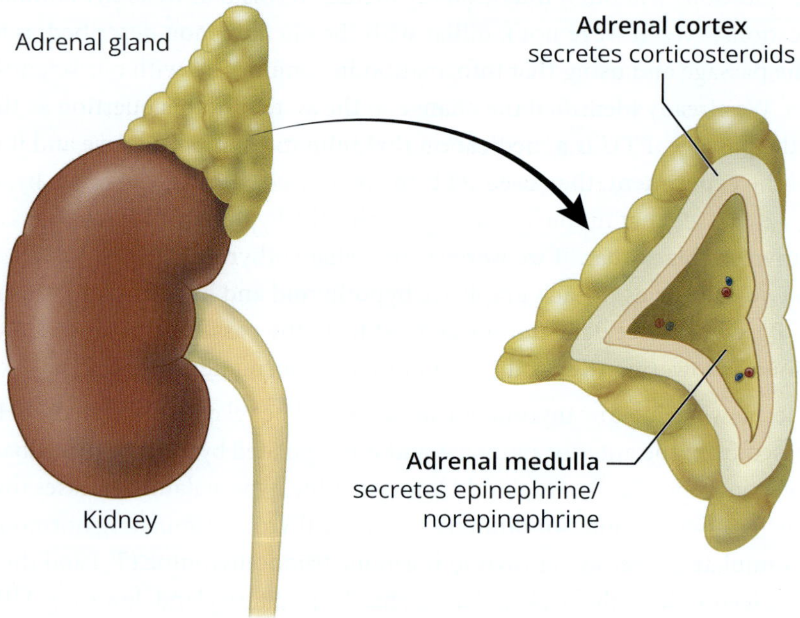

Figure 5.13 The Adrenal Gland

Glucocorticoids

Glucocorticoids are steroid hormones that regulate glucose levels. In addition, these hormones also affect protein metabolism. The two glucocorticoids most likely to be tested on the MCAT are **cortisol** and **cortisone**. These hormones raise blood glucose by increasing gluconeogenesis and decreasing protein synthesis. Cortisol and cortisone can also decrease inflammation and immunologic responses. Cortisol is known as a stress hormone because it is released in times of physical or emotional stress. This increases blood sugar and provides a ready source of fuel in case the body must react quickly to a dangerous stimulus.

Glucocorticoid release is under the control of adrenocorticotropic hormone (ACTH) as described earlier. Corticotropin-releasing factor (CRF) from the hypothalamus promotes release of adrenocorticotropic hormone (ACTH) from the anterior pituitary, which promotes release of glucocorticoids from the adrenal cortex.

REAL WORLD

Many people who suffer from joint pain are treated with glucocorticoid injections into the joint space to decrease inflammation. In addition, glucocorticoids are used to treat systemic inflammation caused by allergic reactions or autoimmune disease.

Mineralocorticoids

Mineralocorticoids are used in salt and water homeostasis; their most profound effects are on the kidneys. The most noteworthy mineralocorticoid is **aldosterone**, which increases sodium reabsorption in the distal convoluted tubule and collecting duct of the nephron. Water follows the sodium cations into the bloodstream, increasing blood volume and pressure. Since water and sodium ions flow together, plasma osmolarity remains unchanged; this is in contrast to ADH, which only increases water reabsorption (decreasing plasma osmolarity). Aldosterone also decreases the reabsorption of potassium and hydrogen ions in these same segments of the nephron, promoting their excretion in the urine.

Unlike the glucocorticoids, aldosterone is primarily under the control of the **renin–angiotensin–aldosterone** system, as shown in Figure 5.14. Decreased blood pressure causes the **juxtaglomerular cells** of the kidney to secrete **renin**, which cleaves an inactive plasma protein, **angiotensinogen** (released by the liver), to its active form, **angiotensin I**. Angiotensin I is then converted to **angiotensin II** by **angiotensin-converting enzyme** (**ACE**) in the lungs. Angiotensin II stimulates the adrenal cortex to secrete aldosterone. Once blood pressure is restored, the stimulus pushing the release of renin is diminished, thus serving as the negative feedback mechanism for this system.

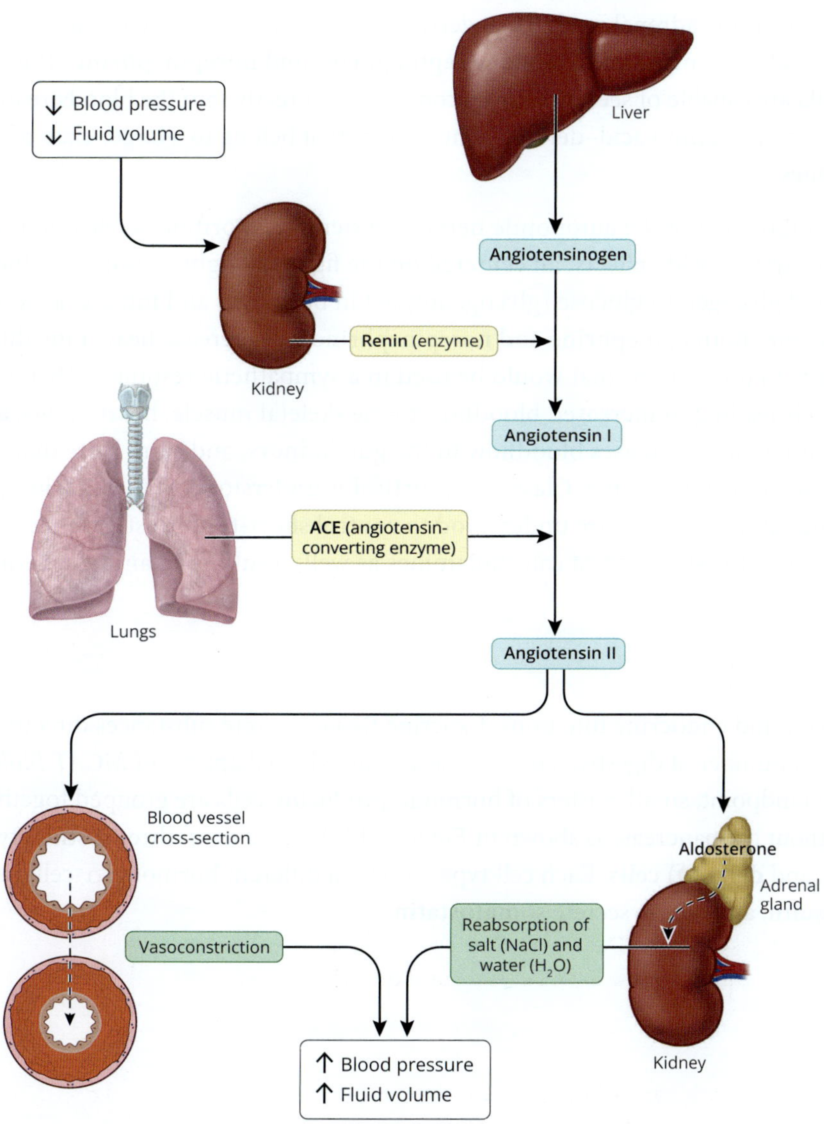

Figure 5.14 The Renin–Angiotensin–Aldosterone System

REAL WORLD

In addition to stimulating the secretion of aldosterone, which increases blood volume and hence blood pressure, angiotensin II also increases blood pressure directly through a powerful vasoconstrictive effect and increases heart rate. Angiotensin-converting enzyme (ACE) inhibitors block the conversion of angiotensin I to angiotensin II, inhibiting vasoconstriction. Therefore, ACE inhibitors are frequently prescribed for the treatment of high blood pressure and congestive heart failure. In the latter case, vasodilation helps reduce vascular resistance, decreasing the pressure against which the failing heart must pump. ACE inhibitors' generic names end with *–pril* (*lisinopril, enalapril, ramipril*).

Cortical Sex Hormones

The adrenal glands also make **cortical sex hormones** (**androgens** and **estrogens**). Because the testes already secrete large quantities of androgens, adrenal testosterone plays a relatively small role in male physiology. But because the ovaries secrete far smaller amounts of androgens, females are much more sensitive to disorders of cortical sex hormone production. For example, certain enzyme deficiencies in the synthetic pathways of other adrenal cortex hormones result in excess androgen production in the adrenal cortex. Such a deficiency would result in no obvious phenotypic effects in a male fetus; however, a genotypic female may be born with ambiguous or masculinized genitalia due to the presence of excess cortical sex hormones. Males can be affected by similar disorders if they lead to excessive production of estrogens.

MNEMONIC

Functions of the corticosteroids:

The 3 **S**'s

- **S**alt (mineralocorticoids)
- **S**ugar (glucocorticoids)
- **S**ex (cortical sex hormones)

Adrenal Medulla

Nestled inside the adrenal cortex is the adrenal medulla. A derivative of the nervous system, this organ is responsible for the production of the sympathetic hormones **epinephrine** and **norepinephrine**. The specialized nerve cells in the medulla are capable of secreting these compounds directly into the bloodstream. Both epinephrine and norepinephrine are amino acid–derivative hormones that belong to a larger class of molecules known as **catecholamines**.

Much like the sympathetic component of the autonomic nervous system, the hormones released from the adrenal medulla have diverse system-wide effects, all centered on the fight-or-flight response. Epinephrine can increase the breakdown of glycogen to glucose (glycogenolysis) in both liver and muscle, as well as increase the basal metabolic rate. Both epinephrine and norepinephrine will increase heart rate, dilate the bronchi, and shunt blood flow to the systems that would be used in a sympathetic response. That is, there is vasodilation of blood vessels leading to increased bloodflow to the skeletal muscle, heart, lungs, and brain. Concurrently, vasoconstriction decreases bloodflow to the gut, kidneys, and skin. Note that the stress response involves both cortisol and epinephrine. Classically, cortisol is understood to mediate long-term (slow) stress responses, while catecholamines are understood to control short-term (fast) stress responses. In fact, cortisol actually increases the synthesis of catecholamines as well, resulting in an increase in catecholamine release.

Pancreas

The pancreas has both exocrine and endocrine functions. Exocrine tissues secrete substances directly into ducts; the pancreas produces a number of digestive enzymes, as discussed in Chapter 9 of *MCAT Biology Review*. From an endocrine standpoint, small clusters of hormone-producing cells are grouped together into **islets of Langerhans** throughout the pancreas, as shown in Figure 5.15. Islets contain three distinct types of cells: **alpha** (α), **beta** (β), and **delta** (δ) **cells**. Each cell type secretes a different hormone: α-cells secrete **glucagon**, β-cells secrete **insulin**, and δ-cells secrete **somatostatin**.

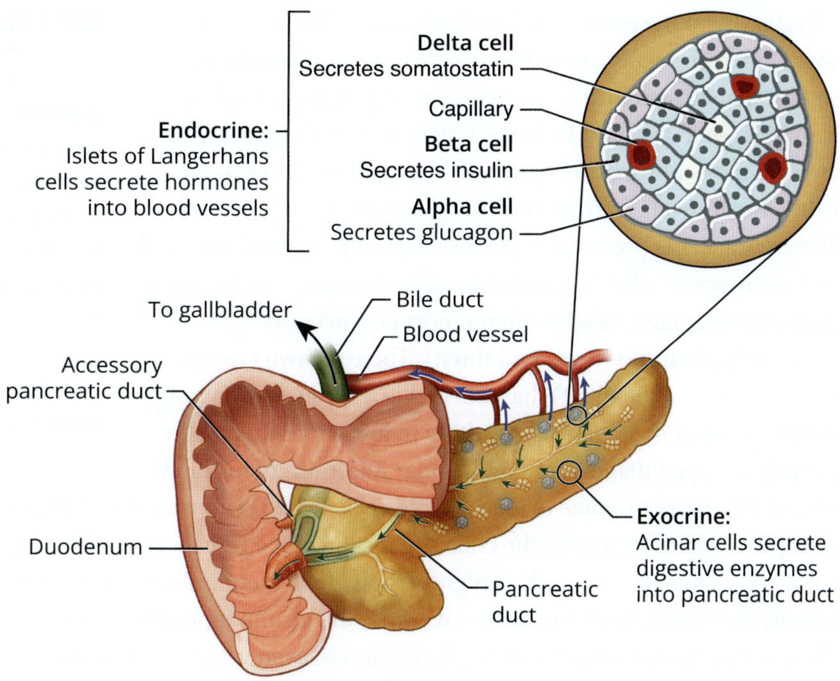

Figure 5.15 Anatomy of the Pancreas
Islets of Langerhans are scattered throughout the pancreas and carry out the endocrine function of the organ.

Glucagon

Glucagon is secreted during times of fasting. When glucose levels are low, glucagon increases glucose production by triggering glycogenolysis, gluconeogenesis, and the degradation of protein and fat. In addition to low blood glucose concentrations, certain gastrointestinal hormones (such as cholecystokinin and gastrin) increase glucagon release from α-cells. When blood glucose concentrations are high, glucagon release is inhibited.

> **MNEMONIC**
>
> **Glucagon** levels are high when **glucose** is **gone**.

Insulin

Insulin is antagonistic to glucagon and is therefore secreted when blood glucose levels are high, as shown in Figure 5.16. Insulin induces muscle and liver cells to take up glucose and store it as glycogen for later use. In addition, because it is active when glucose levels are high, insulin stimulates anabolic processes such as fat and protein synthesis.

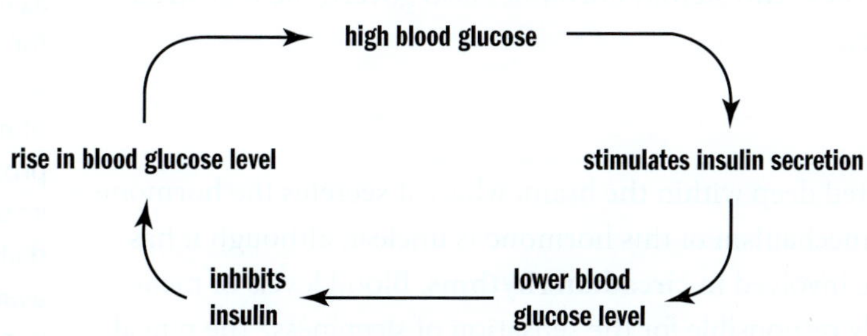

Figure 5.16 Insulin Has a Direct Relationship with Blood Glucose Concentration
When blood glucose levels are high, insulin levels rise, causing cells to take up glucose from the blood; when blood glucose levels are low, insulin levels remain low as well.

In excess, insulin will cause **hypoglycemia**, which is characterized by low blood glucose concentration. Underproduction, insufficient secretion, or insensitivity to insulin all can result in **diabetes mellitus**, which is clinically characterized by **hyperglycemia** (excess glucose in the blood). In the kidneys, excessive glucose in the filtrate will overwhelm the nephron's ability to reabsorb glucose, resulting in its presence in the urine. Because it is an osmotically active particle and does not readily cross the cell membrane, the presence of glucose in the filtrate leads to excess excretion of water and an increase—that is sometimes quite dramatic—in the urine volume. Therefore, patients who have diabetes often report **polyuria** (increased frequency of urination) and **polydipsia** (increased thirst). There are two types of diabetes mellitus. **Type I** (insulin-dependent) diabetes mellitus is caused by autoimmune destruction of the β-cells of the pancreas, resulting in low or absent insulin production. People who have type I diabetes require regular injections of insulin to prevent hyperglycemia and to permit uptake of glucose into cells. **Type II** (non-insulin-dependent) diabetes mellitus is the result of receptor-level resistance to the effects of insulin. Type II diabetes mellitus is partially inherited and partially due to environmental factors, such as high-carbohydrate diets and obesity. Certain pharmaceutical agents can be taken orally to help the body more effectively use the insulin it produces. These individuals require insulin only when their bodies can no longer control glucose levels, even when aided by these medications.

KEY CONCEPT

Insulin decreases plasma glucose. Glucagon increases plasma glucose. Growth hormone, glucocorticoids, and epinephrine are also capable of increasing plasma glucose. These hormones that raise blood glucose levels are commonly called counterregulatory hormones.

Somatostatin

Somatostatin is an inhibitor of both insulin and glucagon secretion. High blood glucose and amino acid concentrations stimulate its secretion. Somatostatin is also produced by the hypothalamus, where it decreases growth hormone secretion in addition to its effects on insulin and glucagon.

Gonads

Because reproductive endocrinology is discussed in detail in Chapter 2 of *MCAT Biology Review*, we offer only a brief overview in this chapter. The **testes** secrete testosterone in response to stimulation by gonadotropins (LH and FSH). Testosterone causes sexual differentiation of the male during gestation and also promotes the development and maintenance of secondary sex characteristics in males, such as axillary and pubic hair, deepening of the voice, and muscle growth.

The **ovaries** secrete estrogen and progesterone in response to gonadotropins. Estrogen is involved in development of the female reproductive system during gestation and also promotes the development and maintenance of secondary sex characteristics in females, such as axillary and pubic hair, breast growth, and body fat redistribution. These two steroid hormones also govern the menstrual cycle as well as pregnancy.

Pineal Gland

The **pineal gland** is located deep within the brain, where it secretes the hormone **melatonin**. The precise mechanism of this hormone is unclear, although it has been demonstrated to be involved in **circadian rhythms**. Blood levels of melatonin are at least partially responsible for the sensation of sleepiness. The pineal gland receives projections directly from the retina, but is not involved in vision; it is hypothesized that the pineal gland responds to decreases in light intensity by releasing melatonin.

REAL WORLD

Melatonin has enjoyed somewhat of a wonder drug status over the past decade as it is touted as a remedy for everything from jet lag to aging. Certainly, one effect of melatonin is to cause profound drowsiness, hence its use in "resetting" one's daily rhythm. Melatonin is available over the counter in health food stores, but the long-term effects of melatonin therapy are currently unknown.

Other Organs

In addition to the organs listed above, specific cells and tissues in other organs exhibit endocrine functions. In the gastrointestinal tract, endocrine tissue can be found in both the stomach and intestine. Many gastrointestinal peptides have been identified; important ones include secretin, gastrin, and cholecystokinin. The specific functions of these hormones are discussed in Chapter 9 of *MCAT Biology Review*, but as we might expect for the digestive system, the stimulus for release of most of these peptides is the presence of specific nutrients.

The kidneys play a role in water balance. As mentioned earlier, ADH increases water permeability in the collecting duct, and the renin–angiotensin–aldosterone system increases sodium and water reabsorption in the distal convoluted tubule and collecting duct. The kidneys also produce **erythropoietin**, which stimulates bone marrow to increase production of erythrocytes (red blood cells). It is secreted in response to low oxygen levels in the blood.

The heart releases **atrial natriuretic peptide** (**ANP**) to help regulate salt and water balance. When cells in the atria are stretched from excess blood volume, they release ANP. This hormone promotes excretion of sodium and therefore increases urine volume. This effect is functionally antagonistic to aldosterone because it lowers blood volume and pressure, and has no effect on blood osmolarity.

The thymus, located directly behind the sternum, releases **thymosin**, which is important for proper T-cell development and differentiation. The thymus atrophies by adulthood, and thymosin levels drop accordingly. The function of T-cells is discussed in Chapter 8 of *MCAT Biology Review*.

A full list of hormones and their actions can be found in Table 5.1 below.

Source	Hormone	Type	Action
Anterior pituitary	Follicle-stimulating hormone (FSH)	Peptide	Stimulates follicle maturation in females; spermatogenesis in males
	Luteinizing hormone (LH)	Peptide	Stimulates ovulation in females; testosterone synthesis in males
	Adrenocorticotropic hormone (ACTH)	Peptide	Stimulates the adrenal cortex to synthesize and secrete glucocorticoids
	Thyroid-stimulating hormone (TSH)	Peptide	Stimulates the thyroid to produce thyroid hormones
	Prolactin	Peptide	Stimulates milk production and secretion
	Endorphins	Peptide	Decrease sensation of pain; can promote euphoria
	Growth hormone (GH)	Peptide	Stimulates bone and muscle growth; raises blood glucose levels
Hypothalamus (released by posterior pituitary)	Antidiuretic hormone (ADH; vasopressin)	Peptide	Stimulates water reabsorption in kidneys by increasing permeability of collecting duct
	Oxytocin	Peptide	Stimulates uterine contractions during labor and milk secretion during lactation; may promote bonding behavior

Table 5.1 Major Hormones in Humans

Thyroid (follicular cells)	Triiodothyronine (T_3) and thyroxine (T_4)	Amino acid-derivative	Stimulate metabolic activity
Thyroid (parafollicular or C cells)	Calcitonin	Peptide	Decreases blood calcium concentrations
Parathyroids	Parathyroid hormone (PTH)	Peptide	Increases blood calcium concentrations
Adrenal cortex	Glucocorticoids (cortisol and cortisone)	Steroid	Increase blood glucose concentrations; decrease protein synthesis; anti-inflammatory
	Mineralocorticoids (aldosterone)	Steroid	Increase water reabsorption in the kidneys by increasing sodium reabsorption; promote potassium and hydrogen ion excretion
Adrenal medulla	Epinephrine and norepinephrine	Amino acid-derivative	Increase blood glucose concentrations and heart rate; dilate bronchi; alter blood flow patterns
Pancreas (α-cells)	Glucagon	Peptide	Stimulates glycogen breakdown (glycogenolysis); increases blood glucose concentrations
Pancreas (β-cells)	Insulin	Peptide	Lowers blood glucose concentrations and promotes anabolic processes
Pancreas (δ-cells)	Somatostatin	Peptide	Suppresses secretion of glucagon and insulin
Testis (and adrenal cortex)	Testosterone	Steroid	Induces the development and maintenance of male reproductive system and male secondary sex characteristics
Ovary (and placenta)	Estrogen	Steroid	Induces the development and maintenance of female reproductive system and female secondary sex characteristics
	Progesterone	Steroid	Promotes maintenance of the endometrium
Pineal gland	Melatonin	Peptide	Involved in circadian rhythms
Kidney	Erythropoietin	Peptide	Stimulates bone marrow to produce erythrocytes
Heart (atria)	Atrial natriuretic peptide (ANP)	Peptide	Promotes salt and water excretion
Thymus	Thymosin	Peptide	Stimulates T-cell development

Table 5.1 (Continued)

MCAT CONCEPT CHECK 5.2

Before you move on, assess your understanding of the material with these questions.

1. For each of the hypothalamic releasing hormones listed below, what hormone(s) does each affect in the anterior pituitary? On which organ does each pituitary hormone act? What hormone(s) are released by the target organs?

Hypothalamic Releasing Hormone	Hormone(s) from Anterior Pituitary	Target Organ	Hormone(s) Released by Target Organ
Gonadotropin-releasing hormone (GnRH)			
Corticotropin-releasing factor (CRF)			
Thyroid-releasing hormone (TRH)			
Dopamine			N/A
Growth hormone–releasing hormone (GHRH)			N/A

2. Which two hormones are primarily involved in calcium homeostasis? Where does each come from, and what effect does each have on blood calcium concentrations?

   •

   •

3. Which endocrine tissue synthesizes catecholamines? What are the two main catecholamines it produces?

4. Which two pancreatic hormones are the major drivers of glucose homeostasis? Where does each come from, and what effect does each have on blood glucose concentrations?

   •

   •

5. Which three hormones are primarily involved in water homeostasis? Where does each come from, and what effect does each have on blood volume and osmolarity?

- ______________________________

- ______________________________

- ______________________________

Conclusion

The endocrine system is unique because its organs are not anatomically related. Hormones are produced in a wide variety of locations and can have far-reaching effects throughout the entire organism. The endocrine system allows for integration and execution of the homeostatic parameters that are necessary to ensure proper functioning of the body. For example, we learned that calcium levels are maintained within a narrow concentration range in the plasma by the antagonistic actions of calcitonin and parathyroid hormone (and vitamin D). Each hormone manipulates the steady state of the organism. As you continue your study of the human body, you will find that the endocrine system has effects on every system of the body by regulating fuel metabolism, blood flow, growth, and development.

In the last section of this chapter, there was a small note on erythropoietin, the hormone that stimulates the production of red blood cells in the bone marrow. Don't interpret this brief mention as an indication that it is relatively unimportant. In fact, every cell of the body (except red blood cells themselves) needs a constant supply of oxygen to accomplish its function. Our bodies take in this oxygen through the respiratory system and then distribute the oxygen to tissues via the circulatory system. In the next two chapters, we will explore each of these systems separately. Recognize, however, that this division is artificial; indeed, like the body as a whole, the respiratory and circulatory systems are inseparable as they serve a common function: providing oxygen for every working cell in the body.

GO ONLINE

You've reviewed the content, now test your knowledge and critical thinking skills by completing a test-like passage set in your online resources!

CONCEPT SUMMARY

Mechanisms of Hormone Action

- Endocrine signaling involves the secretion of **hormones** directly into the bloodstream. The hormones travel to distant target tissues, where they bind to receptors and induce a change in gene expression or cell function.
- **Peptide hormones** are composed of amino acids and are derived from larger precursor proteins that are cleaved during posttranslational modification.
  - Peptide hormones are polar and cannot pass through the plasma membrane.
  - These hormones bind to extracellular receptors, where they trigger the transmission of a **second messenger**.
  - Each step of the **signaling cascade** can induce **amplification** of the signal.
  - Peptide hormones exert effects that usually have rapid onset but are short lived.
  - These hormones are water-soluble, so they travel freely in the bloodstream and do not require a special carrier.
- **Steroid hormones** are derived from cholesterol.
  - Steroid hormones are minimally polar and can pass through the plasma membrane.
  - These hormones bind to and promote a conformational change in cytosolic or intranuclear receptors; the hormone–receptor complex binds to DNA, altering the transcription of a particular gene.
  - Steroid hormones exert effects that usually have slow onset but are long-lived.
  - Because these hormones are lipid-soluble, they cannot dissolve in the bloodstream and must be carried by specific proteins.
- **Amino acid–derivative hormones** are modified amino acids.
  - Their chemistry shares some features with peptide hormones and some features with steroid hormones; different amino acid–derivative hormones share different features with these other hormone classes.
  - Common examples are epinephrine, norepinephrine, triiodothyronine, and thyroxine.
- Hormones can be classified by their target tissues.
  - **Direct hormones** have major effects on non-endocrine tissues.
  - **Tropic hormones** have major effects on other endocrine tissues.

Endocrine Organs and Hormones

- The hypothalamus is the bridge between the nervous and endocrine systems.
  - The release of hormones from the hypothalamus is mediated by a number of factors, including projections from other parts of the brain, chemo- and baroreceptors in the blood vessels, and negative feedback from other hormones.
  - In **negative feedback**, the final hormone (or product) of a pathway inhibits hormones (or enzymes) earlier in the pathway, maintaining **homeostasis**.

  - The hypothalamus stimulates the anterior pituitary gland through paracrine release of hormones into the hypophyseal portal system, which directly connects the two organs.
  - **Gonadotropin-releasing hormone** (**GnRH**) promotes the release of follicle-stimulating hormone (FSH) and luteinizing hormone (LH).
  - **Growth hormone–releasing hormone** (**GHRH**) promotes the release of growth hormone.
  - **Thyroid-releasing hormone** (**TRH**) promotes the release of thyroid-stimulating hormone (TSH).
  - **Corticotropin-releasing factor** (**CRF**) promotes the release of adrenocorticotropic hormone (ACTH).
  - **Prolactin-inhibiting factor** (**PIF** or **dopamine**) inhibits the release of prolactin.
  - Interactions with the posterior pituitary occur via the axons of nerves projected by the hypothalamus. Antidiuretic hormone (ADH or vasopressin) and oxytocin are synthesized in the hypothalamus and then travel down these axons to the posterior pituitary, where they are released into the bloodstream.
- The **anterior pituitary** releases hormones in response to stimulation from the hypothalamus. Four of these (FSH, LH, ACTH, and TSH) are tropic hormones, while three (prolactin, endorphins, and growth hormone) are direct hormones.
  - **Follicle-stimulating hormone** (**FSH**) promotes the development of ovarian follicles in females and spermatogenesis in males.
  - **Luteinizing hormone** (**LH**) promotes ovulation in females and testosterone production in males.
  - **Adrenocorticotropic hormone** (**ACTH**) promotes the synthesis and release of glucocorticoids from the adrenal cortex.
  - **Thyroid-stimulating hormone** (**TSH**) promotes the synthesis and release of triiodothyronine and thyroxine from the thyroid.
  - **Prolactin** promotes milk production.
  - **Endorphins** decrease perception of pain and can produce euphoria.
  - **Growth hormone** (**GH**) promotes growth of bone and muscle and shunts glucose to these tissues. It raises blood glucose concentrations.
- The **posterior pituitary** releases two hormones produced in the hypothalamus.
  - **Antidiuretic hormone** (**ADH** or **vasopressin**) is secreted in response to low blood volume or increased blood osmolarity and increases reabsorption of water in the collecting duct of the nephron, increasing blood volume and decreasing blood osmolarity.
  - **Oxytocin** is secreted during childbirth and promotes uterine contractions. It also promotes milk ejection and may be involved in bonding behavior. It is unusual in that it has a **positive feedback** loop, not negative.
- The **thyroid** is located at the base of the neck in front of the trachea; it produces three key hormones.
  - **Triiodothyronine** (T_3) and **thyroxine** (T_4) are produced by **follicular cells** and contain iodine. They increase basal metabolic rate and alter the utilization of glucose and fatty acids. Thyroid hormones are required for proper neurological and physical development in children.
  - **Calcitonin** is produced by **parafollicular** (**C**) **cells**. It decreases plasma calcium concentration by promoting calcium excretion in the kidneys, decreasing calcium absorption in the gut, and promoting calcium storage in bone.

- The **parathyroid glands** release **parathyroid hormone (PTH)**, which increases blood calcium concentration.
    - PTH decreases excretion of calcium by the kidneys and increases bone resorption directly to increase blood calcium concentration.
    - PTH activates vitamin D, which is necessary for calcium and phosphate absorption from the gut.
    - PTH promotes resorption of phosphate from bone and reduces reabsorption of phosphate in the kidney, but vitamin D promotes absorption of phosphate from the gut; these two effects on phosphate concentration somewhat cancel each other out.
- The **adrenal cortex** produces three classes of steroid hormones.
    - **Glucocorticoids** such as **cortisol** and **cortisone** increase blood glucose concentration, reduce protein synthesis, inhibit the immune system, and participate in the stress response. Glucocorticoid release is stimulated by ACTH.
    - **Mineralocorticoids** such as **aldosterone** promote sodium reabsorption in the distal convoluted tubule and collecting duct, thus increasing water reabsorption. Aldosterone also increases potassium and hydrogen ion excretion. Aldosterone activity is regulated by the **renin–angiotensin–aldosterone system**, not ACTH.
    - **Cortical sex hormones** include **androgens** (like **testosterone**) and **estrogens** in both males and females.
- The **adrenal medulla** is derived from the nervous system and secretes catecholamines into the bloodstream.
    - **Catecholamines** include **epinephrine** and **norepinephrine**, which are involved in the fight-or-flight (sympathetic) response.
    - These hormones promote glycogenolysis, increase the basal metabolic rate, increase heart rate, dilate the bronchi, and alter blood flow.
- The endocrine **pancreas** produces hormones that regulate glucose homeostasis.
    - **Glucagon** is produced by **α-cells** and raises blood glucose levels by stimulating protein and fat degradation, glycogenolysis, and gluconeogenesis.
    - **Insulin** is produced by **β-cells** and lowers blood glucose levels by stimulating glucose uptake by cells and promoting anabolic processes, like glycogen, fat, and protein synthesis.
    - **Somatostatin** is produced by **δ-cells** and inhibits insulin and glucagon secretion.
- The gonads produce hormones that are involved in the development and maintenance of the reproductive systems and secondary sex characteristics.
    - The **testes** secrete **testosterone**.
    - The **ovaries** secrete **estrogen** and **progesterone**.
- The **pineal gland** releases **melatonin**, which helps to regulate **circadian rhythms**.
- Other organs may release hormones, even if they are not primarily considered part of the endocrine system.
    - Cells in the stomach and intestine produce hormones like **secretin**, **gastrin**, and **cholecystokinin**.
    - The kidneys secrete **erythropoietin**, which stimulates bone marrow to produce erythrocytes (red blood cells) in response to low oxygen levels in the blood.
    - The atria of the heart secrete **atrial natriuretic peptide (ANP)**, which promotes excretion of salt and water in the kidneys in response to stretching of the atria (high blood volume).
    - The thymus secretes **thymosin**, which is important for proper T-cell development and differentiation.

ANSWERS TO CONCEPT CHECKS

5.1

1.

Criterion	Peptide Hormones	Steroid Hormones
Chemical precursor	Amino acids (polypeptides)	Cholesterol
Location of receptor	Extracellular (cell membrane)	Intracellular or intranuclear
Mechanism of action	Stimulates a receptor (usually a G protein–coupled receptor), affecting levels of second messengers (commonly cAMP). Initiates a signal cascade	Binds to a receptor, induces conformational change, and regulates transcription at the level of the DNA
Method of travel in the bloodstream	Dissolves and travels freely	Binds to a carrier protein
Speed of onset	Quick	Slow
Duration of action	Short lived	Long lived

2. Amino acid–derivative hormones are made by modifying amino acids, such as the addition of iodine to tyrosine (in thyroid hormone production).
3. Direct hormones are secreted into the bloodstream and travel to a target tissue, where they have direct effects. Tropic hormones cause secretion of another hormone that then travels to the target tissue to cause an effect.

5.2

1.

Hypothalamic Releasing Hormone	Hormone(s) from Anterior Pituitary	Target Organ	Hormone(s) Released by Target Organ
Gonadotropin-releasing hormone (GnRH)	Follicle-stimulating hormone (FSH) and luteinizing hormone (LH)	Gonads (testes or ovaries)	Testosterone (testes) or estrogen and progesterone (ovaries)
Corticotropin-releasing factor (CRF)	Adrenocortico-tropic hormone (ACTH)	Adrenal cortex	Glucocorticoids (cortisol and cortisone)
Thyroid-releasing hormone (TRH)	Thyroid-stimulating hormone (TSH)	Thyroid	Triiodothyronine (T_3), thyroxine (T_4)
Dopamine	Prolactin*	Breast tissue	N/A
Growth hormone–releasing hormone (GHRH)	Growth hormone	Bone, muscle	N/A
*Note that a *decrease* in dopamine from the hypothalamus promotes prolactin secretion.			

2. Calcitonin from the parafollicular (C-) cells of the thyroid decreases blood calcium concentration. Parathyroid hormone from the parathyroid glands increases blood calcium concentration.
3. The adrenal medulla synthesizes catecholamines, including epinephrine and norepinephrine.
4. Glucagon from the α-cells of the pancreas increases blood glucose concentration. Insulin from the β-cells of the pancreas decreases blood glucose concentration.
5. Antidiuretic hormone (ADH or vasopressin) from the hypothalamus (released by the posterior pituitary) increases blood volume and decreases blood osmolarity. Aldosterone from the adrenal cortex increases blood volume with no effect on blood osmolarity. Atrial natriuretic peptide (ANP) from the heart decreases blood volume with no effect on blood osmolarity.

SCIENCE MASTERY ASSESSMENT EXPLANATIONS

1. **C**

Unlike the other hormones listed here, ADH is not secreted by the adrenal cortex and is therefore not a *–corticoid.* Rather, ADH is a peptide hormone produced by the hypothalamus and released by the posterior pituitary that promotes water reabsorption. The other associations are all correct.

2. **D**

A hormone that directly stimulates a non-endocrine target tissue is referred to as a direct hormone. Glancing at the answer choices, we notice that all of the hormones are secreted by the anterior pituitary gland. The direct hormones secreted by the anterior pituitary are prolactin, endorphins, and growth hormone (GH). All of the other answer choices are tropic hormones. The tropic hormones of the anterior pituitary include follicle-stimulating hormone (FSH), luteinizing hormone (LH), adrenocorticotropic hormone (ACTH), and thyroid-stimulating hormone (TSH).

3. **A**

The parathyroid glands secrete parathyroid hormone (PTH), a hormone that functions to increase blood calcium levels. An increase in synthetic activity of the parathyroid glands would lead to an increase in PTH and, therefore, an increase in blood calcium levels through three mechanisms: increased calcium reabsorption in the kidneys (decreased excretion), increased bone resorption, and increased absorption of calcium from the gut (via activation of vitamin D).

4. **B**

Peptide hormones are composed of chains of amino acids and, though they vary in size, are generally too large, charged, and polar to cross the cell membrane. Instead, these hormones bind to extracellular receptors and rely on second messengers to mediate their effects. All of these observations justify **(B)**.

5. **B**

Inflammation of the thyroid or iodine deficiency can cause hypothyroidism, in which the thyroid hormones are undersecreted or not secreted at all. Hypothyroidism in newborn infants causes cretinism, which is characterized by poor neurological and physical development (including intellectual disabilities, short stature, and coarse facial features). While iodine deficiency can result in a swelling of the thyroid gland (called a goiter), which can also be seen in causes of hyperthyroidism, iodine deficiency does not cause hyperthyroidism, eliminating **(D)**. Galactorrhea, **(A)**, is associated with prolactin; gigantism, **(C)**, is associated with growth hormone.

6. **C**

The hypothalamic–pituitary–thyroid axis includes the secretion of thyroid-releasing hormone (TRH) from the hypothalamus triggering the secretion of thyroid-stimulating hormone (TSH) from the anterior pituitary, which stimulates the secretion of triiodothyronine (T_3) and thyroxine (T_4) from the thyroid. Overproduction of TRH would promote overproduction of TSH, eliminating **(B)**. Destruction of the follicular cells that produce T_3 and T_4 would remove negative feedback, allowing TSH levels to rise, eliminating **(A)** and **(D)**. High levels of T_4 would cause too much negative feedback and lower TSH levels, making **(C)** the correct answer.

7. **B**

Steroid hormones are nonpolar cholesterol derivatives and bind to internal receptors. Importantly, as cholesterol derivatives, these hormones generally lack nitrogen and are composed primarily of carbon, hydrogen, and oxygen. All of these factors support **(B)** as the right answer. By contrast, **(A)** can be eliminated because peptide hormones would localize to the cell surface. And, while amino acid derivatives can signal like steroid hormones, **(C)** can be eliminated since the chemical composition given in the question stem indicates a lack of nitrogen. **(D)** can be eliminated since the term "direct" refers to the hormone target, and data about the target of the hormone are not given in this question stem.

8. **B**

Pancreatic somatostatin secretion is increased by high blood glucose or amino acid levels, leading to decreased insulin and glucagon secretion, eliminating **(A)** and **(D)**. Somatostatin is thus always an inhibitory hormone, confirming **(B)**. The stimuli for somatostatin release include high blood glucose or amino acids, as mentioned above, as well as high levels of certain gastrointestinal hormones, as discussed in Chapter 9 of *MCAT Biology Review*—but not cortisol, eliminating **(C)**.

9. **C**

β-cells are responsible for insulin production. The function of insulin is to lower blood glucose levels by promoting the influx of glucose into cells and by stimulating anabolic processes, such as glycogenesis or fat and protein synthesis. Thus, destruction of the β-cells would result in a cessation of insulin production, which would lead to hyperglycemia, or high blood glucose concentration.

10. **D**

The stimulus for renin production is low blood pressure, which causes the juxtaglomerular cells of the kidney to produce renin, an enzyme that converts the plasma protein angiotensinogen to angiotensin I. Angiotensin I is then converted to angiotensin II by an enzyme in the lungs; angiotensin II then stimulates the adrenal cortex to secrete aldosterone. Aldosterone helps to restore blood volume by increasing sodium reabsorption in the kidney, leading to an increase in water reabsorption. This removes the initial stimulus for renin production. Thus, **(A)**, **(B)**, and **(C)** correctly describe the renin–angiotensin–aldosterone system, while **(D)** describes the stimulus for erythropoietin secretion.

11. **B**

The question stem indicates that the newly discovered hormone functions as a first messenger, stimulating the conversion of ATP to cAMP; cAMP functions as a second messenger, triggering a signaling cascade in the cell. Hormones that act via second messengers and are relatively large in size (short peptides or complex polypeptides) are peptide hormones. This hormone could be a tropic hormone, but it is also entirely possible for it to be a direct hormone; thus, **(D)** can be eliminated.

12. **B**

Regardless of the cause, the low levels of calcium in the blood require treatment. While other therapies are more frequently used to treat hypocalcemia (low blood calcium levels), such as calcium gluconate or calcium chloride, administration of parathyroid hormone would also raise blood calcium concentration. Calcitonin would be a poor choice in this case, as this hormone lowers blood calcium concentrations, eliminating **(A)**. Aldosterone and thymosin play no role in calcium homeostasis, eliminating **(C)** and **(D)**.

13. **C**

Both oxytocin and vasopressin (another name for antidiuretic hormone) end with the suffix *–in*; this should hint that they are peptide or amino acid–derivative hormones. These two hormones are both synthesized by the hypothalamus, but released by the posterior pituitary. Remember that the posterior pituitary does not actually synthesize any hormones itself; rather, it contains the axons that originate in cells in the hypothalamus and is the site of release for these hormones.

14. **C**

Dopamine is used in a number of neurological systems; most relevant to the endocrine system is the fact that dopamine secretion prevents prolactin release. Thus, an individual taking medications that block dopamine receptors would lose this inhibition on prolactin release and have elevated prolactin levels.

15. **D**

The question stem states that an infant who is genotypically female is born with ambiguous genitalia, meaning that the genitalia do not appear to be specifically female or specifically male. In a genotypic female, this indicates that the infant was exposed to androgens during the fetal period. In addition, the infant is also losing sodium, causing hyponatremia. This indicates two issues: excess androgens and a lack of aldosterone, a hormone required for proper reuptake of sodium in the kidneys. Both of these hormones are synthesized in the adrenal cortex, making **(D)** the correct answer. Note that neither of these hormones is regulated by the hypothalamic–pituitary–adrenal axis, eliminating **(A)** and **(B)**.

GO ONLINE
Consult your online resources for additional practice.

SHARED CONCEPTS

Behavioral Sciences Chapter 5
Motivation, Emotion, and Stress

Biochemistry Chapter 3
Nonenzymatic Protein Function and Protein Analysis

Biochemistry Chapter 8
Biological Membranes

Biochemistry Chapter 12
Bioenergetics and Regulation of Metabolism

Biology Chapter 4
The Nervous System

Biology Chapter 10
Homeostasis

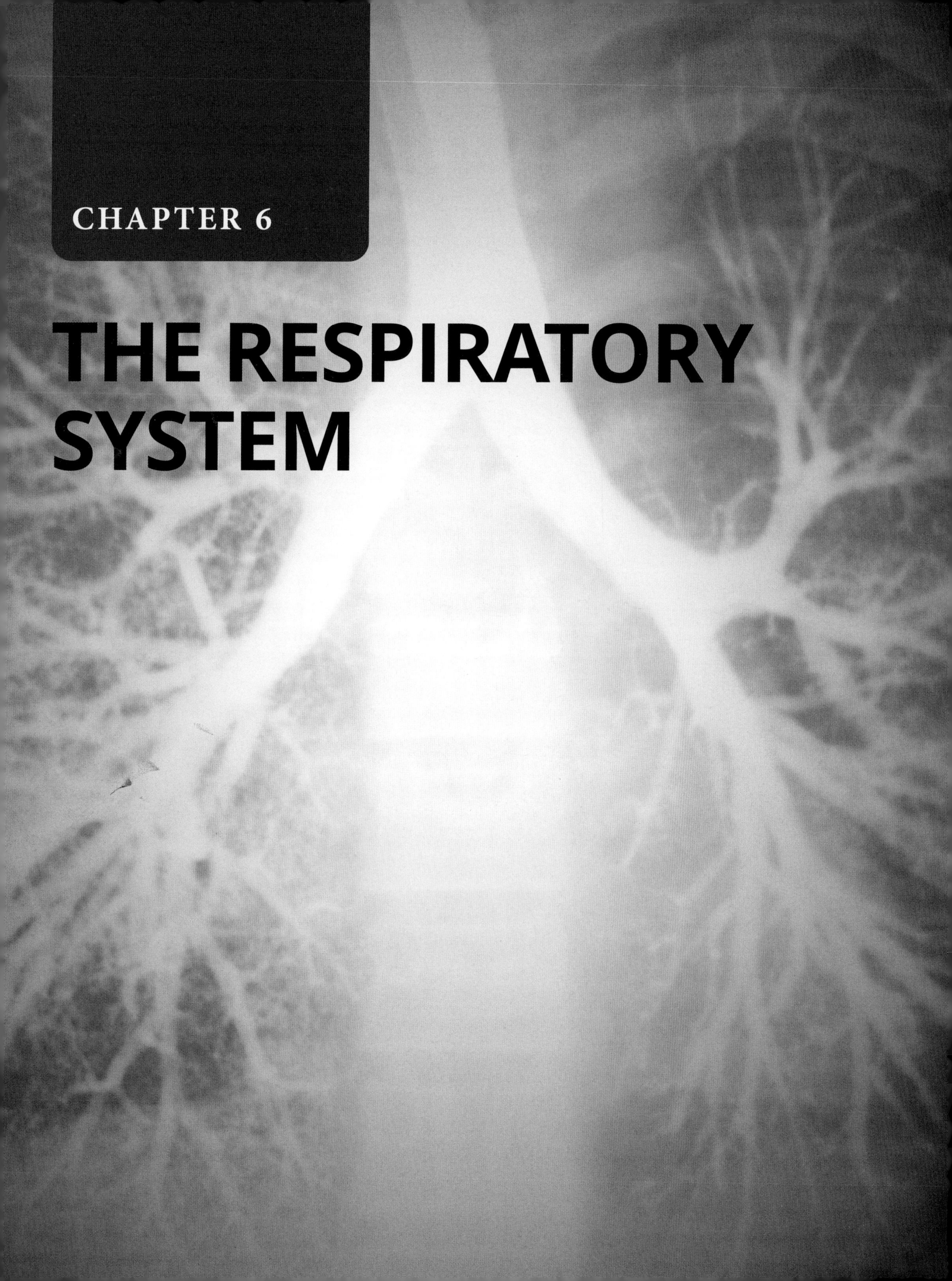

CHAPTER 6

THE RESPIRATORY SYSTEM

SCIENCE MASTERY ASSESSMENT

Every pre-med knows this feeling: there is so much content I have to know for the MCAT! How do I know what to do first or what's important?

While the high-yield badges throughout this book will help you identify the most important topics, this Science Mastery Assessment is another tool in your MCAT prep arsenal. This quiz (which can also be taken in your online resources) and the guidance below will help ensure that you are spending the appropriate amount of time on this chapter based on your personal strengths and weaknesses. Don't worry though—skipping something now does not mean you'll never study it. Later on in your prep, as you complete full-length tests, you'll uncover specific pieces of content that you need to review and can come back to these chapters as appropriate.

How to Use This Assessment

If you answer 0–7 questions correctly:

Spend about 1 hour to read this chapter in full and take limited notes throughout. Follow up by reviewing **all** quiz questions to ensure that you now understand how to solve each one.

If you answer 8–11 questions correctly:

Spend 20–40 minutes reviewing the quiz questions. Beginning with the questions you missed, read and take notes on the corresponding subchapters. For questions you answered correctly, ensure your thinking matches that of the explanation and you understand why each choice was correct or incorrect.

If you answer 12–15 questions correctly:

Spend less than 20 minutes reviewing all questions from the quiz. If you missed any, then include a quick read-through of the corresponding subchapters, or even just the relevant content within a subchapter, as part of your question review. For questions you answered correctly, ensure your thinking matches that of the explanation and review the Concept Summary at the end of the chapter.

1. All of the following facilitate gas exchange in the lungs EXCEPT:
   A. thin alveolar walls.
   B. multiple subdivisions of the respiratory tree.
   C. differences in the partial pressures of O_2 and CO_2.
   D. active transporters in alveolar cells.

2. Which of the following associations correctly pairs a stage of respiration with the muscle actions occurring during that stage?
   A. Inhalation—diaphragm relaxes
   B. Inhalation—internal intercostal muscles contract
   C. Exhalation—diaphragm contracts
   D. Exhalation—external intercostal muscles relax

3. Total lung capacity is equal to the vital capacity plus the:
   A. tidal volume.
   B. expiratory reserve volume.
   C. residual volume.
   D. inspiratory reserve volume.

4. The intrapleural pressure is necessarily lower than the atmospheric pressure during:
   A. inhalation, because the expansion of the chest cavity causes compression of the intrapleural space, decreasing its pressure.
   B. inhalation, because the expansion of the chest cavity causes expansion of the intrapleural space, decreasing its pressure.
   C. exhalation, because the compression of the chest cavity causes compression of the intrapleural space, decreasing its pressure.
   D. exhalation, because the compression of the chest cavity causes expansion of the intrapleural space, decreasing its pressure.

5. A patient presents to the emergency room with a stab wound to the left side of the chest. On a chest X-ray, blood is noted to be collecting in the chest cavity, causing collapse of both lobes of the left lung. The blood is most likely located between:
   A. the parietal pleura and the chest wall.
   B. the parietal pleura and the visceral pleura.
   C. the visceral pleura and the lung.
   D. the alveolar walls and the lung surface.

6. Each of the following statements regarding the anatomy of the respiratory system is true EXCEPT:
   A. the epiglottis covers the glottis during swallowing to ensure that food does not enter the trachea.
   B. the trachea and bronchi are lined by ciliated epithelial cells.
   C. the pharynx contains two vocal cords, which are controlled by skeletal muscle and cartilage.
   D. the nares are lined with vibrissae, which help filter out particulate matter from inhaled air.

7. Which of the following is a correct sequence of passageways through which air travels during inhalation?
   A. Pharynx → trachea → bronchioles → bronchi → alveoli
   B. Pharynx → trachea → larynx → bronchi → alveoli
   C. Larynx → pharynx → trachea → bronchi → alveoli
   D. Pharynx → larynx → trachea → bronchi → alveoli

8. Idiopathic pulmonary fibrosis (IPF) is a disease in which scar tissue forms in the alveolar walls, making the lung tissue significantly more stiff. Which of the following findings would likely be detected through spirometry in a patient with IPF?
   I. Decreased total lung capacity
   II. Decreased inspiratory reserve volume
   III. Increased residual volume
   A. I only
   B. II only
   C. I and II only
   D. I, II, and III

9. Studies have indicated that premature babies are often deficient in lysozyme. What is a possible consequence of this deficiency?
   A. Respiratory distress and alveolar collapse shortly after birth
   B. Increased susceptibility to certain infections
   C. Inability to humidify air as it passes through the nasal cavity
   D. Slowing of the respiratory rate in response to acidemia

10. Some forms of pneumonia cause an excess of fluids such as mucus or pus to build up within an entire lobe of the lung. How will this affect the diffusion of gases within the affected area?
   - **A.** Carbon dioxide can diffuse out, but oxygen will not be able to enter the blood.
   - **B.** Oxygen can diffuse into the blood, but carbon dioxide cannot diffuse out.
   - **C.** No change in diffusion will occur.
   - **D.** No diffusion will occur in the affected area.

11. Some people with anxiety disorders respond to stress by hyperventilating. It is recommended that they breathe into a paper bag and then rebreathe this air. Why is this treatment appropriate?
   - **A.** Hyperventilation causes an increase in blood carbon dioxide, and breathing the air in the bag helps to readjust blood levels of carbon dioxide.
   - **B.** Hyperventilation causes a decrease in blood carbon dioxide, and breathing the air in the bag helps to readjust blood levels of carbon dioxide.
   - **C.** Hyperventilation causes an increase in blood oxygen, and breathing the air in the bag helps to readjust blood levels of oxygen.
   - **D.** Hyperventilation causes a decrease in blood oxygen, and breathing the air in the bag helps to readjust blood levels of oxygen.

12. A patient presents to the emergency room with an asthma attack. The patient has been hyperventilating for the past hour and has a blood pH of 7.52. The patient is given treatment and does not appear to respond, but a subsequent blood pH reading is 7.41. Why might this normal blood pH NOT be a reassuring sign?
   - **A.** The patient's kidneys may have compensated for the alkalemia.
   - **B.** The normal blood pH reading is likely inaccurate.
   - **C.** The patient may be descending into respiratory failure.
   - **D.** The patient's blood should ideally become acidemic for some time to compensate for the alkalemia.

13. Premature infants with respiratory distress are often placed on ventilators. Often, the ventilators are set to provide positive end-expiratory pressure. Why might this setting be useful for a premature infant?
   - **A.** Premature infants lack surfactant.
   - **B.** Premature infants lack lysozyme.
   - **C.** Premature infants cannot thermoregulate.
   - **D.** Premature infants are unable to control pH.

14. In emphysema, the alveolar walls are destroyed, decreasing the recoil of the lung tissue. Which of the following changes may be seen in a patient with emphysema?
   - **A.** Increased residual volume
   - **B.** Decreased total lung capacity
   - **C.** Increased blood concentration of oxygen
   - **D.** Decreased blood concentration of carbon dioxide

15. Allergic reactions occur due to an overactive immune response to a substance. Which cells within the respiratory tract play the largest role in the generation of allergic reactions?
   - **A.** Alveolar epithelial cells
   - **B.** Macrophages
   - **C.** Mast cells
   - **D.** Ciliated epithelial cells

Answer Key

1. **D** (See section 6.2)
2. **D** (See section 6.1)
3. **C** (See section 6.1)
4. **B** (See section 6.1)
5. **B** (See section 6.1)
6. **C** (See section 6.1)
7. **D** (See section 6.1)
8. **B** (See section 6.1)
9. **B** (See section 6.2)
10. **D** (See section 6.2)
11. **B** (See section 6.2)
12. **C** (See section 6.2)
13. **A** (See section 6.1)
14. **A** (See section 6.1)
15. **C** (See section 6.2)

The relevant section of the chapter to review for each question is given in parentheses after the correct answer. Detailed explanations can be found at the end of the chapter.

CHAPTER 6

THE RESPIRATORY SYSTEM

In This Chapter

CHAPTER PROFILE

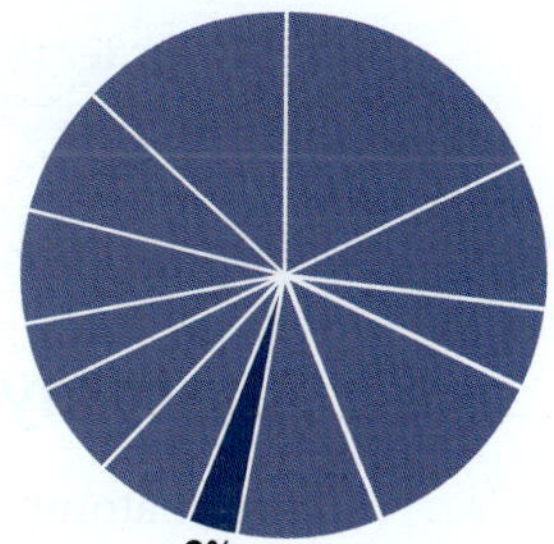

The content in this chapter should be relevant to about 3% of all questions about biology on the MCAT.

This chapter covers material from the following AAMC content category:

3B: Structure and integrative functions of the main organ systems

Introduction

Coughing. Fever. Shortness of breath. Hypoxia. All are symptoms of a number of pulmonary diseases, from a flareup of *chronic obstructive pulmonary disease* (COPD), to *Streptococcus pneumoniae* (pneumococcal) pneumonia, to a type of hypersensitivity pneumonitis known as *extrinsic allergic alveolitis* (EAA). This last example is a bit more esoteric and can be brought on by hypersensitivity to anything from dried grass, to rat urine, to mold that grows in hot tubs—what is sometimes called *hot tub lung*. Not all cases of hot tub lung are severe, but certainly none are enjoyable. They are often misdiagnosed as asthma or bronchitis and may be treated with steroids, which quell the immune system and reduce inflammation. Because hot tub lung can potentially go away by itself, antibiotic therapy is not always recommended. As a physician, you may end up simply having to tell your patients that the best way to avoid hot tub lung is to make sure that the tub is cleaned properly and routinely before use.

The lesson here isn't to avoid hot tubs. It's that the lungs are essential, sensitive organs with delicate membranes that must be protected. Many types of stressors (pathogens, particles, or chemicals) can irritate them and cause respiratory distress. In this chapter, we'll look at the structure of the lungs and the microanatomy of respiration. We'll also talk about the mechanics of breathing, as well as the overall function of the lungs.

MCAT EXPERTISE

You may be surprised at the low percentage of questions associated with this chapter, given that this chapter touches on several classic MCAT topics including pressure, gases, and equilibrium. And you may see questions on your MCAT that relate to the work done on air in the lungs, for example. However, such a question would depend much more on your general knowledge of work, energy, and gases (regardless of context) than your knowledge of the respiratory system specifically.

6.1 Anatomy and Mechanism of Breathing

LEARNING OBJECTIVES

After Chapter 6.1, you will be able to:

- Identify the muscles involved in inhalation and exhalation
- Explain the purpose and function of surfactant
- Recall the mathematical relationships between vital capacity, inspiratory reserve volume, expiratory reserve volume, and tidal volume
- Predict how the brain will alter respiratory rate in response to changing blood levels of O_2 and CO_2
- Order the structures in the pathway that air uses to enter the body, from the nares to the alveoli

The lungs are located in the **thoracic cavity**, the structure of which is specially designed to perform breathing.

Anatomy

The anatomy of the respiratory system is summarized in Figure 6.1. Gas exchange occurs in the lungs. Air enters the respiratory tract through the external **nares** of the nose and then passes through the nasal cavity, where it is filtered by mucous membranes and nasal hairs (**vibrissae**).

KEY CONCEPT

The nose and mouth serve several important roles in breathing by removing dirt and particulate matter from the air and warming and humidifying it before it reaches the lungs.

Next, air passes into the pharynx and the larynx. The **pharynx** resides behind the nasal cavity and at the back of the mouth; it is a common pathway for both air destined for the lungs and food destined for the esophagus. In contrast, the **larynx** lies below the pharynx and is only a pathway for air. To keep food out of the respiratory tract, the opening of the larynx (**glottis**) is covered by the **epiglottis** during swallowing. The larynx contains two **vocal cords** that are maneuvered using skeletal muscle and cartilage. From the larynx, air passes into the cartilaginous **trachea** and then into one of the two mainstem **bronchi**. The bronchi and trachea contain **ciliated pseudostratified columnar epithelial cells** to catch and remove particulate that have made it past the mucous membranes in the nose and mouth.

In the **lungs**, the bronchi continue to divide into smaller structures known as **bronchioles**, which divide further until they end in the tiny balloon-like structures in which gas exchange occurs (**alveoli**). Each alveolus, as shown in Figure 6.2, is coated with **surfactant**, a detergent that lowers surface tension and prevents the alveolus from collapsing on itself. A network of capillaries surrounds each alveolus to carry oxygen and carbon dioxide. The branching and minute size of the alveoli allow for an exceptionally large surface area for gas exchange—approximately 100 m^2 in total.

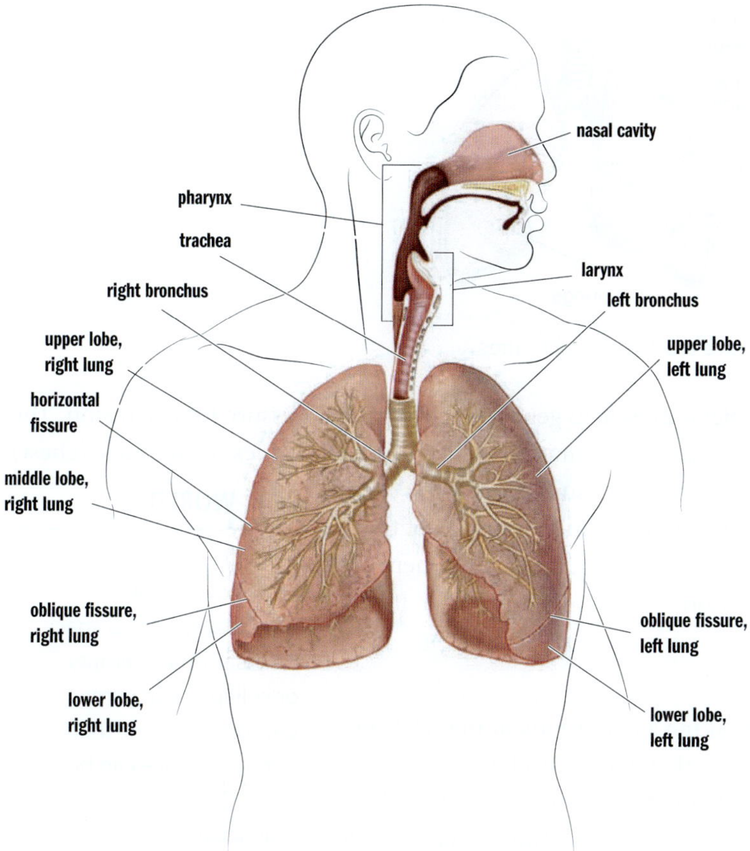

Figure 6.1 Anatomy of the Respiratory System

REAL WORLD

The left lung has a small indentation, making it slightly smaller than the right lung. It also contains only two lobes, while the right lung contains three. Why might this be? It is due to the position of the heart in the thoracic cavity.

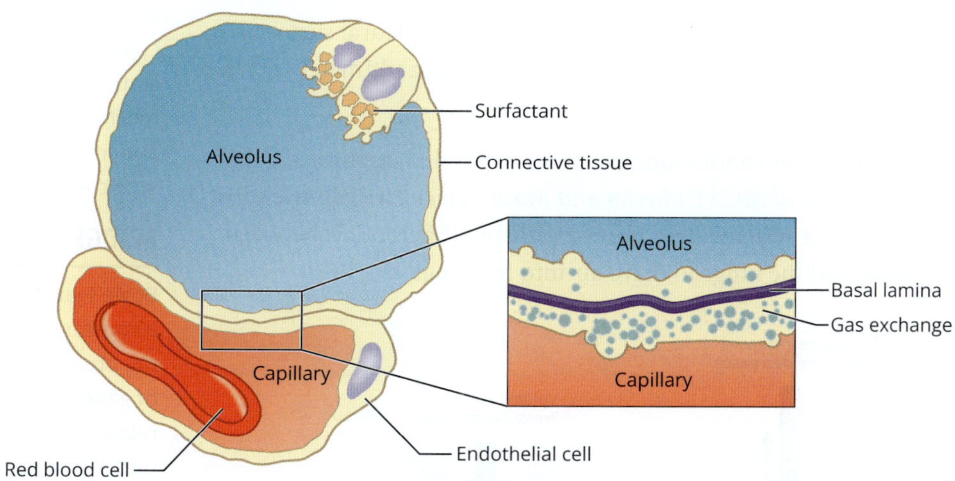

Figure 6.2 Alveolus

The lungs themselves are contained in the thoracic cavity, which also contains the heart. The chest wall forms the outside of the thoracic cavity. Membranes known as **pleurae** surround each lung, as shown in Figure 6.3. The pleura forms a closed sac against which the lung expands. The surface adjacent to the lung is the **visceral pleura**, and the outer part is the **parietal pleura**.

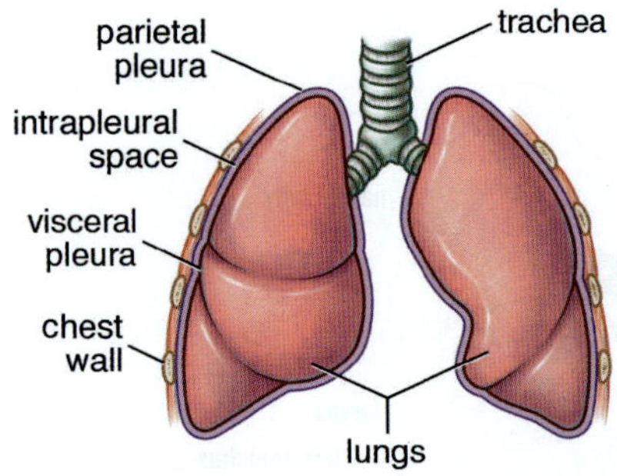

Figure 6.3 Lung Membranes

The lungs do not fill passively, and require skeletal muscle to generate the negative pressure for expansion. The most important of these muscles is the **diaphragm**, a thin, muscular structure that divides the thoracic (chest) cavity from the abdominal cavity. The diaphragm is under somatic control, even though breathing itself is under autonomic control. In addition, muscles of the chest wall, back, and neck may also participate in breathing, especially when breathing is labored due to a pathologic condition.

Breathing

Before we discuss breathing itself, it is worth taking a closer look at the relationship between the pleurae and the lungs. Imagine that you have a large, partially deflated balloon. Now, imagine taking your fist and pushing it against the balloon so that the balloon comes up and surrounds your hand. This is analogous to a lung and its pleura. Our fist is the lung, and the balloon represents both pleural layers. The side directly touching our fist is the visceral pleura, and the outer layer is the parietal pleura, which is associated with the chest wall in real life. The space within the sac is referred to as the **intrapleural space**, which contains a thin layer of fluid. This pleural fluid helps lubricate the two pleural surfaces. The pressure differentials that can be created across the pleura ultimately drive breathing, as we explore in the next section.

Let's turn to the mechanics of ventilation, which are grounded in physics. As discussed in Chapters 2 and 3 of *MCAT Physics and Math Review*, we can use pressure to do useful work in a system. Here, we use pressure differentials between the intrapleural space and the lungs to drive air into the lungs.

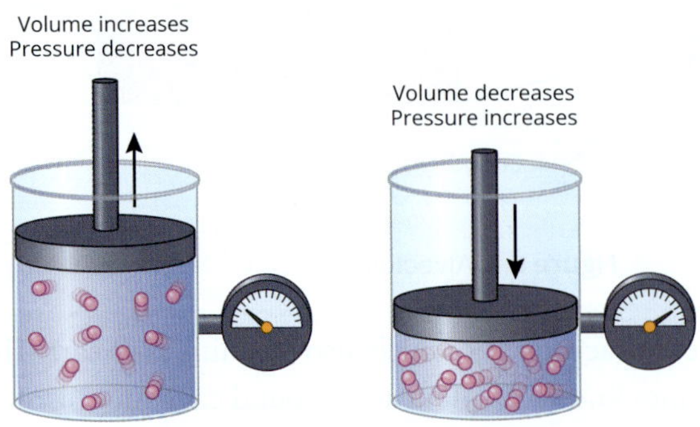

Figure 6.4 Boyle's Law

REAL WORLD

The intrapleural space is an example of a potential space—a space that is normally empty or collapsed. In some pathologic states, that potential space can be expanded by fluid or air that accumulates between the two pleural layers. For example, in a pleural effusion, fluid accumulates in the intrapleural space. In a pneumothorax, air collects here. Each of these states disturbs the normal mechanics of the breathing apparatus and can cause atelectasis, or lung collapse.

BRIDGE

Boyle's law states that, at a constant temperature, the pressure and volume of gases are inversely related. This is the principle underlying negative-pressure breathing: as the chest wall expands, volume increases and pressure decreases in the lungs, and air is drawn into the lungs. See Figure 6.4 for an illustration of this concept.

Inhalation

Inhalation is an active process. We use our diaphragm as well as the **external intercostal muscles** (one of the layers of muscles between the ribs) to expand the thoracic cavity, as shown in Figure 6.5. As the diaphragm flattens and the chest wall expands outward, the **intrathoracic volume** (the volume of the chest cavity) increases. Specifically, because the intrapleural space most closely abuts the chest wall, its volume increases first. Can we predict what will happen to intrapleural pressure? From our understanding of Boyle's law, an increase in intrapleural volume leads to a *decrease* in intrapleural pressure.

Now we have low pressure in the intrapleural space. What about inside the lungs? The gas in the lungs is initially at atmospheric pressure, which is now higher than the pressure in the intrapleural space. The lungs will therefore expand into the intrapleural space, and the pressure in the lungs will drop. Air will then be sucked in from a higher-pressure environment—the outside world. This mechanism is referred to as **negative-pressure breathing** because the driving force is the lower (relatively negative) pressure in the intrapleural space compared with the lungs.

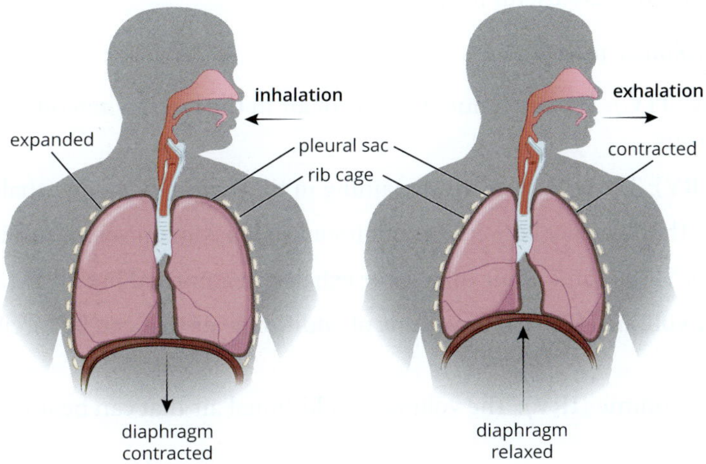

Figure 6.5 Stages of Ventilation
The diaphragm contracts during inhalation and relaxes during exhalation.

Exhalation

Unlike inhalation, exhalation does not have to be an active process. Simple relaxation of the external intercostal muscles will reverse the processes we discussed in the last paragraph. As the diaphragm and external intercostals relax, the chest cavity decreases in volume. What will happen to pressure in the intrapleural space? It will go up, again explained by Boyle's law. Alveolar (intrapulmonary) pressure rises above atmospheric pressure, while intrapleural pressure stays negative relative to both, creating a pressure gradient that drives air out of the lungs. Now pressure in the intrapleural space is higher than in the lungs, which is still at atmospheric pressure. Thus, air will be pushed out, resulting in exhalation. During active tasks, we can speed this process up by using the **internal intercostal muscles** and abdominal muscles, which oppose the external intercostals and pull the rib cage down. This actively decreases the volume of the thoracic cavity. Finally, recall that surfactant prevents the complete collapse of the alveoli during exhalation by reducing surface tension at the alveolar surface.

KEY CONCEPT

Inhalation and exhalation require different amounts of energy expenditure. Muscle contraction is required to create the negative pressure in the thoracic cavity that forces air into the lungs during inspiration. Expiration during calm states is entirely due to elastic recoil of the lungs and the musculature. During more active states, the muscles can be used to force air out and speed up the process of ventilation.

Remember the balloon analogy from before. The lungs have a resilient, elastic quality and are attached via the pleurae to the chest wall. The chest wall expands on inhalation, pulling the lungs with it and creating the pressure differential required for inhalation. As the chest wall relaxes, the lungs recoil due to the intrinsic elastic quality of the lungs and surface tension in the alveoli, accentuating the relaxation process. When the lungs recoil, their volume becomes smaller, and the pressure increases. Now the pressure inside the lungs is higher than the outside pressure, and exhalation occurs. Note that the indirect connection of the lungs to the chest wall also prevents them from collapsing completely on recoil, like surfactant.

REAL WORLD

Emphysema is a disease characterized by the destruction of the alveolar walls. This results in reduced elastic recoil of the lungs, making the process of exhalation extremely difficult. Most cases of emphysema are caused by cigarette smoking.

Lung Capacities and Volumes

In pulmonology (the medical field associated with the lungs and breathing), we frequently must assess lung capacities and volumes. One instrument used to measure these quantities is a **spirometer**. While a spirometer cannot measure the amount of air remaining in the lung after complete exhalation (residual volume), it provides a number of measures that are useful in clinical medicine.

Commonly tested lung volumes include:

- **Total lung capacity** (TLC): The maximum volume of air in the lungs when one inhales completely; usually around 6 to 7 liters
- **Residual volume** (RV): The volume of air remaining in the lungs when one exhales completely
- **Vital capacity** (VC): The difference between the minimum and maximum volume of air in the lungs (TLC – RV)
- **Tidal volume** (TV): The volume of air inhaled or exhaled in a normal breath
- **Expiratory reserve volume** (ERV): The volume of additional air that can be forcibly exhaled after a normal exhalation
- **Inspiratory reserve volume** (IRV): The volume of additional air that can be forcibly inhaled after a normal inhalation

These different lung volumes and capacities can be seen in Figure 6.6.

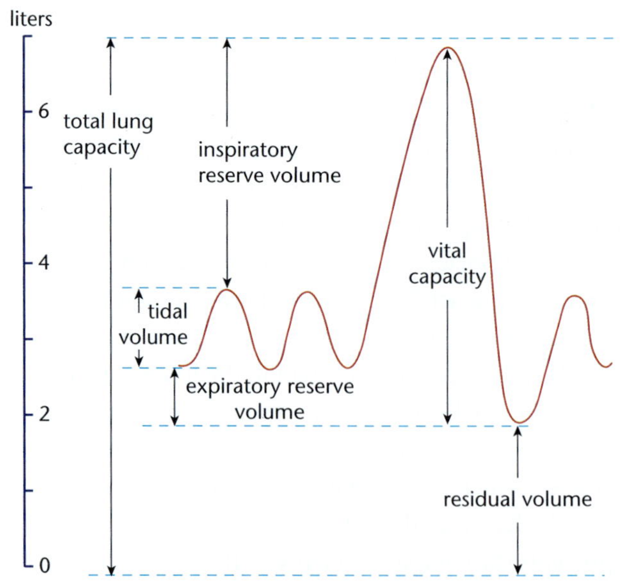

Figure 6.6 Lung Volumes

Regulation of Breathing

Breathing requires input from our nervous control center. Ventilation is primarily regulated by a collection of neurons in the medulla oblongata called the **ventilation center** that fire rhythmically to cause regular contraction of respiratory muscles. These neurons contain **chemoreceptors** that are primarily sensitive to carbon dioxide concentration. As the partial pressure of carbon dioxide in the blood rises (**hypercarbia** or **hypercapnia**), the **respiratory rate** will increase so that more carbon dioxide is exhaled, causing carbon dioxide levels in the blood to fall. These cells also respond to changes in oxygen concentration, although this tends to have significance only during periods of significant **hypoxemia** (low oxygen concentration in the blood).

We can, to a limited extent, control our breathing consciously. We can choose to breathe more rapidly or slowly; however, extended periods of hypoventilation would lead to increased carbon dioxide levels and an override by the medulla oblongata (which would jump-start breathing). The opposite process (hyperventilation) would blow off too much carbon dioxide and ultimately inhibit ventilation.

MCAT CONCEPT CHECK 6.1

Before you move on, assess your understanding of the material with these questions.

1. List the structures in the respiratory pathway, from where air enters the nares to the alveoli.

____

2. Which muscle(s) are involved in inhalation? Exhalation?
   - Inhalation:

   ____

   - Exhalation:

   ____

3. What is the purpose of surfactant?

____

4. What is the mathematical relationship between vital capacity (VC), inspiratory reserve volume (IRV), expiratory reserve volume (ERV), and tidal volume (TV)?

____

5. If blood levels of CO_2 become too low, how does the brain alter the respiratory rate to maintain homeostasis?

____

6.2 Functions of the Respiratory System

LEARNING OBJECTIVES

After Chapter 6.2, you will be able to:

- Describe the mechanisms used in the respiratory system to prevent infection
- Recall the chemical equation for the bicarbonate buffer system
- Predict how blood pH will change in response to changing concentrations of O_2 or CO_2

No organ system functions alone. The lungs function in gas exchange, but this is only part of the respiratory story. The lungs are lined with a tremendous number of capillaries that can also be used in thermoregulation. The lungs also represent a pathway into the body and serve an immune function to prevent invaders from gaining access to the bloodstream. Finally, the lungs also allow for control of blood pH by controlling carbon dioxide concentrations. Therefore, the lungs are integrated with many other body systems, including the cardiovascular, immune, renal, and nervous systems.

Gas Exchange

Gas exchange is, of course, the primary function of the lungs. Each alveolus is surrounded by a network of capillaries. The capillaries bring deoxygenated blood from the **pulmonary arteries**, which originate from the right ventricle of the heart. The walls of the alveoli are only one cell thick, which facilitates the diffusion of carbon dioxide from the blood into the lungs, and oxygen into the blood. The oxygenated blood returns to the left atrium of the heart via the **pulmonary veins**.

The driving force for gas exchange is the pressure differential of the gases. When it initially arrives at the alveoli, blood has a relatively low partial pressure of oxygen and a relatively high partial pressure of carbon dioxide, facilitating transfer of each down its respective concentration gradient, as shown in Figure 6.7. Because the gradient between the blood and air in the lungs is already present as the blood enters the lungs, no energy is required for gas transfer.

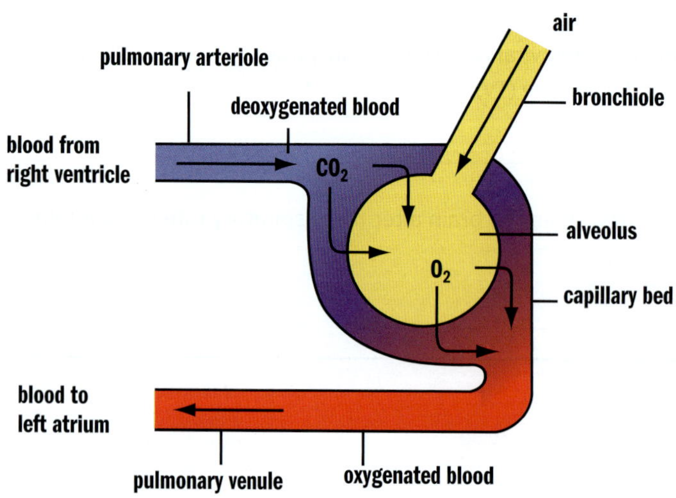

Figure 6.7 Gas Exchange in the Alveolus

REAL WORLD

Diffusion of gases occurs across a very thin membrane between the alveolus and the capillary. However, certain diseases may cause fibrosis, or scarring, of this membrane, resulting in less effective diffusion. Other diseases may cause a limitation of ventilation (gas flow) or perfusion (blood flow) to the lung. All of these mechanisms can cause hypoxia—low blood oxygen levels—although they accomplish that same end result through different means.

KEY CONCEPT

O_2 in the alveoli flows down its partial pressure gradient from the alveoli into the pulmonary capillaries, where it can bind to hemoglobin for transport. Meanwhile, CO_2 flows down its partial pressure gradient from the capillaries into the alveoli for expiration.

How would our respiratory systems adjust if we moved to higher altitudes where less oxygen is available? First, we would breathe more rapidly to try to avoid hypoxia; second, the binding dynamics of hemoglobin to oxygen would be altered to facilitate the unloading of oxygen at the tissues. As we will discuss in Chapter 7 of *MCAT Biology Review*, the natural response of hemoglobin to the decreased carbon dioxide concentration in the environment would actually be to *decrease* the unloading of oxygen to tissues, so other mechanisms must counteract and override this phenomenon. In the short term, the body can optimize oxygen delivery through measures like increasing the respiratory and heart rates. In the long term, the body could produce more red blood cells or develop more blood vessels (vascularization), which would facilitate the distribution of oxygen to tissues.

Thermoregulation

In order to maximize gas exchange, there is a tremendous surface area over which the alveoli and capillaries interact. Because the entire respiratory tract is highly vascular, it can also be used for **thermoregulation**, or the regulation of body temperature. Heat—the transfer of thermal energy—is regulated via the body surfaces by **vasodilation** and **vasoconstriction**. As capillaries expand, more blood can pass through these vessels, and a larger amount of thermal energy can be dissipated. As capillaries contract, less blood can pass through them, conserving thermal energy. Nasal and tracheal capillaries are most frequently used for these purposes within the respiratory system. While these capillary beds provide a mechanism for thermoregulation, humans predominantly regulate temperature using capillaries and sweat glands in the skin, or rapid muscle contraction (shivering). The respiratory system can also transfer heat to the environment through evaporation of water in mucous secretions. Other animals, such as dogs, take advantage of this cooling mechanism by **panting**.

Immune Function

As mentioned above, the lungs provide a large interface for the body to interact with the outside world. While this is important for gas exchange and thermoregulation, it also comes with potential risks—pathogens such as bacteria, viruses, and fungi can cause infections in the lung, or can gain access to the body through the rich vascularity of the alveolar membranes. By necessity, the lungs must be able to fight off potential invaders. The first line of defense is the nasal cavity, which has small hairs (vibrissae) that help to trap particulate matter and potentially infectious particles. The nasal cavity also contains an enzyme called ***lysozyme***. Also found in tears and saliva, lysozyme is able to attack the peptidoglycan walls of gram-positive bacteria. The internal airways are lined with mucus, which traps particulate matter and larger invaders. Underlying cilia then propel the mucus up the respiratory tract to the pharynx, where it can be expelled or swallowed; this mechanism is called the **mucociliary escalator** (Figure 6.8).

MCAT EXPERTISE

The division within the sciences is largely artificial; the MCAT often contains questions that integrate multiple science disciplines. A question located in the *Biological and Biochemical Foundations of Living Systems* section may require knowledge of general chemistry. In fact, 10% of this section is chemistry: 5% general chemistry and 5% organic chemistry.

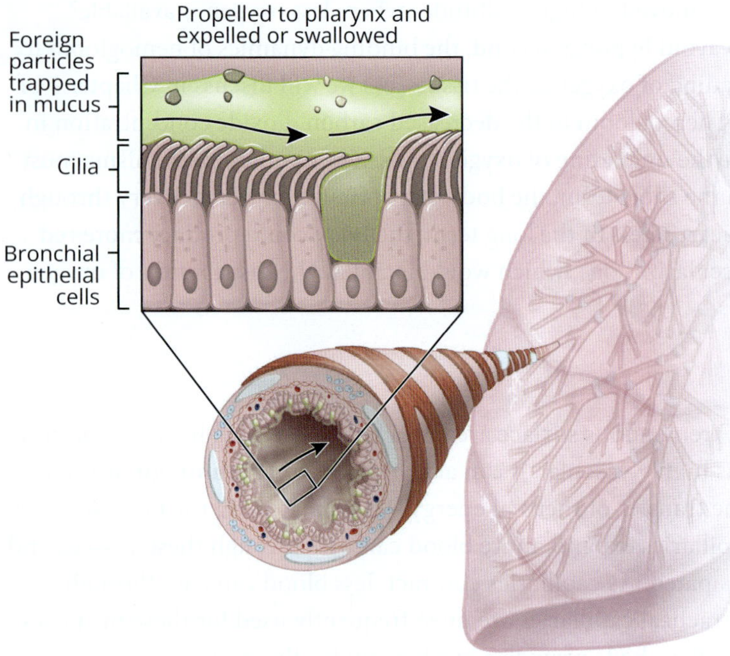

Figure 6.8 Mucociliary Escalator

The lungs, especially the alveoli, also contain numerous immune cells, including macrophages. **Macrophages** can engulf and digest pathogens and signal to the rest of the immune system that there is an invader. Mucosal surfaces also contain IgA antibodies that help to protect against pathogens that contact the mucous membranes. Finally, **mast cells** also populate the lungs. These cells have preformed antibodies on their surfaces. When the right substance attaches to the antibody, the mast cell releases inflammatory chemicals into the surrounding area to promote an immune response. Unfortunately, these antibodies are often reactive to substances such as pollen and molds, so mast cells also provide the inflammatory chemicals that mediate allergic reactions.

Control of pH

The respiratory system plays a role in pH balance through the **bicarbonate buffer system** in the blood:

$$CO_2\,(g) + H_2O\,(l) \rightleftharpoons H_2CO_3\,(aq) \rightleftharpoons H^+\,(aq) + HCO_3^-\,(aq)$$

Questions regarding the bicarbonate buffer system are MCAT favorites, and you are very likely to see it in some form on Test Day. This equation represents an opportunity for the MCAT to test understanding of basic chemistry concepts, such as Le Châtelier's principle, as well as how disturbances in pH may affect respiration.

The body attempts to maintain a pH between 7.35 and 7.45. When the pH is lower, and hydrogen ion concentration is higher (**acidemia**), acid-sensing chemoreceptors just outside the blood–brain barrier send signals to the brain to increase the respiratory rate. Further, an increasing hydrogen ion concentration will cause a shift in the bicarbonate buffer system, generating additional carbon dioxide. As described earlier, the respiratory centers in the brain are

REAL WORLD

Pneumonia is an infection of the lung most often caused by bacteria or viruses. *Atypical pneumonia*, commonly called walking pneumonia (because the infection does not require hospitalization and does not leave the patient bedridden), is often caused by a very small bacterium called *Mycoplasma pneumoniae*. This bacterium causes a prolonged cough because it damages epithelial cells lining the lung and paralyzes the cilia lining the respiratory tract. The lack of cilia makes it much more difficult to clear mucus from the lungs. The cough lasts until the respiratory epithelial cells have recovered and the cilia are once again functional.

REAL WORLD

Metabolic acidosis—a condition of excess acid by any mechanism besides hypoventilation—is a common occurrence in medicine. Anaerobic respiration can generate lactic acid; individuals with type 1 diabetes mellitus can produce ketoacids when they are hypoinsulinemic; certain poisons, like methanol and formaldehyde, can produce organic acids. In each of these cases, one of the primary methods of compensation is increasing respiration rate.

sensitive to this increasing partial pressure of carbon dioxide and will also promote an increase in respiratory rate.

As the respiratory rate increases, more carbon dioxide is blown off. This will also push the buffer equation to the left, but notice the difference: the shift to the left in the previous paragraph was caused by an increase in hydrogen ion concentration, which elevated the concentration of carbon dioxide. Here, the removal of carbon dioxide causes a shift to the left that allows the hydrogen ion concentration to drop back to normal.

If the blood is too basic (**alkalemia**), then the body will seek to increase acidity. How can the lungs contribute to this? If the respiratory rate is slowed, then more carbon dioxide will be retained, shifting the buffer equation to the right and producing more hydrogen ions and bicarbonate ions. This results in a lower pH.

Overall, the lungs play a role in the immediate adjustment of carbon dioxide levels and, by extension, hydrogen ion levels. However, as seen in Figure 6.9, the lungs do not work alone to maintain proper pH. The kidneys also play a role by modulating secretion and reabsorption of H^+ and bicarbonate (HCO_3^-) within the nephron. This is a much slower response, however, and represents long-term compensation. For more information on kidney function and homeostasis, see Chapter 10 of *MCAT Biology Review*.

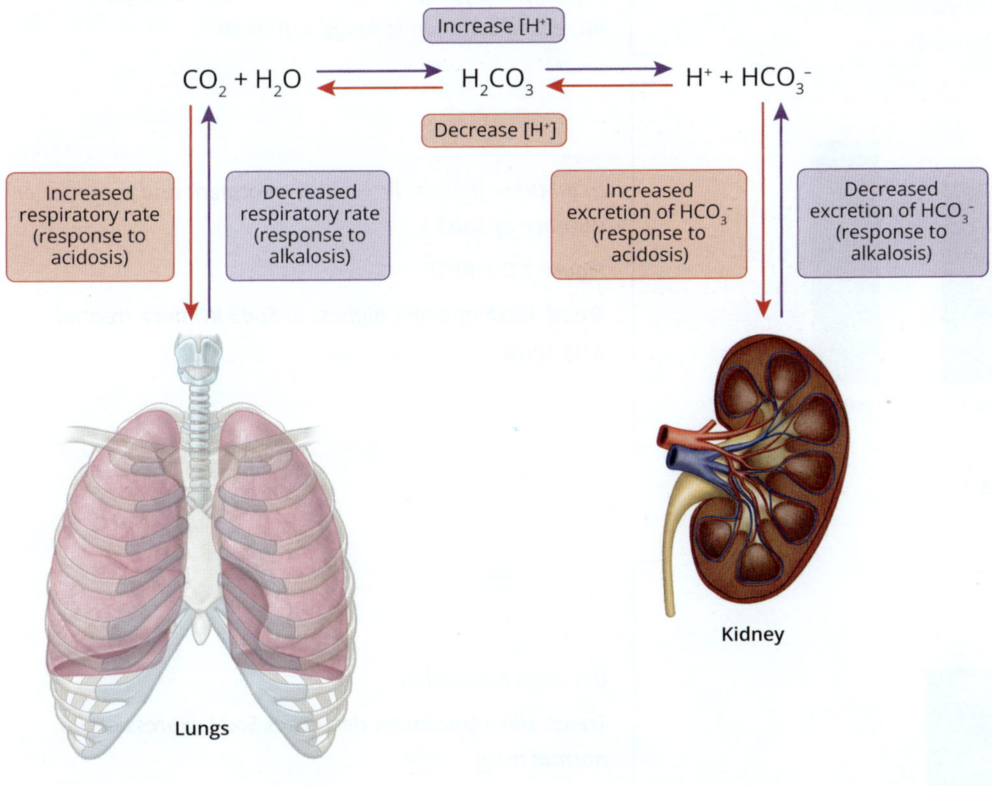

Figure 6.9 Bicarbonate Buffer System

BRIDGE

If H^+ is an acid and HCO_3^- is a base, then why doesn't increasing both of them yield a constant pH? The reason is that H^+ is a strong acid, while HCO_3^- is a weak base. Just like a titration, discussed in Chapter 10 of *MCAT General Chemistry Review*, this combination will shift the pH of the solution toward the acidic range.

KEY CONCEPT

This equation is essential to Test Day success:

$$CO_2(g) + H_2O\,(l) \rightleftharpoons H_2CO_3\,(aq) \rightleftharpoons H^+\,(aq) + HCO_3^-\,(aq)$$

It is likely to be tested in both the *Biological and Biochemical Foundations of Living Systems* and the *Chemical and Physical Foundations of Biological Systems* sections.

BIOLOGY GUIDED EXAMPLE WITH EXPERT THINKING

Chronic inhalation of crystalline silica has been shown to result in silicosis and pulmonary fibrosis and may also play a role in the development of pulmonary hypertension. The mechanism by which these pathologies develop is not clearly understood, but oxidant/antioxidant imbalances have been suggested.

Background info: silica damages the lungs, maybe through oxidants

Extracellular superoxide dismutase (Sod3) is one of the most abundant antioxidant enzymes in the pulmonary vasculature.

Researcher thought process: this enzyme is most prevalent in the blood vessels around the lungs, so let's test it first!

To study the role of Sod3 in the development of silica-mediated pathologies, scientists injected a crystalline silica suspension into the trachea of WT and Sod3–/– mice.

Experimental set up: compare silica-induced lung pathologies between WT and Sod3–/– (knockout) mice

28 days later, a pressure catheter was inserted into the right ventricle through the jugular vein to measure the right ventricular systolic pressure (RVSP) (Figure 1). Elevated RVSP is associated with pulmonary hypertension.

Exp 1: measured RVSP; high RVSP = pulmonary hypertension

Following the RVSP measurement, mice were sacrificed. mRNA was extracted from lung tissue and assayed for Sod3 expression (Figure 2).

Exp 2: measuring Sod3 gene expression

Lung sections were stained with Mason's trichrome to visualize collagen, a marker of pulmonary fibrosis (Figure 3).

Exp 3: quantifying collagen content in the lungs; increased collagen in lungs = fibrosis

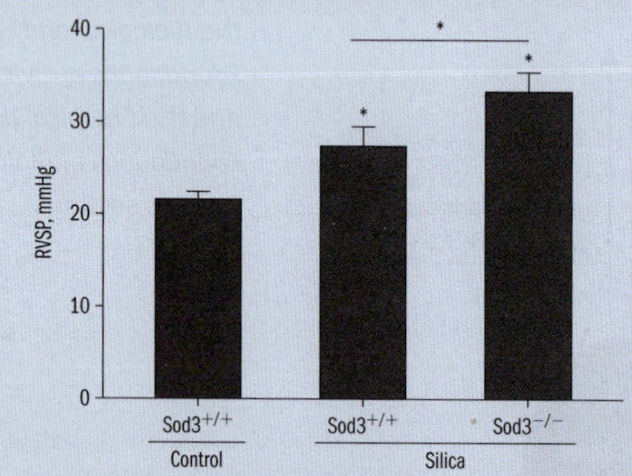

Figure 1

In all three figures, IV = silica treatment and presence or absence of Sod3

Figure 1 DV: RVSP

Trend: RVSP appears highest in Sod3 KO mice treated with silica

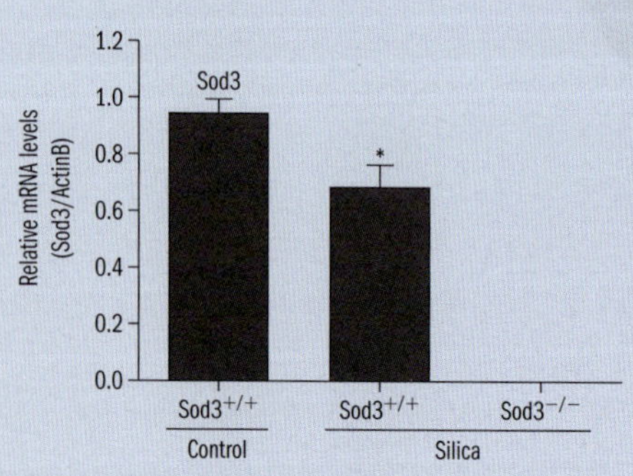

Figure 2

DV: Sod3 expression

Trend: silica treatment decreases Sod3 expression in normal mice

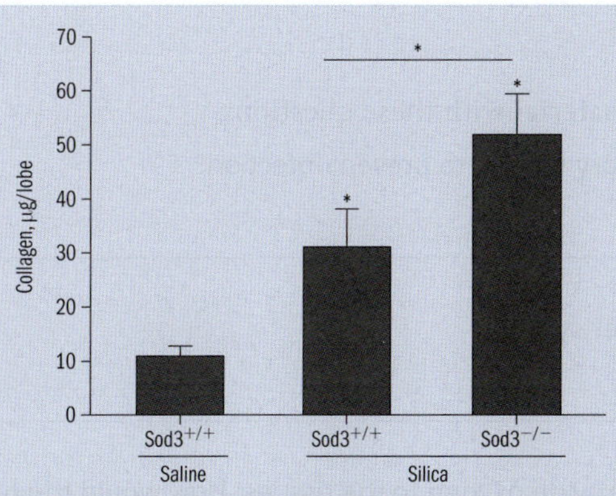

Figure 3

DV: collagen in lungs

Trend: highest in Sod3 KO mice treated with silica

Adapted from Zelko, I. N., Zhu, J., & Roman, J. (2018). Role of SOD3 in silica-related lung fibrosis and pulmonary vascular remodeling. *Respiratory Research*, *19*(1), 221. doi:10.1186/s12931-018-0933-6.

Based on the findings of this study, does Sod3 protect against or exacerbate crystalline silica-induced pathologies?

This question is really testing our understanding of how the presence or absence of Sod3 affects the development of silica-induced lung pathologies. Finding an answer will require a strong understanding of the experimental design and careful analysis of the data. Let's start with the experimental design. Paragraph 2 tells us that we have three experimental groups: normal mice not treated with silica, normal mice treated with silica, and Sod3 knockout (KO) mice treated with silica. The normal mice lacking treatment serve as a negative control, whereas the normal mice treated with silica serve as the positive control. Paragraph 1 tells us that crystalline silica has already been shown to cause pulmonary fibrosis and silicosis, so we should expect to see indicators of these pathologies in normal mice treated with silica, but not in the untreated mice. If Sod3 has a protective role, deleting it should lead to an increase in lung damage. If Sod3 exacerbates silica-induced lung damage, deleting it should lead to a decrease in lung damage.

Time to analyze the data! Figure 1 shows that in normal mice, exposure to silica leads to an increase in RVSP, indicating a potential role for silica in the development of pulmonary hypertension. Furthermore, deletion of Sod3 leads to a greater elevation in RVSP, suggesting that Sod3 may have a protective role. Figure 2 shows the expression of the Sod3 transcript in lung tissue. The Sod3 KO mice show no expression, which is consistent with a gene knockout. We also note that the silica exposure leads to a decrease in Sod3 expression. Figure 3 shows an elevation in collagen content in the lungs of silica-treated mice compared to untreated mice. This elevation is significantly higher in Sod3 KO mice. Taken together, these results suggest that Sod3 protects against both silica-induced pulmonary fibrosis and pulmonary hypertension.

Because knockout of Sod3 lead to an increase in pulmonary fibrosis and pulmonary hypertension after exposure to crystalline silica, Sod3 most likely serves a protective role in the lungs against silica-mediated damage.

MCAT CONCEPT CHECK 6.2

Before you move on, assess your understanding of the material with these questions.

1. What are some of the mechanisms used in the respiratory system to prevent infection?

___

2. What is the chemical equation for the bicarbonate buffer system?

___

3. Respiratory failure refers to inadequate ventilation to provide oxygen to the tissues. How would the pH change in respiratory failure?

___

Conclusion

As we learn about the human body, it may be easy to reduce the complex and varied functions of the lungs to breathing and providing a supply of oxygen. The lungs do indeed perform gas exchange, which relies on differences in partial pressures of gases between the alveoli and the blood. Oxygen is taken up by the blood, while carbon dioxide is released for exhalation. Inhalation and exhalation also require pressure differentials created by anatomical structures such as the chest wall, diaphragm, pleurae, and lungs.

However, the lungs are so much more than just *bags of air*; gas exchange is not the only function of the respiratory system. The respiratory system also serves essential roles in thermoregulation, immunity, and pH regulation. As we go through the individual systems within the human body, take special note of how each system is integrated with the other systems. One of the more clear connections is the binding of oxygen to hemoglobin in the lungs and in the rest of the circulatory system—a concept we will expand upon in the next chapter, along with the effects of altitude, pH, and chemicals on this binding.

▶ GO ONLINE

You've reviewed the content, now test your knowledge and critical thinking skills by completing a test-like passage set in your online resources!

CONCEPT SUMMARY

Anatomy and Mechanism of Breathing

- Air is drawn in through the **nares**, and through the nasal cavity and **pharynx**, where it is warmed and humidified. It is filtered by nasal hairs (**vibrissae**) and mucous membranes. It then enters the **larynx**, followed by the **trachea**. The trachea divides into two mainstem **bronchi**, which divide into **bronchioles**, which divide into continually smaller passages until they reach the alveoli.
- **Alveoli** are small sacs that interface with the pulmonary capillaries, allowing gases to diffuse across a one-cell-thick membrane.
- **Surfactant** in the alveoli reduces surface tension at the liquid–gas interface, preventing collapse.
- The pleurae cover the lungs and line the chest wall.
  - The **visceral pleura** lies adjacent to the lung itself.
  - The **parietal pleura** lines the chest wall.
  - The **intrapleural space** lies between these two layers and contains a thin layer of fluid that lubricates the two pleural surfaces.
- The **diaphragm** is a thin skeletal muscle that helps to create the pressure differential required for breathing.
- Inhalation is an active process.
  - The diaphragm and **external intercostal muscles** expand the thoracic cavity, increasing the volume of the intrapleural space. This decreases the intrapleural pressure.
  - This pressure differential ultimately expands the lungs, dropping the pressure within and drawing in air from the environment. This mechanism is termed **negative-pressure breathing**.
- Exhalation may be passive or active.
  - In passive exhalation, relaxation of the muscles of inspiration and elastic recoil of the lungs allow the chest cavity to decrease in volume, reversing the pressure differentials seen in inhalation.
  - In active exhalation, the internal intercostal muscles and abdominal muscles can be used to forcibly decrease the volume of the thoracic cavity, pushing out air.
- A **spirometer** can be used to measure lung capacities and volumes.
  - **Total lung capacity** (TLC) is the maximum volume of air in the lungs when one inhales completely.
  - **Residual volume** (RV) is the volume of air remaining in the lungs when one exhales completely.
  - **Vital capacity** (VC) is the difference between the minimum and maximum volume of air in the lungs.
  - **Tidal volume** (TV) is the volume of air inhaled or exhaled in a normal breath.
  - **Expiratory reserve volume** (ERV) is the volume of additional air that can be forcibly exhaled after a normal exhalation.
  - **Inspiratory reserve volume** (IRV) is the volume of additional air that can be forcibly inhaled after a normal inhalation.
- Ventilation is regulated by the **ventilation center**, a collection of neurons in the medulla oblongata.
  - **Chemoreceptors** respond to carbon dioxide concentrations, increasing the respiratory rate when there is a high concentration of carbon dioxide in the blood (**hypercarbia** or **hypercapnia**).

  - The ventilation center can also respond to low oxygen concentrations in the blood (**hypoxemia**) by increasing ventilation rate.
  - Ventilation can also be controlled consciously through the cerebrum, although the medulla oblongata will override the cerebrum during extended periods of hypo- or hyperventilation.

Functions of the Respiratory System

- The lungs perform gas exchange with the blood through simple diffusion across concentration gradients.
  - Deoxygenated blood with a high carbon dioxide concentration is brought to the lungs via the **pulmonary arteries**.
  - Oxygenated blood with a low carbon dioxide concentration leaves the lungs via the **pulmonary veins**.
- The large surface area of interaction between the alveoli and capillaries allows the respiratory system to assist in thermoregulation through **vasodilation** and **vasoconstriction** of capillary beds.
- The respiratory system must be protected from potential pathogens.
  - Multiple mechanisms, including vibrissae, mucous membranes, and the **mucociliary escalator**, help filter the incoming air and trap particulate matter.
  - **Lysozyme** in the nasal cavity and saliva attacks peptidoglycan cell walls of gram-positive bacteria.
  - **Macrophages** can engulf and digest pathogens and signal to the rest of the immune system that there is an invader.
  - Mucosal surfaces are covered with IgA antibodies.
  - **Mast cells** have antibodies on their surface that, when triggered, can promote the release of inflammatory chemicals. Mast cells are often involved in allergic reactions as well.
- The respiratory system is involved in pH control through the bicarbonate buffer system.
  - When blood pH decreases, respiration rate increases to compensate by blowing off carbon dioxide. This causes a left shift in the buffer equation, reducing hydrogen ion concentration.
  - When blood pH increases, respiration rate decreases to compensate by trapping carbon dioxide. This causes a right shift in the buffer equation, increasing hydrogen ion concentration.

ANSWERS TO CONCEPT CHECKS

6.1

1. Nares $\longrightarrow$ nasal cavity $\longrightarrow$ pharynx $\longrightarrow$ larynx $\longrightarrow$ trachea $\longrightarrow$ bronchi $\longrightarrow$ bronchioles $\longrightarrow$ alveoli
2. Inhalation uses the diaphragm and external intercostal muscles; in labored breathing, muscles of the neck and back may also be involved. Passive exhalation uses the recoil of these same muscles; active exhalation also uses the internal intercostal muscles and abdominal muscles.
3. Surfactant reduces surface tension at the air–liquid interface in the alveoli. This prevents their collapse.
4. Vital capacity is the sum of the inspiratory reserve volume, expiratory reserve volume, and tidal volume: $VC = IRV + ERV + TV$
5. When CO_2 levels become too low, the brain can decrease the respiratory rate in order to raise CO_2 levels.

6.2

1. Immune mechanisms in the respiratory system include vibrissae in the nares, lysozyme in the mucous membranes, the mucociliary escalator, macrophages in the lungs, mucosal IgA antibodies, and mast cells.
2. $CO_2\ (g) + H_2O\ (l) \rightleftharpoons H_2CO_3\ (aq) \rightleftharpoons H^+\ (aq) + HCO_3^-\ (aq)$
3. In respiratory failure, ventilation slows, and less carbon dioxide is blown off. As this occurs, the buffer equation shifts to the right, and more hydrogen ions are generated. This results in a lower pH of the blood.

SCIENCE MASTERY ASSESSMENT EXPLANATIONS

1. **D**

Gas exchange in the lungs relies on passive diffusion of oxygen and carbon dioxide. This is accomplished easily because there is always a difference in the partial pressures of these two gases and because the subdivision of the respiratory tree creates a large surface area of interaction between the alveoli and the circulatory system. In addition, the thin alveolar walls allow for fast diffusion and gas exchange. Therefore, **(A)**, **(B)**, and **(C)** can be eliminated. **(D)** is the correct answer because active transport is not used in the gas exchange process in the lungs.

2. **D**

The muscles involved in ventilation are the diaphragm, which separates the thoracic cavity from the abdominal cavity, and the intercostal muscles. During inhalation, the diaphragm contracts and flattens, while the external intercostal muscles contract, pulling the rib cage up and out. These actions cause an overall increase in the volume of the thoracic cavity. During exhalation, both the diaphragm and the external intercostals relax, causing a decrease in the volume of the thoracic cavity because of the recoil of these tissues. In forced exhalation, the internal intercostals and abdominal muscles may contract to force out air. Thus, the only correct association from the given answers is **(D)**.

3. **C**

Total lung capacity is equal to the vital capacity (the maximum volume of air that can be forcibly inhaled and exhaled from the lungs) plus the residual volume (the air that always remains in the lungs, preventing the alveoli from collapsing).

4. **B**

During inhalation, the chest cavity expands, causing expansion of the intrapleural space. According to Boyle's law, an increase in volume at a constant temperature is accompanied by a decrease in pressure. When the intrapleural pressure (and, by extension, the alveolar pressure) is less than atmospheric pressure, air enters the lungs. During exhalation, these pressure gradients reverse; the volume of the chest cavity decreases, causing intrapleural pressure to increase (become less negative), which in turn raises the alveolar pressure above atmospheric pressure. This pressure gradient drives air out of the lungs, but the intrapleural pressure itself remains lower than the atmospheric pressure.

5. **B**

The intrapleural space, bounded by the parietal and visceral pleurae, is a potential space. As such, it is normally collapsed and contains a small amount of fluid. However, introduction of fluid or air into the intrapleural space can fill the space, causing collapse of the lung. The other options listed are too firmly apposed to permit blood to collect in these spaces.

6. **C**

The pharynx, which lies behind the nasal cavity and oral cavity, is a common pathway for food entering the digestive system and air entering the respiratory system. It is the larynx that contains the vocal cords, not the pharynx.

7. **D**

Air enters the respiratory tract through the external nares (nostrils) and travels through the nasal cavities. It then passes through the pharynx and into the larynx. Ingested food also passes through the pharynx on its way to the esophagus; to ensure that food does not accidentally enter the larynx, the epiglottis covers the larynx during swallowing. After the larynx, air goes to the trachea, which eventually divides into two bronchi, one for each lung. The bronchi branch into smaller bronchioles, which terminate in clusters of alveoli. From the given sequences, only **(D)** correctly describes the sequence of the passages through which air travels.

8. **B**

In a patient with IPF, the increased stiffness of the lungs would likely decrease the volume of air the individual could inhale, which would decrease both the total lung capacity and inspiratory reserve volume. However, spirometry cannot measure the total lung capacity accurately because it cannot determine the residual volume—the volume of air left in the lungs when an individual has maximally exhaled. Because the residual volume makes up a portion of the total lung capacity (total lung capacity = vital capacity + residual volume), a spirometer cannot be used to determine the total lung capacity. Therefore, while Statement I is a true statement about individuals with IPF, it cannot appear in the answer choice. Finally, increased stiffness of the lungs would be expected to decrease the residual volume, not increase it; further, residual volume, as described above, cannot be measured with a spirometer.

9. **B**

Lysozyme is an enzyme present in the nasal cavity, saliva, and tears that degrades peptidoglycan, preventing infection by gram-positive bacteria. Thus, premature infants who lack lysozyme are more likely to suffer from infections with these organisms.

10. **D**

If an area of the lung becomes filled with mucus and inflammatory cells, the area will not be able to participate in gas exchange. Because no air will enter or leave the area, the concentration gradient will no longer exist, and neither oxygen nor carbon dioxide will be able to diffuse across the alveolar wall.

11. **B**

When people hyperventilate, their respiratory rate increases. When the respiratory rate increases, more carbon dioxide is blown off. This causes a shift to the left in the bicarbonate buffer equation, and the blood becomes more alkaline. Breathing into the bag allows some of this carbon dioxide to be returned to the bloodstream in order to maintain the proper pH.

12. **C**

When a patient who has an asthma attack does not respond to treatment and has been hyperventilating for over an hour, the patient may become fatigued and may not be able to maintain hyperventilation. In this case, the patient's breathing rate starts to decrease, and the patient fails to receive adequate oxygen. By extension, carbon dioxide is trapped in the blood, and the pH begins to drop. Despite the fact that this pH is normal at the moment, this patient is crashing and may start demonstrating acidemia in the near future. While the kidneys should compensate for alkalemia, this is a slow process and would not normalize the blood pH within an hour; further, adequate compensation by the kidneys would actually be a reassuring sign, eliminating **(A)**. There is no evidence to suggest that the measurement was inaccurate, eliminating **(B)**. Finally, after treatment, the patient should return to a normal blood pH with adequate ventilation and would not be expected to overcompensate by becoming acidemic, eliminating **(D)**.

13. **A**

This question requires a few different levels of thinking. The question stem states that premature infants often require ventilation using positive end-expiratory pressures. While you are not expected to know ventilator settings for the MCAT, you should be able to decode what this phrase means: at the end of expiration, the ventilator will provide a higher pressure than normal, which forces extra air into the alveoli. This pressure must be used to prevent alveolar collapse, which should remind you that surfactant serves the same purpose by reducing surface tension. Thus, it makes sense that if premature babies lack surfactant, providing extra air pressure at the end of expiration would be beneficial.

14. **A**

The intrinsic elastic properties of the lung are important during exhalation as the passive recoil of lung tissue helps decrease lung volume. With decreased recoil, the patient will have difficulty exhaling completely, increasing the residual volume. The total lung capacity would be expected to increase in this case because there would be less recoil opposing inhalation, eliminating **(B)**. With decreased alveolar surface area, one would expect decreased gas exchange, which would decrease blood concentrations of oxygen while increasing blood concentrations of carbon dioxide, eliminating **(C)** and **(D)**.

15. **C**

Allergic reactions occur when a substance binds to an antibody and promotes an overactive immune response with inflammatory chemicals. The antibody is already attached to a mast cell. Thus, when the substance binds to the antibody, the mast cell can release the inflammatory mediators that cause allergic reactions.

GO ONLINE

Consult your online resources for additional practice.

SHARED CONCEPTS

Biology Chapter 7
The Cardiovascular System

Biology Chapter 10
Homeostasis

General Chemistry Chapter 6
Equilibrium

General Chemistry Chapter 8
The Gas Phase

General Chemistry Chapter 10
Acids and Bases

Physics and Math Chapter 3
Thermodynamics

CHAPTER 7

THE CARDIOVASCULAR SYSTEM

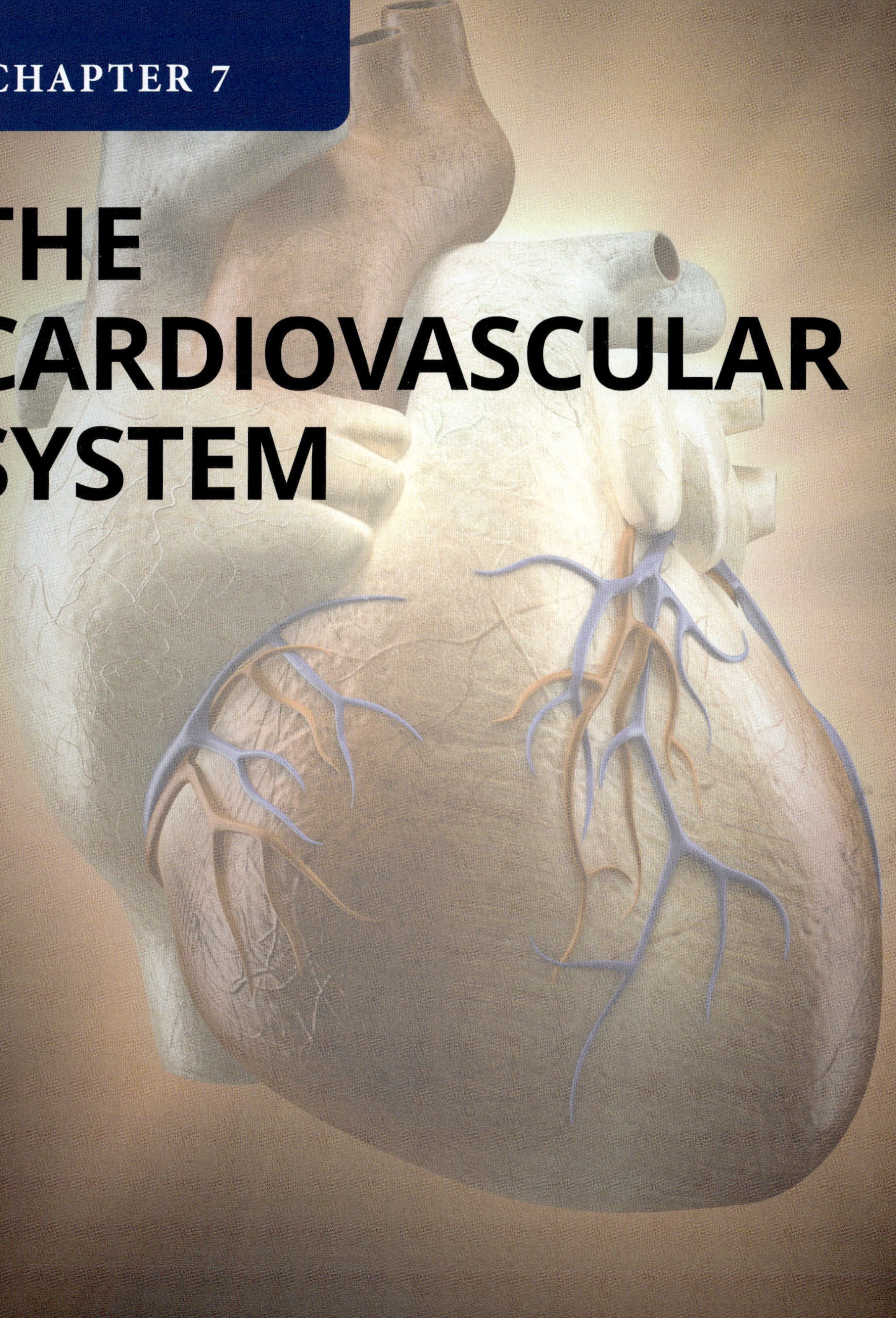

SCIENCE MASTERY ASSESSMENT

Every pre-med knows this feeling: there is so much content I have to know for the MCAT! How do I know what to do first or what's important?

While the high-yield badges throughout this book will help you identify the most important topics, this Science Mastery Assessment is another tool in your MCAT prep arsenal. This quiz (which can also be taken in your online resources) and the guidance below will help ensure that you are spending the appropriate amount of time on this chapter based on your personal strengths and weaknesses. Don't worry though—skipping something now does not mean you'll never study it. Later on in your prep, as you complete full-length tests, you'll uncover specific pieces of content that you need to review and can come back to these chapters as appropriate.

How to Use This Assessment

If you answer 0–7 questions correctly:

Spend about 1 hour to read this chapter in full and take limited notes throughout. Follow up by reviewing **all** quiz questions to ensure that you now understand how to solve each one.

If you answer 8–11 questions correctly:

Spend 20–40 minutes reviewing the quiz questions. Beginning with the questions you missed, read and take notes on the corresponding subchapters. For questions you answered correctly, ensure your thinking matches that of the explanation and you understand why each choice was correct or incorrect.

If you answer 12–15 questions correctly:

Spend less than 20 minutes reviewing all questions from the quiz. If you missed any, then include a quick read-through of the corresponding subchapters, or even just the relevant content within a subchapter, as part of your question review. For questions you answered correctly, ensure your thinking matches that of the explanation and review the Concept Summary at the end of the chapter.

CHAPTER 7

THE CARDIOVASCULAR SYSTEM

1. Which of the following is a FALSE statement regarding erythrocytes?
   - **A.** Erythrocytes contain hemoglobin.
   - **B.** Erythrocytes are anaerobic.
   - **C.** The nuclei of erythrocytes are located in the middle of the biconcave disc.
   - **D.** Erythrocytes are phagocytized in the spleen and liver after a certain period of time.

2. Which of the following is the correct sequence of a cardiac impulse?
   - **A.** SA node → AV node → Purkinje fibers → bundle of His → ventricles
   - **B.** AV node → bundle of His → Purkinje fibers → ventricles → atria
   - **C.** SA node → atria → AV node → bundle of His → Purkinje fibers → ventricles
   - **D.** SA node → AV node → atria → bundle of His → Purkinje fibers → ventricles

3. Hemoglobin's affinity for O_2:
   - **A.** increases in exercising muscle tissue.
   - **B.** decreases as blood P_aCO_2 decreases.
   - **C.** decreases as blood pH decreases.
   - **D.** is higher in maternal blood than in fetal blood.

4. Which of the following correctly traces the circulatory pathway?
   - **A.** Superior vena cava → right atrium → right ventricle → pulmonary artery → lungs → pulmonary veins → left atrium → left ventricle → aorta
   - **B.** Superior vena cava → left atrium → left ventricle → pulmonary artery → lungs → pulmonary veins → right atrium → right ventricle → aorta
   - **C.** Aorta → right atrium → right ventricle → pulmonary artery → lungs → pulmonary veins → left atrium → left ventricle → superior vena cava
   - **D.** Superior vena cava → right atrium → right ventricle → pulmonary veins → lungs → pulmonary artery → left atrium → left ventricle → aorta

5. At the venous end of a capillary bed, the osmotic pressure:
   - **A.** is greater than the hydrostatic pressure.
   - **B.** results in a net outflow of fluid.
   - **C.** is significantly higher than the osmotic pressure at the arterial end.
   - **D.** causes proteins to enter the interstitium.

6. A patient's chart indicates a cardiac output of 7500 mL per minute and a stroke volume of 50 mL. What is the patient's pulse, in beats per minute?
   - **A.** 50
   - **B.** 100
   - **C.** 150
   - **D.** 400

7. An unconscious patient is rushed into the emergency room and needs an immediate blood transfusion. Because there is no time to check the patient's medical history or determine blood type, which type of blood should the patient receive?
   - **A.** AB^+
   - **B.** AB^-
   - **C.** O^+
   - **D.** O^-

8. Which of the following is true regarding arteries and veins?
   - **A.** Arteries are thin-walled, muscular, and elastic, whereas veins are thick-walled and inelastic.
   - **B.** Arteries always conduct oxygenated blood, whereas veins always carry deoxygenated blood.
   - **C.** The blood pressure in the aorta is always higher than the pressure in the superior vena cava.
   - **D.** Arteries facilitate blood transport by using skeletal muscle contractions, whereas veins make use of the pumping of the heart to push blood.

9. At any given time, there is more blood in the venous system than the arterial system. Which of the following features of veins allows for this?
   - **A.** Relative lack of smooth muscle in the wall
   - **B.** Presence of valves
   - **C.** Proximity of veins to lymphatic vessels
   - **D.** Thin endothelial lining

10. Which of the following is involved in the body's primary blood-buffering mechanism?
    A. Fluid intake
    B. Absorption of nutrients in the gastrointestinal system
    C. Carbon dioxide produced from metabolism
    D. Hormones released by the kidneys

11. Due to kidney disease, a person is losing albumin into the urine. What effect is this likely to have within the capillaries?
    A. Increased oncotic pressure
    B. Increased hydrostatic pressure
    C. Decreased oncotic pressure
    D. Decreased hydrostatic pressure

12. The tricuspid valve prevents backflow of blood from the:
    A. left ventricle into the left atrium.
    B. aorta into the left ventricle.
    C. pulmonary artery into the right ventricle.
    D. right ventricle into the right atrium.

13. The world record for the longest-held breath is 22 minutes and 0 seconds. If a sample were taken from this individual during the last minute of breath-holding, which of the following might be observed?
    A. Increased hemoglobin affinity for oxygen
    B. Decreased P_aCO_2
    C. Increased hematocrit
    D. Decreased pH

14. A person has a heart attack that primarily affects the wall between the two ventricles. Which portion of the electrical conduction system is most likely affected?
    A. AV node
    B. SA node
    C. Bundle of His
    D. Left ventricular muscle

15. Which vascular structure creates the most resistance to blood flow?
    A. Aorta
    B. Arterioles
    C. Capillaries
    D. Veins

Answer Key

1. **C** (See section 7.2)
2. **C** (See section 7.1)
3. **C** (See section 7.3)
4. **A** (See section 7.1)
5. **A** (See section 7.3)
6. **C** (See section 7.1)
7. **D** (See section 7.2)
8. **C** (See section 7.1)
9. **A** (See section 7.1)
10. **C** (See section 7.3)
11. **C** (See section 7.3)
12. **D** (See section 7.1)
13. **D** (See section 7.3)
14. **C** (See section 7.1)
15. **B** (See section 7.3)

The relevant section of the chapter to review for each question is given in parentheses after the correct answer. Detailed explanations can be found at the end of the chapter.

CHAPTER 7

THE CARDIOVASCULAR SYSTEM

In This Chapter

CHAPTER PROFILE

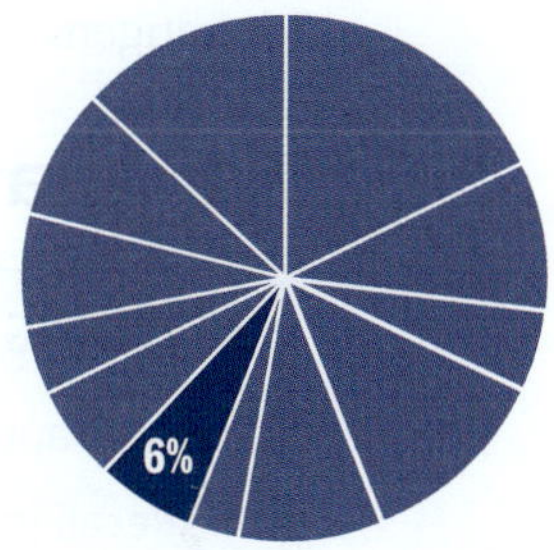

The content in this chapter should be relevant to about 6% of all questions about biology on the MCAT.

This chapter covers material from the following AAMC content category:

3B: Structure and integrative functions of the main organ systems

Introduction

As late as the 19th century, physicians adhered to a doctrine of health known as *humoralism.* This theory, developed by Greek and Roman physicians and philosophers and adopted by Islamic physicians, remained dominant in medical thought and practice until it was displaced by modern medical research in the 1800s. The theory of humoralism holds that the human body is composed of four fluids or substances called humors: black bile, yellow bile, phlegm, and blood. In the healthy state, these four humors are in balance, but excess or deficiency of any one of them would cause illness, disease, and even maladaptive personality characteristics. Over the course of a lifetime the levels of each of the four humors would rise and fall in accordance with diet and activity, resulting in maladies reflective of the imbalance. Treatments were intended to restore this balance.

Perhaps one of the most well-known treatments associated with humoralism is the practice of bloodletting. Because many diseases were associated with an excess of blood, physicians would withdraw significant amounts of blood from their patients to restore balance to the four humors. Methods for bloodletting were many, and some were dramatic—including drawing blood from major veins in the arm or neck and puncturing arteries. Devices known as scarificators were developed to cut into the superficial vessels. Most famously, leeches were used (especially in the early 19th century) to draw out excess blood. In fact, in the early decades of the 1800s, hundreds of millions of leeches were used by European physicians; in the 1830s, France alone imported about 40 million leeches per year for medical treatments.

While the humoral theory has been completely discredited by modern science, some practices associated with humoralism are still being used, albeit based on very different medical understanding and for different purposes. For example, new research has shown that medicinal leeches can be used effectively in microsurgery to help prevent blood coagulation, and in reconstructive surgery to stimulate circulation to the reattached tissue.

The cardiovascular system is one of the most commonly tested organ systems on the MCAT. It serves a variety of functions, including the movement of respiratory gases, nutrients, and wastes. We will review the structures and functional anatomy of the cardiovascular system and then discuss blood and its functional components. We'll also trace the pathways created by the electrically excitable cells that initiate and spread contractions through the heart. A quick recap of genetics and inheritance will help explain the consequences of ABO and Rh antigens. In addition, the binding of oxygen and carbon dioxide to hemoglobin will be discussed in detail.

7.1 Anatomy of the Cardiovascular System High Yield

LEARNING OBJECTIVES

After Chapter 7.1, you will be able to:

- Recall the names of the chambers and valves of the heart
- Describe the chain of events in the conduction system of the heart that leads to heartbeat generation
- Identify autonomic inputs into the heart and their effects
- Distinguish between arteries, capillaries, and veins
- Explain why the right side of the heart is less muscular than the left side
- Trace the flow of blood through the heart:

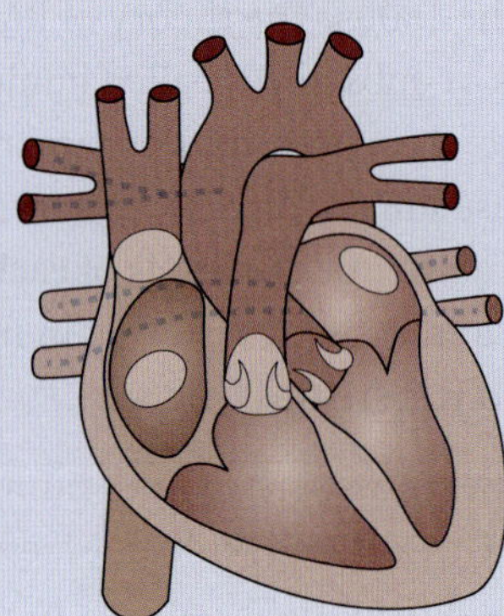

The **cardiovascular system** consists of a muscular four-chambered **heart**, **blood vessels**, and **blood**, as shown in Figure 7.1. The heart acts as a pump, distributing blood through the vasculature. The vasculature consists of arteries, capillaries, and veins. After blood travels through veins, it is returned to the right side of the heart where it is pumped to the lungs to be reoxygenated. Then, the oxygenated blood returns to the left side of the heart where it is once again pumped to the rest of the body.

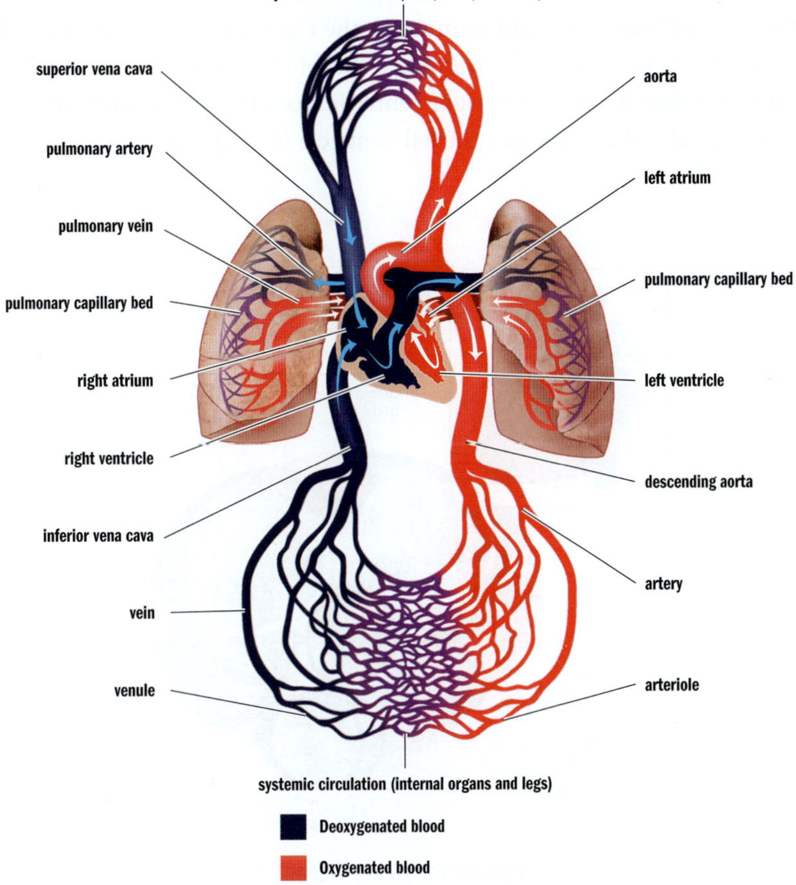

Figure 7.1 Anatomy of the Cardiovascular System

The Heart

The **heart** is a four-chambered structure composed predominantly of cardiac muscle. We often speak of the heart as a pump, supporting a single circulatory system. However, the heart is actually composed of two pumps supporting two different circulations in series. The right side of the heart accepts deoxygenated blood returning from the body and moves it to the lungs by way of the pulmonary arteries; this constitutes the first pump (**pulmonary circulation**). The second pump is the left side of the heart, which receives oxygenated blood from the lungs by way of the pulmonary veins and forces it out to the body through the aorta (**systemic circulation**).

Each side of the heart consists of an atrium and a ventricle. The **atria** are thin-walled structures where blood is received from either the **venae cavae** (deoxygenated blood entering the right side of the heart) or the **pulmonary veins** (oxygenated blood entering the left side of the heart). The atria contract to push blood into the **ventricles**. After the ventricles fill, they contract to send blood to the lungs (right ventricle) and the systemic circulation (left ventricle). Note that the ventricles are far more muscular than the atria, allowing for more powerful contractions that are necessary to push blood through the rest of the body.

The atria are separated from the ventricles by the **atrioventricular (AV) valves**. Likewise, the ventricles are separated from the vasculature by the **semilunar valves**. These valves allow the heart muscle to create the pressure within the

MNEMONIC

Atrioventricular valves:

LAB RAT

Left **A**trium = **B**icuspid

Right **A**trium = **T**ricuspid

ventricles necessary to propel the blood forward within the circulation, while also preventing backflow of blood (Figure 7.2). The valve between the right atrium and the right ventricle is known as the **tricuspid valve** (three leaflets), while the valve between the left atrium and the left ventricle is known as the **mitral** or **bicuspid valve** (two leaflets). The valve that separates the right ventricle from the pulmonary circulation is known as the **pulmonary valve,** while the valve that separates the left ventricle from the aorta is known as the **aortic valve**. Both semilunar valves have three leaflets.

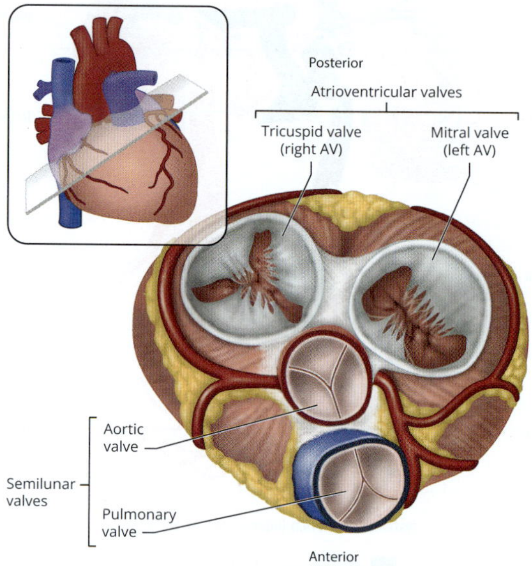

Figure 7.2 Heart Valves

One of the central themes in biology is something that we've touched on already in previous chapters: structure and function are related. The right and left sides of the heart are two different pumps, with the right side of the heart pumping blood to the lungs, and the left side of the heart pumping blood into the systemic circulation. Blood leaving the left side of the heart must travel a considerable distance, so blood pressure must be maintained as far away as the feet. Thus, the left side of the heart is more muscular than the right side of the heart. In fact, if the right side of the heart were as muscular as the left and pumped blood as forcefully, this would damage the lungs.

Electrical Conduction in the Heart

The coordinated, rhythmic contraction of cardiac muscle originates in an electrical impulse generated by and traveling through a pathway formed by four electrically excitable structures, as shown in Figure 7.3. This commonly tested pathway consists of, in order of excitation: the sinoatrial (SA) node, the atrioventricular (AV) node, the bundle of His (AV bundle) and its branches, and the Purkinje fibers. Impulse initiation occurs at the **SA node**, which generates 60–100 signals per minute without requiring any neurological input. This small collection of cells is located in the wall of the right atrium. As the depolarization wave spreads from the SA node, it causes the two atria to contract simultaneously. While most ventricular filling is passive (that is, blood moves from the atria to the ventricles based solely on ventricular relaxation), atrial **systole** (contraction) results in an increase in atrial pressure that forces a little more

KEY CONCEPT

Cardiac muscle has myogenic activity, meaning that it can contract without any neurological input. The SA node generates about 60–100 beats per minute, even if all innervation to the heart is cut. The neurological input to the heart is important in speeding up and slowing the rate of contraction, but not generating it in the first place.

blood into the ventricles. This additional volume of blood is called the **atrial kick** and accounts for about 5–30 percent of cardiac output. Next, the signal reaches the **AV node**, which sits at the junction of the atria and ventricles. The signal travels slower through the AV node, which allows the ventricles to fill completely before they contract. The signal then travels down the **bundle of His** and its branches, embedded in the **interventricular septum** (wall), and to the **Purkinje fibers**, which distribute the electrical signal through the ventricular muscle. The muscle cells are connected by **intercalated discs**, which contain many gap junctions directly connecting the cytoplasm of adjacent cells. This allows for coordinated ventricular contraction.

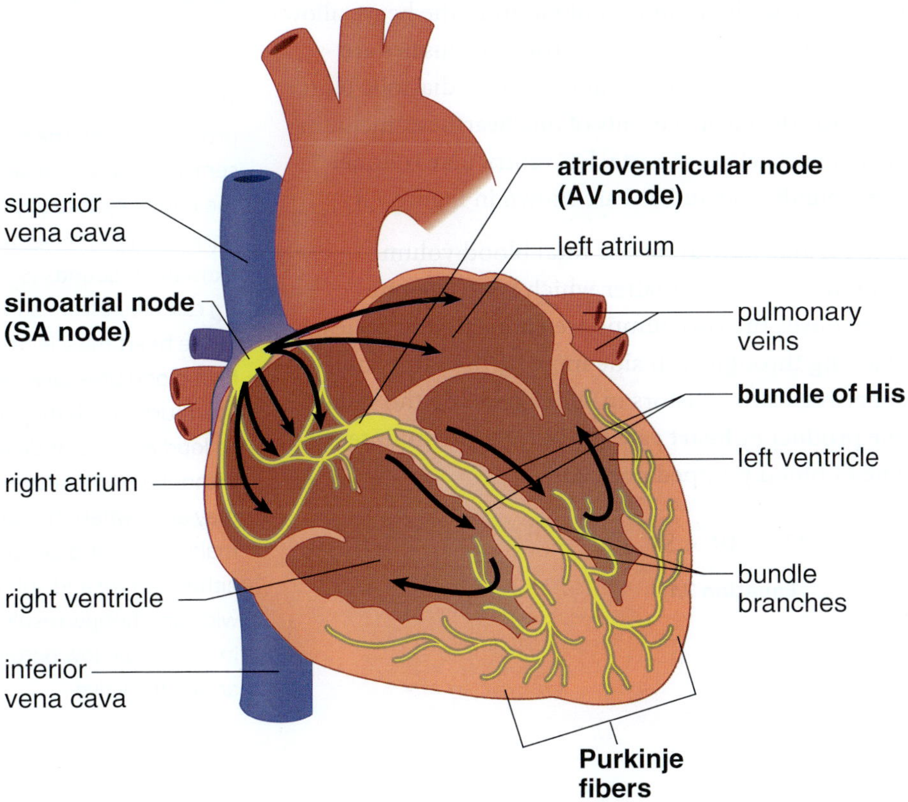

Figure 7.3 Electrical Conduction System of the Heart
Electrical impulses travel from the SA node to the AV node, through the bundle of His, and finally to the Purkinje fibers.

The SA node has an intrinsic rhythm of 60–100 signals per minute, so the normal human heart rate is 60–100 beats per minute. Highly conditioned athletes may have heart rates significantly lower than 60, in the range of 40–50 beats per minute. Stress, exercise, excitement, surprise, or danger can cause the heart rate to rise significantly above 100.

The circulatory system is under autonomic control. The autonomic system consists of the sympathetic ("fight-or-flight") and parasympathetic ("rest-and-digest") branches, controls the heart and affects the vasculature. Sympathetic signals speed up the heart rate and increase the contractility of cardiac muscle, while parasympathetic signals, provided by the **vagus nerve**, slow down the heart rate.

REAL WORLD

The heart's electrical impulses can be detected on the body's surface by placing electrodes on the skin on opposite sides of the heart. A recording of these currents is called an electrocardiogram (ECG or EKG; the *K*, by the way, reflects the German spelling). Electrocardiograms are incredibly powerful tools for assessing the status of a patient's heart. A normal EKG is shown below.

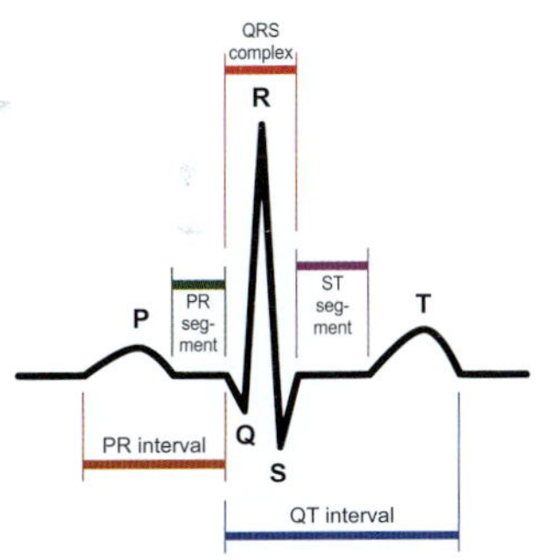

Depolarization precedes cardiac muscle contraction, so the electrical spikes of the EKG occur just before a cardiac contractile event. The P-wave occurs immediately before the atria contract, and the QRS complex occurs just before the ventricles contract. The T-wave represents ventricular repolarization.

Contraction

The heart is a muscle that must contract in order to move blood. Each heartbeat is composed of two phases, known as systole and diastole. During **systole**, ventricular contraction and closure of the AV valves occurs and blood is pumped out of the ventricles. During **diastole**, the ventricles are relaxed, the semilunar valves are closed, and blood from the atria fills the ventricles. Contraction of the ventricles generates a higher pressure during systole, whereas their relaxation during diastole causes the pressure to decrease. The elasticity of the walls of the large arteries, which stretch to receive the volume of blood from the heart, allows the vessels to maintain sufficient pressure while the ventricular muscles are relaxed. In fact, if it weren't for the elasticity of the large arteries, diastolic blood pressure would plummet to zero. The normal events of one heartbeat, including pressures in the left atrium, left ventricle, and aorta; left ventricular volume; normal and pathologic heart sounds; and an EKG are shown in Figure 7.4.

A measure to be aware of is **cardiac output**, or the total blood volume pumped by a ventricle in a minute. Does it matter which ventricle one chooses? As mentioned previously, the two pumps are connected in series, so the volumes of blood passing through each side must be the same, much like the electrical current between two resistors in series must be the same. Cardiac output (CO) is the product of **heart rate** (HR, beats per minute) and **stroke volume** (SV, volume of blood pumped per beat):

$$CO = HR \times SV$$

Equation 7.1

REAL WORLD

The rhythmic impulses we hear when we listen to someone's heart with a stethoscope (*lub dub*) are referred to as the heart sounds. The first sound, S_1, is produced when the two AV valves close at the start of systole to prevent backflow into the atria. The second sound, S_2, is produced when the two semilunar valves close at the end of systole to prevent backflow into the ventricles. Extra heart sounds (S_3 and S_4) can result from stiffness of the heart muscle or high blood pressure. Heart murmurs, which may be so loud as to be audible without a stethoscope, may arise when the valves malfunction and become either narrow and stiff or wide and floppy, resulting in abnormal flow patterns across the valve.

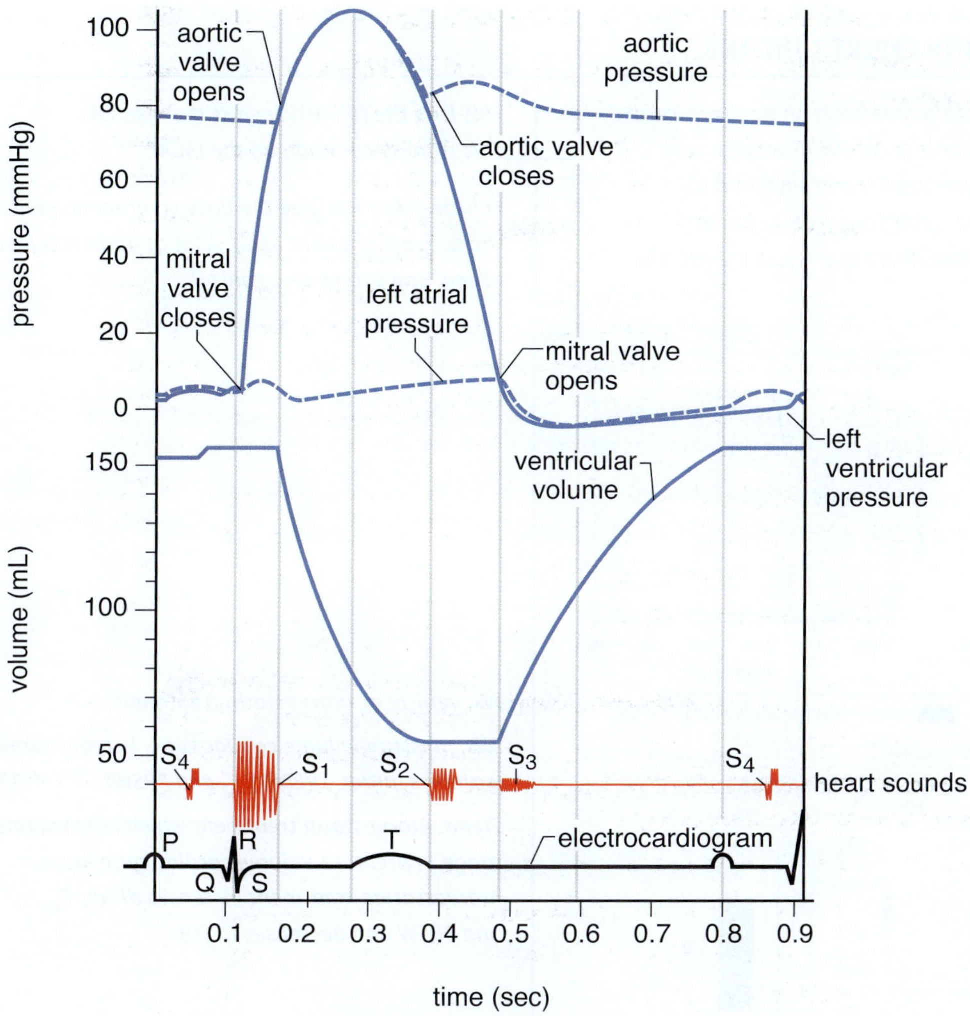

Figure 7.4 The Cardiac Cycle
The MCAT will not expect a thorough understanding of every detail of this diagram; it is more important to see how the changes in valves (open or closed), pressures, and volumes are related.

For humans, cardiac output is about 5 liters per minute. During periods of exercise or rest, the autonomic nervous system will increase (sympathetic) or decrease (parasympathetic) cardiac output, respectively.

REAL WORLD

There is a limit to how fast the heart can beat and still pump blood effectively. Because the heart fills with blood when it is relaxing (diastole), the faster it beats, the less time there is for blood to enter the heart during relaxation. Thus, a faster heartbeat means diminishing returns in terms of the amount of blood supplied to the body. A dangerous condition called ventricular tachycardia (often abbreviated *v-tach*) features a very rapid rate of ventricular contraction. The heart in v-tach cannot properly fill with blood and, paradoxically, stops pumping blood despite its fast rate. Systemic pressures drop precipitously. Death will result unless the heart is forced out of this abnormal rhythm.

BIOLOGY GUIDED EXAMPLE WITH EXPERT THINKING

To further investigate the effects of atorvastatin on post-myocardial infarction recovery, left ventricular myocardial infarction was artificially induced in rats. Rats were randomly assigned to atorvastatin or vehicle treatment. After four weeks, the left ventricles of all rats were examined. Results are summarized in Figures 1A–F below.

This isn't the full article, just the results! This is fairly common on the MCAT.

Vehicle means to give the base solution without the active ingredient itself. A lot of times it is just saline, and serves as a control.

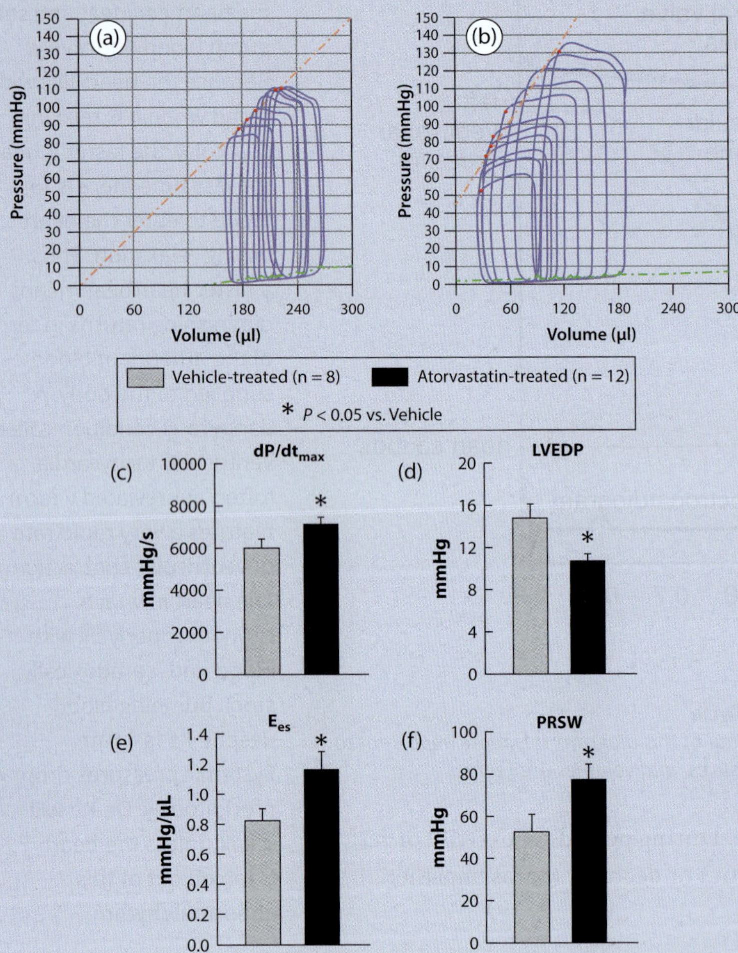

IVs: vehicle or atorvastatin treatment

DVs: pressure-volume cardiac cycle, hemodynamic variables (dP/dt, LVEDP, E_{es}, and PRSW)

Trend: Atorvastatin treatment widens the volume range in pressure-volume cardiac cycle loops. Atorvastating treatment increases dP/dt, E_{es}, and PRSW and decreases LVEDP.

Figure 1 Representative pressure-volume cardiac cycle loops from a vehicle-treated rat (a) and an atorvastatin-treated rat (b) recorded during preload manipulation by a brief period of inferior vena cava occlusion. Panels (c)–(f) illustrate the quantitative analysis of hemodynamic variables of the rats including dP/dt (c), LV end-diastolic pressure (d), end-systolic elastance (e), and preload recruitable stroke work (f).

Adapted from Tang X-L, Sanganalmath SK, Sato H, Bi Q, Hunt G, Vincent RJ, et al. (2011) Atorvastatin therapy during the peri-infarct period attenuates left ventricular dysfunction and remodeling after myocardial infarction. *PLoS One* 6(9): e25320. https://doi.org/10.1371/journal.pone.0025320.

Which treatment condition is correlated with a greater stroke volume in rats following myocardial infarction?

This question asks us to interpret the given figure in order to determine which condition is associated with a particular outcome. The MCAT will require us to bring in testable content knowledge, but it will also expect us to know how to use logical reasoning to analyze an experiment.

The first step is to think about what the question is asking for us to analyze from within the given passage and figure. We know from our outside content knowledge that stroke volume is defined as the volume of blood pumped per heartbeat. Simply speaking, all we need to do is to identify what information on the figure is related to the volume of blood pumped.

If we're not sure how to do this, a good place to start is to look at the units of each graph in the figure. In a novel figure, units can serve as a great clue as to what the figure is about. Since we're looking for stroke volume, we should be looking for units of volume like liters or cm^3. Parts (c) through (f) have units of pressure per seconds, pressure, or pressure per volume, which are not what we are looking for. We'll need to refer to images (a) and (b), both of which have a unit of volume on their *x*-axes.

According to the figure label, graph (a) shows the vehicle-treated rat, and graph (b) shows the atorvastatin-treated rat. The label also tells us that these graphs show pressure-volume cardiac cycle loops of two rats, one in each condition. Now we must relate these graphs to stroke volume. Remember that stroke volume is the volume of blood pumped per heartbeat. In other words, it is the amount of blood pumped after one cardiac cycle. On a pressure-volume graph, a cardiac cycle is seen here as a rectangular loop, with the height and width of the loop representing the pressure change and volume change, respectively. Looking at the two graphs in the figure, we must compare the changes in the volume of the loops of the two conditions. Even without explicitly measuring the dimensions, we can see that the atorvastatin graph has much wider loops, and thus a greater stroke volume.

Based on parts (a) and (b) of Figure 1, we can reasonably conclude that treatment with atorvastatin is correlated with greater stroke volume in rats post-infarction as compared to the control (vehicle) treatment.

The Vasculature

In order to deliver blood to the entire body, the circulatory system utilizes vessels of different sizes. The three major types of vessels are arteries, veins, and capillaries. Blood travels away from the heart in **arteries**, the largest of which is the aorta (in the systemic circulation). Major arteries, such as the common carotids, subclavians, and renal arteries, branch off of the aorta to distribute the bloodflow toward different peripheral tissues. Arteries then undergo further divisions and name changes as they divert blood to specific tissues and organs until, upon reaching their target, they branch into **arterioles**, which ultimately lead to **capillaries** that perfuse the tissues. There is also a set of coronary arteries at the base of the aorta that sends blood to perfuse the heart musculature. On the venous side of a capillary network, the capillaries join together into **venules**, which join to form **veins**. Venous blood empties into the superior and inferior venae cavae for entry into the right side of the heart. All blood vessels are lined with **endothelial cells**. This special type of cell helps to maintain the vessel by releasing chemicals that aid in vasodilation and vasoconstriction. In addition, endothelial cells can allow white blood cells to pass through the vessel wall and into the tissues during an inflammatory response. Finally, endothelial cells release certain chemicals when damaged that are involved in the formation of blood clots to repair the vessel and stop bleeding.

Cross sections of the different blood vessels are shown in Figure 7.5. Don't worry about the names of the layers; simply be able to recognize that the same types of cells comprise the different vessels and that arteries have much more smooth muscle than veins.

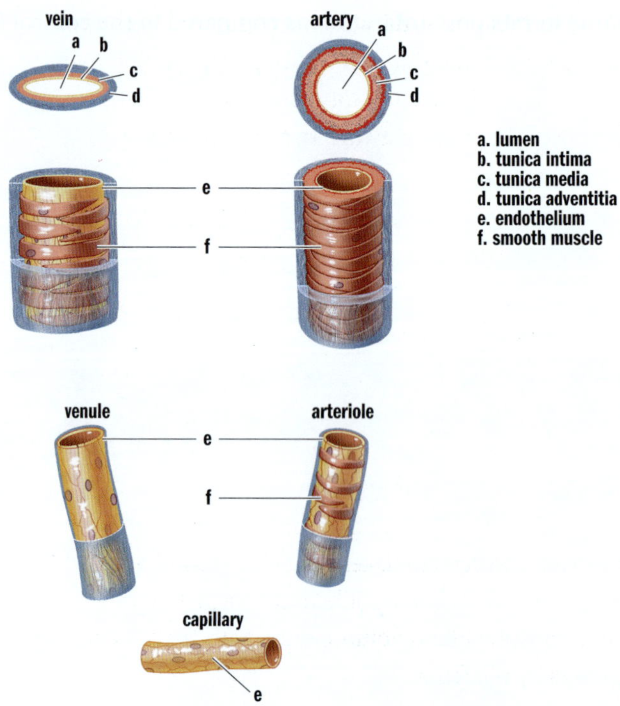

Figure 7.5 Structure of Blood Vessels

MNEMONIC

Arteries carry blood **a**way from the heart.

REAL WORLD

A heart attack, or myocardial infarction, is caused by a lack of bloodflow through the coronary arteries, which results in decreased oxygen delivery to the cardiac muscle itself. Anaerobic respiration cannot produce enough ATP to keep up with demand, so the muscle tissue begins to die. A person suffering a heart attack is often given a β-blocker, which blocks the sympathetic stimulation of the heart, resulting in lower heart rate and lower contractility. With a β-blocker, the heart does not work as hard, so its oxygen demand is diminished, which helps to prevent further damage to cardiac tissue.

Arteries

Arteries move blood away from the heart to the lungs and other parts of the body. Most arteries contain oxygenated blood; in fact, only the pulmonary arteries and umbilical arteries contain deoxygenated blood. Smaller, muscular arteries are known as arterioles.

Arteries are highly muscular and elastic, creating tremendous resistance to the flow of blood. This is one of the reasons why the left side of the heart must generate much higher pressures: to overcome the resistance caused by systemic arteries. After arteries are filled with blood, the elastic recoil from their walls maintains a high pressure and forces blood forward.

Capillaries

Capillaries are vessels with a single endothelial cell layer and are so small that red blood cells must pass through the capillaries in a single-file line. The thin wall of the capillary allows easy diffusion of gases (O_2 and CO_2), nutrients (most notably, glucose), and wastes (ammonia and urea, among others). Capillaries are therefore the interface for communication of the circulatory system with the tissues. Remember, too, that blood also carries hormones, so capillaries allow endocrine signals to arrive at their target tissues.

Capillaries can be quite delicate. When capillaries are damaged, blood can leave the capillaries and enter the interstitial space. If this occurs in a closed space, it results in a bruise.

Veins

Veins are thin-walled, inelastic vessels that transport blood to the heart. Except for the pulmonary and umbilical veins, all veins carry deoxygenated blood. **Venules** are smaller venous structures that connect capillaries to the larger veins of the body.

The smaller amount of smooth muscle in the walls of veins gives them less recoil than arteries. Furthermore, veins are able to stretch to accommodate larger quantities of blood. Indeed, three-fourths of our total blood volume may be in venous circulation at any one time. Note that, even though the volume of arterial blood is normally much less than the volume of venous blood, the total volume passing through either side of the heart per unit time (cardiac output) is the same.

Given that the heart is located in the chest, bloodflow in most veins is upward from the lower body back to the heart, against gravity. In the inferior vena cava, this translates into a large amount of blood in a vertical column. The pressure at the bottom of this venous column in the large veins of the legs can be quite high. In fact, it can exceed systolic pressure (120 mmHg), going as high as 200 mmHg or more. Thus, veins have both structures and processes to push the blood forward and prevent backflow. For example, Figure 7.6 shows that the body's larger veins contain valves; as blood flows forward in the veins, the valves open. When blood tries to move backward, the valves will slam shut. Failure of the venous valves can result in the formation of varicose veins, which are distended where blood has pooled. People who are pregnant are especially susceptible to the formation of varicose veins due to an increase in the total blood volume during pregnancy and compression of the inferior vena cava by the fetus.

REAL WORLD

Blood clots may form in the deep veins of the legs as a result of injury, inactivity (blood stasis), or a hypercoagulable state (a tendency for the blood to clot excessively). The clots may dislodge and travel through the right atrium and right ventricle, through the pulmonary artery, and into the lungs. Such clots, called pulmonary emboli (or, more specifically, thromboemboli), block segments of the pulmonary arteries and produce rapid, labored breathing and chest pain. Death may occur if the thromboemboli are large.

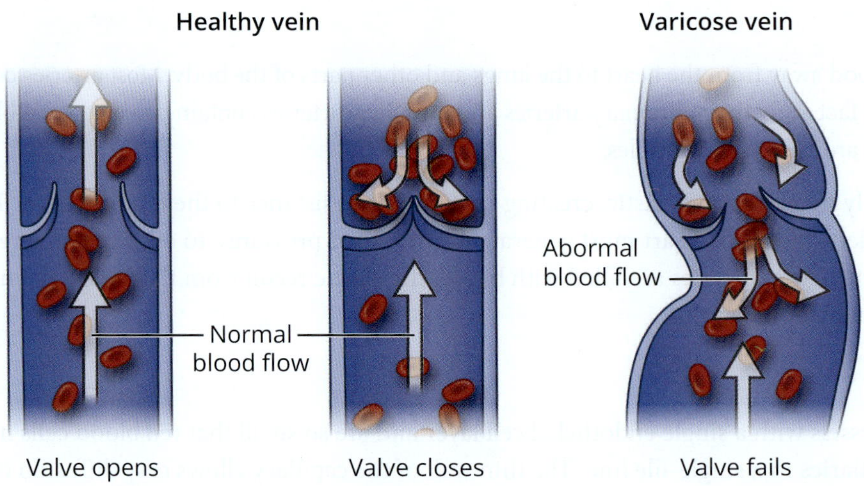

Figure 7.6 Vein Valves

In addition to high pressure in the lower extremities, the small amount of smooth muscle also creates a challenge for propelling blood forward. Thus, the veins must rely on an external force to generate the pressure to push blood toward the heart. Most veins are surrounded by skeletal muscles, which squeeze the veins as the muscles contract, forcing the blood up against gravity in much the same way that squeezing the bottom of a tube of toothpaste causes the contents to be expelled through the top of the tube. This is why sitting motionless for long periods of time, such as in the cramped middle seat on a long transoceanic flight or after surgery, can increase the risk of blood clot formation in the veins of the legs and pelvis. Blood pools in the lower extremities, and sluggish blood coagulates more easily. A clot in the deep veins of the leg is called a deep vein thrombosis (DVT). This clot may become dislodged and travel through the right side of the heart to the lungs (known as a *pulmonary embolus*), where it can cause a life-threatening condition called a **pulmonary embolism**.

REAL WORLD

Many patients may be immobile following a surgical procedure or during a long hospital stay. This introduces the threat of DVT and pulmonary emboli, which are very undesirable complications in someone who is already sick. Thus, in hospitals, special wraps are placed on the legs that contract rhythmically in order to prevent pooling of blood and the formation of blood clots. In addition, many patients receive medications like *heparin* or *warfarin* to prevent the formation of clots.

Circulation

Circulation is, by definition, circular. Let's return to the anatomy of the heart and vasculature, shown in Figure 7.1, to trace the flow of blood through the body. A closeup of bloodflow through the heart is also shown in Figure 7.7. Here, we begin with the return of blood to the right atrium. Blood returns to the heart from the body via the venae cavae, which are divided into the **superior vena cava (SVC)** and the **inferior vena cava (IVC)**. The superior vena cava returns blood from the portions of the body above the heart, while the inferior vena cava returns blood from portions of the body below the heart. Deoxygenated blood enters the right atrium, travels through the tricuspid valve, and enters the right ventricle. On contraction, the blood from the right ventricle passes through the pulmonary valve and enters the pulmonary arteries, where it travels to the lungs and breaks up into continuously smaller vessels. Once the blood reaches the capillaries that line the alveoli, it participates in gas exchange, with carbon dioxide leaving the blood and oxygen entering the blood. The blood then travels into pulmonary venules and into the pulmonary veins, which carry the blood to the left side of the heart. Oxygenated blood enters the left atrium, travels through the mitral valve, and enters the left ventricle. On contraction, the blood from the left ventricle passes through the aortic valve and enters the aorta. From the aorta, blood enters arteries, then arterioles, and then capillaries. After gas and nutrient exchange occurs at the capillaries, the blood enters the venules, which lead to the larger veins. The veins then empty into either the SVC or IVC for return to the right side of the heart.

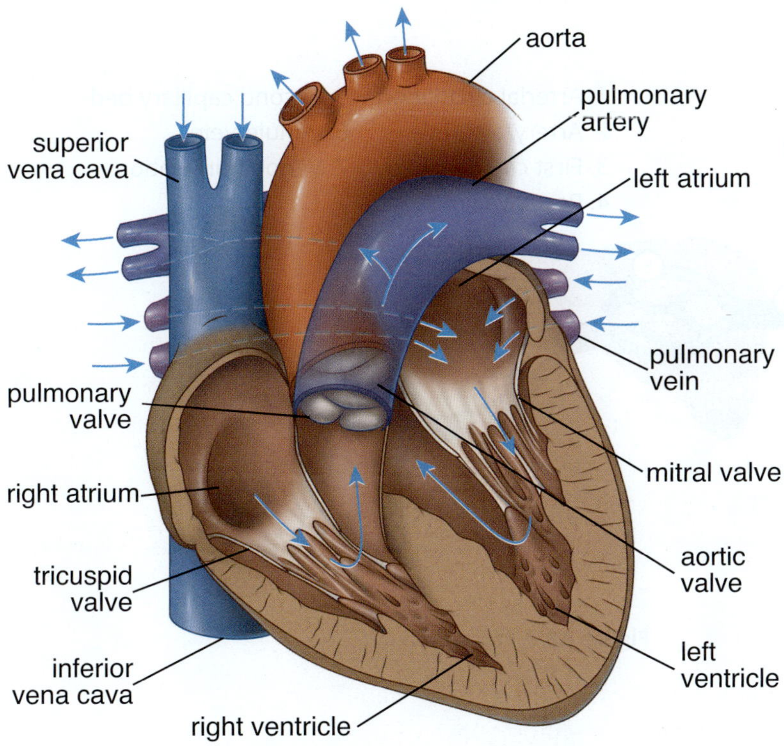

Figure 7.7 Bloodflow through the Heart

REAL WORLD

While *bicuspid valve* is an acceptable alternative name for *mitral valve*, it is rarely used in medicine. Most practitioners will refer to valves by one-letter abbreviations (*M* for mitral). The name *mitral* refers to a *miter*, which is the name for a ceremonial headdress worn by some religious leaders. The two large leaflets of the mitral valve somewhat resemble this headdress.

Written in shorthand, the pathway appears like this:

$$\text{right atrium} \xrightarrow[\text{valve}]{\text{tricuspid}} \text{right ventricle} \xrightarrow[\text{valve}]{\text{pulmonary}} \text{pulmonary artery} \rightarrow \text{lungs} \rightarrow$$

$$\text{pulmonary veins} \rightarrow \text{left atrium} \xrightarrow[\text{valve}]{\text{mitral}} \text{left ventricle} \xrightarrow[\text{valve}]{\text{aortic}} \text{aorta} \rightarrow \text{arteries} \rightarrow$$

$$\text{arterioles} \rightarrow \text{capillaries} \rightarrow \text{venules} \rightarrow \text{veins} \rightarrow \text{venae cavae} \rightarrow \text{right atrium}$$

In most cases, blood will pass through only one capillary bed before returning to the heart. However, there are three **portal systems** in the body, in which blood passes through two capillary beds rather than the usual one. In portal systems, the blood flows through both capillary beds via a **portal vein** before returning to the heart. See Figure 7.8 for a visual representation of a portal system. In the **hepatic portal system**, blood leaving capillary beds in the walls of the gut passes through the hepatic portal vein before reaching the capillary beds in the liver. In the **hypophyseal portal system**, blood leaving capillary beds in the hypothalamus travels to a capillary bed in the anterior pituitary to allow for paracrine secretion of releasing hormones. In the **renal portal system**, blood leaving the glomerulus travels through an efferent arteriole before surrounding the nephron in a capillary network called the vasa recta.

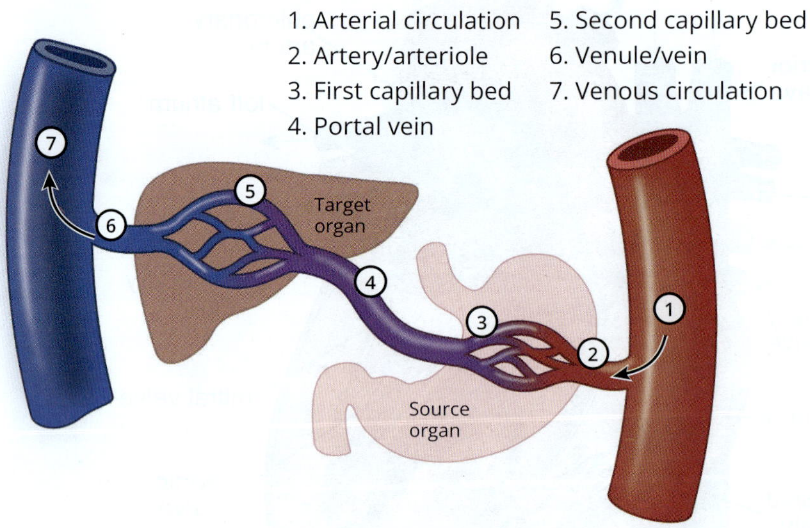

Figure 7.8 A Portal System

MCAT CONCEPT CHECK 7.1

Before you move on, assess your understanding of the material with these questions.

1. Starting from entering the heart from the venae cavae, what are the four chambers through which blood passes in the heart? Which valve prevents backflow into each chamber?

Heart Chamber	Valve That Prevents Backflow

2. Starting with the site of impulse initiation, what are the structures in the conduction system of the heart?

3. Compare and contrast arteries, capillaries, and veins:

Vessel	Carries Blood in Which Direction?	Relative Wall Thickness	Smooth Muscle Present?	Contains Valves?
Artery				
Capillary				
Vein				

4. Why does the right side of the heart contain less cardiac muscle than the left side?

5. If all autonomic input to the heart were cut, what would happen?

7.2 Blood

LEARNING OBJECTIVES

After Chapter 7.2, you will be able to:

- Recall the components of plasma
- Predict compatible blood types given a blood type
- Identify the purpose of hematocrit measurements, as well as the relevant unit of measurement
- Recognize the different types of leukocytes and their functions
- Describe how platelets are produced
- Distinguish between cell types within blood that contain or do not contain a nucleus

Now that we have examined the pump and the pipes through which blood travels, let's take a look at this fluid.

Composition

In the pathology lab, we frequently study the composition of the blood using a centrifuge. By spinning the blood at a rapid rate, we can separate this complex fluid into three main layers based on density. By volume, blood is about 55% liquid and 45% cells, as shown in Figure 7.9. **Plasma** is the liquid portion of blood, an aqueous mixture of nutrients, salts, respiratory gases, hormones, and blood proteins. Plasma can be further refined via the removal of clotting factors into serum. The cellular portion of blood consists of three major categories: **erythrocytes**, **leukocytes**, and **platelets**. All blood cells are formed from hematopoietic stem cells, which originate in the bone marrow.

REAL WORLD

Serum (plural sera) is used in a variety of medical testing procedures such as antibody testing and blood typing. Serum is considered preferable to plasma for many applications due to the lack of clotting factors and fibrinogens.

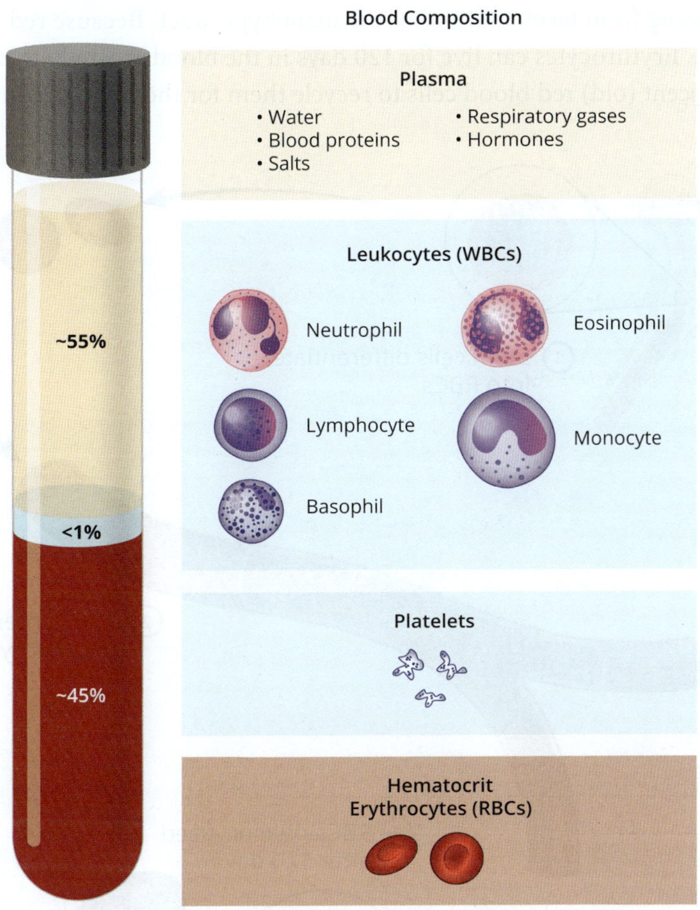

Figure 7.9 The Composition of Blood

Erythrocytes—Red Blood Cells

In the body, oxygen and nutrients are delivered to the peripheral tissues, and carbon dioxide and other wastes (such as hydrogen ions and ammonia) are picked up from the peripheral tissues and delivered to the organs that process this waste: the lungs, liver, and kidneys. The **erythrocyte** or **red blood cell** is a specialized cell designed for oxygen transport. Oxygen does not simply dissolve in the cytoplasm of the red blood cell—remember, molecular oxygen is nonpolar and therefore has low solubility in aqueous environments. Rather, each erythrocyte contains about 250 million molecules of **hemoglobin**, each of which can bind four molecules of oxygen. Therefore, each red blood cell can carry approximately 1 billion molecules of oxygen.

Red blood cells are unique in a number of ways, and their modifications reflect the special role they play in the human body. Red blood cells are biconcave, or indented on both sides, which serves a dual purpose. First, this shape assists them in traveling through tiny capillaries. Second, it increases the cell's surface area, which increases gas exchange. Red blood cells are also unique in that, when they mature, the nuclei, mitochondria, and other membrane-bound organelles are lost. The loss of organelles makes space for the molecules of hemoglobin. In addition, the loss of mitochondria in particular means that the red blood cell does not consume the oxygen it is carrying before it is delivered to peripheral tissues. In other words, red blood cells do not carry out oxidative phosphorylation to generate ATP; rather, they rely entirely on glycolysis for

ATP, with lactic acid (arising from fermentation) as the main byproduct. Because red blood cells lack nuclei, they are unable to divide. Erythrocytes can live for 120 days in the bloodstream before cells in the liver and spleen phagocytize senescent (old) red blood cells to recycle them for their parts (Figure 7.10).

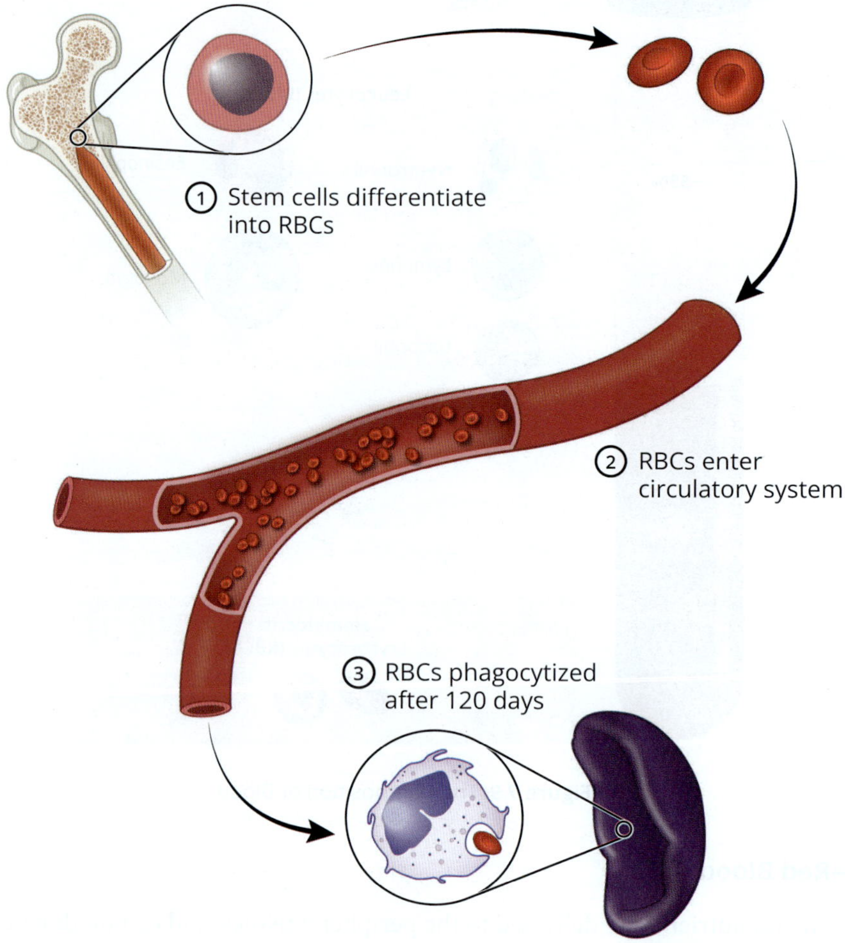

Figure 7.10 Erythrocyte Life Cycle

In medicine, a complete blood count measures the quantity of each cell type in the blood. For red blood cells, two commonly given measures are the hemoglobin and hematocrit. Hemoglobin, of course, measures the quantity of hemoglobin in the blood, giving a result in grams per deciliter. **Hematocrit** is a measure of how much of the blood sample consists of red blood cells, given as a percentage. A normal hemoglobin is considered to be between 13.5 and 17.5 $\frac{g}{dL}$ for phenotypical males and between 12.0 and 16.0 $\frac{g}{dL}$ for phenotypical females. A normal hematocrit is considered to be between 41 and 53% for males and between 36 and 46% for females. For example, a patient may have a hemoglobin of 13.8 $\frac{g}{dL}$ and a hematocrit of 41.2%. The difference between male and female hematocrit levels is resultant of a couple factors: (1) Males usually have more testosterone, which increases the rate of red blood cell production, raising hematocrit; and (2) females often menstruate once a month, which lowers hematocrit.

Leukocytes—White Blood Cells

Leukocytes or **white blood cells** usually comprise less than 1 percent of total blood volume. This translates into about 4,500–11,000 leukocytes per microliter of blood, which is a small number relative to the erythrocyte concentration. This number can massively increase under certain conditions when we need more white blood cells, most notably during infection. White blood cells are a crucial part of the immune system, acting as our defenders against pathogens, foreign cells, cancer, and other materials not recognized as *self*. Let's briefly discuss five basic types of leukocytes, which are all categorized into two classes: granulocytes and agranulocytes.

The granular leukocytes or **granulocytes** (**neutrophils**, **eosinophils**, and **basophils**) are so named because they contain cytoplasmic granules that are visible by microscopy. These granules contain a variety of compounds that are toxic to invading microbes; these compounds can be released through exocytosis. Granular leukocytes are involved in inflammatory reactions, allergies, pus formation, and destruction of bacteria and parasites. The specific functions of the three granulocytes are discussed in Chapter 8 of *MCAT Biology Review*.

The agranulocytes, which do not contain granules that are released by exocytosis, consist of **lymphocytes** and **monocytes**. Lymphocytes are important in the **specific immune response**, the body's targeted fight against particular pathogens, such as viruses and bacteria. Some lymphocytes act as primary responders against an infection, while others function to maintain a long-term memory bank of pathogen recognition. These cells, in a very real sense, help our body learn from experience and are prepared to mount a fast response upon repeated exposure to familiar pathogens. Many vaccines work by training these cells. Through exposure to a weakened pathogen, or an antigenic protein (a protein that can be recognized by the immune system) of the pathogen, memory cells can be created. For example, most children in the United States receive the varicella (chickenpox) vaccine, which includes a live but weakened strain of the varicella-zoster virus that causes chickenpox. When the vaccine is administered, the virus is recognized as foreign and an immune response is activated. During this process, certain immune cells form a memory of the virus; in other words, our body learns to remember the virus and prepares itself to ward off the virus if it appears again later in life.

Lymphocyte maturation takes place in one of three locations. Lymphocytes that mature in the bone marrow are referred to as B-cells, and those that mature in the thymus are called T-cells. B-cells are responsible for antibody generation, whereas T-cells kill virally infected cells and activate other immune cells. The details of these two components of the specific immune response are discussed in Chapter 8 of *MCAT Biology Review*.

The other agranulocytes are monocytes, which phagocytize foreign matter such as bacteria. Most organs of the body contain a collection of these phagocytic cells; once they leave the bloodstream and enter an organ, monocytes are renamed **macrophages**. Each organ's macrophage population may have a specific name, as well. In the central nervous system, for example, they are called **microglia**; in the skin, they are called **Langerhans cells**; in bone, they are called **osteoclasts**.

Thrombocytes—Platelets

As seen in Figure 7.11, **thrombocytes** or **platelets** are cell fragments or shards released from cells in bone marrow known as **megakaryocytes**. Their function is to assist in blood clotting and they are present in high concentrations (150,000–400,000 per microliter of blood). The enzymatic reactions involved in the formation of a clot (the clotting cascade) will be discussed shortly.

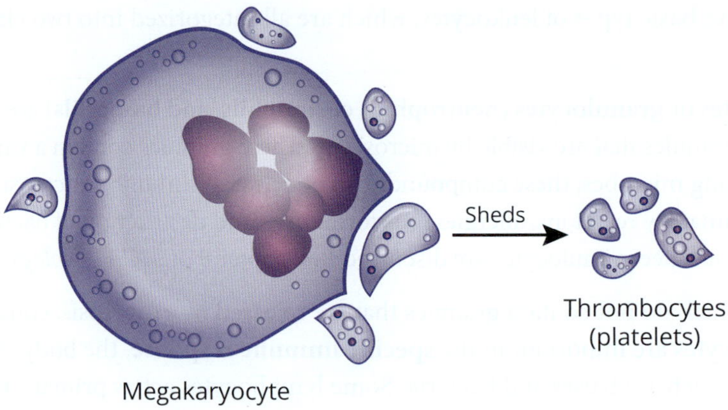

Figure 7.11 Megakaryocyte to Platelet

As mentioned above, all of the cellular elements of blood originate in the bone marrow. The production of blood cells and platelets is called **hematopoiesis**, and is triggered by a number of hormones, growth factors, and cytokines. The most notable of these are **erythropoietin**, which is secreted by the kidney and stimulates mainly red blood cell development **(erythropoiesis)**, and **thrombopoietin**, which is secreted by the liver and kidney and stimulates mainly platelet development **(thrombopoiesis)**. The hematopoietic pathways are shown in Figure 7.12.

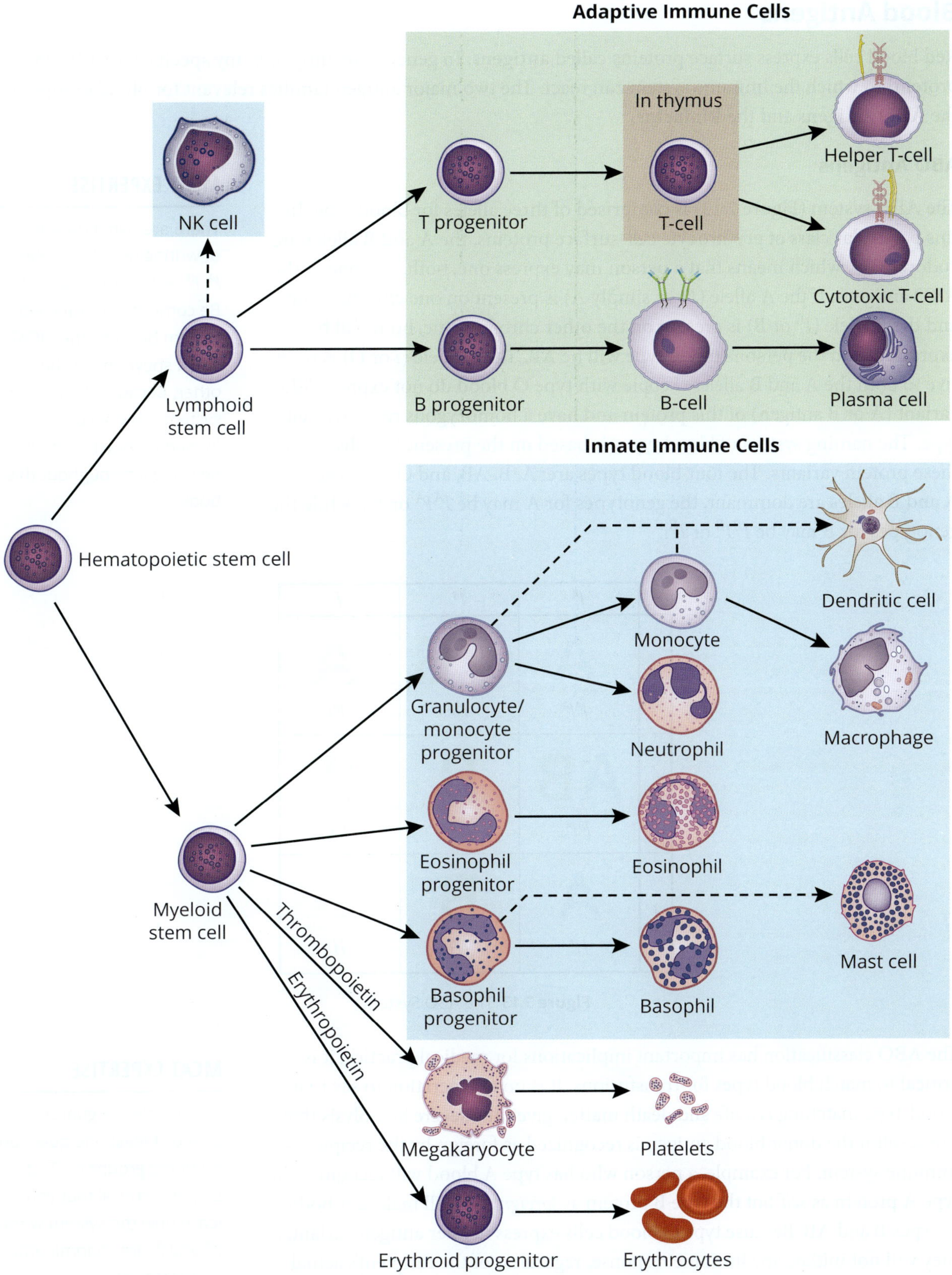

Figure 7.12 Hematopoiesis

Blood Antigens

Red blood cells express surface proteins called **antigens**. In general, an antigen is any specific target (usually a protein) to which the immune system can react. The two major antigen families relevant for blood groups are the **ABO antigens** and the **Rh factor**.

ABO Antigens

The ABO system (Figure 7.13) is comprised of three alleles for blood type. In this particular class of erythrocyte cell-surface proteins, the A and B alleles are codominant, which means that a person may express one, both, or none of the ABO antigens. If the A allele (I^A or simply A) is present on one chromosome and the B allele (I^B or B) is present on the other chromosome, both will be expressed, and the person's blood type will be AB. The O allele (i or O) is recessive to both the A and B alleles. People with type O blood do not express either variant (A or B antigen) of this protein and have a homozygous recessive genotype. The naming system of blood types is based on the presence or absence of these protein variants. The four blood types are: A, B, AB, and O. Because the A and B alleles are dominant, the genotypes for A may be I^AI^A or I^Ai, while the genotypes for B may be I^BI^B or I^Bi.

MCAT EXPERTISE

There are two different ways of writing the ABO alleles: I^A, I^B, and i; or A, B, and O. Be comfortable using either system because the MCAT could show one or the other. Because the former system is more common in medical practice, we'll be using it throughout this book.

	I^A	I^B	i
I^A	A I^AI^A	AB I^AI^B	A I^Ai
I^B	AB I^BI^A	B I^BI^B	B I^Bi
i	A iI^A	B iI^B	O ii

Figure 7.13 The ABO System

The ABO classification has important implications for medical practice; it is critical to match blood types for transfusions. It is no exaggeration to say that blood-type matching is a life and death matter, given the severe hemolysis that can result if the donor blood antigen is recognized as foreign by the recipient's immune system. For example, a person who has type A blood will recognize the type A protein as *self* but the type B protein as *foreign* and will make antibodies to types B and AB. Because type O blood cells express neither antigen variant, they will not initiate any immune response, regardless of the recipient's actual blood type; people with type O blood are therefore considered **universal donors** because their blood will not cause ABO-related hemolysis in any recipient.

MCAT EXPERTISE

You are almost guaranteed to see at least one question on blood groups on Test Day. It is critical that you learn how the system works (I^A and I^B are codominant, i is recessive).

However, a recipient who is type O will produce both anti-A *and* anti-B antibodies and can only receive type O blood. On the other hand, people with type AB blood are considered **universal recipients** because they can receive blood from all blood types: no blood antigen is foreign to individuals who have AB blood, so no adverse reactions will occur upon transfusion. A more thorough description of each blood type is given in Table 7.1. Note that whole blood is almost never given in a transfusion; rather, packed red blood cells (with no plasma) are generally given. Thus, we care only about the donor's red blood cell antigens (and not the plasma antibodies) when determining whether hemolysis will occur.

Another important point needs to be made here about antibodies. Antibodies are created in response to an antigen, and they specifically target that antigen. You would not expect to have antibodies to the Ebola virus if you had never been exposed to it. This is true for the Rh factor (discussed in detail in the next section) as well—an individual who is Rh-negative would not have anti-Rh antibodies prior to exposure to Rh-positive blood. Why, then, does an individual lacking the A allele automatically have an anti-A antibody? The reason may lie in the gut: research has demonstrated that *E. coli* that inhabit the colon may have proteins that match the A and B alleles. This would serve as a source of exposure and would allow one to develop anti-A (or anti-B) antibodies prior to exposure to another person's blood. This is why ABO compatibility is so important during blood transfusions—giving the wrong ABO blood type would lead to rapid hemolysis.

KEY CONCEPT

Antigens are the stimuli for B-cells to make antibodies. After exposure of a B-cell to its specific antigen, the cell becomes an antibody-producing factory.

Blood Type	Genotype(s)	Antigens Produced	Antibodies Produced	Can Donate to . . .	Can Receive from . . .
A	I^AI^A, I^Ai	A	anti-B	A, AB	A, O
B	I^BI^B, I^Bi	B	anti-A	B, AB	B, O
AB	I^AI^B	A and B	none	AB only	A, B, AB, O (universal recipient)
O	*ii*	none	anti-A and anti-B	A, B, AB, O (universal donor)	O only

Table 7.1 ABO Blood Types

REAL WORLD

The most common blood type in the United States is O^+. The least common is AB^-.

REAL WORLD

In blood bank pathology, the Rh factor is often referred to as D. Note that while the A, B, and D proteins are the most important for blood typing, dozens of other antigens can (and should) be matched as well, including C, E, Kell, Lewis, Duffy, and others. The more antigens that are correctly matched, the lower the probability of hemolysis.

Rh Factor

The **Rh factor** (so named because it was first described in rhesus monkeys) is also a surface protein expressed on red blood cells. Although at one time it was thought to be a single antigen, it has since been found to exist as several variants. When left unmodified, Rh-positive (Rh^+) or Rh-negative (Rh^-) refers to the presence or absence of the D antigen on red blood cells, which is determined by the presence or absence of a functional *RHD* gene. The presence or absence of D can also be indicated with a plus or minus superscript on the ABO blood type (such as O^+ or AB^-). Rh-positivity follows autosomal dominant inheritance; one positive allele is enough for the protein to be expressed.

The Rh factor status is particularly important in obstetric medicine. Exposure to at least a small amount of fetal blood during childbirth is inevitable, no matter how good the obstetrician is. If a person who is pregnant is Rh^- and the fetus is Rh^+, the person will become sensitized to the Rh factor, and the person's immune system will begin making antibodies against it. This is not a problem for the first child; by the time the person starts producing antibodies, the child has already been born. However, any subsequent pregnancy in which the fetus is Rh^+ will present a problem because maternal anti-Rh antibodies can cross the placenta and attack the fetal blood cells, resulting in hemolysis of the fetal cells. This condition is known as **erythroblastosis fetalis** (depicted in Figure 7.14) and can be fatal to the fetus. Today, we can use medicine to prevent this condition. There is less concern with maternal-fetal ABO mismatching because antibodies against AB antigens are of a class called IgM, which does not readily cross the placenta (unlike anti-Rh IgG antibodies, which can).

REAL WORLD

When a person who is Rh^- is pregnant with a first Rh^+ fetus, the risk of erythroblastosis fetalis in subsequent Rh-mismatched pregnancies can usually be avoided by giving the Rh^- parent Rh-immunoglobulin (RhoGAM) during pregnancy and immediately after delivery. Administration of immunoglobulin (which is a type of passive immunization) will absorb the fetus's Rh^+ cells, preventing the production of anti-Rh antibodies by the parent.

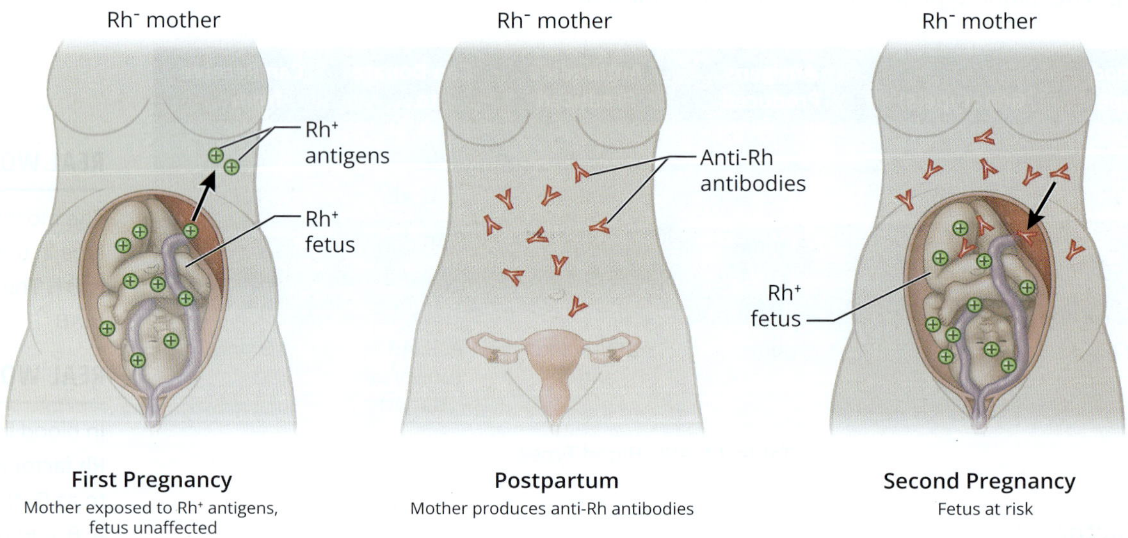

Figure 7.14 Erythroblastosis Fetalis

MCAT CONCEPT CHECK 7.2

Before you move on, assess your understanding of the material with these questions.

1. What are the components of plasma?

___

2. An individual with B^+ blood is in an automobile accident and requires a blood transfusion. What blood types could this person receive? After recovery, the same individual, thankful for the transfusion, decides to donate blood. To which blood types could this person donate?
   - Could receive from:

   ___

   - Could donate to:

   ___

3. What does a hematocrit measure? What are the units for hematocrit?

___

4. Which types of leukocytes are involved in the specific immune response?

___

5. Where do platelets come from?

___

6. Which cell type(s) in blood contain nuclei? Which do not?
   - Contain nuclei:

   ___

   - Do not contain nuclei:

   ___

7.3 Physiology of the Cardiovascular System

LEARNING OBJECTIVES

After Chapter 7.3, you will be able to:

- Predict the impact of changing bloodflow through arteries, capillaries, and veins on blood pressure and heart function
- Recall the bicarbonate buffer chemical equation, including its catalyzing enzyme
- Explain how the oxyhemoglobin dissociation curve can be shifted to the left or right
- Recall the series of events and compounds in a coagulation cascade
- Identify the regions of the body associated with different parts of the oxyhemoglobin dissociation curve:

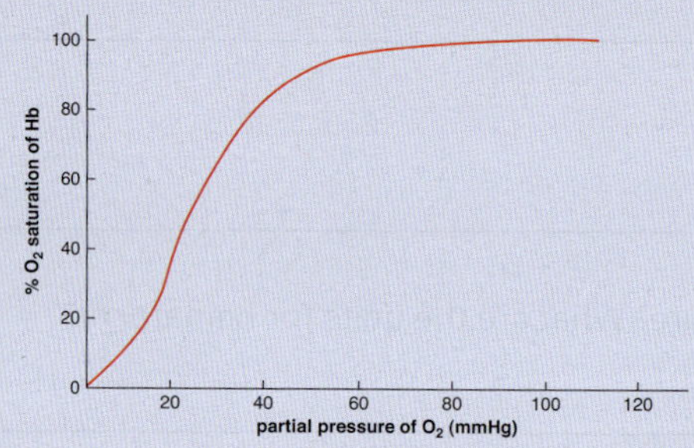

The cardiovascular system transports many compounds, including gases, nutrients, and waste products, to and from the body's tissues via red blood cells and plasma. Furthermore, it serves an important role in immunity through specialized cells, such as leukocytes, which help the body fight localized or systemic pathogens. Capillaries within the body can dilate and constrict to maintain proper body temperature. In addition, the circulatory system mediates the formation of blood clots to repair damaged vessels. These functions reflect the important jobs of the cardiovascular system, which include maintenance of blood pressure, gas and solute exchange, coagulation, and thermoregulation.

Blood Pressure

Before we can even discuss gas and solute exchange, it is important to recognize that, for the circulatory system to serve its predominant functions, blood pressure must be kept sufficiently high to propel blood forward. Blood pressure, therefore, provides healthcare professionals with information regarding the health of the circulatory system. In addition, high blood pressure, or *hypertension*, is a pathological state that may result in damage to the blood vessels and organs. Blood pressure is a measure of the force per unit area exerted on the wall of the blood vessels and is measured with a **sphygmomanometer**. Sphygmomanometers measure the gauge pressure in the systemic circulation, which is the pressure above and beyond atmospheric pressure (760 mmHg at sea level), as discussed in Chapter 4 of *MCAT Physics and Math Review*. Blood pressure is expressed as a ratio of the systolic (ventricular contraction) to diastolic (ventricular relaxation) pressures. Pressure gradually drops from the arterial to venous circulation, with the largest drop occurring across the arterioles, as shown in Figure 7.15. Normal blood pressure is considered to be between 90/60 and 120/80.

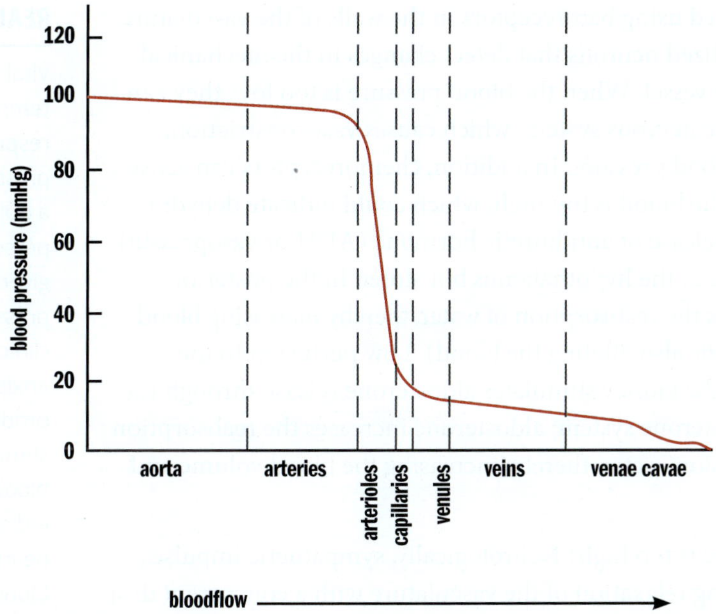

Figure 7.15 Mean Arterial Pressure at Different Locations in the Cardiovascular System

KEY CONCEPT

The largest drop in blood pressure occurs across the arterioles. This is critical because the capillaries are thin-walled and unable to withstand the pressure of the arterial side of the vasculature.

An analogy can be drawn between circulation and an electric circuit. Much like an electromotive force (voltage) drives a current through a given electrical resistance, the pressure gradient across the circulatory system drives cardiac output through a given vascular resistance. This analogy is an important one to remember because the equations of electric circuits can be applied to the cardiovascular system. For example, Ohm's law ($V = IR$) can be translated into the following equation for circulation:

$$\Delta P = \text{CO} \times \text{TPR}$$

Equation 7.2

where ΔP is the pressure differential across the circulation, CO is the cardiac output, and TPR is the total peripheral (vascular) resistance.

It is also important to note that arterioles and capillaries act much like resistors in a circuit. When electricity travels through a wire, the wire itself provides an intrinsic level of resistance that limits the flow of electricity through it. Resistance is based on three factors: resistivity, length, and cross-sectional area. Resistivity has no obvious correlate in physiology, but the other two factors certainly do. The longer a blood vessel is, the more resistance it offers. The larger the cross-sectional area of a blood vessel, the less resistance it offers. In addition, arteries are highly muscular and are able to expand and contract as needed to change vascular resistance and maintain blood pressure. Arterioles can also contract to limit the amount of blood entering a given capillary bed (much like increasing resistance will decrease current flow to a given branch in a circuit). Finally, with the exception of the three portal systems, all systemic capillary beds are in parallel with each other. Therefore, opening capillary beds will decrease vascular resistance (like adding another resistor in parallel) and, assuming the body can compensate, increase cardiac output.

Blood pressure is regulated using baroreceptors in the walls of the vasculature. Baroreceptors are specialized neurons that detect changes in the mechanical forces on the walls of the vessel. When the blood pressure is too low, they can stimulate the sympathetic nervous system, which causes vasoconstriction, thereby increasing the blood pressure. In addition, chemoreceptors can sense when the osmolarity of the blood is too high, which could indicate dehydration. This promotes the release of antidiuretic hormone (ADH or vasopressin), a peptide hormone made in the hypothalamus but stored in the posterior pituitary, which increases the reabsorption of water, thereby increasing blood volume and pressure (while also diluting the blood). Low perfusion to the juxtaglomerular cells of the kidney stimulates aldosterone release through the renin–angiotensin–aldosterone system; aldosterone increases the reabsorption of sodium and, by extension, water, thereby increasing the blood volume and pressure.

So, what if blood pressure is too high? Neurologically, sympathetic impulses could decrease, permitting relaxation of the vasculature with a concurrent drop in blood pressure. Within the heart, specialized atrial cells are able to secrete a hormone called **atrial natriuretic peptide** (**ANP**). This hormone aids in the loss of salt within the nephron, acting as a natural diuretic with loss of fluid. Interestingly, ANP is a fairly weak diuretic. Some fluid is lost, but it is often not enough to counter the effects of a high-salt diet on blood pressure. Indeed, the human body has many different ways to raise blood pressure, but very few ways to lower it.

REAL WORLD

Vital signs include temperature, heart rate, respiratory rate, and blood pressure. They provide a quick snapshot of a person's condition at a given moment. High blood pressure may indicate clinical hypertension, anxiety, catecholamine-producing tumors, or stimulant use, while low blood pressure may indicate hemorrhage, a heart attack, sepsis (severe bloodstream infection), or neurological damage. These are very broad differential diagnoses; however, vital signs combined with a quick clinical history provide a way for clinicians to identify the patients that require immediate intervention.

Gas and Solute Exchange

Blood pressure ensures sufficient forward flow of blood through the system. However, what happens when the blood reaches the capillaries? Here, oxygen and nutrients diffuse out of the blood into tissues, while waste products like carbon dioxide, hydrogen ions, urea, and ammonia diffuse into the blood. In addition, hormones are secreted into the capillaries, travel with the circulation, and diffuse into their target tissue. Ions and fluid must also be returned to the blood to ensure that no area becomes too swollen with fluid. Regardless of the substance being exchanged, there is one fundamental concept to be considered in this process: concentration gradients. In each case, one side of the capillary wall has a higher concentration of a given substance than the other. This allows for movement of gases and solutes by diffusion.

Oxygen

Oxygen is carried primarily by **hemoglobin** in the blood, which is shown in Figure 7.16. Hemoglobin is a protein composed of four cooperative subunits, each of which has a prosthetic heme group that binds to an oxygen molecule. The binding of oxygen occurs at the heme group's central iron atom (Fe^{2+}), which can undergo changes in its oxidation state. The binding or releasing of oxygen to or from the iron atom in the heme group is an oxidation–reduction reaction. It is also important to note that some oxygen does diffuse into the blood and dissolve into the plasma, but this amount is negligible compared to the quantity of oxygen bound to hemoglobin. The level of oxygen in the blood is often measured as the partial pressure of O_2 within the blood, or P_aO_2. A normal P_aO_2 is approximately 70–100 mmHg. However, taking this measurement is inconvenient because it involves taking a sample of blood from an artery. By contrast, **oxygen saturation**—that is, the percentage of hemoglobin molecules carrying oxygen—is easily measured using a finger probe. A healthy oxygen saturation level is above 97 percent.

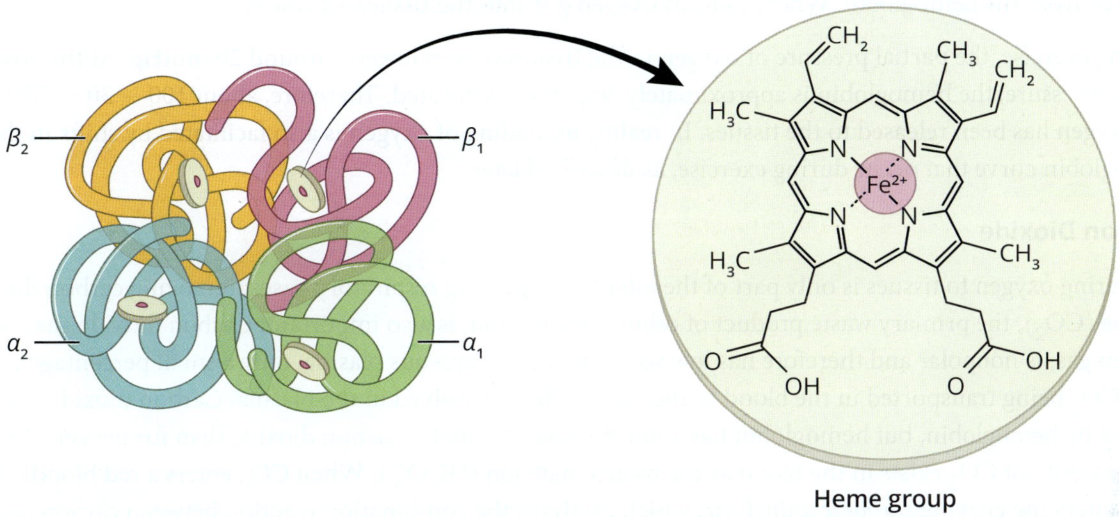

Figure 7.16 Hemoglobin and the Heme Group

In the lungs, oxygen diffuses into the alveolar capillaries. As the first oxygen binds to a heme group, it induces a conformational shift in the shape of hemoglobin from taut to relaxed. This shift increases hemoglobin's affinity for oxygen, making it easier for subsequent molecules of oxygen to bind to the remaining three unoccupied heme groups. As other heme groups acquire an oxygen molecule, the affinity continues to increase, thus creating a positive feedback-like (spiraling forward) mechanism. Once all of the hemoglobin subunits are bound to oxygen, the removal of one molecule of oxygen will induce a conformational shift, decreasing the overall affinity for oxygen, and making it easier for the other molecules of oxygen to leave the heme groups. This is again a positive feedback process; as oxygen molecules leave hemoglobin, it becomes progressively easier for more oxygen to be removed. This phenomenon is a form of allosteric regulation referred to as **cooperative binding** and results in the classic sigmoidal (*S*-shaped) oxyhemoglobin dissociation curve shown in Figure 7.17.

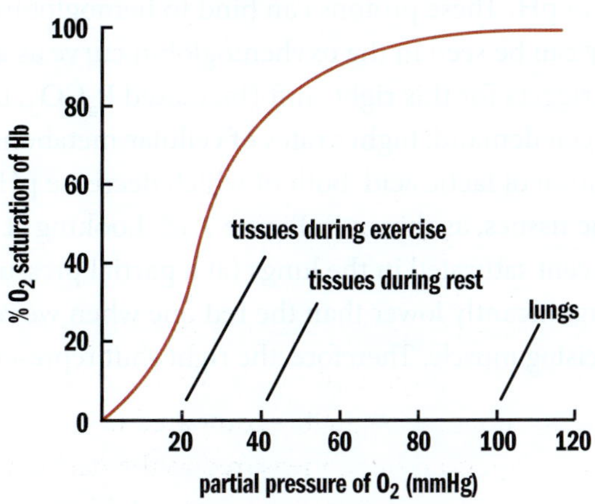

Figure 7.17 Oxyhemoglobin Dissociation Curve

Before looking at shifts in this curve, let's make sure we understand what everything means. According to the curve, the blood is 100 percent saturated in the lungs, at a partial pressure of 100 mmHg O_2. The tissues are at a lower partial pressure of oxygen, around 40 mmHg during rest; at this lower partial pressure, the hemoglobin is approximately 80 percent saturated. Therefore, about $100 - 80 = 20\%$ of the oxygen has been released from the hemoglobin. Where did this oxygen go? Into the tissues, of course.

During exercise, the partial pressure of oxygen in the tissues is even lower—around 20 mmHg. At this lower partial pressure, the hemoglobin is approximately 30 percent saturated. Therefore, about $100 - 30 = 70\%$ of the oxygen has been released to the tissues. In reality, unloading of oxygen is also facilitated by shifts in the hemoglobin curve that occur during exercise, as described later.

Carbon Dioxide

Delivering oxygen to tissues is only part of the job of transporting respiratory gases; removing carbon dioxide gas (CO_2), the primary waste product of cellular respiration, is also important. Carbon dioxide gas, like oxygen gas, is nonpolar and therefore has low solubility in the aqueous plasma; only a small percentage of the total CO_2 being transported in the blood to the lungs will be dissolved in the plasma. Carbon dioxide can be carried by hemoglobin, but hemoglobin has a much lower affinity for carbon dioxide than for oxygen. The vast majority of CO_2 exists in the blood as the bicarbonate ion (HCO_3^-). When CO_2 enters a red blood cell, it encounters the enzyme *carbonic anhydrase*, which catalyzes the combination reaction between carbon dioxide and water to form carbonic acid (H_2CO_3). Carbonic acid, a weak acid, will dissociate into a proton and the bicarbonate anion. The hydrogen ion (proton) and bicarbonate ion both have high solubilities in water, making them a more effective method of transporting metabolic waste products to the lungs for excretion. Upon reaching the alveolar capillaries in the lungs, the same reactions that led to the formation of the proton and bicarbonate anion can be reversed, allowing us to breathe out carbon dioxide:

$$CO_2(g) + H_2O(l) \xrightleftharpoons{\text{Carbonic anhydrase}} H_2CO_3(aq) \rightleftharpoons H^+(aq) + HCO_3^-(aq)$$

This chemical reaction is important, not only because it provides an effective means of ridding the body's tissues of carbon dioxide gas, but also because the concentration of free protons in the blood affects pH; the pH, in turn, can have allosteric effects on the oxyhemoglobin dissociation curve. Increased carbon dioxide production will cause a right shift in the bicarbonate buffer equation (remember Le Châtelier's Principle), resulting in an increase in H^+ and a decrease in pH. These protons can bind to hemoglobin, reducing hemoglobin's affinity for oxygen. This decreased affinity can be seen in the oxyhemoglobin curve as a shift to the right; this is known as the **Bohr effect**. Note that the triggers for this right shift (increased P_aCO_2, increased $[H^+]$, decreased pH) are often associated with oxygen demand; higher rates of cellular metabolism result in increased carbon dioxide production and accumulation of lactic acid, both of which decrease pH. This decreased affinity allows more oxygen to be unloaded at the tissues, as shown in Figure 7.18. Looking at the red and green lines, we see that hemoglobin is nearly 100 percent saturated in the lungs (at a partial pressure of 100 mmHg O_2) for both lines. However, the green line is significantly lower than the red one when we reach a partial pressure of 20 mmHg O_2, around that of exercising muscle. Therefore, the right shift represents greater unloading of oxygen into the tissues.

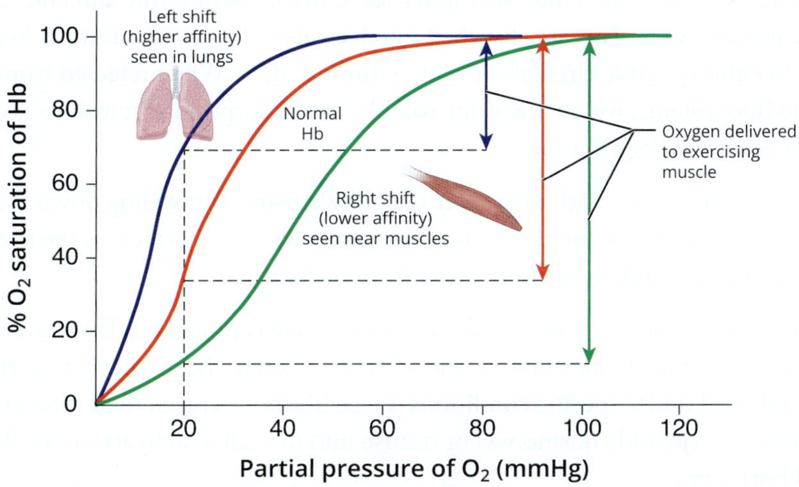

Figure 7.18 Shifts in the Oxyhemoglobin Dissociation Curve

MNEMONIC

Causes of a **right** shift of the oxyhemoglobin curve: **Exercise** is the **right** thing to do.

The following occur during **exercise**:

- Increased P_aCO_2
- Increased $[H^+]$ (decreased pH)
- Increased temperature

Other causes of a right shift in the oxyhemoglobin curve include increased temperature and increased 2,3-bisphosphoglycerate (2,3-BPG), a side product of glycolysis in red blood cells. 2,3-BPG is a convenient signaling molecule. If a cell is in need of more energy, it will increase the rate of glycolysis and the electron transport chain will subsequently work more. Due to this, the cell has an increased need for oxygen, so the byproduct of this process also being the signal to bring in more oxygen from hemoglobin makes this process significantly more efficient.

A left shift, like the blue line in Figure 7.18, may occur due to decreased P_aCO_2, decreased $[H^+]$, increased pH, decreased temperature, and decreased 2,3-BPG. In addition, **fetal hemoglobin** (**HbF**) has a higher affinity for oxygen than **adult hemoglobin** (**HbA**). This should make sense because fetal red blood cells must literally pull oxygen off of maternal hemoglobin and onto fetal hemoglobin.

KEY CONCEPT

Fetal hemoglobin has a higher affinity for oxygen than adult hemoglobin, and therefore has a left-shifted curve compared to adult hemoglobin.

The bicarbonate buffer system is also important because it links the respiratory and renal systems. Disturbances in either of these systems can lead to changes in the pH of the blood. For example, if an individual hyperventilates, excess CO_2 will be blown off, shifting the bicarbonate buffer system to the left and decreasing the concentration of protons. This leads to an increase in pH, or what is known as respiratory alkalosis. The kidney can compensate for this change by increasing excretion of bicarbonate, which brings the pH back to normal. In contrast, in *renal tubular acidosis type I*, the kidney is unable to excrete acid effectively. This leads to a buildup of protons in the blood (metabolic acidosis), which causes the buffer system to shift to the left. The excess CO_2 formed in the process can be exhaled, and the person may increase respiratory rate to compensate, bringing the pH back to normal.

Nutrients, Waste, and Hormones

In addition to respiratory gases, blood also carries nutrients, waste products, and hormones to the appropriate location for use or disposal. As discussed earlier, concentration gradients guide much of the movement of these substances to and from the tissues.

Carbohydrates and amino acids are absorbed into the capillaries of the small intestine and enter the systemic circulation via the hepatic portal system. Fats are absorbed into lacteals in the small intestine, bypassing the hepatic portal circulation to enter systemic circulation via the thoracic duct. When released from intestinal cells, fats are packaged into lipoproteins, which are water-soluble. The absorption of nutrients is covered more extensively in Chapter 9 of *MCAT Biology Review*.

Wastes, such as carbon dioxide, ammonia, and urea, enter the bloodstream by traveling down their respective concentration gradients from the tissues to the capillaries. The blood eventually travels to the kidneys, where these waste products are filtered or secreted for elimination from the body.

Hormones enter the circulation in or near the organ where the hormone is produced. This usually occurs by exocytosis, allowing for secretion of hormones into the bloodstream. Certain hormones are carried by proteins in the blood and are released under specific conditions. Once hormones reach their target tissues, they can activate cell-surface receptors (peptide hormones) or diffuse into the cell to activate intracellular or intranuclear receptors (steroid hormones).

Fluid Balance

In the bloodstream, two pressure gradients are essential for maintaining a proper balance of fluid volume and solute concentrations between the blood and the interstitium (the cells surrounding the blood vessels). These are the opposing but related hydrostatic and osmotic (oncotic) pressures. Figure 7.19 depicts these opposing forces.

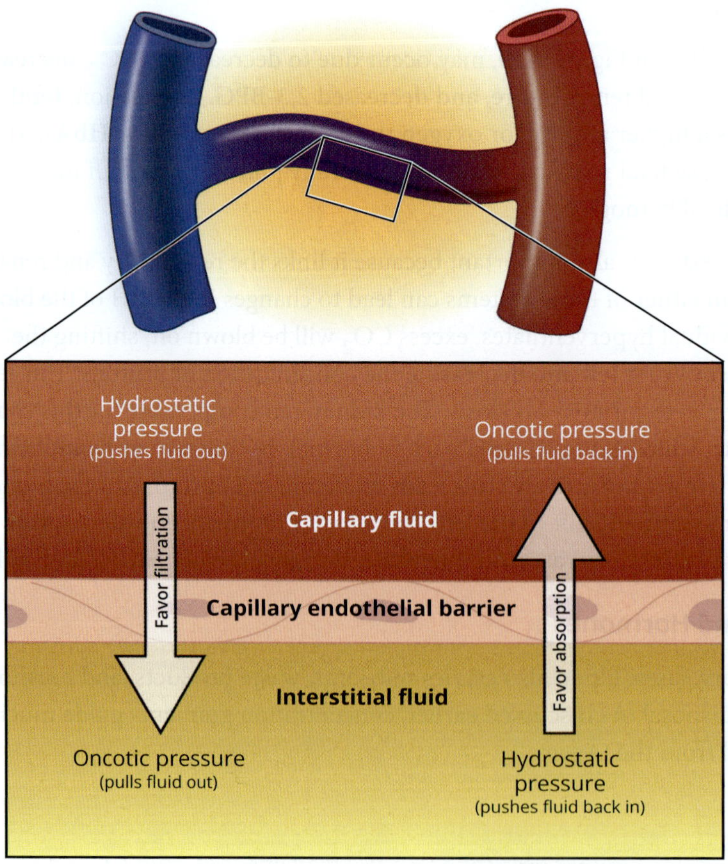

Figure 7.19 Hydrostatic vs. Oncotic Pressure

Hydrostatic pressure is the force per unit area that the blood exerts against the vessel walls. This is generated by the contraction of the heart and the elasticity of the arteries, and can be measured upstream in the large arteries as blood pressure. Hydrostatic pressure pushes fluid out of the bloodstream and into the interstitium through the capillary walls, which are somewhat leaky by design. Think about a water balloon with little holes on the surface. As the water balloon is filled with more water there is a greater outward pressure exerted on the balloon and there would be an increase in the amount of water pushed out of the little holes. **Osmotic pressure**, on the other hand, is the "sucking" pressure generated by solutes as they attempt to draw water into the bloodstream. Because most of this osmotic pressure is attributable to plasma proteins, it is usually called **oncotic pressure**.

At the arteriole end of a capillary bed, hydrostatic pressure (pushing fluid out) is much larger than oncotic pressure (drawing fluid in), and there is a net efflux of water from the circulation, as shown in Figure 7.20. As fluid moves out of the vessels, the hydrostatic pressure drops significantly, but the osmotic pressure stays about the same. Therefore, at the venule end of the capillary bed, hydrostatic pressure (pushing fluid out) has dropped below oncotic pressure (drawing fluid in), and there is a net influx of water back into the circulation.

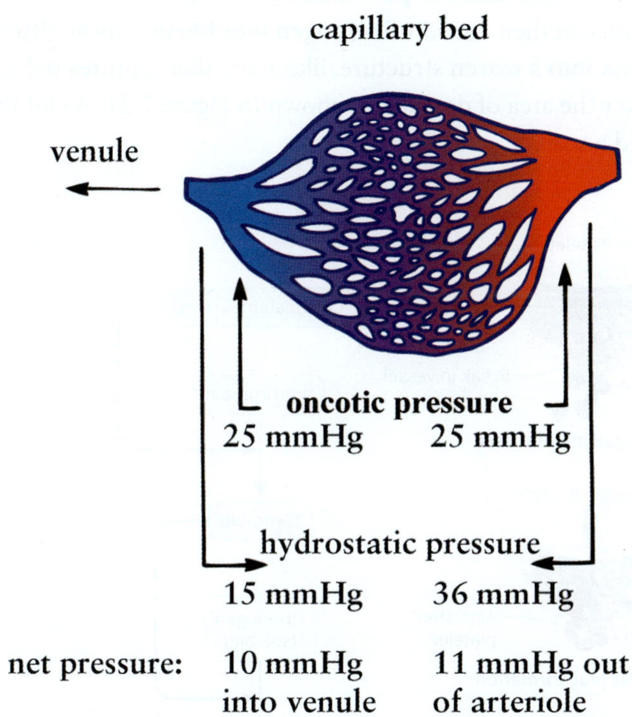

Figure 7.20 Starling Forces at a Capillary Bed

KEY CONCEPT

Hydrostatic pressure *pushes* fluid *out* of vessels and is dependent on blood pressure generated by the heart and the elastic arteries. Osmotic pressure *pulls* fluid back *into* the vessels and is dependent on the number of particles dissolved in the plasma; most are proteins, so we often refer to this as oncotic pressure.

The balance of these opposing pressures, also called **Starling forces**, is essential for maintaining the proper fluid volumes and solute concentrations inside and outside the vasculature. Imbalance of these pressures can result in too much or too little fluid in the tissues. For example, accumulation of excess fluid in the interstitium results in a condition called **edema**. We should note that some interstitial fluid is also taken up by the lymphatic system. Most lymphatic fluid (**lymph**) is returned to the central circulatory system by way of a channel called the **thoracic duct**. Blockage of lymph nodes by infection or surgery can also result in edema. Although you do not need to learn or memorize the Starling equation, which quantifies the net filtration rate between two fluid compartments, you should understand that the movement of solutes and fluid at the capillary level is governed by pressure differentials, just like the movement of carbon dioxide and oxygen in the lungs.

Coagulation

We have now covered most of the functions of red blood cells and plasma. We've briefly touched on white blood cells, which we'll explore more extensively in Chapter 8 of *MCAT Biology Review*. This leaves us with platelets, which protect the vascular system in the event of damage by forming a clot. **Clots** are composed of both coagulation factors (proteins) and platelets, and they prevent (or at least minimize) blood loss. When the endothelium of a blood vessel is damaged, it exposes the underlying connective tissue, which contains collagen and a protein called **tissue factor**. When platelets come into contact with exposed collagen, they sense this as evidence of injury. In response, they release their contents and begin to aggregate, or clump together. Simultaneously, **coagulation factors**, most of which are secreted by the liver, sense tissue factor and initiate a complex activation cascade. While the details of the coagulation cascade are beyond the scope of the MCAT, it is important to know that the endpoint of the cascade is the activation of **prothrombin** to form **thrombin** by ***thromboplastin***. Thrombin can then convert **fibrinogen** into **fibrin**. Fibrin ultimately forms small fibers that aggregate and cross-link into a woven structure, like a net, that captures red blood cells and other platelets, forming a stable clot over the area of damage, as shown in Figure 7.21. A clot that forms on a surface vessel that has been cut is called a scab.

REAL WORLD

Certain genetic diseases, such as hemophilia, cause malfunctions in the cascade of clotting reactions and increase the risk of life-threatening blood loss from even relatively minor injuries. Hemophilia A is the most common form and, as a sex-linked trait, is far more common in genotypical males than genotypical females.

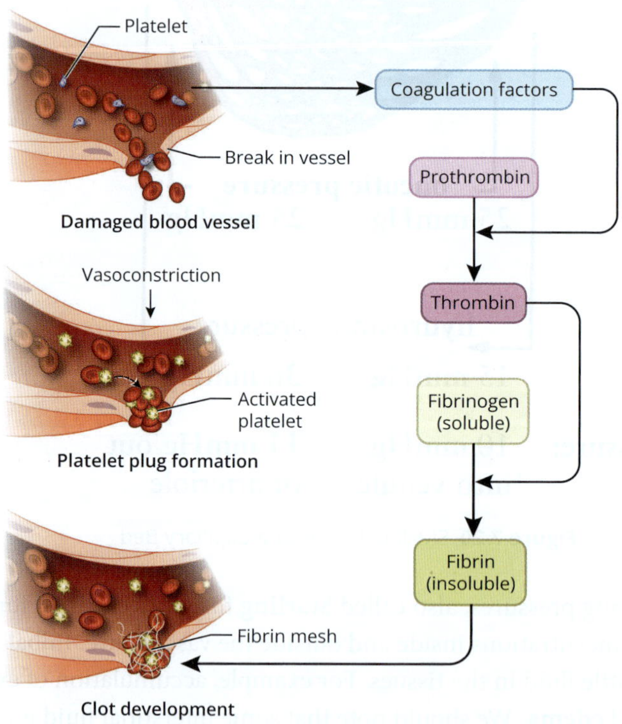

Figure 7.21 Thrombus (Clot) Formation Pathway

Thrombus formation, or blood clotting, occurs when blood vessels are injured and when blood flow is stagnant or sluggish. Sluggish blood flow can contribute to thrombus formation because it allows clotting factors to accumulate in an area. The process begins when platelets attach to the matrix that becomes exposed when the endothelial cells lining blood vessels are disrupted. This attachment then activates quiescent $\alpha_{IIb}\beta_3$ integrin molecules, causing them to adhere to circulating proteins—including fibrinogen, which forms bridges to additional platelets. Together the cells and proteins ultimately form a network of cells and fibers dense enough to plug the injury and prevent blood loss until the wound can be repaired.

Ultimately, the clot will have to be broken down. This task is accomplished predominantly by **plasmin**, which is generated from **plasminogen**.

MCAT CONCEPT CHECK 7.3

Before you move on, assess your understanding of the material with these questions.

1. In bacterial sepsis (overwhelming bloodstream infection), a number of capillary beds throughout the body open simultaneously. What effect would this have on the blood pressure? Besides the risk of infection, why might sepsis be dangerous for the heart?

   ___

2. What is the chemical equation for the bicarbonate buffer system? What enzyme catalyzes this reaction?

   ___

3. Where should you look on the oxyhemoglobin dissociation curve to determine the amount of oxygen that has been delivered to tissues?

   ___

4. What direction does the oxyhemoglobin dissociation curve shift as a result of exercise? What physiological changes cause this shift and why?

   ___

5. Exposure of which subendothelial compounds start the coagulation cascade? What protein helps stabilize the clot?

   - Starts the cascade:

   ___

   - Stabilizes the clot:

   ___

Conclusion

The cardiovascular system is one of the most commonly tested MCAT topics. You should be familiar with its basic structure: a system with two pumps in series. The right ventricle pumps blood into the pulmonary circulation, while the left ventricle pumps blood into the systemic circulation. We discussed the myogenic activity of cardiac muscle and the pathway that electricity follows in the heart through the SA node, AV node, bundle of His, and Purkinje fibers. The movement of blood through the vascular system is a result of the heart's pumping to generate pressure. Blood pressure is a measure of the blood's force per unit area on the vessel walls and is recorded as a gauge pressure (pressure above and beyond atmospheric pressure). We discussed the differences in structure between arteries, capillaries, and veins, and how these anatomical differences are reflective of their different functions. We then reviewed the composition of blood along with the three major blood cell types. We examined the ABO and Rh antigen systems, which frequently appear on the MCAT due to their widespread clinical relevance. The blood's ability to carry oxygen and carbon dioxide was also described; recall that carbon dioxide is primarily carried as bicarbonate ions in the blood. The conversion of carbon dioxide to and from this ion is accomplished by the enzyme carbonic anhydrase.

In this chapter, we focused on the functions of red blood cells, plasma, and platelets. We briefly examined the immune system, which is primarily driven by the actions of white blood cells and their products. Immunology is considered one of the most challenging courses in medical school, as you'll learn about dozens of cytokines, clusters of differentiation (CD), and specialized cell types. In the next chapter, we'll focus on the basics of immunology, discussing the major components of the innate (nonspecific) and adaptive (specific) immune responses.

GO ONLINE

You've reviewed the content, now test your knowledge and critical thinking skills by completing a test-like passage set in your online resources!

CONCEPT SUMMARY

Anatomy of the Cardiovascular System

- The **cardiovascular system** consists of a muscular four-chambered heart, blood vessels, and blood.
- The **heart** is composed of **cardiac muscle** and supports two different circulations: the **pulmonary circulation** and the **systemic circulation**.
  - Each side of the heart consists of an **atrium** and a **ventricle**.
  - The atria are separated from the ventricles by the **atrioventricular valves** (**tricuspid** on the right, bicuspid [mitral] on the left).
  - The ventricles are separated from the vasculature by the **semilunar valves** (**pulmonary** on the right, **aortic** on the left).
  - The pathway of blood is: right atrium $\xrightarrow[\text{valve}]{\text{tricuspid}}$ right ventricle $\xrightarrow[\text{valve}]{\text{pulmonary}}$ pulmonary artery → lungs → pulmonary veins → left atrium $\xrightarrow[\text{valve}]{\text{mitral}}$ left ventricle $\xrightarrow[\text{valve}]{\text{aortic}}$ aorta → arteries → arterioles → capillaries → venules → veins → venae cavae → right atrium
  - The left side of the heart contains more muscle than the right side because the systemic circulation has a much higher resistance and pressure.
  - Electrical conduction of the heart starts at the **sinoatrial (SA) node** and then goes to the **atrioventricular (AV) node**. From the AV node, electrical impulses travel to the **bundle of His** before traveling through the **Purkinje fibers**.
  - **Systole** refers to the period during ventricular contraction when the AV valves are closed. During **diastole**, the heart is relaxed and the semilunar valves are closed.
  - The **cardiac output** is the product of **heart rate** and **stroke volume**.
  - The sympathetic nervous system increases the heart rate and contractility. The parasympathetic nervous system decreases heart rate.
- The vasculature consists of arteries, veins, and capillaries.
  - **Arteries** are thick, highly muscular structures with an elastic quality. This allows for recoil and helps to propel blood forward within the system. Small muscular arteries are **arterioles**, which control flow into capillary beds.
  - **Capillaries** have walls that are one cell thick, making them so narrow that red blood cells must travel through them single file. Capillaries are the sites of gas and solute exchange.
  - **Veins** are inelastic, thin-walled structures that transport blood to the heart. They are able to stretch in order to accommodate large volumes of blood but do not have recoil capability. Veins are compressed by surrounding skeletal muscles and have **valves** to maintain one-way flow. Small veins are called **venules**.

- A portal system is one in which blood passes through two capillary beds in series.
  - In the **hepatic portal system**, blood travels from the gut capillary beds to the liver capillary bed via the hepatic portal vein.
  - In the **hypophyseal portal system**, blood travels from the capillary bed in the hypothalamus to the capillary bed in the anterior pituitary.
  - In the **renal portal system**, blood travels from the glomerulus to the vasa recta through an efferent arteriole.

Blood

- Blood is composed of cells and plasma, an aqueous mixture of nutrients, salts, respiratory gases, hormones, and blood proteins.
- **Erythrocytes** (**red blood cells**) lack mitochondria, a nucleus, and organelles in order to make room for **hemoglobin**, a protein that carries oxygen. Common measurements include hemoglobin concentration and **hematocrit**, the percentage of blood composed of erythrocytes.
- **Leukocytes** (**white blood cells**) are formed in the bone marrow. They are a crucial part of the immune system.
  - Granular leukocytes such as neutrophils, eosinophils, and basophils play a role in nonspecific immunity.
  - Agranulocytes, including lymphocytes and monocytes, also play a role in immunity, with lymphocytes playing a large role in specific immunity.
- **Thrombocytes** (**platelets**) are cell fragments from **megakaryocytes** that are required for coagulation.
- Blood antigens include the surface antigens A, B, and O, as well as Rh factor (D).
  - The I^A (*A*) and I^B (*B*) alleles are codominant, while the *i* (*O*) allele is recessive. People have antibodies for any AB alleles they do not have.
  - Positive Rh factor is dominant. An Rh-negative individual will only create anti-Rh antibodies after exposure to Rh-positive blood.

Physiology of the Cardiovascular System

- **Blood pressure** refers to the force per unit area that is exerted on the walls of blood vessels by blood. It is divided into systolic and diastolic components.
  - It must be high enough to overcome the resistance created by arterioles and capillaries, but low enough to avoid damaging the vasculature and surrounding structures.
  - It can be measured with a **sphygmomanometer**.
  - Blood pressure is maintained by baroreceptor and chemoreceptor reflexes. Low blood pressure promotes **aldosterone** and **antidiuretic hormone** (**ADH** or **vasopressin**) release. High blood osmolarity also promotes ADH release. High blood pressure promotes **atrial natriuretic peptide** (**ANP**) release.
- Gas and solute exchange occurs at the level of the capillaries and relies on the existence of concentration gradients to facilitate diffusion across the capillary walls. Capillaries are also leaky, which aids in the transport of gases and solutes.

- **Starling forces** consist of **hydrostatic pressure** and **osmotic (oncotic) pressure**. Hydrostatic pressure is the pressure of the fluid within the blood vessel, while osmotic pressure is the "sucking" pressure drawing water toward solutes. Oncotic pressure is osmotic pressure due to proteins. Hydrostatic pressure forces fluid out at the arteriolar end of a capillary bed; oncotic pressure draws it back in at the venule end.
- Oxygen is carried by hemoglobin, which exhibits **cooperative binding**. In the lungs, there is a high partial pressure of oxygen, resulting in loading of oxygen onto hemoglobin. In the tissues, there is a low partial pressure of oxygen, resulting in unloading. With cooperative binding, each successive oxygen bound to hemoglobin increases the affinity of the other subunits, while each successive oxygen released decreases the affinity of the other subunits.
- Carbon dioxide is largely carried in the blood in the form of carbonic acid, or bicarbonate and hydrogen ions. Carbon dioxide is nonpolar and not particularly soluble, while bicarbonate, hydrogen ions, and carbonic acid are polar and highly soluble.
- A high P_aCO_2, high $[H^+]$, low pH, high temperature, and high concentration of 2,3-BPG can cause a right shift in the **oxyhemoglobin dissociation curve**, reflecting a decreased affinity for oxygen.
- In addition to the opposites of the causes of a right shift, a left shift can also be seen in the dissociation curve for fetal hemoglobin compared to adult hemoglobin.
- Nutrients, wastes, and hormones are carried in the bloodstream to tissues for use or disposal.

- **Coagulation** results from an activation cascade.
  - When the endothelial lining of a blood vessel is damaged, the collagen and **tissue factor** underlying the endothelial cells are exposed. This results in a cascade of events known as the **coagulation cascade**, ultimately resulting in the formation of a clot over the damaged area.
  - Platelets bind to the collagen and are stabilized by **fibrin**, which is activated by **thrombin**.
  - Clots can be broken down by **plasmin**.

ANSWERS TO CONCEPT CHECKS

7.1

1.

Heart Chamber	Valve That Prevents Backflow
Right atrium	Tricuspid valve
Right ventricle	Pulmonary valve
Left atrium	Mitral (bicuspid) valve
Left ventricle	Aortic valve

2. Sinoatrial (SA) node → atrioventricular (AV) node → bundle of His (AV bundle) and its branches → Purkinje fibers

3.

Vessel	Carries Blood Which Direction?	Relative Wall Thickness	Smooth Muscle Present?	Contains Valves?
Artery	Away from heart	Thick	Yes, a lot	No
Capillary	From arterioles to venules	Very thin (one cell layer)	No	No
Vein	Toward heart	Thin	Yes, a little	Yes

4. The right side of the heart pumps blood into a lower-resistance circuit and must do so at lower pressures; therefore, it requires less muscle. The left side of the heart pumps blood into a higher-resistance circuit at higher pressures; therefore, it requires more muscle.
5. If all autonomic innervation to the heart were lost, the heart would continue beating at the intrinsic rate of the pacemaker (SA node). The individual would be unable to modify heart rate via the sympathetic or parasympathetic nervous system, but the heart would not stop beating.

7.2

1. Plasma is an aqueous mixture of nutrients, salts, respiratory gases, hormones, and blood proteins (clotting proteins, immunoglobulins, and so on).
2. A person with B^+ blood could receive B^+, B^-, O^+, or O^- blood. A person with B^+ blood could donate to people with B^+ or AB^+ blood.
3. Hematocrit measures the percentage of a blood sample occupied by red blood cells. It is measured in percentage points.
4. Lymphocytes are involved in specific immune defense.
5. Platelets are cellular fragments or shards that are given off by megakaryocytes in the bone marrow.
6. Only leukocytes (including neutrophils, eosinophils, basophils, monocytes/macrophages, and lymphocytes) contain nuclei. Erythrocytes and platelets do not.

7.3

1. Opening up more capillary beds (which are in parallel) will decrease the overall resistance of the circuit. The cardiac output will therefore increase in an attempt to maintain constant blood pressure. This is a risk to the heart because the increased demand on the heart can eventually tire it, leading to a heart attack or a precipitous drop in blood pressure.
2. The bicarbonate buffer system equation is

$$CO_2\ (g) + H_2O\ (l) \rightleftharpoons H_2CO_3\ (aq) \rightleftharpoons H^+\ (aq) + HCO_3^-\ (aq).$$

   The combining of carbon dioxide and water is catalyzed by carbonic anhydrase.
3. The amount of oxygen delivery can be seen as a drop in the *y*-value (percent hemoglobin saturation) on an oxyhemoglobin dissociation curve. For example, if the blood is 100% saturated while in the lungs (at 100 mmHg O_2) and only 80% saturated while in tissues (at 40 mmHg O_2), then 20% of the oxygen has been released to tissues.
4. The oxyhemoglobin curve shifts to the right during exercise in response to increased arterial CO_2, increased $[H^+]$, decreased pH, and increased temperature. This right shift represents hemoglobin's decreased affinity for oxygen, which allows more oxygen to be unloaded at the tissues.
5. The coagulation cascade can be started by the exposure of collagen and tissue factor to platelets and coagulation factors. The clot is stabilized by fibrin.

SCIENCE MASTERY ASSESSMENT EXPLANATIONS

1. **C**

Erythrocytes, or red blood cells, are produced in the red bone marrow and circulate in the blood for about 120 days, after which they are phagocytized in the spleen and the liver, eliminating **(D)**. Red blood cells have a disc-like shape and lose their membranous organelles (like mitochondria and nuclei) during maturation. This makes **(C)** the correct answer. Erythrocytes are filled with hemoglobin; their lack of mitochondria makes their metabolism solely anaerobic, eliminating **(A)** and **(B)**.

2. **C**

An ordinary cardiac contraction originates in, and is regulated by, the sinoatrial (SA) node. The impulse travels through both atria, stimulating them to contract simultaneously. The impulse then arrives at the atrioventricular (AV) node, which momentarily slows conduction, allowing for completion of atrial contraction and ventricular filling. The impulse is then carried by the bundle of His and its branches through the Purkinje fibers in the walls of both ventricles, generating a strong contraction.

3. **C**

According to the Bohr effect, decreasing the pH in the blood decreases hemoglobin's affinity for O_2. This makes **(C)** the correct answer. The affinity is generally lowered in exercising muscle to facilitate unloading of oxygen to tissues, eliminating **(A)**. A decrease in the P_aCO_2 would cause a decrease in $[H^+]$ or increased pH—which increases hemoglobin's affinity for O_2, eliminating **(B)**. Finally, **(D)** is incorrect because hemoglobin's affinity for O_2 is higher in fetal blood than in adult blood.

4. **A**

Blood drains from the superior and inferior venae cavae into the right atrium. It passes through the tricuspid valve and into the right ventricle, and then through the pulmonary valve into the pulmonary artery, which leads to the lungs. Oxygenated blood returns to the left atrium via the pulmonary veins. It flows through the mitral valve into the left ventricle. From the left ventricle, it is pumped through the aortic valve into the aorta for distribution throughout the body.

5. **A**

The exchange of fluid is greatly influenced by the differences in the hydrostatic and osmotic pressures of blood and tissues. The osmotic (oncotic) pressure remains relatively constant; however, the hydrostatic pressure at the arterial end is greater than the hydrostatic pressure at the venous end. As a result, fluid moves out of the capillaries at the arterial end and back in at the venous end. Fluid is reabsorbed at the venous end because the osmotic pressure exceeds the hydrostatic pressure. Proteins should not cross the capillary wall under normal circumstances.

6. **C**

The first step in solving this problem is to define cardiac output: cardiac output = heart rate × stroke volume. We can therefore divide the cardiac output by the stroke volume to determine heart rate:

$$HR = \frac{CO}{SV} = \frac{7500\ \frac{mL}{min}}{50\ \frac{mL}{beat}} = 150\ \frac{beats}{min}$$

Note that this heart rate is actually pathologically fast; a normal heart rate is considered to be between 60 and 100 beats per minute.

7. **D**

Without knowing a patient's blood type, the only type of transfusion that we can safely give is O^-. People with O^- blood are considered universal donors because their blood cells contain no surface antigens. Therefore, O^- blood can be given to anyone without potentially life-threatening consequences from ABO or Rh incompatibility.

8. **C**

The only answer choice that correctly describes arteries and veins is **(C)**; the pressure in the aorta usually ranges between 120 and 80 mmHg, depending on whether the heart is in systole or diastole, whereas the pressure in the superior vena cava is near zero. **(A)** is incorrect because arteries are thick-walled and veins are thin-walled. **(B)** is also incorrect; this relationship is reversed in pulmonary and umbilical circulation. **(D)** is reversed as well; arteries make use of the pumping of the heart and the "snapping back" of their elastic walls to transport blood, whereas venous blood is propelled along by skeletal muscle contractions.

9. **A**

The relative lack of smooth muscle in venous walls allows stretching to store most of the blood in the body. Valves in the veins allow for one-way flow of blood toward the heart, not stretching. Both arteries and veins are close to lymphatic vessels, which has no bearing on their relative difference in volume. Both arteries and veins have a single-cell endothelial lining.

10. **C**

Carbon dioxide is a byproduct of metabolism in cells that later combines with water to form bicarbonate in a reaction catalyzed by carbonic anhydrase. This system is blood plasma's most important buffer system. Food and fluid absorption are not significant sources of buffering, eliminating **(A)** and **(B)**. While the kidneys can be involved in acid–base balance, they carry out this function through their filtration, secretion, and reabsorption mechanisms, not through hormone release, eliminating **(D)**.

11. **C**

In circulation, plasma proteins play an important role in generating osmotic (oncotic) pressure. This allows water that is displaced at the arterial end of a capillary bed by hydrostatic pressure to be reabsorbed at the venule end. Loss of these plasma proteins would cause a decrease in the plasma osmotic (oncotic) pressure.

12. **D**

The atrioventricular valves are located between the atria and the ventricles on both sides of the heart. Their role is to prevent backflow of blood into the atria. The valve on the right side of the heart has three cusps and is called the tricuspid valve. It prevents backflow of blood from the right ventricle into the right atrium.

13. **D**

Holding one's breath for a prolonged period would result in a drop in oxygenation and an increase in P_aCO_2. The increased carbon dioxide would associate with water to form carbonic acid, which would dissociate into a proton and a bicarbonate anion. Further, the low oxygen saturation would eventually lead to anaerobic metabolism in some tissues, causing an increase in lactic acid. These would all lead to a decreased pH.

14. **C**

The cardiac conduction system starts at the SA node, which is located near the top of the right atrium, and continues down to the AV node, which is located between the two AV valves. The bundle of His is located within the wall between the ventricles, and is likely to be affected if the wall between the ventricles has been damaged by a heart attack. This may affect the left ventricle, but the left ventricular muscle itself is not part of the cardiac conduction system.

15. **B**

The greatest amount of resistance is provided by the arterioles. Arterioles are highly muscular and have the ability to contract and dilate in order to regulate blood pressure.

GO ONLINE

Consult your online resources for additional practice.

EQUATIONS TO REMEMBER

(7.1) **Cardiac output:** $CO = HR \times SV$

(7.2) **Ohm's law applied to circulation:** $\Delta P = CO \times TPR$

SHARED CONCEPTS

Biochemistry Chapter 9
Carbohydrate Metabolism I

Biology Chapter 6
The Respiratory System

Biology Chapter 8
The Immune System

General Chemistry Chapter 12
Electrochemistry

Physics and Math Chapter 4
Fluids

Physics and Math Chapter 6
Circuits

CHAPTER 8

THE IMMUNE SYSTEM

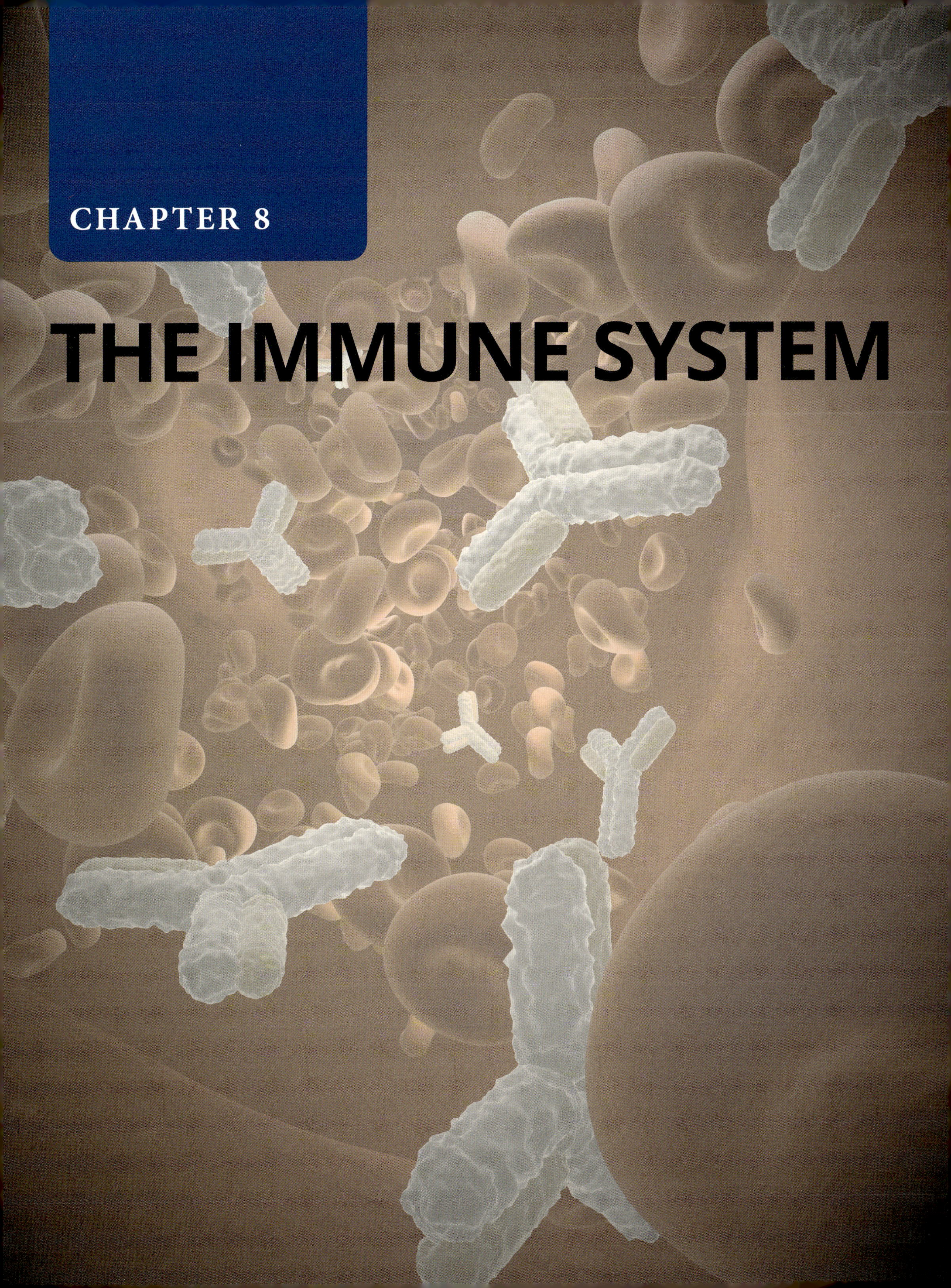

SCIENCE MASTERY ASSESSMENT

Every pre-med knows this feeling: there is so much content I have to know for the MCAT! How do I know what to do first or what's important?

While the high-yield badges throughout this book will help you identify the most important topics, this Science Mastery Assessment is another tool in your MCAT prep arsenal. This quiz (which can also be taken in your online resources) and the guidance below will help ensure that you are spending the appropriate amount of time on this chapter based on your personal strengths and weaknesses. Don't worry though—skipping something now does not mean you'll never study it. Later on in your prep, as you complete full-length tests, you'll uncover specific pieces of content that you need to review and can come back to these chapters as appropriate.

How to Use This Assessment

If you answer 0–7 questions correctly:

Spend about 1 hour to read this chapter in full and take limited notes throughout. Follow up by reviewing **all** quiz questions to ensure that you now understand how to solve each one.

If you answer 8–11 questions correctly:

Spend 20–40 minutes reviewing the quiz questions. Beginning with the questions you missed, read and take notes on the corresponding subchapters. For questions you answered correctly, ensure your thinking matches that of the explanation and you understand why each choice was correct or incorrect.

If you answer 12–15 questions correctly:

Spend less than 20 minutes reviewing all questions from the quiz. If you missed any, then include a quick read-through of the corresponding subchapters, or even just the relevant content within a subchapter, as part of your question review. For questions you answered correctly, ensure your thinking matches that of the explanation and review the Concept Summary at the end of the chapter.

1. In DiGeorge syndrome, the thymus can be completely absent. The absence of the thymus would leave an individual unable to mount specific defenses against which of the following types of pathogens?
   A. Viruses
   B. Bacteria
   C. Parasites
   D. Fungi

2. Which of the following are NOT involved in cell-mediated immunity?
   A. Memory cells
   B. Plasma cells
   C. Cytotoxic cells
   D. Suppressor cells

3. The lymphatic system:
   A. transports hormones throughout the body.
   B. transports chylomicrons to the circulatory system.
   C. causes extravasation of fluid into tissues.
   D. is the site of mast cell activation.

4. Which of the following are involved in antibody production?
   A. Plasma cells
   B. Memory cells
   C. Helper T-cells
   D. Cytotoxic cells

5. Which of the following is NOT true of the innate immune system?
   A. Includes macrophages to mediate inflammation
   B. Is always active against infection
   C. Recognizes unique features of a pathogen
   D. Contains cells derived from a hematopoietic stem cell

6. Which of the following is an example of adaptive immunity?
   A. PRRs recognize that a pathogen is an invasive parasite and eosinophils are recruited to the area.
   B. Complement is activated, causing osmotic instability in a bacterium.
   C. Memory B-cells generated through vaccination are activated when their antigen is encountered.
   D. Dendritic cells sample bacteria within a laceration and travel to the lymph nodes to present the antigen.

7. Which of the following is true regarding passive and active immunity?
   A. Active immunity requires weeks to build, whereas passive immunity is acquired immediately.
   B. Active immunity is short lived, whereas passive immunity is long lived.
   C. Active immunity may be acquired during pregnancy through the placenta.
   D. Passive immunity may be acquired through vaccination.

8. Where are most self-reactive T-cells eliminated?
   A. Spleen
   B. Lymph nodes
   C. Bone marrow
   D. Thymus

9. What is the response of the immune system to downregulation of MHC molecules on somatic cells?
   A. B-cells are activated and antibodies are released.
   B. T-cells are activated, resulting in a cytotoxic response.
   C. Natural killer cells induce apoptosis of affected cells.
   D. Macrophages engulf the pathogen and display its antigens.

10. Which of the following correctly indicates the response of $CD8^+$ T-cells when activated?

A. Secretion of cytotoxic chemicals
B. Causing isotype switching
C. Presentation of antigens
D. Activation of B-cells

11. Lymphoma is cancer of the cells of lymphoid lineage. These cells often reside within lymph nodes. What type of cell is NOT likely to cause a lymphoma?

A. $CD8^+$ T-cells
B. B-cells
C. Macrophages
D. T_h1 cells

12. Upon encountering an antigen, only T-cells with a specific T-cell receptor are activated. This is an example of:

A. innate immunity.
B. a cytotoxic T-cell response.
C. humoral immunity.
D. clonal selection.

13. Which cell type is a phagocyte that attacks bacterial pathogens in the bloodstream?

A. Neutrophils
B. Eosinophils
C. Basophils
D. Dendritic cells

14. What type of immunity is likely to be affected by removal of the spleen?

A. Cytotoxic immunity
B. Humoral immunity
C. Innate immunity
D. Passive immunity

15. Which of the following is NOT an example of a nonspecific defense mechanism?

A. Skin provides a physical barrier against invasion.
B. Macrophages engulf and destroy foreign particles.
C. An inflammatory response is initiated in response to physical damage.
D. Cytotoxic T-cells destroy cells displaying foreign antigens.

Answer Key

1. **A** (See section 8.3)
2. **B** (See section 8.3)
3. **B** (See section 8.4)
4. **A** (See section 8.3)
5. **C** (See section 8.1)
6. **C** (See section 8.3)
7. **A** (See section 8.3)
8. **D** (See section 8.3)
9. **C** (See section 8.2)
10. **A** (See section 8.3)
11. **C** (See section 8.4)
12. **D** (See section 8.3)
13. **A** (See section 8.3)
14. **B** (See section 8.3)
15. **D** (See section 8.2)

The relevant section of the chapter to review for each question is given in parentheses after the correct answer. Detailed explanations can be found at the end of the chapter.

CHAPTER 8

THE IMMUNE SYSTEM

In This Chapter

CHAPTER PROFILE

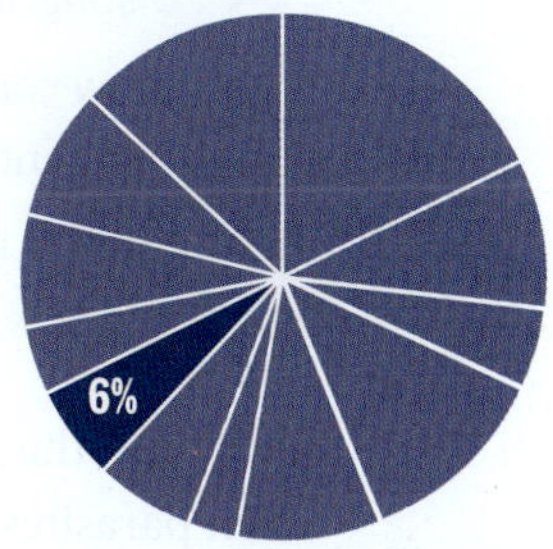

The content in this chapter should be relevant to about 6% of all questions about biology on the MCAT.

This chapter covers material from the following AAMC content category:

3B: Structure and integrative functions of the main organ systems

Introduction

Over the past few decades, the public's imagination has been captured by alarming reports of "flesh-eating" bacteria and diseases. While these bacteria do not actually eat flesh, that doesn't make them any less dangerous. "Flesh-eating" bacteria cause a condition called *necrotizing fasciitis*, a serious disease that requires aggressive medical and surgical treatment including intravenous antibiotics, surgical debridement (removal) of the necrotic tissue, and sometimes even amputation. Many different types of bacteria, including group A *Streptococcus*, *Clostridium perfringens*, and methicillin-resistant *Staphylococcus aureus* (MRSA), can cause necrotizing fasciitis. The massive destruction of skin, muscle, and connective tissue by the release of bacterial toxins called superantigens is life-threatening. These superantigens cause the immune system to become nonspecifically overactivated. Necrotizing fasciitis is dangerous not only because of the bacteria and subsequent inflammatory response, but also because the destruction of skin—a nonspecific immune defense—leaves the body susceptible to superinfection (infection with another pathogen).

In this chapter, we will consider this type of nonspecific defense, as well as specific immune defenses. The human body relies on the interaction between the innate (nonspecific) and adaptive (specific) immune systems in order to protect itself from disease. However, the immune system is not always perfect in its responses. Sometimes the immune system may become nonspecifically overactivated, as is the case with necrotizing fasciitis, or it may become activated against the same human it is supposed to protect. We will discuss the individual parts of the immune system and how these parts work together to protect from disease. In addition, we will discuss the concept of autoimmunity, or disease that results from immune attack against oneself. We'll briefly touch on vaccines, which take advantage of our understanding of the immune system to protect us from life-threatening infections. The immune system is largely integrated with the lymphatic system, which will be discussed in this chapter as well.

8.1 Structure of the Immune System

LEARNING OBJECTIVES

After Chapter 8.1, you will be able to:

- Distinguish between innate and adaptive immunity
- Draw comparisons between B- and T-cells, including their development, maturation, functions, specificity, and control mechanisms
- Identify immune cells as granulocytes or agranulocytes

Each day, the human body is exposed to numerous bacteria, viruses, fungi, and even parasites. Yet our bodies are able to protect us from infection most of the time. Even when we do get sick, the immune system is usually able to contain and eliminate the infection.

Innate and Adaptive Immunity

In order to fight infection, the human body has two different divisions of the immune system: innate and adaptive immunity, compared in Figure 8.1. **Innate immunity** is composed of defenses that are always active against infection, but lack the ability to target specific invaders; for this reason, it is also called **nonspecific immunity**. **Adaptive** or **specific immunity** refers to the defenses that target a specific pathogen. This system is slower to act, but can maintain immunological memory of an infection to mount a faster attack in subsequent infections.

MCAT EXPERTISE

The immune system is a topic where cell biology, biochemistry, anatomy, and biology interact. Thus, it is a topic that allows the MCAT to ask questions that integrate these four topics. As we discuss these complex ideas, focus on the big picture first, creating a mental image to help you put these concepts together. Then go back and plug in the details. This approach will foster your ability to associate structure with function and to think critically about the topic on Test Day.

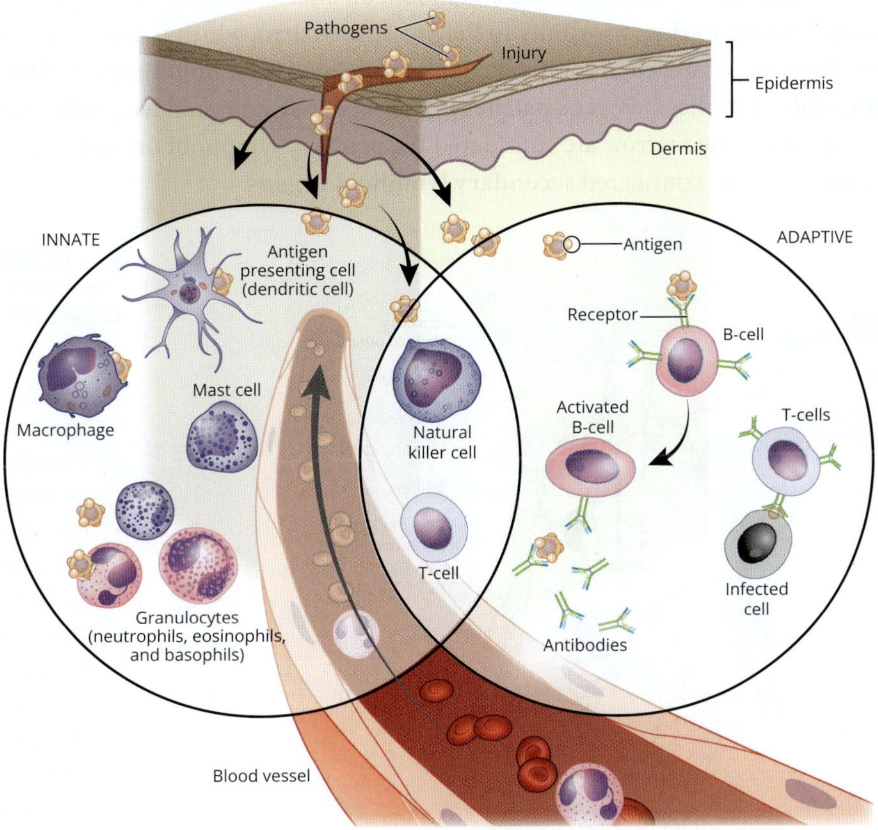

Figure 8.1 Divisions of the Immune System

Anatomy

The immune system is not housed in a single organ, as shown in Figure 8.2. The structure and components that serve as nonspecific defenses often serve functions in other organ systems. The **bone marrow** produces all of the **leukocytes** (**white blood cells**) that participate in the immune system through the process of hematopoiesis, discussed in Chapter 7 of *MCAT Biology Review*. The **spleen** is a location of blood storage and activation of **B-cells**, which turn into **plasma cells** to produce antibodies as part of adaptive immunity. Note that when B-cells leave the bone marrow, they are considered mature but naïve (because they have not yet been exposed to an antigen). Because these antibodies dissolve and act in the blood (rather than within cells), this division of adaptive immunity is called **humoral immunity**. **T-cells**, another class of adaptive immune cells, mature in the **thymus**, a small gland just in front of the pericardium, the sac that protects the heart. The thymus is biggest at puberty, and then begins to shrink and becomes less active as the individual gets older, which partially explains why the elderly have weaker immune systems. T-cells are the agents of **cell-mediated immunity** because they coordinate the immune system and directly kill virally infected cells. Finally, **lymph nodes**, a major component of the lymphatic system,

REAL WORLD

Lay people not involved in medicine often say that their "glands" are swollen when they feel a sensation of fullness around the throat. From a biological standpoint, lymph nodes are not glands—they do not secrete products into the bloodstream (endocrine) or ducts (exocrine). What they are actually experiencing is known medically as *lymphadenopathy*, or the swelling of the lymph nodes that occurs with activation of the immune system.

provide a place for immune cells to communicate and mount an attack; B-cells can be activated here as well. Other immune tissue is found in close proximity to the digestive system, which is a site of potential invasion by pathogens. These tissues are commonly called **gut-associated lymphoid tissue** (GALT) and include the **tonsils** and **adenoids** in the head, **Peyer's patches** in the small intestine, and lymphoid aggregates in the **appendix**. The thymus and bone marrow are considered the **primary lymphoid organs**, while the other structures mentioned above are considered **secondary lymphoid organs**.

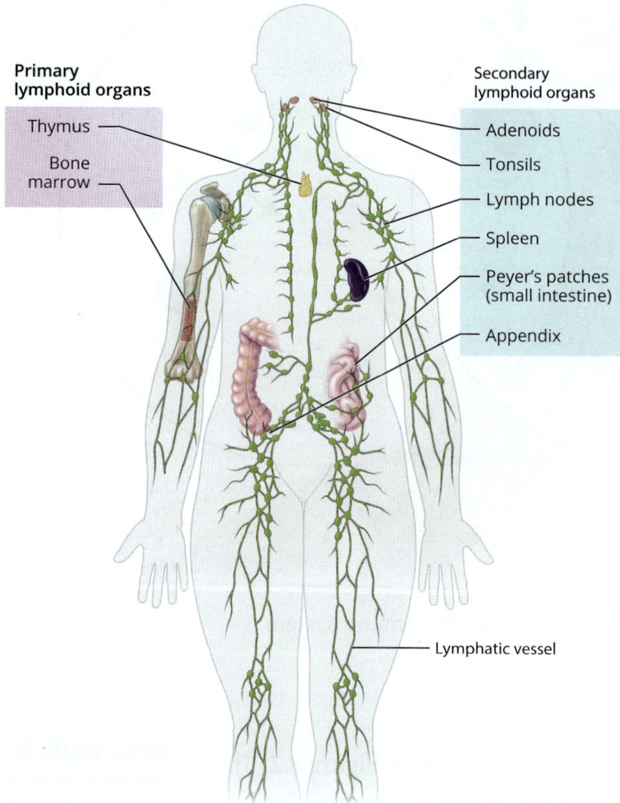

Figure 8.2 Anatomy of the Immune and Lymphatic Systems

KEY CONCEPT

Organs of the immune system:

- Lymph nodes filter lymph and are a site where immune responses can be mounted.
- Bone marrow is the site of immune cell production.
- The thymus is the site of T-cell maturation.
- The spleen acts as a storage area for white blood cells and platelets, a recycling center for red blood cells, and a filter of blood for the immune system.

Leukocytes are produced in the bone marrow through hematopoiesis, shown in Figure 8.3. (Note: This is the same image shown in Figure 7.12, but is copied here for convenience.) Leukocytes are divided into two groups of cells: **granulocytes** and **agranulocytes**. These names refer to the presence or absence of **granules** in the cytoplasm. These granules contain toxic enzymes and chemicals, which can be released by exocytosis, and are particularly effective against bacterial, fungal, and parasitic pathogens. Both granulocytes and agranulocytes come from a common precursor: **hematopoietic stem cells**. Remember from Chapter 7 of *MCAT Biology Review* that hematopoietic stem cells are also the cell type that gives rise to red blood cells and platelets. Granulocytes include cells such as **neutrophils**, **eosinophils**, and **basophils**. The names of these cells actually refer to the way that the cells appear after staining with certain chemicals. Agranulocytes include the **lymphocytes**, which are responsible for antibody production, immune system modulation, and targeted killing of infected cells. **Monocytes**, which are phagocytic cells in the bloodstream, are also considered agranulocytes. They become **macrophages** in tissues; many tissues have resident populations of macrophages with specific names (such as **microglia** in the central nervous system, **Langerhans cells** in the skin, and **osteoclasts** in bone).

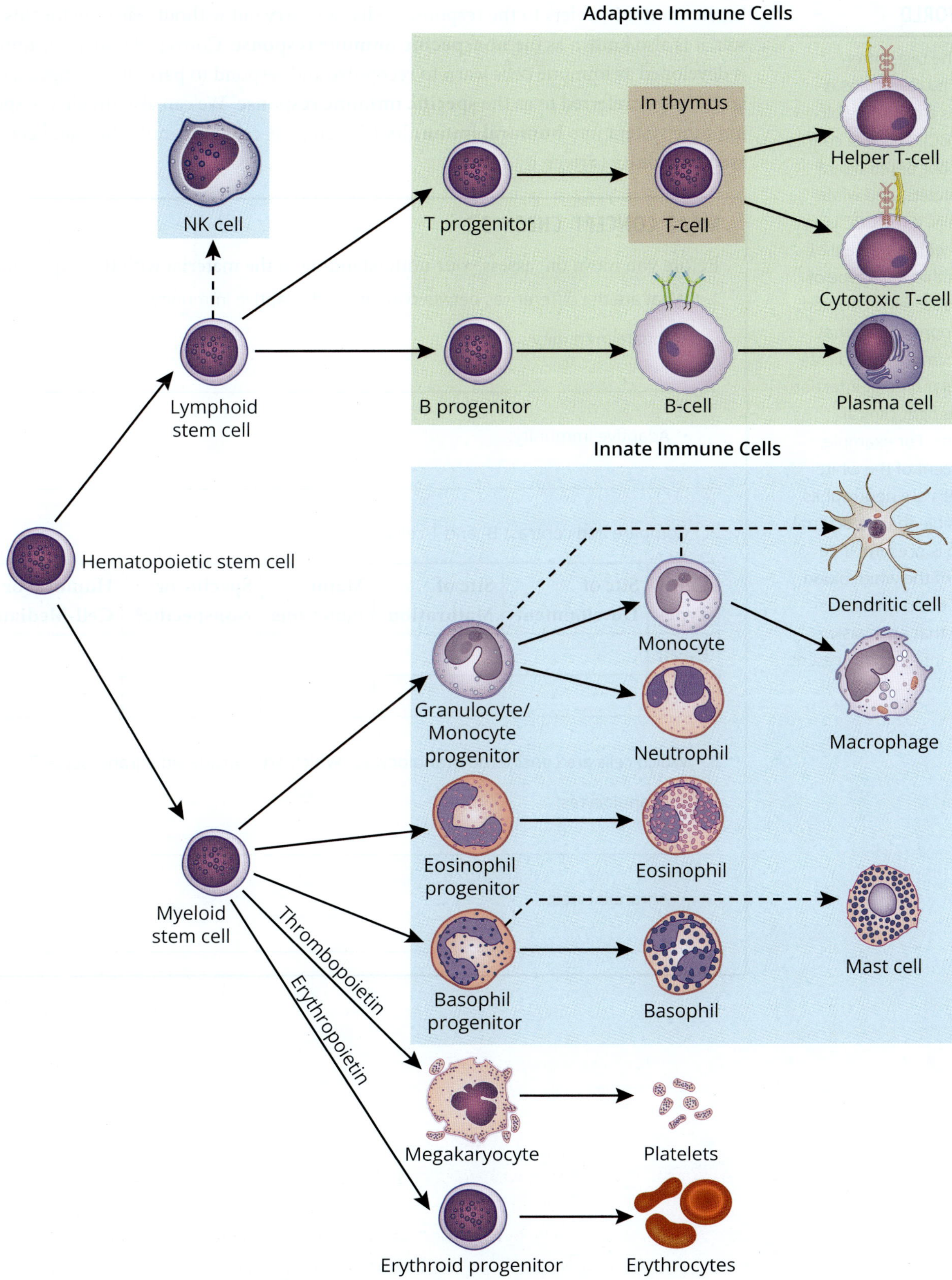

Figure 8.3 Hematopoiesis

Innate immunity refers to the responses cells can carry out without learning; for this reason, it is also known as the **nonspecific immune response**. Conversely, adaptive immunity is developed as immune cells learn to recognize and respond to particular antigens, and is often aptly referred to as the **specific immune response**. We can also divide the specific immune system into **humoral immunity** (driven by B-cells and antibodies) and **cell-mediated immunity** (driven by T-cells).

REAL WORLD

One of the tests often ordered by physicians is known as a complete blood count (CBC). This test counts the number of red blood cells, platelets, and white blood cells. If the CBC is ordered with a *differential*, it means that each type of white blood cell is counted. Any cell populations that are abnormal may indicate a particular type of infection given the right clinical conditions. For example, if 90 percent of the white blood cells are neutrophils, it is possible that a bacterial infection is present. If 20 percent of the white blood cells are eosinophils, it is possible that an invasive parasitic infection is present.

MCAT CONCEPT CHECK 8.1

Before you move on, assess your understanding of the material with these questions.

1. What are the differences between innate and adaptive immunity?
   - Innate immunity:

   ____

   - Adaptive immunity:

   ____

2. Compare and contrast B- and T-cells:

Cell Type	Site of Development	Site of Maturation	Major Functions	Specific or Nonspecific?	Humoral or Cell-Mediated?
B-cell					
T-cell					

3. Which cells are considered granulocytes? Which are considered agranulocytes?
   - Granulocytes:

   ____

   - Agranulocytes:

   ____

8.2 The Innate Immune System

LEARNING OBJECTIVES

After Chapter 8.2, you will be able to:

- Describe the immunologic functions of each of the noncellular nonspecific immune defenses, including defensins and mucus
- Identify the immune cell type used for antigen presentation
- Differentiate between MHC-I and MHC-II
- Recall the stimuli required for activating natural killer cells, neutrophils, eosinophils, basophils, and mast cells

The innate immune system consists of cells and structures that offer nonspecific protection.

Noncellular Nonspecific Defenses

Our first line of defense is the **skin** (**integument**). In Chapter 10 of *MCAT Biology Review*, we will discuss the specific homeostatic functions of the skin; for now, we'll focus on how skin protects the body. The skin provides a physical barrier between the outside world and our internal organs, preventing most bacteria, viruses, fungi, and parasites from entering the body. Additionally, antibacterial enzymes called **defensins** can be found on the skin. Sweat also has antimicrobial properties. The skin is an important first line of defense: a cut or abrasion on the skin provides an entry point for pathogens into the body. Deeper wounds allow pathogens to penetrate deeper into the body.

As discussed in Chapter 6 of *MCAT Biology Review* and as shown in Figure 8.4, the respiratory system also has mechanisms to prevent pathogens from entering the body. The respiratory passages are mucous membranes, lined with cilia to trap particulate matter and push it up toward the oropharynx, where it can be swallowed or expelled. The upper respiratory tract has many twists and turns so foreign entities have high chances of bumping into the mucus which prevents bacteria, viruses, or particles like dust from gaining access to the lung tissue below. Several other mucous membranes, including those around the eye and in the oral cavity, produce a nonspecific bacterial enzyme called **lysozyme**, which is secreted in tears and saliva, respectively.

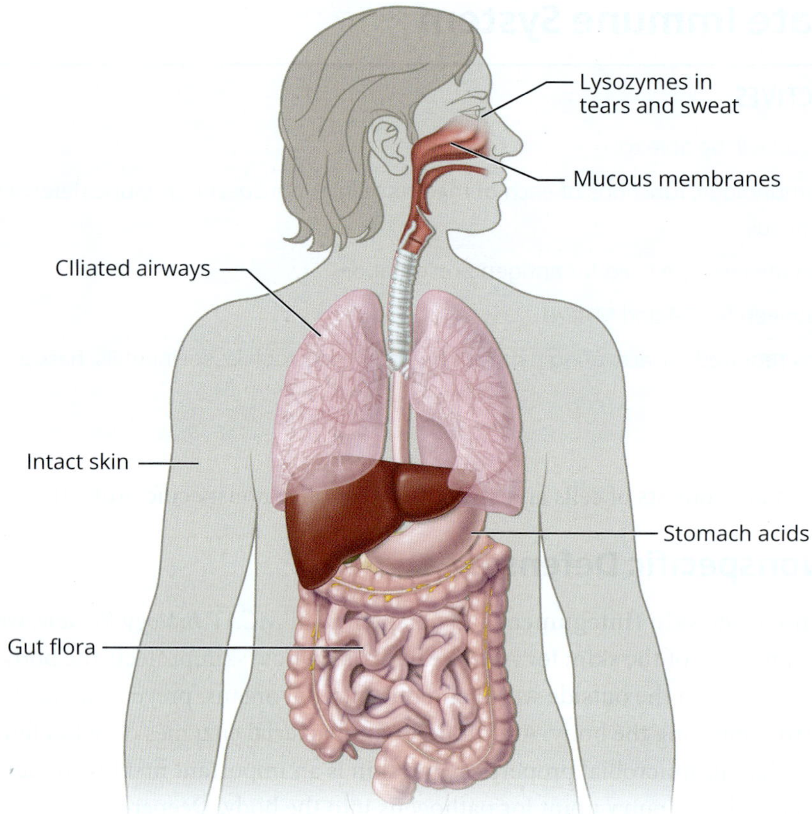

Figure 8.4 Noncellular Nonspecific Defenses

The Gastrointestinal Tract

The gastrointestinal tract also plays a role in nonspecific immunity. First, the stomach secretes acid, resulting in the elimination of most pathogens. In addition, the gut is colonized by bacteria. Most of these bacteria lack the necessary characteristics to cause infection. Because there is already such a large bacterial population in the gut, many potential invaders are not able to compete and are thus kept at bay. Many antibiotics reduce the population of gut flora, providing an opportunity for the growth of pathogens resistant to that antibiotic.

Complement

The **complement** system consists of a number of proteins in the blood that act as a nonspecific defense against bacteria. Complement can be activated through a **classical pathway** (which requires the binding of an antibody to a pathogen) or an **alternative pathway** (which does not require antibodies), as summarized in Table 8.1. The complement proteins punch holes in the cell walls of bacteria, making them osmotically unstable. Despite the association with antibodies, complement is considered a nonspecific defense because it cannot be modified to target a specific organism over others.

REAL WORLD

The GI tract of a newborn baby is particularly susceptible to infection because the newborn's immune system is underdeveloped and the GI tract is not yet colonized. Breast milk contains a family of antibodies that are particularly effective on mucosal surfaces and help to defend newborn babies against gastrointestinal infections.

Pathway	Trigger	Immunity Type
Classical pathway	Antigen-antibody complexes (IgG or IgM)	Requires adaptive immunity
Alternative pathway	Spontaneous activation on pathogen surfaces	Fully innate

Table 8.1 Complement Activation Pathways

Interferons

To protect against viruses, cells that have been infected with viruses produce **interferons**, proteins that prevent viral replication and dispersion. Interferons cause nearby cells to decrease production of both viral and cellular proteins. They also decrease the permeability of these cells, making it harder for a virus to infect them. In addition, interferons upregulate MHC class I and class II molecules, resulting in increased antigen presentation and better detection of the infected cells by the immune system, as described in the next section. Interferons are responsible for many "flu-like" symptoms that occur during viral infection, including malaise, tiredness, muscle soreness, and fever.

Cells of the Innate Immune System

So, what happens when bacteria, viruses, fungi, or parasites breach noncellular defenses? The cells of the innate immune system are always poised and ready to attack.

Macrophages

Macrophages, a type of agranulocyte, reside within the tissues. These cells derive from blood-borne **monocytes** and can become a **resident population** within a tissue (becoming a permanent, rather than transient, cell group in the tissue). Many of these resident macrophages are highlighted throughout *MCAT Biology Review*, including microglia in the central nervous system, Langerhans cells in the skin, and osteoclasts in bone. When a bacterial invader enters a tissue, the macrophages become activated. The activated macrophage does three things. First, it phagocytizes the invader through endocytosis. Then, it digests the invader using enzymes. Finally, it presents little pieces of the invader (mostly peptides) to other cells using a protein called **major histocompatibility complex** (**MHC**). MHC binds to a pathogenic peptide (also called an **antigen**) and carries it to the cell surface, where it can be recognized by cells of the adaptive immune system. In addition, macrophages release **cytokines**, chemical substances that stimulate inflammation and recruit additional immune cells to the area.

MHC molecules come in two main classes: class I and class II. All nucleated cells in the body display **MHC class I** molecules. Any protein produced within a cell can be loaded onto MHC-I and sent to the surface of the cell by the Golgi apparatus, as shown in Figure 8.5. This allows the immune system to monitor the health of these cells and to detect if the cells have been infected with a virus or another intracellular pathogen; only those cells that are infected would be expected to present an unfamiliar (nonself) protein on their surfaces. Therefore, the MHC-I pathway is often called the **endogenous pathway** because it binds antigens that come from inside the cell. Cells that have been invaded by intracellular pathogens can then be killed by a certain group of T-cells (cytotoxic T-lymphocytes) to prevent infection of other cells.

REAL WORLD

MHC molecules are highly variable among humans, but can usually be divided into particular subtypes. People with certain MHC subtypes have different susceptibility to disease, and individuals with certain subtypes are considerably more susceptible to autoimmune diseases. It is also important to match the MHC types of the donor and recipient as closely as possible during transplants to avoid rejection.

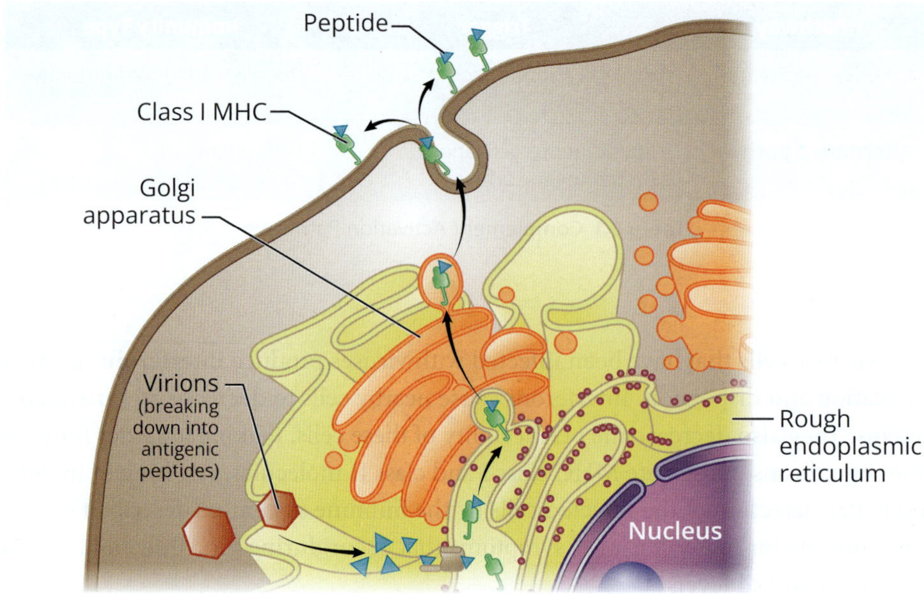

Figure 8.5 Endogenous Pathway for Antigen Presentation (MHC Class I)
MHC-I exists in all nucleated cells.

MHC class II molecules are mainly displayed by professional **antigen-presenting cells** like macrophages, as shown in Figure 8.6. Remember that these phagocytic cells pick up pathogens from the environment, process them, and then present them on MHC-II. An antigen is a substance (usually a pathogenic protein) that can be targeted by an antibody. While antibody production is the domain of the adaptive immune system, it is important to understand that cells of the innate immune system also present antigens. Because these antigens originated outside the cell, the MHC-II pathway is often called the **exogenous pathway**. The presentation of an antigen by an immune cell may result in the activation of both the innate and adaptive immune systems. Professional antigen-presenting cells include macrophages, **dendritic cells** in the skin, some B-cells, and certain activated epithelial cells.

KEY CONCEPT

Major histocompatibility complex molecules are joined with antigens. The MHC–antigen complex then goes to the cell surface to display the antigen. This allows the immune system to monitor the health of cells. MHC-I is in all nucleated cells and presents endogenous antigens. MHC-II is in antigen-presenting cells and presents exogenous antigens.

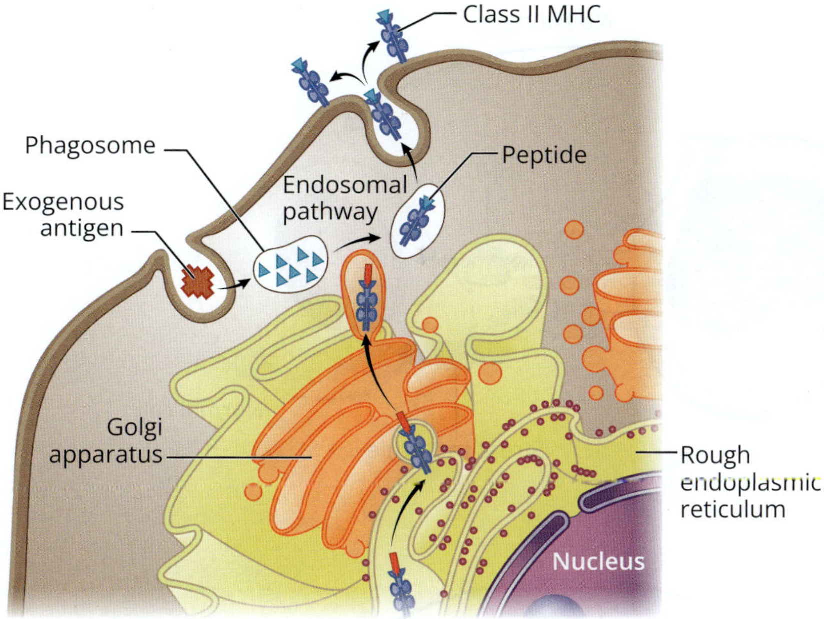

Figure 8.6 Exogenous Pathway for Antigen Presentation (MHC Class II)
MHC-II exists only in professional antigen-presenting cells, like macrophages, dendritic cells, some B-cells, and some activated epithelial cells.

Macrophages and dendritic cells also have special receptors known as **pattern recognition receptors** (**PRR**), the best-described of which are **toll-like receptors** (**TLR**). PRRs are able to recognize the category of the invader (bacterium, virus, fungus, or parasite). They specifically recognize **pathogen-associated molecular patterns (PAMPs)**. These are highly repeated characteristics in pathogenic invaders and can range from recognizable patterns in viral genetic information to the lipopolysaccharide (LPS) of bacteria. This allows for the production of appropriate cytokines to recruit the right type of immune cells; each immune cell has different weapons that can target particular groups of pathogens.

Natural Killer Cells

In the arms race between the human immune system and pathogens, some pathogens have found ways to avoid certain defenses. For example, some viruses cause downregulation of MHC molecules, making it harder for T-cells to recognize the presence of an infection. **Natural killer** (**NK**) **cells**, a type of nonspecific lymphocyte, are able to detect the downregulation of MHC and induce apoptosis in these virally infected cells, as seen in Figure 8.7. Cancer cells may also downregulate MHC production, so NK cells also offer protection from the growth of cancer as well. To a degree, we can think of NK cells as a train conductor checking the passenger's tickets. The NK cells navigate the body verifying that cells have uninhibited MHC-1 complexes (their tickets) and removing them if they do not have them.

KEY CONCEPT

The innate immune cells are nonspecific and form the first line of defense against pathogens.

Innate Immunity

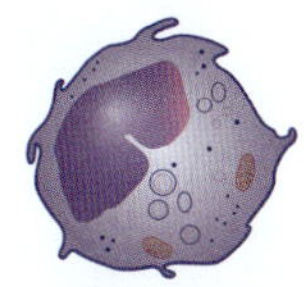

Macrophages envelop pathogens and break them down.

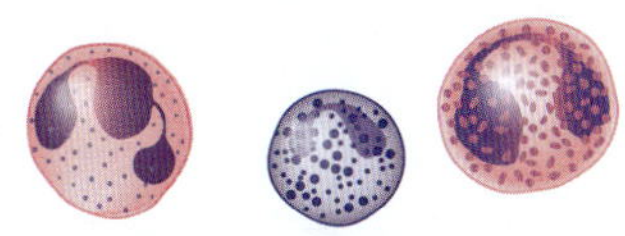

Granulocytes contain granules and also contribute to inflammation. The three types of granulocytes are neutrophils, eosinophils, and basophils.

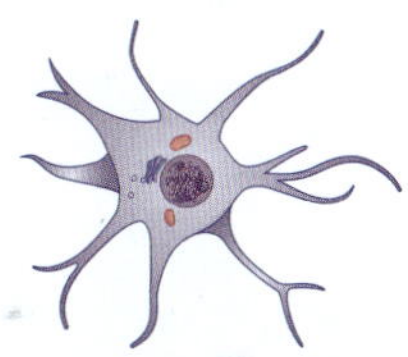

Dendritic cells induce adaptive immune cells to attack pathogens by presenting them with antigens from those pathogens.

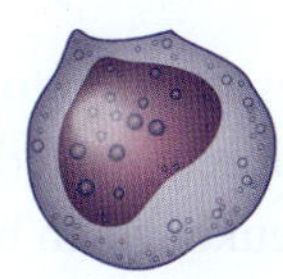

Natural killer cells destroy cancer cells and body cells infected with pathogens.

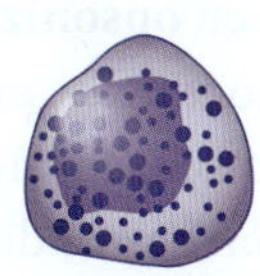

Mast cells release histamine and other inflammatory agents.

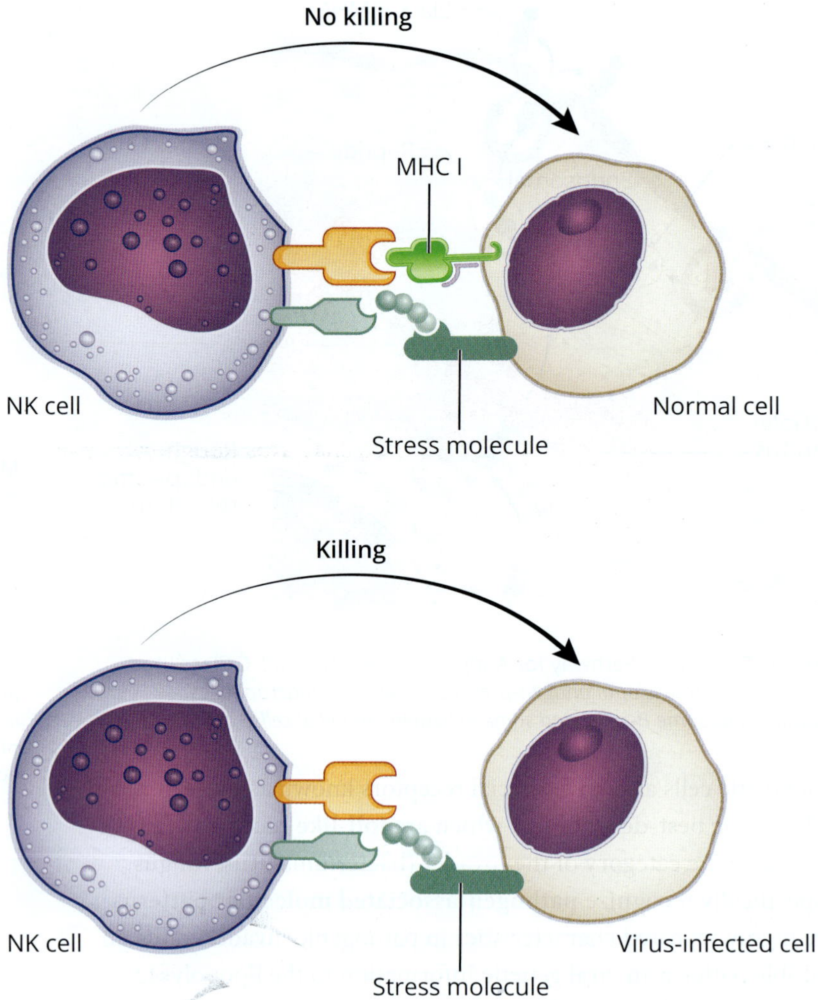

Figure 8.7 Natural Killer Cell Activation

Granulocytes

In addition to macrophages, the granulocytes, which include neutrophils, eosinophils, and basophils (and closely related mast cells), are also involved in nonspecific defense. **Neutrophils** are the most populous leukocyte in blood and are very short lived (a bit more than five days). These cells are phagocytic, like macrophages, and target bacteria. Neutrophils can follow bacteria using chemotaxis—the movement of a motile cell or an organism according to chemical stimuli; in this case, the neutrophil senses products given off by bacteria, moving up the concentration gradient to the source. Neutrophils can also detect bacteria once they have been **opsonized** (marked with an antibody from a B-cell). Other cells, like natural killer cells, macrophages, monocytes, and eosinophils, also contain receptors for antibodies and can attack opsonized bacteria. Dead neutrophil collections are responsible for the formation of **pus** during an infection.

Eosinophils contain bright red-orange granules and are primarily involved in allergic reactions and invasive parasitic infections. Upon activation, eosinophils are recruited to sites of inflammation, where they release a variety of bioactive mediators, including granule proteins, as well as cytokines, chemokines, and lipid mediators. This results in vasodilation and increased leakiness of the blood

KEY CONCEPT

Histamine causes inflammation by inducing vasodilation and the movement of fluid and cells from the bloodstream into tissues.

vessels, allowing additional immune cells (especially monocytes and neutrophils) to move out of the bloodstream and into the tissue. The process of **inflammation** (see Figure 8.8) is particularly useful against extracellular pathogens, including bacteria, fungi, and parasites.

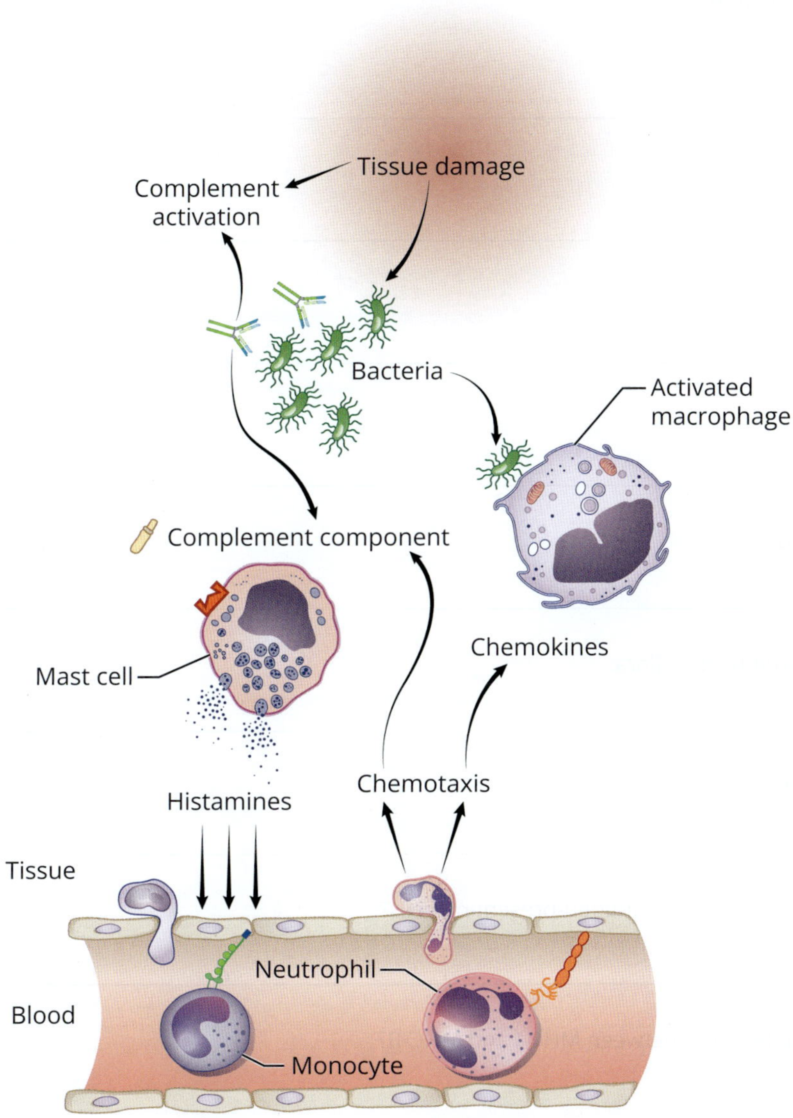

Figure 8.8 Immune and Inflammatory Response

Finally, **basophils** contain large purple granules and are involved in allergic responses. They are the least populous leukocyte in the bloodstream under normal conditions. **Mast cells** are closely related to basophils, but have smaller granules and exist in the tissues, mucosa, and epithelium. Both basophils and mast cells release large amounts of histamine in response to allergens, leading to inflammatory responses.

MCAT CONCEPT CHECK 8.2

Before you move on, assess your understanding of the material with these questions.

1. For each of the noncellular nonspecific immune defenses listed below, provide a brief description of its immunologic function:
   - Skin:

   - Defensins:

   - Lysozyme:

   - Mucus:

   - Stomach acid:

   - Normal gastrointestinal flora:

   - Complement:

   ---
2. Which cells are professional antigen-presenting cells?

   ---
3. What are the differences between MHC-I and MHC-II?
   - MHC-I:

   - MHC-II:

   ---

4. What stimulus activates each of the following types of cells?
   - Natural killer cells:

   ____

   - Neutrophils:

   ____

   - Eosinophils:

   ____

   - Basophils and mast cells:

   ____

8.3 The Adaptive Immune System High Yield

LEARNING OBJECTIVES

After Chapter 8.3, you will be able to:

- Recall the major classes of lymphocytes and their functions
- Describe the three main effects that circulating antibodies can have on a pathogen
- Describe the effects of positive and negative selection on T-cell maturation
- Explain why the secondary response to a pathogen is more efficient than the primary response
- Differentiate between passive and active immunity
- Explain how antibodies become specific for a given antigen

The adaptive immune system can identify specific invaders and mount an attack against that pathogen. The response is variable and depends on the identity of the pathogen. The adaptive immune system can be divided into two divisions: humoral immunity and cell-mediated (cytotoxic) immunity. Each involves the identification of the specific pathogen and organization of an appropriate immune response.

Cells of the Adaptive Immune System

The adaptive immune system consists mainly of two types of lymphocytes, B-cells and T-cells. B-cells govern the humoral response, while T-cells mount the cell-mediated response. All cells of the immune system are created in the bone marrow, but B- and T-cells mature in different locations. B-cells mature in the bone marrow and spleen (although the B in their name originally stood for the bursa of Fabricius, an organ found in birds), and T-cells mature in the thymus. When we are exposed to a pathogen, it may take a few days for the physical symptoms to be relieved. This occurs because the adaptive immune response takes time to form specific defenses against the pathogen.

KEY CONCEPT

B-cells mature in the **b**one marrow. **T**-cells mature in the **t**hymus.

Humoral Immunity

Humoral immunity, which involves the production of **antibodies**, may take as long as a week to become fully effective after initial infection. These antibodies are specific to the antigens of the invading microbe. Antibodies are produced by B-cells, which are lymphocytes that originate and mature in the bone marrow and are activated in the spleen and lymph nodes.

Antibodies (also called **immunoglobulins** [**Ig**]) can carry out many different jobs in the body (see Figure 8.9). Just as antigens can be displayed on the surface of cells or can float freely in blood, chyle (lymphatic fluid), or air, so too can antibodies be present on the surface of a cell or secreted into body fluids. When an antibody binds to an antigen, the response will depend on the location. For antibodies secreted into body fluids, there are four main possibilities: first, once bound to a specific antigen, antibodies may attract other leukocytes to phagocytize those antigens immediately. This is called opsonization, as described earlier. Second, antibodies may cause pathogens to clump together or **agglutinate**, forming large insoluble complexes that can be phagocytized. Third, antibodies can block the ability of a pathogen to invade tissues, essentially neutralizing it. Fourth, antibodies can trigger the complement cascade system. For cell-surface antibodies, the binding of antigen to a B-cell causes activation of that cell, resulting in its proliferation and formation of plasma and memory cells, as described later in this chapter. In contrast, when antigen binds to antibodies on the surface of a mast cell, it causes **degranulation** (exocytosis of granule contents), releasing histamine and causing an inflammatory allergic reaction.

KEY CONCEPT

The adaptive immune cells target invaders with greater specificity, but respond slower since they are replicated in response to an antigen.

Adaptive Immunity

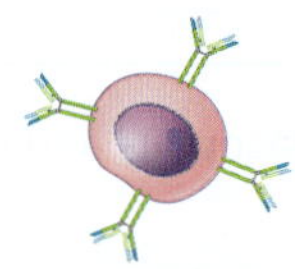

B-cells respond to antigens by dividing and making antibodies that can neutralize pathogens directly or indirectly with the help of other leukocytes.

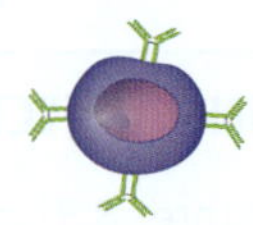

T-cells have a variety of functions in adaptive immune response. Cytotoxic T-cells detect specific antigens and destroy the infected cells that present them. Suppressor and helper T-cells play coordinating roles in immune response. Memory T-cells prepare for potential reinfections.

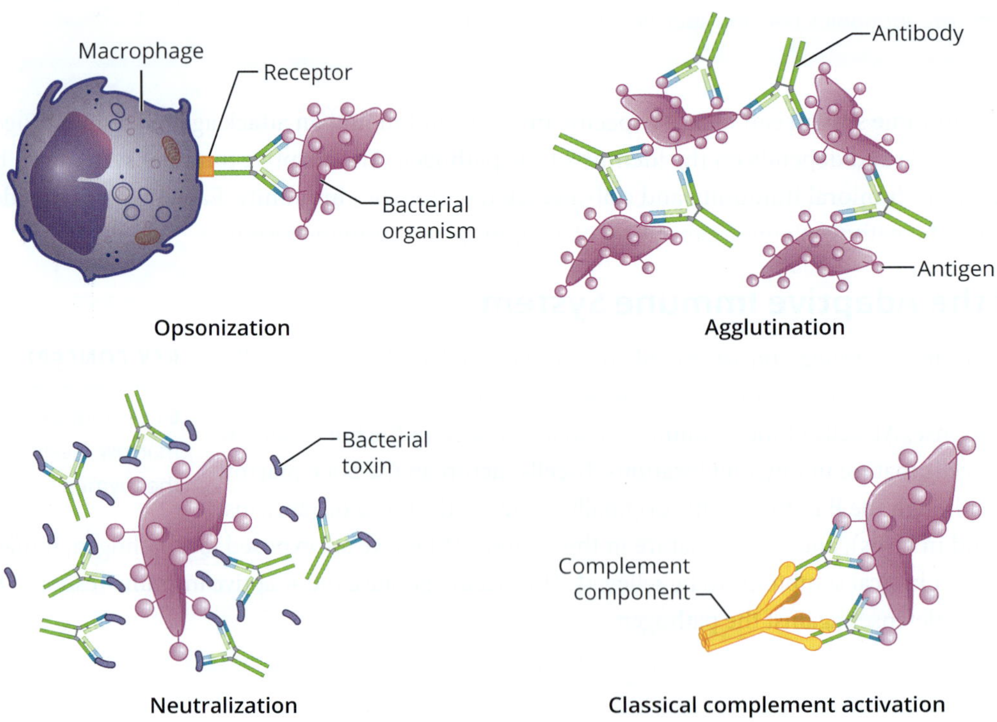

Figure 8.9 Antibody Functions

Antibodies are Y-shaped molecules that are made up of two identical **heavy chains** and two identical **light chains**, as shown in Figure 8.10. Disulfide linkages and noncovalent interactions hold the heavy and light chains together. Each antibody has an **antigen-binding region** at the end of which is called the **variable region (domain)**, at the tips of the Y. The branches of the Y are known as the **fragment antigen binding region (Fab region)**. Within this region, there are specific polypeptide sequences that will bind one, and only one, specific antigenic sequence. Part of the reason it takes so long to initiate the antibody response is that each B-cell undergoes **hypermutation** of its antigen-binding region, trying to find the best match for the antigen. Only those B-cells that can bind the antigen with high affinity survive, providing a mechanism for generating specificity called **clonal selection**. The remaining part of the antibody molecule is known as the **constant region (domain)**, also known as the **fragment crystallizable region (Fc region)**. It is this region that cells such as natural killer cells, macrophages, monocytes, and eosinophils have receptors for, and that can initiate the complement cascade. Each B-cell makes only one type of antibody, but we have many B-cells, so our immune system can recognize many antigens. Further, antibodies come in five different isotypes (IgM, IgD, IgG, IgE, and IgA). While the specific purposes of each antibody isotype is outside the scope of the MCAT, you should know that the different types can be used at different times during the adaptive immune response, for different types of pathogens, or in different locations in the body. Cells can change which isotype of antibody they produce when stimulated by specific cytokines in a process called **isotype switching**.

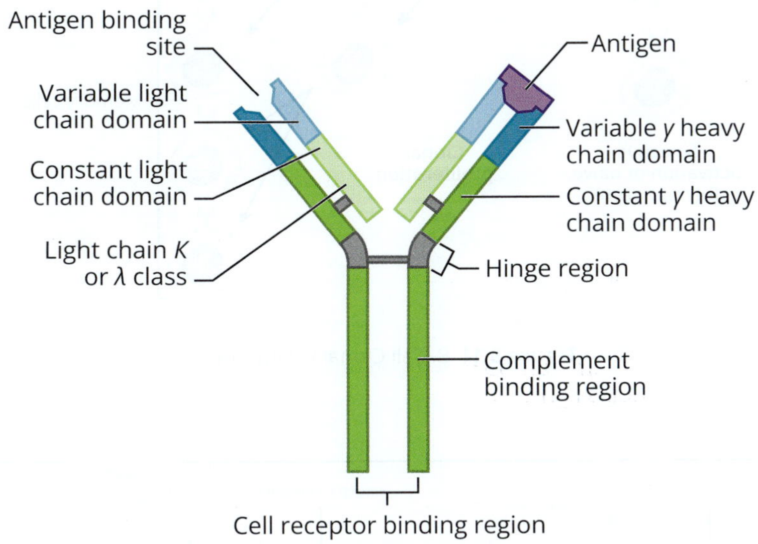

Figure 8.10 Structure of an Antibody Molecule

Not all B-cells that are generated actively or constantly produce antibodies. Antibody production is an energetically expensive process, and there is no reason to expend energy to produce antibodies that are not needed. Instead, **naïve** B-cells (those that have not yet been exposed to an antigen) wait in the lymph nodes for their particular antigen to come along. Upon exposure to the correct antigen, a B-cell will proliferate and produce two types of daughter cells. **Plasma cells** produce large amounts of antibodies, whereas **memory B-cells** stay in the lymph node, awaiting reexposure to the same antigen. This initial activation takes approximately seven to ten days and is known as the **primary response**. The plasma cells will eventually die, but the memory cells may last the lifetime of the organism. If the same antigen is ever presented again, the memory cells rapidly proliferate and differentiate into plasma cells to produce antibodies specific to the source of that antigen (see Figure 8.11). This immune response, called the **secondary response**, will be more rapid and robust. This can be seen in Figure 8.12. The development of these lasting memory cells is the basis of the efficacy of

vaccination. The goal of vaccination is to give an individual's immune system exposure to a pathogen's antigens without actually having to contract the disease in its fullness. This allows antigen-presenting cells to carry the antigens to the lymph nodes where memory cells can be developed and used in case of a future infection with the actual disease.

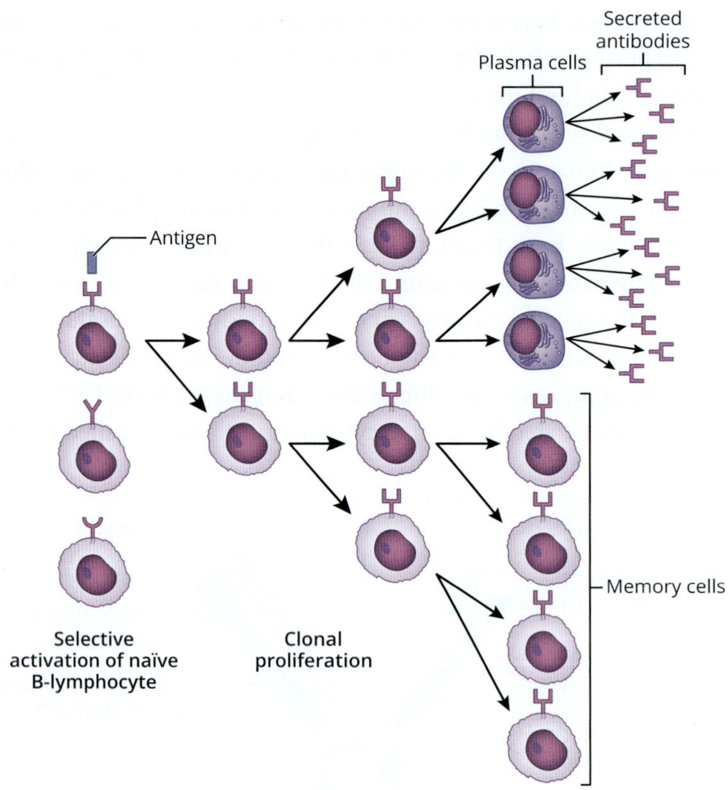

Figure 8.11 B-Cell Clonal Proliferation

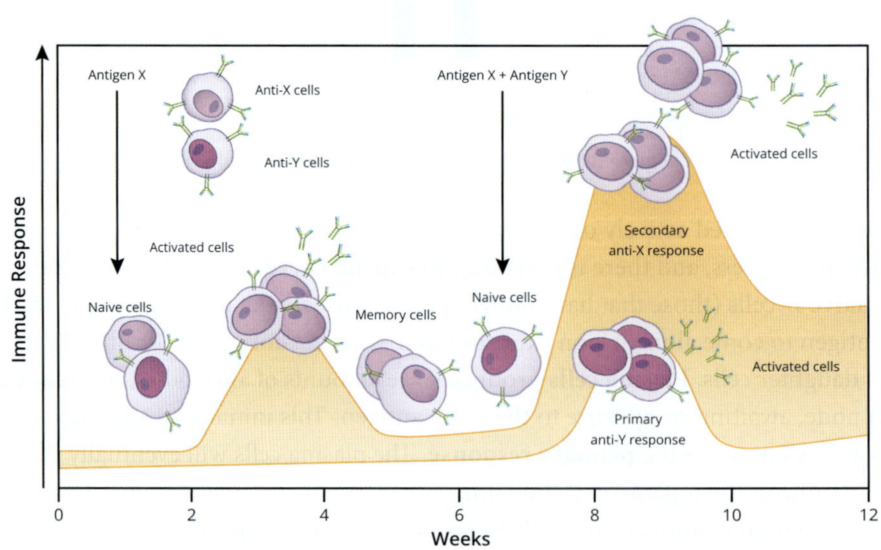

Figure 8.12 Primary vs. Secondary Immune Response

Cytotoxic Immunity

Whereas humoral immunity is based on the activity of B-cells, cell-mediated immunity involves the T-cells. T-cells mature in the thymus, where they undergo both positive and negative selection (see Figure 8.13). **Positive selection** refers to allowing only the maturation of cells that can respond to the presentation of antigen on MHC (cells that cannot respond to MHC undergo apoptosis because they will not be able to respond in the periphery). **Negative selection** refers to causing apoptosis in cells that are self-reactive (activated by proteins produced by the organism itself). The maturation of T-cells is facilitated by **thymosin**, a peptide hormone secreted by thymic cells. Once the T-cell has left the thymus, it is mature but naïve. Upon exposure to antigen, T-cells will also undergo clonal selection so that only those with the highest affinity for a given antigen proliferate.

REAL WORLD

"CD" in immunology stands for *cluster of differentiation* and includes cell-surface markers that can be detected by the lab technique called flow cytometry; these markers give an indication of the types of leukocytes under investigation, how many are present, and their state of maturity.

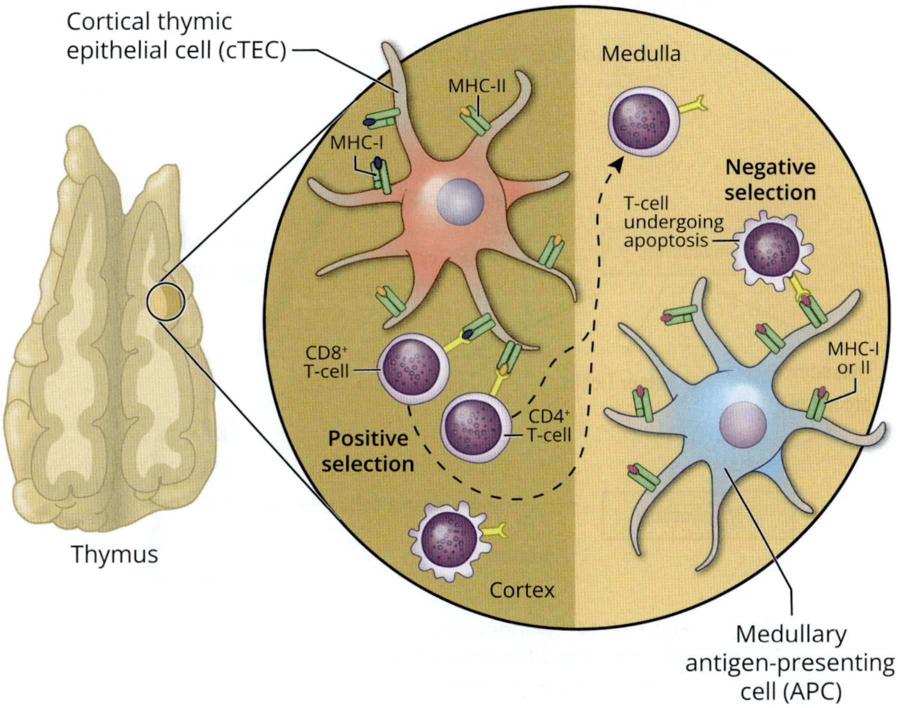

Figure 8.13 Positive and Negative Selection in the Maturation of T-Cells

There are three major types of T-cells: helper T-cells, suppressor T-cells, and killer (cytotoxic) T-cells. **Helper T-cells (T_h)**, also called **$CD4^+$ T-cells**, coordinate the immune response by secreting chemicals known as **lymphokines**. These molecules are capable of recruiting other immune cells (such as plasma cells, cytotoxic T-cells, and macrophages) and increasing their activity. The loss of these cells, as occurs in **human immunodeficiency virus (HIV)** infection, prevents the immune system from mounting an adequate response to infection; in advanced HIV infection, also called **acquired immunodeficiency syndrome (AIDS)**, even weak pathogens can cause devastating consequences. $CD4^+$ T-cells respond to antigens presented on MHC-II molecules. Because MHC-II presents exogenous antigens, $CD4^+$ T-cells are most effective against bacterial, fungal, and parasitic infections.

KEY CONCEPT

$CD4^+$ T-cells are better at fighting extracellular infections, while $CD8^+$ T-cells are better at targeting intracellular infections.

Cytotoxic T-cells (T_c or **CTL**, for cytotoxic T-lymphocytes), also called **CD8$^+$ T-cells**, are capable of directly killing virally infected cells by injecting toxic chemicals that promote apoptosis into the infected cell. CD8$^+$ T-cells respond to antigens presented on MHC-I molecules. Because MHC-I presents endogenous antigens, CD8$^+$ T-cells are most effective against viral (and intracellular bacterial or fungal) infections.

Suppressor or **regulatory T-cells** (T_{reg}) also express CD4, but can be differentiated from helper T-cells because they also express a protein called *Foxp3*. These cells help to tone down the immune response once infection has been adequately contained. These cells also turn off self-reactive lymphocytes to prevent autoimmune diseases: this is termed **self-tolerance.**

Finally, **memory T-cells** can be generated. Similar to memory B-cells, these cells lie in wait until the next exposure to the same antigen. When activated, they carry out a more robust and rapid response.

A summary of the different types of lymphocytes in adaptive (specific) immunity is shown in Figure 8.14.

MNEMONIC

CD × MHC = 8

CD4$^+$ cells respond to MHC-II **(4 × 2 = 8)**

CD8$^+$ cells respond to MHC-I **(8 × 1 = 8)**

REAL WORLD

Many suppressor T-cells were formerly self-reactive T-cells that have been turned off. When a suppressor T-cell inactivates another lymphocyte, it can either target it for destruction or promote its conversion into another suppressor T-cell.

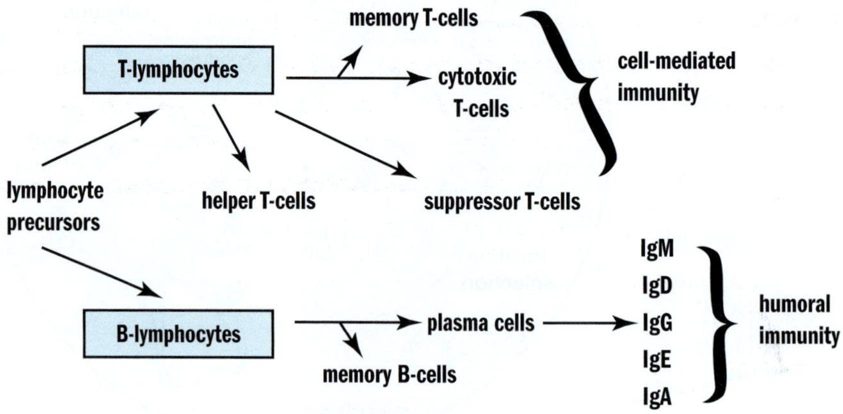

Figure 8.14 Lymphocytes of Specific Immunity
This diagram shows the differentiation of lymphocyte precursors and the cell types involved in specific immunity.

Activation of the Adaptive Immune System

It is important to note that the innate and adaptive immune systems are not really disparate entities that function separately. The proper functioning of the entire immune system depends on the interactions between these two systems. There are five types of infectious pathogens: bacteria, viruses, fungi, parasites (including protozoa, worms, and insects), and prions (for which there are no immune defenses). While the immune system's response depends on the specific identity of the pathogen, we present two classic examples in Figure 8.15: a bacterial (extracellular pathogen) infection and a viral (intracellular pathogen) infection. Keep in mind that this categorization is imperfect; for example, some bacteria, like *Mycobacterium tuberculosis* and *Listeria monocytogenes*, are actually intracellular pathogens.

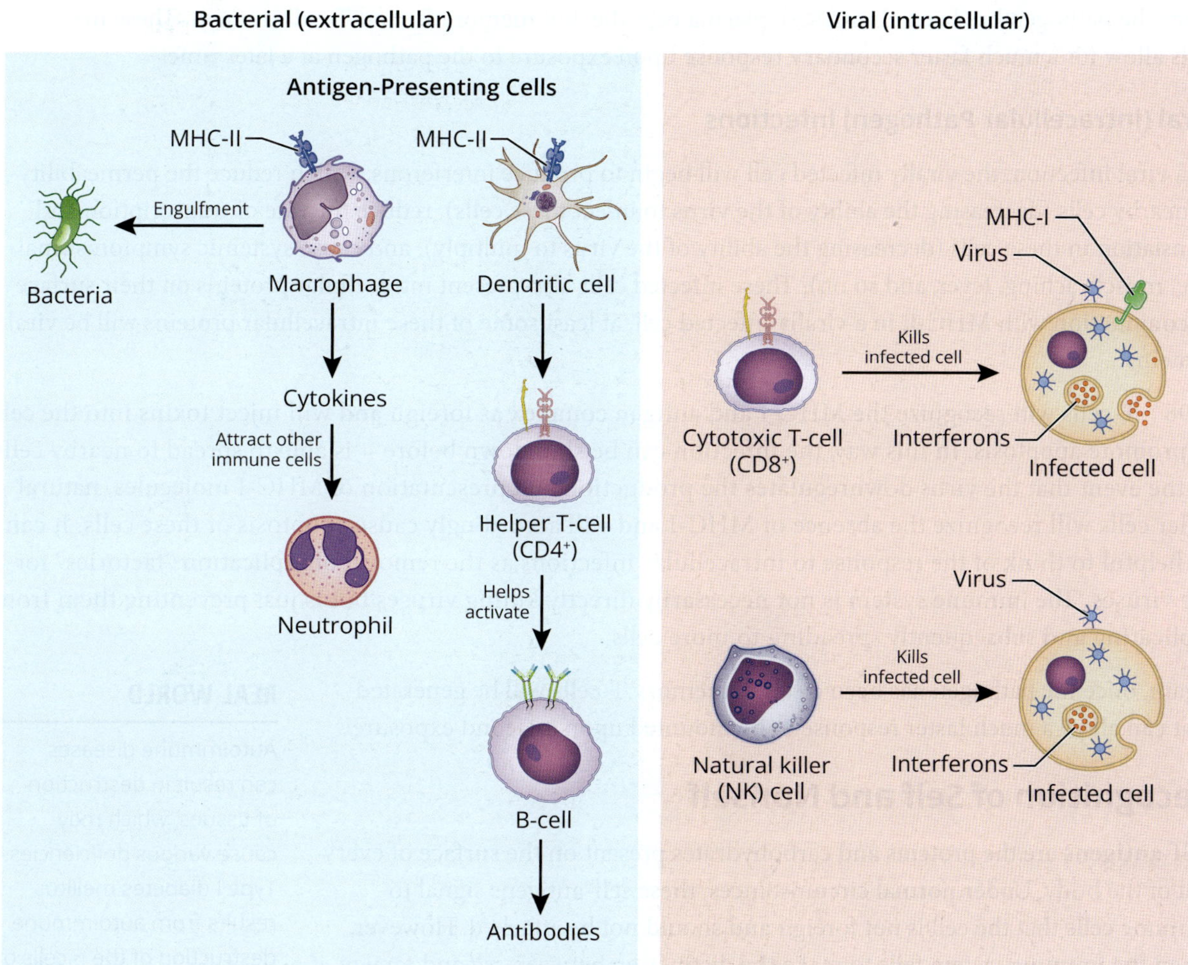

Figure 8.15 Bacterial vs. Viral Infection Response

Bacterial (Extracellular Pathogen) Infections

Macrophages are like the sentinels of the human body, always on the lookout for potential invaders. Let's say a person suffers a laceration and bacteria are introduced into the body via this laceration. First, macrophages (and other antigen-presenting cells) engulf the bacteria and subsequently release inflammatory mediators. These cells also digest the bacteria and present antigens from the pathogen on their surfaces in conjunction with MHC-II. The cytokines attract inflammatory cells, including neutrophils and additional macrophages. Mast cells are activated by the inflammation and degranulate, resulting in histamine release and increased leakiness of the capillaries. This augments the ability of the immune cells to leave the bloodstream to travel to the affected tissue. The dendritic cell then leaves the affected tissue and travels to the nearest lymph node, where it presents the antigen to B-cells. B-cells that produce the correct antibody proliferate through clonal selection to create plasma cells and memory cells. Antibodies then travel through the bloodstream to the affected tissue, where they tag the bacteria for destruction.

At the same time, dendritic cells are also presenting the antigen to T-cells, activating a T-cell response. In particular, $CD4^+$ T-cells are activated. These cells come in two types, called T_h1 and T_h2. T_h1 cells release interferon gamma (IFN-γ), which activates macrophages and increases their ability to kill bacteria. T_h2 cells help activate B-cells and are more common in parasitic infections.

After the pathogen has been eliminated, plasma cells die, but memory B- and T-cells remain. These memory cells allow for a much faster secondary response upon exposure to the pathogen at a later time.

Viral (Intracellular Pathogen) Infections

In a viral infection, the virally infected cell will begin to produce interferons, which reduce the permeability of nearby cells (decreasing the ability of the virus to infect these cells), reduce the rate of transcription and translation in these cells (decreasing the ability of the virus to multiply), and cause systemic symptoms (malaise, muscle aching, fever, and so on). These infected cells also present intracellular proteins on their surface in conjunction with MHC-I; in a virally infected cell, at least some of these intracellular proteins will be viral proteins.

$CD8^+$ T-cells will recognize the MHC-I and antigen complex as foreign and will inject toxins into the cell to promote apoptosis. In this way, the infection can be shut down before it is able to spread to nearby cells. In the event that the virus downregulates the production and presentation of MHC-I molecules, natural killer cells will recognize the absence of MHC-I and will accordingly cause apoptosis of these cells. It can be helpful to think of the response to intracellular infections as the removal of replication "factories" for the viruses. The immune system is not necessarily directly killing viruses but is just preventing them from replicating and subsequently spreading to more cells.

Again, once the pathogen has been cleared, memory T-cells will be generated that can allow a much faster response to be mounted upon a second exposure.

REAL WORLD

Autoimmune diseases can result in destruction of tissues, which may cause various deficiencies. Type I diabetes mellitus results from autoimmune destruction of the β-cells of the pancreas. This results in an inability to produce insulin, characterized by high blood sugars and excessive utilization of fats and proteins for energy. Other examples of autoimmune diseases include multiple sclerosis, myasthenia gravis, psoriasis, systemic lupus erythematosus, rheumatoid arthritis, Graves' disease, and Guillain–Barré syndrome.

Recognition of Self and Nonself

Self-antigens are the proteins and carbohydrates present on the surface of every cell of the body. Under normal circumstances, these self-antigens signal to immune cells that the cell is not foreign and should not be attacked. However, when the immune system fails to make the distinction between *self* and *foreign*, it may attack cells expressing particular self-antigens, a condition known as **autoimmunity**. Note that autoimmunity is only one potential problem with immune functioning: another problem arises when the immune system misidentifies a foreign antigen as dangerous when, in fact, it is not. Pet dander, pollen, and peanuts are not inherently threatening to human life, yet some people's immune systems are hypersensitive to these antigens and become overactivated when these antigens are encountered. This is called an allergic reaction. Allergies and autoimmunity are part of a family of immune reactions classified as **hypersensitivity reactions**.

The human body strives to prevent autoimmune reactions very early in T-cell and B-cell maturation processes. T-cells are educated in the thymus. Part of this education involves the elimination of T-cells that respond to self-antigens, called negative selection. Immature B-cells that respond to self-antigens are eliminated before they leave the bone marrow. However, this process is not perfect, and occasionally a cell that responds to self-antigens is allowed to survive. Most autoimmune diseases can be treated with a number of therapies; one common example is administration of **glucocorticoids** (modified versions of cortisol), which have potent immunosuppressive qualities.

Immunization

Often, diseases can have significant, long-term consequences. Infection with the poliovirus, for example, can cause permanent paralysis. Polio used to be a widespread illness; however, today we hardly hear about outbreaks of polio because of a highly effective vaccination program that led to the elimination of polio from many parts of the world.

Immunization can be achieved in an active or passive fashion. In **active immunity**, the immune system is stimulated to produce antibodies against a specific pathogen. The means by which we are exposed to this pathogen may either be natural or artificial. Through natural exposure, antibodies are generated by B-cells once an individual becomes infected. Artificial exposure (through vaccines) also results in the production of antibodies; however, the individual never experiences true infection. Instead, the individual receives an injection or intranasal spray containing an antigen that will activate B-cells to produce antibodies to fight the specific infection. The antigen may be a weakened or killed form of the microbe, or it may be a part of the microbe's protein structure.

Immunization may also be achieved passively. **Passive immunity** results from the transfer of antibodies to an individual. The immunity is transient because only the antibodies, and not the plasma cells that produce them, are given to the individual. Natural examples are the transfer of antibodies across the placenta during pregnancy to protect the fetus and the transfer of antibodies from a mother to her nursing infant through breast milk. In some cases of exposure, such as to the rabies virus or tetanus, intravenous immunoglobulin may be given to prevent the pathogen from spreading.

REAL WORLD

In 1998, a paper published in *The Lancet* claimed to have found a link between vaccines and autism. This paper was withdrawn from *The Lancet* after it was demonstrated that the primary author had an undisclosed conflict of interest and that the results were scientifically inaccurate. In fact, no well-designed scientific study has yet shown this link to exist. Nevertheless, reporting of this unsubstantiated connection in the lay media has influenced some parents and guardians to avoid immunizing their children. Since 1998, outbreaks of measles and mumps in the United States and other industrialized nations have raised concerns about the resurgence of illnesses that were previously thought to have been eliminated from these countries. Vaccines do carry risks, including rare cases of encephalitis (brain inflammation) and Guillain–Barré syndrome (an autoimmune disease in which the myelin of peripheral nerves is attacked), but so too do the pathogens these vaccines protect against.

BIOLOGY GUIDED EXAMPLE WITH EXPERT THINKING

The development of immune-mediated liver failure during viral hepatitis has recently been linked to the action of $CD8^+$ T-cells. Several effector mechanisms have been identified in preclinical models, including the cytokines interferon (IFN) and tumor necrosis factor (TNF), as well as apoptosis-inducing molecules such as Fas Ligand (FasL) and perforin-1 (Prf1). To better study these factors, a mouse model of acute hepatitis was developed by immunizing mice with OVA epitope (a short peptide sequence derived from the protein ovalbumin) and then infected with recombinant adenovirus expressing OVA peptide 30 days later. Acute liver damage was observed, marked by an increase in serum alanine aminotransferase (sALT), a marker of liver damage, and a decrease in body weight.

Topic: $CD8^+$ T-cells and hepatitis

These are all components of the immune system that may lead to immune-mediated liver failure

New model to study immune-mediated liver damage during acute hepatitis

Damage to liver = elevated sALT, decrease in body weight

To study the contribution of FasL and TNF to liver pathology, mice were injected with Anti-FasL, anti-TNF, or IgG control antibodies before adenovirus challenge. Researchers measured sALT levels and body weight in the days post challenge (Figure 1). To better elucidate the role of perforin-1, OVA-specific T-cells (OT-1 cells) with either WT perforin or perforin-1 KO (OT-1 x Prf1-/- cells), were injected into naive mice prior to adenovirus challenge. Serum ALT and weight measurements were taken following infection (Figure 2).

Exp 1: test FasL and TNF contribution, antibodies added that will prevent factors from exerting their normal biological function

Exp 2: test role of perforin-1, add T-cells with and without perforin-1, measure sALT and body mass

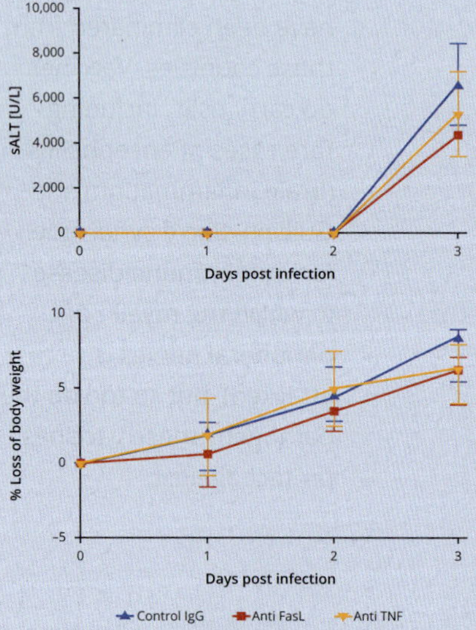

Figure 1

Figure 1 = antibody study

IV: antibody treatment

DVs: sALT levels and % loss of body weight

Trend: in both graphs, the three groups have overlapping error bars

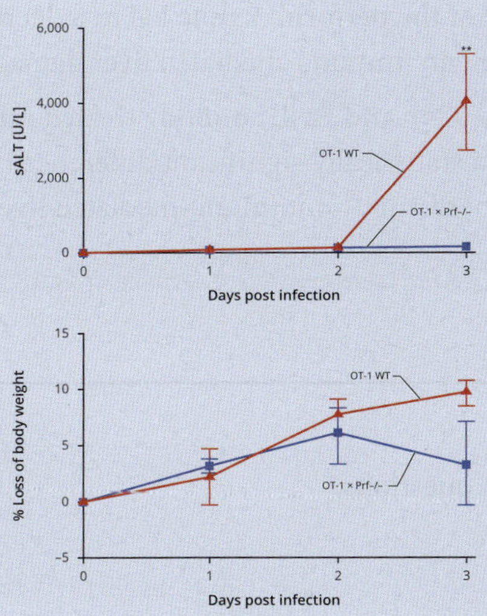

Figure 2

Figure 2 = cell transfer study

IV: presence or absence of perforin-1

DVs: same as previous

Trends: mice given perforin-1 knockout cells have no increase in sALT and lose less weight compared to controls

Adapted from Welz, M., Eickhoff, S., Abdullah, Z., Trebicka, J., Gartlan, K. H., Spicer, J. A., & Kastenmüller, W. (2018). Perforin inhibition protects from lethal endothelial damage during fulminant viral hepatitis. *Nature Communications*, *9*(1), 4805. doi:10.1038/s41467-018-07213-x.

Based on the results, which of the three parameters tested, FAS Ligand, Tumor Necrosis Factor, or Perforin, is most likely involved in the destruction of liver tissue during acute infection?

This question is really testing our understanding of the experimental design and comprehension of the results. Let's start with the experimental design. Paragraph 1 tells us that there are four main factors that are believed to be involved in immune-mediated liver damage: FasL, TNF, perforin-1, and INF. To test the involvement of these factors, the researchers designed a new experimental model. They first injected mice with OVA peptide to induce a primary immune response and the development of memory cells. Thirty days later, the researchers infected the mice with adenovirus expressing OVA. This will result in activation of memory cells and a secondary immune response, which the researchers showed was able to induce immune-controlled liver damage.

In the first experiment, the mice were injected with antibodies against FasL and TNF prior to adenovirus infection. These antibodies will bind to FasL and TNF, rendering them unable to function, similar to knocking out the gene (but significantly cheaper than developing transgenic mice!). Figure 1 shows the results. We notice that there is no significant difference in sALT levels nor body weight loss between mice treated with the control antibody and mice treated with either FasL or TNF antibody. We see the same increase in sALT and the same decrease in weight loss, indicating that removing TNF and FasL function did not prevent liver damage. This suggests that these two factors are not required for the immune-mediated liver damage.

In the second experiment, we test the involvement of perforin-1. The experimental setup is slightly different. Instead of injecting OVA peptide, OVA specific T-cells were injected into mice. Two different types of cells were used, normal and perforin-1 knockout. The mice were then infected with adenovirus as before. This enables us to examine the contribution of perforin-1 in liver damage. Figure 2 shows the results of the experiment. We can note that there is a significant difference in sALT levels between control and perforin-1 knockout (KO) cells. There is no elevation in sALT in the knockout cells, whereas there is an increase in control cells. This suggests that perforin-1 contributes to liver damage. Furthermore, mice given perforin-1 KO cells lose less weight compared to mice given control cells. Because a knockout of the perforin-1 gene led to a decrease in immune-mediated liver damage in mice, perforin-1 plays an important role in immune-mediated liver damage.

Because the results show no significant difference between the control and TNF and FasL antibody treated mice, TNF and FasL do not play a role in immune-mediated liver damage. However, a statistically significant difference between control and perforin-1 knockout cells was observed, indicating a role for perforin-1 in immune-mediated liver damage.

MCAT CONCEPT CHECK 8.3

Before you move on, assess your understanding of the material with these questions.

1. For each of the lymphocytes listed below, what are its main functions?
   - Plasma cell:
   - Memory B-cell:
   - Helper T-cell:
   - Cytotoxic T-cell:
   - Suppressor (regulatory) T-cell:
   - Memory T-cell:
2. What are the three main effects circulating antibodies can have on a pathogen?
   -
   -
   -

3. How do antibodies become specific for a given antigen?

---

4. A T-cell appropriately passes through positive selection, but then inappropriately passes through negative selection. What will this T-cell be reactive toward?

---

5. Which cells account for the fact that the secondary response to a pathogen is much more rapid and robust than the primary response?

---

6. What is the difference between active and passive immunity?
    - Active immunity:

    - Passive immunity:

8.4 The Lymphatic System

LEARNING OBJECTIVES

After Chapter 8.4, you will be able to:

- Predict how a blockage of flow from a lymph node would impact the lymphatic system and the body as a whole
- Describe the factors and structures linking lymphatic and cardiovascular circulation

The immune system and the lymphatic system are intimately related. B-cells proliferate and develop within the lymphatic system, especially the lymph nodes. This system also serves other functions for the body.

Structure

The lymphatic system, along with the cardiovascular system, is a type of circulatory system. It is made up of one-way vessels that become larger as they move toward the center of the body. These vessels carry lymphatic fluid (**lymph**) and most join to form a large **thoracic duct** in the posterior chest, which then delivers the fluid into the left subclavian vein (near the heart).

Lymph nodes are small, bean-shaped structures along the lymphatic vessels. Lymph nodes contain a lymphatic channel, as well as an artery and a vein. The lymph nodes provide a space for the cells of the immune system to be exposed to possible pathogens.

REAL WORLD

Certain cancers, especially breast cancer, are prone to spread via lymphatic channels. Mastectomy, a surgery that removes the breast, is one of the treatments for breast cancer. In order to ensure that all of the cancer has been removed, local lymph nodes are often removed at the same time.

Function

The lymphatic system serves many different purposes for the body by providing a secondary system for circulation.

Equalization of Fluid Distribution

At the capillaries, fluid leaves the bloodstream and goes into the tissues. The quantity of fluid that leaves the tissues at the arterial end of the capillary bed depends on both hydrostatic and oncotic pressures (Starling forces). Remember that the oncotic pressure of the blood draws water back into the vessel at the venule end, once hydrostatic pressure has decreased. Because the net pressure drawing fluid in at the venule end is slightly less than the net pressure pushing fluid out at the arterial end, about 10–20% of fluid remains in the tissues. Lymphatic vessels drain these tissues and subsequently return the fluid to the bloodstream. A depiction of lymphatic vessels can be observed in Figure 8.16.

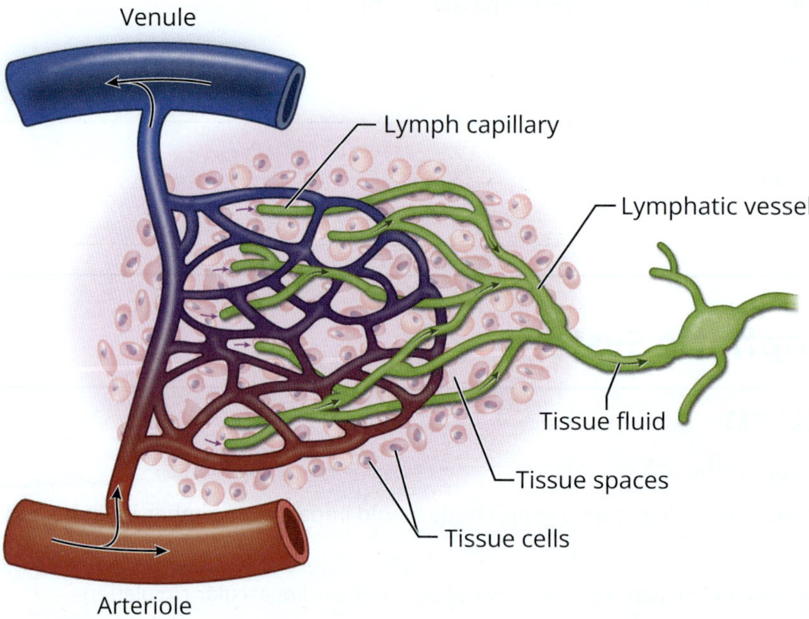

Figure 8.16 The Lymphatic System in Relation to Tissues and Blood Circulation

The lymphatics offer some protection against pathology. For example, if the blood has a low concentration of albumin (a key plasma protein), the oncotic pressure of the blood is decreased, and less water is driven back into the bloodstream at the venule end. Thus, this fluid will collect in the tissues. Provided that the lymphatic channels are not blocked, much of this fluid may eventually return to the bloodstream via the lymphatics. Only when the lymphatics are overwhelmed does **edema** occur—swelling due to fluid collecting in tissue.

Transportation of Biomolecules

Lipids (fats) are large molecules and cannot easily diffuse directly into the small capillaries in the digestive system, so the body must use another way to get fats into circulation. The lymphatic system can transport fats from the digestive system into the bloodstream. **Lacteals,** small lymphatic vessels, are located at the center of each villus in the small intestine. Fats, packaged into **chylomicrons** by intestinal mucosal cells, enter the lacteal for transport. Lymphatic fluid carrying many chylomicrons takes on a milky white appearance and is called **chyle**. This process is depicted in Figure 8.17.

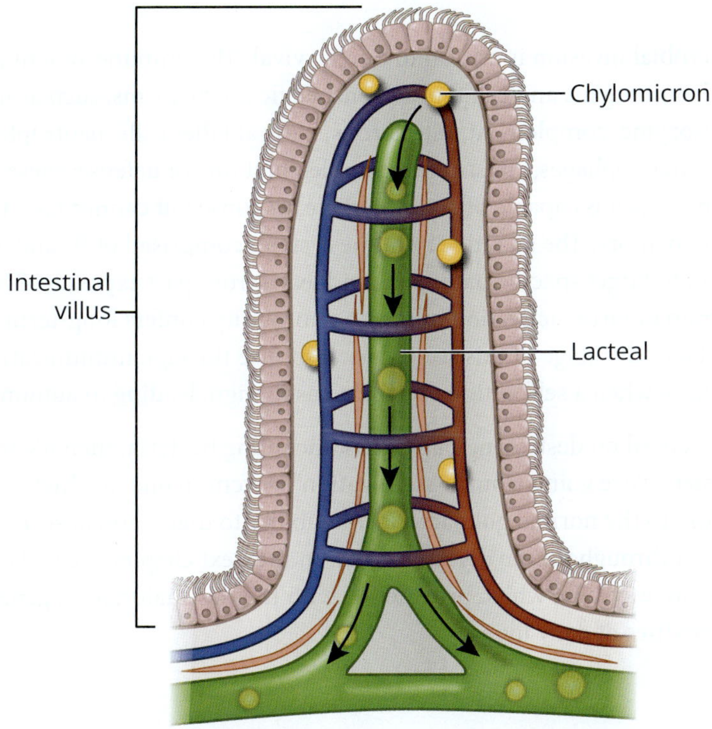

Figure 8.17 Lymphatic Transport of Fat in the Digestive System

Immunity

As stated previously in this chapter, lymph nodes are a place for antigen-presenting cells and lymphocytes to interact. B-cells proliferate and mature in the lymph nodes in collections called **germinal centers**.

MCAT CONCEPT CHECK 8.4

Before you move on, assess your understanding of the material with these questions.

1. *Filariasis* is the name for an infection with a member of a certain group of parasites, most notably *Wuchereria bancrofti*. This parasite resides in lymph nodes and causes blockage of flow. If an individual had a *W. bancrofti* infection in the lymph nodes of the thigh, what would likely happen?

____

____

2. What structure is primarily responsible for returning materials from lymphatic circulation to the cardiovascular system?

____

Conclusion

The ability to fend off microbial invasion is critical to our survival. The immune system is throughout the body and involves multiple different organs and cell types. Nonspecific mechanisms, such as intact skin, mucous membranes, defensins, lysozyme, complement, interferons, natural killer cells, neutrophils, eosinophils, basophils, and monocytes/macrophages, constitute a complex first line of defense; these mechanisms comprise the innate immune system, which is capable of an immediate response but cannot target a specific pathogen or maintain immunologic memory. The adaptive immune system, comprised of B- and T-cells (lymphocytes), allows our immune system to target specific pathogens and learn from past exposure. Thus, once we are infected with a certain strain of virus, activation of specific immunity confers long-term protection against that particular virus. We take advantage of this secondary response through immunization, and we can see the problems specificity can have when a self-antigen is labeled as foreign, leading to autoimmune disease.

If the immune system is focused on destroying pathogens, including bacteria, then it's an interesting transition we make in the next chapter. We're going from a "sterilization" system to one in which bacterial colonization is the norm. From oral flora to the normal gut bacteria, our ability to digest and absorb nutrients is intimately linked to symbiotic bacteria throughout the digestive tract. In the next chapter, we will explore the anatomy and physiology of the digestive system, which provides us with the raw materials to generate energy, build proteins, and carry out activities of daily living.

GO ONLINE

You've reviewed the content, now test your knowledge and critical thinking skills by completing a test-like passage set in your online resources!

CONCEPT SUMMARY

Structure of the Immune System

- The immune system can be divided into innate and adaptive immunity.
    - **Innate immunity** is composed of defenses that are always active, but that cannot target a specific invader and cannot maintain immunologic memory; also called **nonspecific immunity**.
    - **Adaptive immunity** is composed of defenses that take time to activate, but that target a specific invader and can maintain immunologic memory; also called **specific immunity**.
- The immune system is dispersed in the body.
    - Immune cells come from the **bone marrow**.
    - The **spleen** and **lymph nodes** are sites where immune responses can be mounted, and in which B-cells are activated.
    - The **thymus** is the site of T-cell maturation.
    - **Gut-associated lymphoid tissue (GALT)** includes the **tonsils** and **adenoids**.
- **Leukocytes**, or white blood cells, are involved in immune defenses.

The Innate Immune System

- Many of the nonspecific defenses are noncellular.
    - The **skin** acts as a physical barrier and secretes antimicrobial compounds, like **defensins**.
    - **Mucus** on mucous membranes traps pathogens; in the respiratory system, the mucus is propelled upward by cilia and can be swallowed or expelled.
    - Tears and saliva contain **lysozyme**, an antibacterial compound.
    - The stomach produces acid, killing most pathogens. Colonization of the gut helps prevent overgrowth by pathogenic bacteria through competition.
    - The **complement** system can punch holes in the cell walls of bacteria, making them osmotically unstable.
    - **Interferons** are given off by virally infected cells and help prevent viral replication and dispersion to nearby cells.
- Many of the nonspecific defenses are also cellular.
    - **Macrophages** ingest pathogens and present them on **major histocompatibility complex** (MHC) molecules. They also secrete **cytokines**.
    - **MHC class I (MHC-I)** is present in all nucleated cells and displays **endogenous antigen** (proteins from within the cell) to cytotoxic T-cells ($CD8^+$ cells).
    - **MHC class II (MHC-II)** is present in professional antigen-presenting cells (macrophages, dendritic cells, some B-cells, and certain activated epithelial cells) and displays **exogenous antigen** (proteins from outside the cell) to helper T-cells ($CD4^+$ cells).
    - **Dendritic cells** are antigen-presenting cells in the skin.
    - **Natural killer cells** attack cells not presenting MHC molecules, including virally infected cells and cancer cells.
    - **Granulocytes** include neutrophils, eosinophils, and basophils.

- **Neutrophils** ingest bacteria, particularly opsonized bacteria (those marked with antibodies). They can follow bacteria using **chemotaxis**.
- **Eosinophils** are used in allergic reactions and invasive parasitic infections. They release **histamine**, causing an inflammatory response.
- **Basophils** are used in allergic reactions. **Mast cells** are related cells found in the skin.

The Adaptive Immune System

- **Humoral immunity** is centered on antibody production by plasma cells, which are activated **B-cells**.
  - **Antibodies** target a particular **antigen**. They contain two heavy chains and two light chains. They have a **constant region** and a **variable region**; the tip of the variable region is the **antigen-binding region**.
  - When activated, the antigen-binding region undergoes **hypermutation** to improve the specificity of the antibody produced. Cells may be given signals to switch **isotypes** of antibody (IgM, IgD, IgG, IgE, IgA).
  - Circulating antibodies can **opsonize** pathogens (mark them for destruction), cause **agglutination** (clumping) into insoluble complexes that are ingested by phagocytes, or neutralize pathogens.
  - Cell-surface antibodies can activate immune cells or mediate allergic reactions.
  - **Memory B-cells** lie in wait for a second exposure to a pathogen and can then mount a more rapid and vigorous immune response (**secondary response**).
- **Cell-mediated** (**cytotoxic**) **immunity** is centered on the functions of **T-cells**.
  - T-cells undergo maturation in the thymus through **positive selection** (only selecting for T-cells that can react to antigen presented on MHC) and **negative selection** (causing apoptosis in self-reactive T-cells). The peptide hormone **thymosin** promotes T-cell development.
  - **Helper T-cells** (**T_h** or **$CD4^+$**) respond to antigen on MHC-II and coordinate the rest of the immune system, secreting **lymphokines** to activate various arms of immune defense. **T_h1 cells** secrete **interferon gamma**, which activates macrophages. **T_h2 cells** activate B-cells, primarily in parasitic infections.
  - **Cytotoxic T-cells** (**T_c**, **CTL**, or **$CD8^+$**) respond to antigen on MHC-I and kill virally infected cells.
  - **Suppressor** (**regulatory**) **T-cells** (**T_{reg}**) tone down the immune response after an infection and promote self-tolerance.
  - **Memory T-cells** serve a similar function to memory B-cells.
- In **autoimmune** conditions, a self-antigen is identified as foreign, and the immune system attacks the body's own cells.
- In **allergic** reactions, nonthreatening exposures incite an inflammatory response.
- Immunization is a method of inducing **active immunity** (activation of B-cells that produce antibodies to an antigen) prior to exposure to a particular pathogen.
- **Passive immunity** is the transfer of antibodies to an individual.

The Lymphatic System

- The **lymphatic system** is a circulatory system that consists of one-way vessels with intermittent lymph nodes.
- The lymphatic system connects to the cardiovascular system via the **thoracic duct** in the posterior chest.
- The lymphatic system equalizes fluid distribution, transports fats and fat-soluble compounds in **chylomicrons**, and provides sites for mounting immune responses.

ANSWERS TO CONCEPT CHECKS

8.1

1. Innate immunity consists of defenses that are always active against pathogens, but that are not capable of targeting specific invaders. It takes longer to mount a response with adaptive immunity, but the response targets a specific pathogen and maintains immunologic memory of the infection to mount a faster response during subsequent infections.

2.

Cell Type	Site of Development	Site of Maturation	Major Functions	Specific or Nonspecific?	Humoral or Cell-Mediated?
B-cell	Bone marrow	Bone marrow (but are activated in spleen or lymph nodes)	Produce antibodies	Specific	Humoral
T-cell	Bone marrow	Thymus	Coordinate immune system and directly kill infected cells	Specific	Cell-mediated

3. Granulocytes include neutrophils, eosinophils, and basophils. Agranulocytes include B- and T-cells (lymphocytes) and monocytes (macrophages).

8.2

1. Skin provides a physical barrier and secretes antimicrobial enzymes. Defensins are examples of antibacterial enzymes on the skin. Lysozyme is antimicrobial and is present in tears and saliva. Mucus is present on mucous membranes and traps incoming pathogens; in the respiratory system, cilia propel the mucus upward so it can be swallowed or expelled. Stomach acid is an antimicrobial substance in the digestive system. The normal gastrointestinal flora provides competition, making it hard for pathogenic bacteria to grow in the gut. Complement is a set of proteins in the blood that can create holes in bacteria.
2. Professional antigen-presenting cells include macrophages, dendritic cells in the skin, some B-cells, and certain activated epithelial cells.
3. MHC-I is found in all nucleated cells and presents pieces of proteins (peptides) created within the cell (endogenous antigens); this can allow for detection of cells infected with intracellular pathogens (especially viruses). MHC-II is only found in antigen-presenting cells and presents proteins that result from the digestion of extracellular pathogens that have been brought in by endocytosis (exogenous antigens).
4. Natural killer cells are activated by cells that do not present MHC (such as virally infected cells and cancer cells). Neutrophils are activated by bacteria, especially those that have been opsonized (tagged with an antibody on their surface). Eosinophils are activated by invasive parasites and allergens. Basophils and mast cells are activated by allergens.

8.3

1. Plasma cells form from B-cells exposed to antigen and produce antibodies. Memory B-cells also form from B-cells exposed to antigen and lie in wait for a second exposure to a given antigen to mount a rapid, robust response. Helper T-cells coordinate the immune system through lymphokines and respond to antigen bound to MHC-II. Cytotoxic T-cells directly kill virally infected cells and respond to antigen bound to MHC-I. Suppressor (regulatory) T-cells quell the immune response after a pathogen has been cleared and promote self-tolerance. Memory T-cells, like memory B-cells, lie in wait until a second exposure to a pathogen to mount a rapid, robust response.
2. Circulating antibodies can mark a pathogen for destruction by phagocytic cells (opsonization), cause agglutination of the pathogen into insoluble complexes that can be taken up by phagocytic cells, or neutralize the pathogen by preventing it from invading tissues.
3. B-cells originally mature in the bone marrow and have some specificity at that point; however, antibodies that can respond to a given antigen undergo hypermutation, or rapid mutation of their antigen-binding sites. Only those B-cells that have the highest affinity for the antigen survive and proliferate, increasing the specificity for the antigen over time.
4. Positive selection occurs when T-cells in the thymus that are able to respond to antigen presented on MHC are allowed to survive (those that do not respond undergo apoptosis). Negative selection occurs when T-cells that respond to self-antigens undergo apoptosis before leaving the thymus. A T-cell that appropriately passes through positive selection, but then inappropriately passes through negative selection will be reactive to self-antigens.
5. Memory cells allow the immune system to carry out a much more rapid and robust secondary response.
6. Active immunity refers to the stimulation of the immune system to produce antibodies against a pathogen. Passive immunity refers to the transfer of antibodies to prevent infection, without stimulation of the plasma cells that produce these antibodies.

8.4

1. Fluid would be unable to return from the lower leg, and edema would result. This infection leads to *elephantiasis*, severe swelling of the limb with thickening of the skin.
2. The thoracic duct carries lymphatic fluid into the left subclavian vein.

SCIENCE MASTERY ASSESSMENT EXPLANATIONS

1. **A**

T-lymphocytes, which mature in the thymus, are the only specific defense against intracellular pathogens. While some bacteria, fungi, and parasites can live intracellularly, viruses—by definition—must replicate within cells. The absence of T-cells would leave an individual unable to fight viral infections with specific defenses.

2. **B**

The lymphocytes involved in cell-mediated immunity are the T-lymphocytes, or T-cells. There are four types of T-cells, each playing a different role in cell-mediated immunity: cytotoxic T-cells, helper T-cells, memory T-cells, and suppressor T-cells. Thus, from the answer choices, the only cells not involved in cell-mediated immunity are the plasma cells, which are differentiated immunoglobulin-secreting B-lymphocytes involved in humoral immunity. **(B)** is therefore the correct answer.

3. **B**

The main function of the lymphatic system is to collect excess interstitial fluid and return it to the circulatory system, maintaining the balance of body fluids. However, this is not one of the answer choices. In addition, the lymphatic system accepts chylomicrons from the small intestine and delivers them to the cardiovascular circulation. Transport of hormones is a function of the cardiovascular system, eliminating **(A)**. The lymphatic system absorbs fluid that has been pushed into tissues, but does not cause the extravasation of the fluid, eliminating **(C)**. Mast cells reside in (and are activated in) the skin and mucous membranes, eliminating **(D)**.

4. **A**

Antibodies are produced by plasma cells derived from B-lymphocytes. The other cells are all types of T-lymphocytes, although memory B-cells can also exist. Upon secondary antigen exposure, memory B-cells rapidly proliferate and differentiate into plasma cells to produce antibodies. Memory B-cells do not directly produce antibodies.

5. **C**

In this question, true statements should be eliminated. The innate immune system does include phagocytes like macrophages, which can activate an inflammatory response to recruit additional immune cells, eliminating **(A)**. The innate immune system acts near entry points into the body and is always active, eliminating **(B)**. Furthermore, all blood cells, including all cells of the immune system, are derived from hematopoietic stem cells in the bone marrow, eliminating **(D)**. By contrast, the innate immune system does not recognize specific antigens on a pathogen, making **(C)** correct.

6. **C**

Adaptive immunity involves the activation of B-cells and T-cells specific to the encountered antigen. Any choice that conforms to this paradigm will be correct. **(C)** indicates that B-cells are activated. Pattern recognition receptors, or PRRs, in **(A)** recognize patterns common to certain pathogens, but do not identify the specific pathogen. Complement is an example of a blood-borne nonspecific defense against bacteria, eliminating **(B)**. Dendritic cells traveling to the lymph nodes **(D)** are a part of the interaction between the innate and adaptive immune systems, but the dendritic cells themselves are nonspecific.

7. **A**

Active immunity refers to the production of antibodies during an immune response. Active immunity may be conferred on an individual by vaccination, such as when an individual is injected with a weakened, inactive, or modified form of a particular antigen that stimulates the immune system to produce antibodies. Active immunity may require weeks to build. Passive immunity, on the other hand, involves the transfer of antibodies through, for example, breast milk. Another example of passive immunity would be during pregnancy, when some maternal antibodies cross the placenta and enter fetal circulation, conferring passive immunity to the fetus. Although passive immunity is acquired immediately, it is very short lived, lasting only as long as the antibodies circulate in blood.

8. **D**

T-cells mature in the thymus, where they are "educated." This education involves the elimination of T-cells with improper binding to MHC–antigen complexes (positive selection) and self-reactive T-cells (negative selection). Thus, self-reactive T-cells are eliminated in the thymus.

9. **C**

Healthy cells exhibit MHC class I molecules. Natural killer cells monitor the expression of MHC molecules on the surface of cells. Viral infection and cancer often cause a reduction in the expression of MHC class I molecules on the cell surface. Natural killer cells detect this lack of MHC and induce apoptosis in the affected cells.

10. **A**

$CD8^+$ T-cells are largely responsible for the cytotoxic immune response. By releasing toxic chemicals into virally infected cells, $CD8^+$ T-cells are able to kill these cells in an effort to contain viral infections. Isotype switching refers to changes in the isotype of antibody produced, which is not caused by $CD8^+$ cells, eliminating **(B)**. Antigens are presented by macrophages, dendritic cells, certain epithelial cells, and some B-cells, eliminating **(C)**. B-cells are not activated by cytotoxic T-lymphocytes, eliminating **(D)**.

11. **C**

Lymphocytes arise from the lymphoid lineage, which includes B-cells and T-cells. Thus, all types of B- and T-cells are capable of causing lymphoma. Macrophages, however, are not lymphocytes and are not likely to cause lymphoma.

12. **D**

When the adaptive immune system encounters an antigen, only the cells with antibodies or T-cell receptors specific to that antigen are activated. This is known as clonal selection. While a T-cell response may be a cytotoxic response, it could also be the activation of helper T-cells; plus, this does not explain the specificity of the response, eliminating **(B)**.

13. **A**

The only phagocytes that attack bacteria on this list are neutrophils and dendritic cells. Dendritic cells are able to sample and present any type of material, and reside in the skin. Neutrophils, on the other hand, are present in the bloodstream and can attack bacteria present there or in tissues. Eosinophils and basophils are involved in the development of allergies; eosinophils also defend against parasites.

14. **B**

The spleen is a location where B-cells mature and proliferate. Therefore, removal of the spleen is likely to result in a reduction of humoral immunity. In fact, many people receive vaccinations prior to removal of the spleen in order to bolster their immunity.

15. **D**

The body employs a number of nonspecific defense mechanisms against foreign invasion. The skin and mucous membranes provide a physical barrier against bacterial invasion. In addition, sweat contains enzymes that attack bacterial cell walls. Certain passages, such as the respiratory tract, are lined with ciliate mucus-coated epithelia, which filter and trap foreign particles. Macrophages engulf and destroy foreign particles. The inflammatory response is initiated in response to physical damage. The only choice that is not a nonspecific defense mechanism is **(D)**, the correct answer. Cytotoxic T-cells are involved in (specific) cell-mediated immunity.

▶ **GO ONLINE**

Consult your online resources for additional practice.

SHARED CONCEPTS

Biochemistry Chapter 3
Nonenzymatic Protein Function and Protein Analysis

Biology Chapter 1
The Cell

Biology Chapter 6
The Respiratory System

Biology Chapter 7
The Cardiovascular System

Biology Chapter 9
The Digestive System

Biology Chapter 10
Homeostasis

CHAPTER 9

THE DIGESTIVE SYSTEM

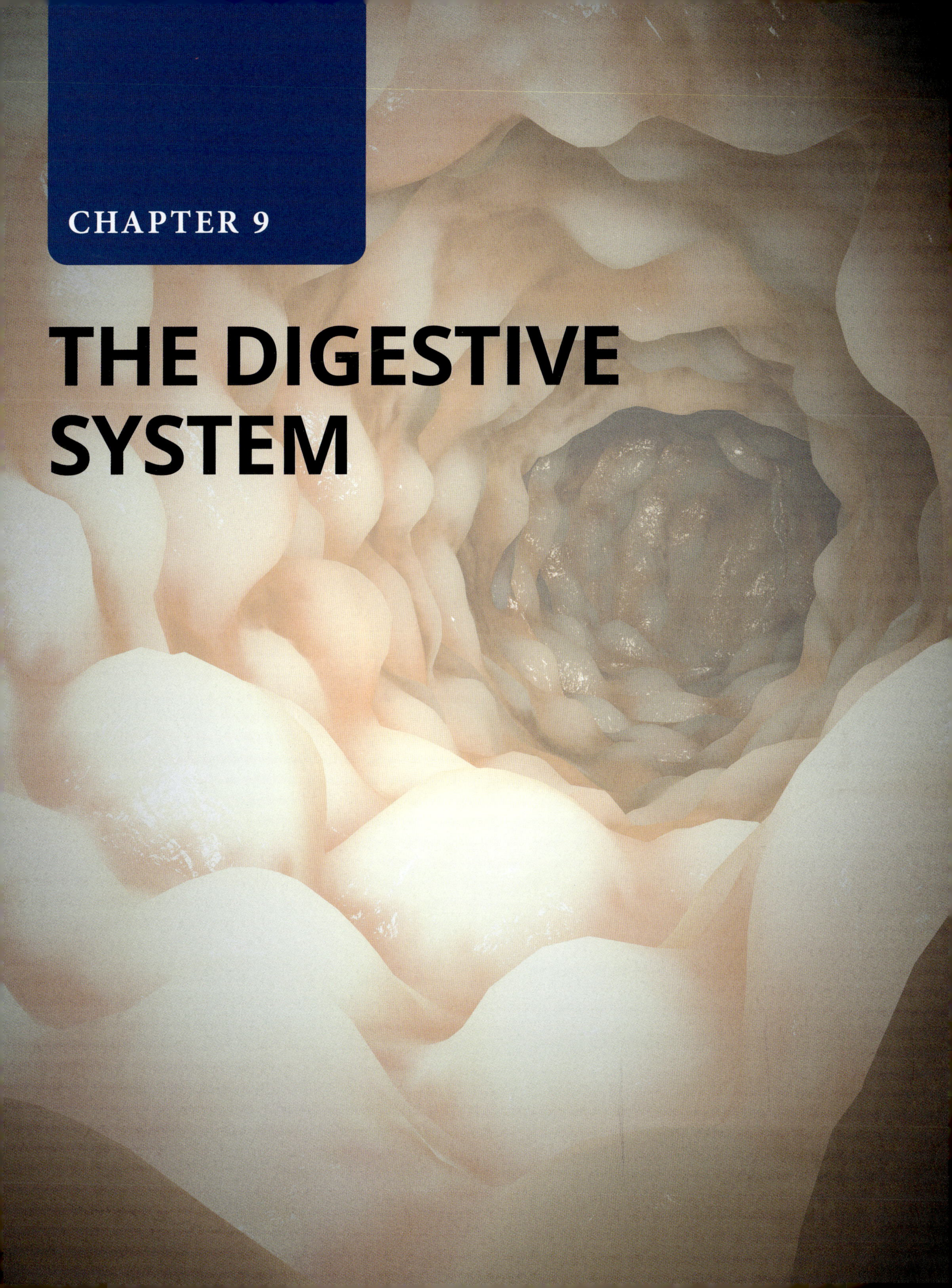

SCIENCE MASTERY ASSESSMENT

Every pre-med knows this feeling: there is so much content I have to know for the MCAT! How do I know what to do first or what's important?

While the high-yield badges throughout this book will help you identify the most important topics, this Science Mastery Assessment is another tool in your MCAT prep arsenal. This quiz (which can also be taken in your online resources) and the guidance below will help ensure that you are spending the appropriate amount of time on this chapter based on your personal strengths and weaknesses. Don't worry though—skipping something now does not mean you'll never study it. Later on in your prep, as you complete full-length tests, you'll uncover specific pieces of content that you need to review and can come back to these chapters as appropriate.

How to Use This Assessment

If you answer 0–7 questions correctly:

Spend about 1 hour to read this chapter in full and take limited notes throughout. Follow up by reviewing **all** quiz questions to ensure that you now understand how to solve each one.

If you answer 8–11 questions correctly:

Spend 20–40 minutes reviewing the quiz questions. Beginning with the questions you missed, read and take notes on the corresponding subchapters. For questions you answered correctly, ensure your thinking matches that of the explanation and you understand why each choice was correct or incorrect.

If you answer 12–15 questions correctly:

Spend less than 20 minutes reviewing all questions from the quiz. If you missed any, then include a quick read-through of the corresponding subchapters, or even just the relevant content within a subchapter, as part of your question review. For questions you answered correctly, ensure your thinking matches that of the explanation and review the Concept Summary at the end of the chapter.

1. Which of the following associations correctly matches a gastric cell with a compound it secretes?
   - **A.** G-cells—HCl
   - **B.** Chief cells—pepsinogen
   - **C.** Parietal cells—alkaline mucus
   - **D.** Mucous cells—intrinsic factor

2. Which of the following is NOT part of the small intestine?
   - **A.** Ileum
   - **B.** Cecum
   - **C.** Jejunum
   - **D.** Duodenum

3. In an experiment, enteropeptidase secretion was blocked. As a direct result, levels of all of the following active enzymes would likely be affected EXCEPT:
   - **A.** trypsin.
   - **B.** aminopeptidase.
   - **C.** chymotrypsin.
   - **D.** carboxypeptidase A.

4. Which of the following INCORRECTLY pairs a digestive enzyme with its function?
   - **A.** Trypsin—hydrolyzes specific peptide bonds
   - **B.** Lactase—hydrolyzes lactose to glucose and galactose
   - **C.** Pancreatic amylase—hydrolyzes starch to maltose
   - **D.** Lipase—emulsifies fats

5. Which of the following correctly lists two organs in which proteins are digested?
   - **A.** Mouth and stomach
   - **B.** Stomach and large intestine
   - **C.** Stomach and small intestine
   - **D.** Small intestine and large intestine

6. Which of the following choices INCORRECTLY pairs a digestive enzyme with its site of secretion?
   - **A.** Sucrase—salivary glands
   - **B.** Carboxypeptidase—pancreas
   - **C.** Trypsin—pancreas
   - **D.** Lactase—duodenum

7. A two-week-old infant is brought to the emergency room. The infant's caregiver reports that the infant has been unable to keep any milk down; shortly after nursing, the infant has sudden projectile vomiting. During exam, an olive-shaped mass can be felt in the infant's upper abdomen. It is determined that there is a constriction in the digestive system that prevents food from reaching the small intestine from the stomach. Which structure is most likely the site of the problem?
   - **A.** Cardiac sphincter
   - **B.** Pyloric sphincter
   - **C.** Ileocecal valve
   - **D.** Internal anal sphincter

8. Many medications have anticholinergic side effects, which block the activity of parasympathetic neurons throughout the body. Individuals who are older may be on many such medications simultaneously, exacerbating the side effects. Which of the following would NOT be expected in an individual taking medications with anticholinergic activity?
   - **A.** Dry mouth
   - **B.** Diarrhea
   - **C.** Slow gastric emptying
   - **D.** Decreased gastric acid production

9. The two graphs below show the relative activities of two enzymes in solutions of varying pH. Which of the following choices correctly identifies the two enzymes?

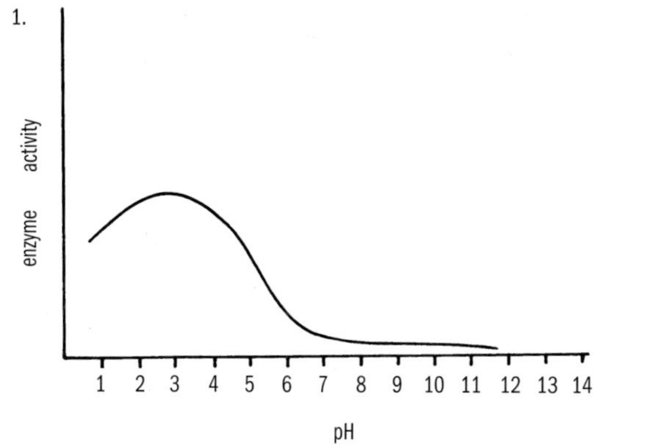

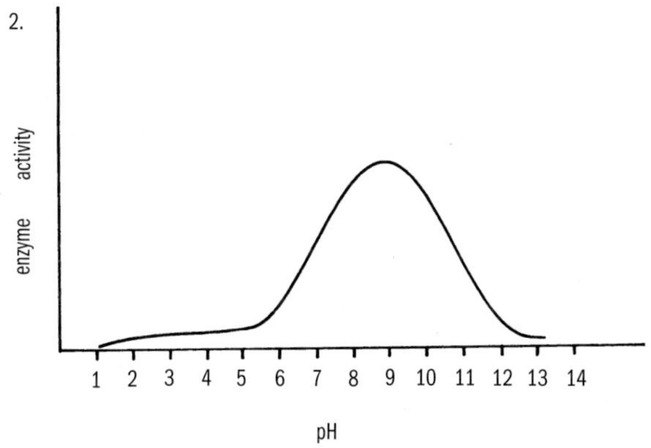

A. 1—chymotrypsin; 2—pepsin
B. 1—pepsin; 2—carboxypeptidase B
C. 1—lactase; 2—aminopeptidase
D. 1—enteropeptidase; 2—amylase

10. Which of the following would NOT likely lead to elevated levels of bilirubin in the blood?
A. Cholangiocarcinoma, a cancer of the bile ducts that can ultimately lead to full occlusion of the duct lumen
B. Autoimmune hemolytic anemia, a disease in which the red blood cells are attacked by antibodies and are lysed
C. Ménétrier's disease, in which rugae thicken and overlying glands lose secretory ability
D. Acetaminophen (Tylenol) overdose, in which the accumulation of toxic metabolites can cause rapid liver failure

11. Which of the following correctly pairs the molecule with its primary site of absorption?
A. Chylomicrons—lacteals
B. Amino acids—large intestine
C. Vitamins A and E—stomach
D. Cholesterol—ascending colon

12. The cleavage of fats into glycerol and fatty acids catalyzed by lipases in the lumen of the duodenum is best described as:
A. mechanical digestion.
B. chemical digestion.
C. intracellular digestion.
D. absorption.

13. Which of the following biomolecules does NOT drain into the liver before arriving at the right side of the heart?
A. Cholecalciferol (vitamin D)
B. Threonine (an amino acid)
C. Fructose (a monosaccharide)
D. Pantothenic acid (vitamin B_5)

14. Which of the following hormones increases feeding behavior?
A. Leptin
B. Cholecystokinin
C. Ghrelin
D. Gastrin

15. Which of the following is likely to be seen in a patient with liver failure?
A. High concentrations of urea in the blood
B. High concentrations of albumin in the blood
C. Low concentrations of ammonia in the blood
D. Low concentrations of clotting factors in the blood

Answer Key

1. **B** (See section 9.2)
2. **B** (See section 9.2)
3. **B** (See section 9.4)
4. **D** (See section 9.2)
5. **C** (See section 9.2)
6. **A** (See section 9.2)
7. **B** (See section 9.2)
8. **B** (See section 9.1)
9. **B** (See section 9.2)
10. **C** (See section 9.3)
11. **A** (See section 9.4)
12. **B** (See section 9.1)
13. **A** (See section 9.3)
14. **C** (See section 9.2)
15. **D** (See section 9.3)

The relevant section of the chapter to review for each question is given in parentheses after the correct answer. Detailed explanations can be found at the end of the chapter.

CHAPTER 9

THE DIGESTIVE SYSTEM

In This Chapter

CHAPTER PROFILE

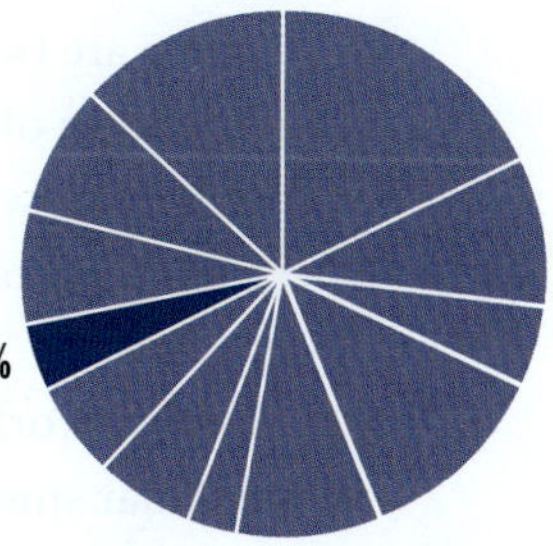

The content in this chapter should be relevant to about 4% of all questions about biology on the MCAT.

This chapter covers material from the following AAMC content category:

3B: Structure and integrative functions of the main organ systems

Introduction

As we continue our survey of organ systems, we now come to the digestive system. As with our previous reviews of other organ systems, we will start with a basic anatomical overview of the organs of digestion (including the accessory organs) and then move on to discuss how these organs function to provide nutrition to the individual. The food we eat is complex, incorporating meats, grains, vegetables and fruits, dairy products, and nuts. The job of the digestive system is to take these complex foods—composed of polysaccharides, fats, and proteins—and turn large macromolecules into smaller, simpler monosaccharides, fatty acids, and amino acids. In order to cleave all of these bonds, the body requires a complex system of mechanical and chemical agents. These compounds can then be absorbed from the gut, transported to the tissues by the circulatory system, and used by cells. In this chapter, we will consider the organs that make up the digestive system as well as the processes by which the foods we eat become the fuel we need for energy, growth, development, and maintenance of other essential activities.

9.1 Anatomy of the Digestive System

LEARNING OBJECTIVES

After Chapter 9.1, you will be able to:

- Describe mechanical and chemical digestion and differentiate between them
- Identify the interactions between the sympathetic and parasympathetic nervous systems and the digestive system
- Trace the path of food through the body, naming major organs and valves in the digestive tract

There are two types of digestion that occur. First, **intracellular digestion**, as a part of **metabolism**, involves the oxidation of glucose and fatty acids for energy. However, our diets do not consist of pure glucose and fatty acids; rather, these substances must be extracted from our food. The process by which these nutrients are obtained from food occurs within the lumen of the **alimentary canal** and is known as **extracellular digestion**. This is technically "outside" the body, because the lumen of the gastrointestinal tract communicates directly with the outside world. The alimentary canal runs from the **mouth** to the **anus** and is sectioned off by **sphincters**, or circular smooth muscles around the canal that can contract to allow compartmentalization of function.

The human digestive tract has specialized sections with different functional roles. The most basic functional distinction is between digestion and absorption. **Digestion** involves the breakdown of food into its constituent organic molecules: starches and other carbohydrates into monosaccharides, lipids (fats) into free fatty acids and glycerol, and proteins into amino acids. Digestion can be subdivided into mechanical and chemical processes. **Mechanical digestion** is the physical breakdown of large food particles into smaller food particles, but does not involve breaking chemical bonds. **Chemical digestion** is the enzymatic cleavage of chemical bonds, such as the peptide bonds of proteins or the glycosidic bonds of starches. The specific mechanical and chemical digestive processes that occur in the major organs of the digestive tract are summarized in Table 9.1. **Absorption** involves the transport of products of digestion from the digestive tract into the circulatory system for distribution to the body's tissues and cells.

Organ	Mechanical Digestion	Chemical Digestion
Mouth	Chewing (mastication) by teeth Tongue mixes food	Salivary amylase breaks down starch into maltose
Stomach	Churning and mixing by muscular contractions	Pepsin breaks down proteins into peptides Hydrochloric acid (HCl) aids enzyme activity
Small intestine	Segmentation (mixes chyme) Peristalsis (moves food along)	Enzymes from pancreas and intestinal lining break down carbohydrates, proteins, and fats: • Amylase → sugars • Proteases → amino acids • Lipase → fatty acids and glycerol

Table 9.1 Mechanical and Chemical Digestion in the Mouth, Stomach, and Small Intestine

The digestive tract, shown in Figure 9.1, begins with the **oral cavity** (mouth) followed by the **pharynx**, a shared pathway for both food entering the digestive system and air entering the respiratory system. From the pharynx, food enters the **esophagus**, which transports it to the **stomach**. From the stomach, food travels to the **small intestine**, and then to the **large intestine**. Finally, waste products of digestion enter the **rectum**, where feces are stored until an appropriate time of release. In addition to the digestive tract itself, the **salivary glands**, **pancreas**, **liver**, and **gallbladder** help to provide the enzymes and lubrication necessary to aid in the digestion of food.

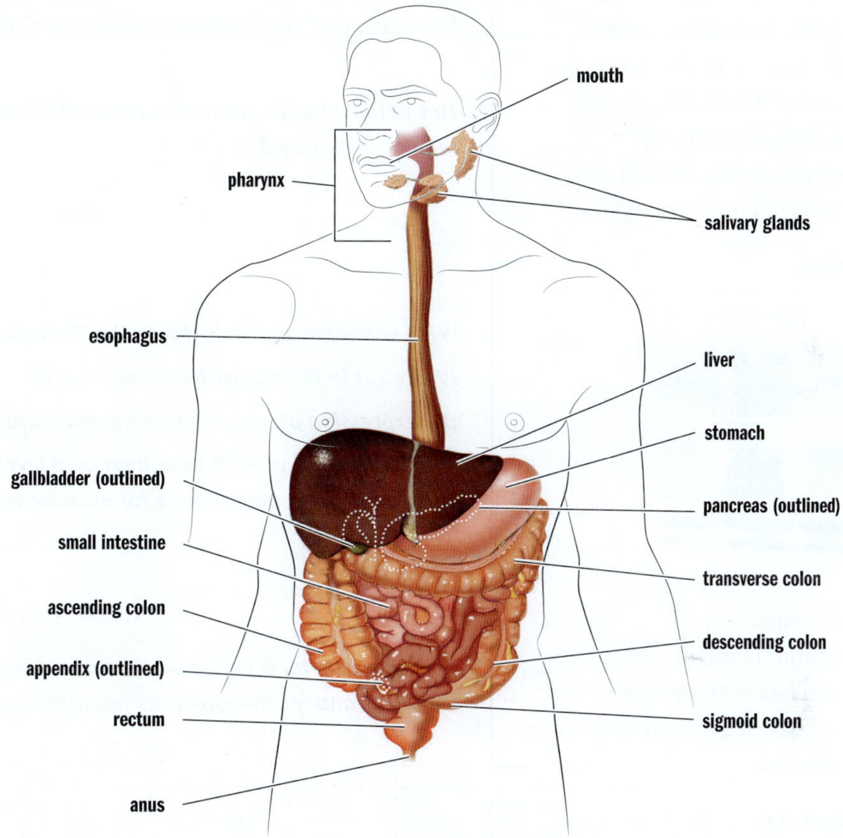

Figure 9.1 Anatomy of the Digestive System

The **enteric nervous system** is a collection of one hundred million neurons that govern the function of the gastrointestinal system. These neurons are present in the walls of the digestive tract and trigger **peristalsis**, or rhythmic contractions of the gut tube, in order to move materials through the system. This system can function independently of the brain and spinal cord, although it is heavily regulated by the autonomic nervous system. The parasympathetic division is involved in stimulation of digestive activities, increasing secretions from exocrine glands and promoting peristalsis. The sympathetic division is involved in the inhibition of these activities. The fact that so often we feel sleepy and lethargic after eating a big meal (often called a *food coma* colloquially) is due, in part, to parasympathetic activity. On the other hand, during periods of high sympathetic activity, bloodflow is decreased to the digestive tract, and gut motility slows significantly.

KEY CONCEPT

All of the glands of the body (except sweat glands) are innervated by the parasympathetic nervous system.

BIOLOGY GUIDED EXAMPLE WITH EXPERT THINKING

Bile acids are crucial for the intestinal absorption of dietary fatty acids, of cholesterol, and of fat-soluble vitamins.

This is just background information

To determine whether the interruption of the enterohepatic circulation of bile acids alters triglyceride and glucose metabolism, researchers

Purpose: determine whether removing bile acids changes metabolism

tested ileal sodium-dependent bile acid transporter (Slc10a2) KO mice.

A new abbreviation "KO" is here, but the next sentence says "knocking out", so I know this must stand for "Knock Out"

Over 95% of intestinal bile acid is absorbed and returned to the liver; thus, knocking out Slc10a2 should dramatically reduce the total pool of bile acid in the body (approx. 80% reduction). In addition, some mice were fed a sucrose-rich (SR) diet to simulate the metabolic stress of an unhealthy diet.

This details the IVs: normal vs reduced bile acids and regular vs sugary diet

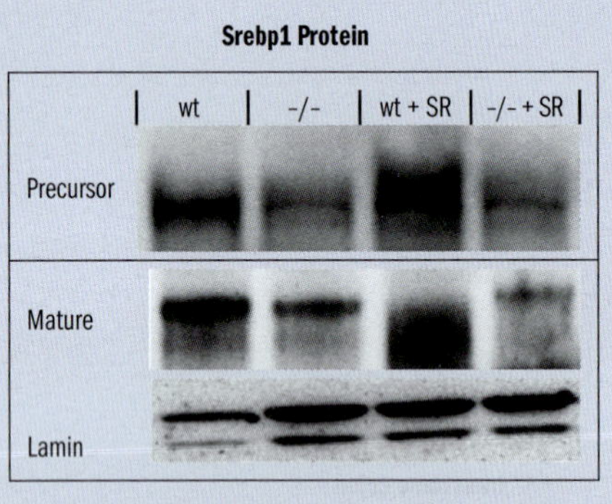

WT is wild-type and -/- is the KO, so SR must be the diet

IV: Srebp1 in WT, KO, with and without SR

DV: expression of precursor and mature protein

Trends: WT mice with SR have increased levels of protein; there is no noticeable change for KO mice with or without SR

Figure 1 Expression of sterol regulatory element-binding protein 1 (Srebp1) Protein Immunoblot. The transcription factor Srebp1c is crucial for optimal activation of most genes in fatty acid synthesis and gluconeogenesis.

This is testing for a new protein involved in fatty acid synthesis and gluconeogenesis (metabolic protein)

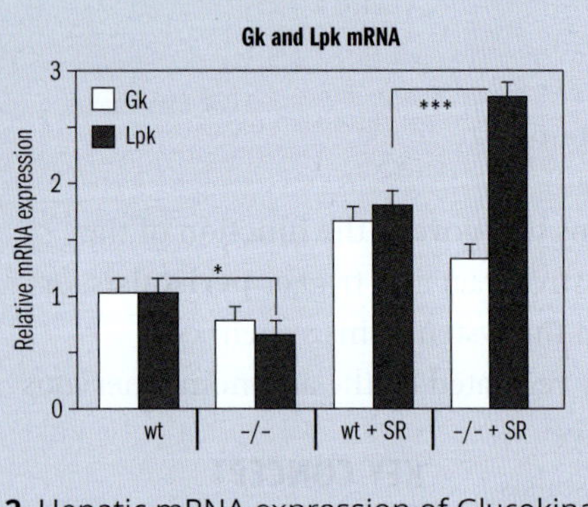

IVs: Gk and Lpk in WT and KO with and without diet (SR)

DV: relative mRNA expression

Trend: Lpk is signficantly lower in KO mice without the diet and significantly higher in KO mice with the diet

Figure 2 Hepatic mRNA expression of Glucokinase (Gk) and Liver Pyruvate Kinase (Lpk)

Adapted from Lundåsen T, Andersson E-M, Snaith M, Lindmark H, Lundberg J, Östlund-Lindqvist A-M, et al. (2012) Inhibition of intestinal bile acid transporter Slc10a2 improves triglyceride metabolism and normalizes elevated plasma glucose levels in mice. *PLoS One* 7(5): e37787. https://doi.org/10.1371/journal.pone.0037787.

Would reducing the total pool of bile acid be a good strategy to combat the hypertriglyceridemia and diabetes induced by an unhealthy diet?

This question asks whether an action, reducing the total pool of bile acid, would have a specified impact on two conditions, hypertriglyceridemia and diabetes. To answer this question, we must assess the data we are given in the article regarding how changing bile acid quantity affects traits and outcomes associated with those conditions.

We should start by making sure we're comfortable with the terms used in the question, relying on either the article or our critical thinking skills to fill our knowledge gaps. Hypertriglyceridemia is a condition when blood triglyceride levels are too high, and diabetes is a condition when blood glucose levels are too high. However, that information wasn't given to us in the passage, and it's not entirely in scope for Test Day—so how could we figure out what we need to know to answer this question? Even if we didn't know this, though, we know the mice were fed food to simulate an unhealthy diet that would supply them with too much sugar, and we should recognize at least diabetes as a metabolic disorder linked with sugar metabolism. We should also recognize that triglycerides are fats, so this is probably a condition involving fat metabolism. Thus, we can assume that any action that lowers blood triglycerides (relating to hypertriglyceridemia) and blood glucose (relating to diabetes) could constitute a potentially beneficial therapy for these two conditions. So, when we look at the data for the experimental mice as compared to controls, we should be looking for changes related to these two metabolic pathways to determine if there are possible treatment implications for reducing bile salt concentrations in order to treat these conditions.

According to the passage, the knockout mice do not have the bile acid transporter, meaning that the pool of available bile acid in their system should be significantly lower. There's also a second variable, diet, which should be simulating mice that are experiencing metabolic stressors in the sucrose-rich condition as compared to normal metabolic function. Figure 1 shows the concentration of a protein involved in fatty acid synthesis in the KO mice versus wild-type mice, with both normal and sucrose-rich diets. In the wild-type mice, we can see that the addition of a metabolically stressful, high-sugar diet (lane 3) leads to a big increase in production of that protein as compared to regular diet (lane 1). However, in the knockout mice, there's no perceivable change from the regular diet (lane 2) to the sucrose-rich diet (lane 4). This is true both for the actual protein and the precursor, which means that the KO mouse is just not transcribing as much of that metabolic protein. The lamin lane down at the bottom seems like it's just a control for protein expression, and it looks pretty much the same across the board, so we can ignore it in our data analysis. Based on this figure, which is all about a metabolic protein in the fatty acid synthesis chain, it looks like the knockout mice just aren't experiencing the same amount of metabolic stress; they're not trying to turn that extra sucrose into fatty acids. Based on this piece of data, it looks like reducing bile acid might be one way to relieve the metabolic stress associated with hypertriglyceridemia, or at least, it's worth more investigation!

Moving on, Figure 2 shows the same conditions, but is measuring mRNA production of two different proteins: glucokinase and pyruvate kinase. Even if we aren't exactly sure of what those enzymes do, they have glucose and pyruvate in their names, so it sounds like they are probably involved in the sugar metabolism pathway. Looking at the figure, we can see in the first two pairs of columns that wild-type mice are expressing more mRNA for both of these proteins than KO mice. After metabolic stress is added, it looks like pyruvate kinase production specifically spikes within the KO mice. That seems to indicate that these mice are responding to the metabolic stress to an even greater extent (in terms of Lpk) than the wild-type mice. Without directly measuring the level of blood glucose, we cannot determine whether that increased metabolic response represents a positive or negative trend. So, unlike the data in Figure 1, it looks like bile salt reduction may not be a good treatment option for diabetic individuals, and we may even need to reevaluate whether it would be truly helpful for those with triglyceridemia, as the energetic processing of fats can't be considered as fully separate from the processing of sugars.

Overall, our takeaway is that we have mixed results. Figure 1 made the reduction of bile salts look like a promising treatment for triglyceridemia, but Figure 2 indicates that reducing bile salts may not be effective in treating diabetes. We can conclude that more data is needed to assess this therapy's effect on sugar and lipid metabolism.

MCAT CONCEPT CHECK 9.1

Before you move on, assess your understanding of the material with these questions.

1. What is the difference between mechanical and chemical digestion?
   - Mechanical digestion:

     ____

   - Chemical digestion:

     ____

2. Trace the path of food through the body, starting with ingestion and ending with excretion of feces:

   ____

3. What effect does the parasympathetic nervous system have on the digestive system? What effect does the sympathetic nervous system have?
   - Parasympathetic nervous system:

     ____

   - Sympathetic nervous system:

     ____

9.2 Ingestion and Digestion

LEARNING OBJECTIVES

After Chapter 9.2, you will be able to:

- Identify the secretory cells of the digestive tract, their secretions, and the function of their secretions
- Explain how bile and pancreatic lipase work together to digest fats
- Recall the key digestive enzymes and hormones produced in saliva, the stomach, and the intestines, and summarize the function of each

To supply the body with nutrients, we must **ingest** (eat) food. Several hormones are involved with feeding behavior, including antidiuretic hormone (ADH or vasopressin), aldosterone, glucagon, ghrelin, leptin, and cholecystokinin. ADH and aldosterone trigger the sensation of thirst, encouraging the behavior of fluid consumption. Glucagon, secreted by the pancreas, and **ghrelin**, secreted by the stomach and pancreas, stimulate feelings of hunger. **Leptin** and **cholecystokinin** do the opposite, stimulating feelings of satiety. Digestion begins in the oral cavity and continues in the stomach and the first part of the small intestine, known as the duodenum.

Oral Cavity

The **oral cavity** plays a role in both mechanical and chemical digestion of food. Mechanical digestion in the mouth involves the breaking up of large food particles into smaller particles using the teeth, tongue, and lips. This process is called **mastication** (chewing). Chewing helps to increase the surface area-to-volume ratio of the food, creating more surface area for enzymatic digestion as it passes through the gut tube. It also moderates the size of food particles entering the lumen of the alimentary canal; food particles that are too large create an obstruction risk in the tract.

KEY CONCEPT

The chemical digestion of carbohydrates occurs in both the mouth and small intestine, with the two amylases targeting complementary starches. Salivary amylase (active in the mouth) has a higher specificity for rapidly soluble starches, while pancreatic amylase (active in the small intestine) has a higher specificity for less soluble, more nonpolar starches.

Chemical digestion is the breakdown of chemical bonds in the macromolecules that make up food. This relies on enzymes from **saliva** produced by the three pairs of **salivary glands**. These three glands, shown in Figure 9.2, are the parotid, sublingual, and submandibular glands. Saliva also aids mechanical digestion by moistening and lubricating food. The salivary glands, like all glands of the digestive tract, are innervated by the parasympathetic nervous system. The presence of food in the oral cavity triggers a neural circuit that ultimately leads to increased parasympathetic stimulation of these glands. Salivation can also be triggered by signals that food is near, such as smell or sight. Saliva contains *salivary amylase*, also known as *ptyalin*, and *lipase*. **Salivary amylase** is capable of hydrolyzing starch into smaller sugars (maltose and dextrins), while **lipase** catalyzes the hydrolysis of lipids. The amount of chemical digestion that occurs in the mouth is minimal, though, because the food does not stay in the mouth for long. Our muscular tongue forms the food into a **bolus**, which is forced back to the pharynx and swallowed.

REAL WORLD

There are three pairs of major salivary glands: the parotid, submandibular, and sublingual glands. Other microscopic salivary glands are scattered throughout the upper digestive system. While the parasympathetic nervous system is responsible for promoting salivation, the sympathetic nervous system has some input into the glands as well. The sympathetic nervous system increases the viscosity of saliva, which is why dry mouth and even a tacky sensation in the mouth occurs during a fight-or-flight response.

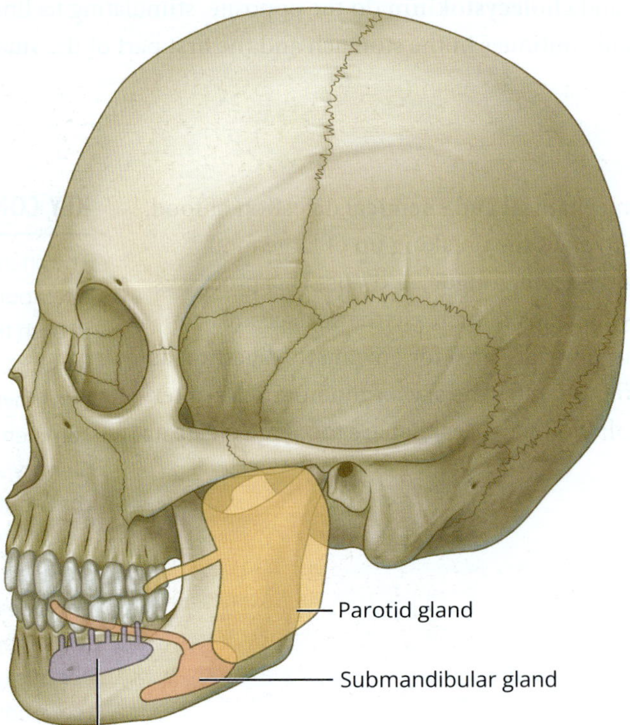

Figure 9.2 Salivary Glands

Pharynx

The **pharynx** is the cavity that leads from the mouth and posterior nasal cavity to the esophagus. The pharynx connects not only to the esophagus, but also to the larynx, which is a part of the respiratory tract. The pharynx can be divided into three parts: the **nasopharynx** (behind the nasal cavity), the **oropharynx** (at the back of the mouth), and the **laryngopharynx** (above the vocal cords). Food is prevented from entering the larynx during swallowing by the **epiglottis**, a cartilaginous structure that folds down to cover the laryngeal inlet. Failure of this mechanism can lead to aspiration of food and choking.

Esophagus

The **esophagus** is a muscular tube that connects the pharynx to the stomach. The top third of the esophagus is composed of skeletal muscle, the bottom third is composed of smooth muscle, and the middle third is a mix of both. What does this mean in terms of nervous control? While the top of the esophagus is under somatic (voluntary) motor control, the bottom—and most of the rest of the gastrointestinal tract, for that matter—is under autonomic (involuntary) nervous control. The rhythmic contraction of smooth muscle that propels food toward the stomach is called **peristalsis**. Under normal circumstances, peristalsis proceeds down the digestive tract. However, certain factors such as exposure to chemicals, infectious agents, physical stimulation in the posterior pharynx, and even cognitive stimulation, can lead to reversal of peristalsis in the process of **emesis (vomiting)**.

Swallowing is initiated in the muscles of the oropharynx, which constitute the **upper esophageal sphincter**. Peristalsis (see Figure 9.3) is simply a series of relaxations and contractions: the smooth muscle constricts on one end of the bolus while the other side relaxes, which results in movement of the bolus. As the bolus approaches the stomach, a muscular ring known as the **lower esophageal sphincter** (**cardiac sphincter**) relaxes and opens to allow the passage of food.

REAL WORLD

Weakness in the lower esophageal sphincter is a key feature of gastroesophageal reflux disease (GERD), which causes classic heartburn symptoms after eating. As food and acid reflux into the lower esophagus, they irritate the less-protected mucosa, stimulating pain receptors. These receptors localize pain poorly, so a general burning sensation is felt in the lower chest—leading to the common term *heartburn*.

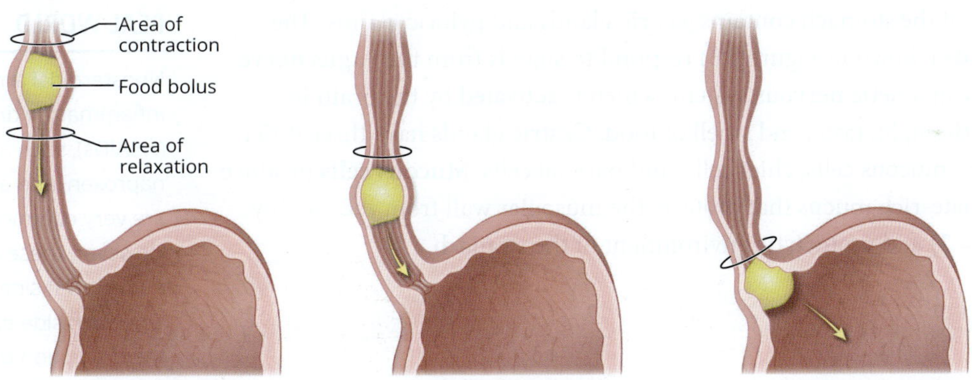

Figure 9.3 Peristalsis

Stomach

There are three main energy sources: carbohydrates, fats, and proteins. As mentioned earlier, the chemical digestion of carbohydrates and fats is initiated in the mouth. No mechanical or chemical digestion takes place in the esophagus, except for the continued enzymatic activity initiated in the mouth by salivary enzymes. Thus, digestion that occurs prior to the entrance of the bolus into the stomach is minimal compared to the digestion that occurs in the stomach and small intestine.

The **stomach** is a highly muscular organ with a capacity of approximately two liters. In humans, the stomach is located in the upper left quadrant of the abdominal cavity, underneath the diaphragm. This organ uses hydrochloric acid and enzymes to digest food, creating a fairly harsh environment. Therefore, its mucosa is quite thick to prevent autodigestion. The stomach can be divided into four main anatomical divisions, as shown in Figure 9.4: the **fundus** and **body**, which contain mostly gastric glands, and the **antrum** and **pylorus,** which contain mostly pyloric glands. The internal curvature of the stomach is called the **lesser curvature**; the external curvature is called the **greater curvature**. The lining of the stomach is thrown into folds called **rugae**.

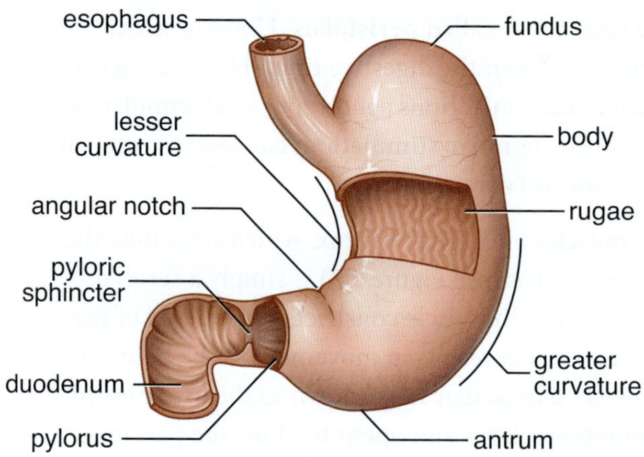

Figure 9.4 Anatomy of the Stomach

The mucosa of the stomach contains gastric glands and pyloric glands. The **gastric glands** (shown in Figure 9.5) respond to signals from the **vagus nerve** of the parasympathetic nervous system, which is activated by the brain in response to the sight, taste, and smell of food. Gastric glands have three different cell types: mucous cells, chief cells, and parietal cells. **Mucous cells** produce the bicarbonate-rich mucus that protects the muscular wall from the harshly acidic (pH = 2) and proteolytic environment of the stomach.

REAL WORLD

Nonsteroidal anti-inflammatory drugs (NSAIDs), such as ibuprofen, naproxen, and aspirin, are very common drugs. However, these drugs are not without side effects. One such side effect is the disruption of mucus production within the stomach. This leaves the mucosa of the stomach unprotected, and irritation results. This irritation can be in the form of *gastritis*, inflammation of the mucosa of the stomach, or *gastric ulcers*, deep wounds in the lining of the stomach.

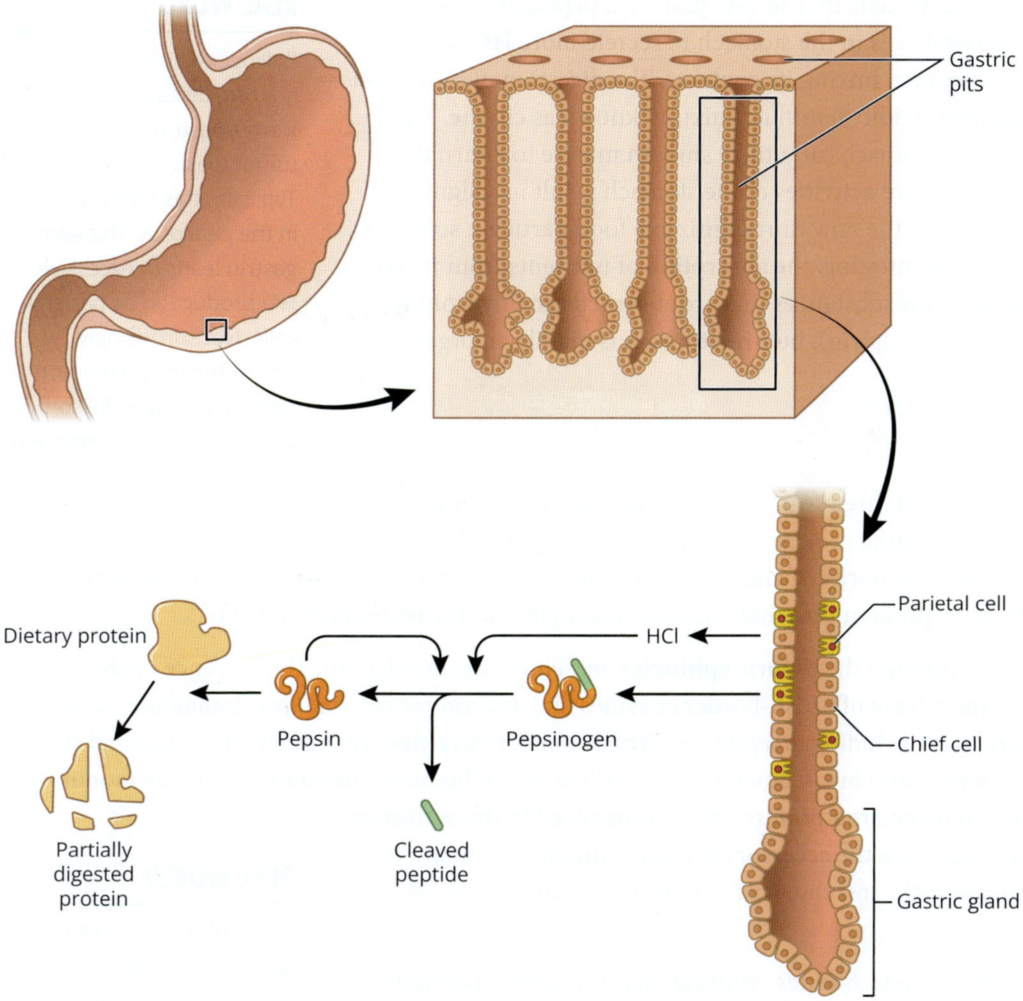

Figure 9.5 Gastric Glands Aiding in Digestion

Gastric juice is a combination of secretions from the other two cell types in the gastric glands: chief cells and parietal cells. The **chief cells** secrete ***pepsinogen***. This is the inactive, **zymogen** form of *pepsin*, a proteolytic enzyme. Hydrogen ions in the stomach, secreted by **parietal cells** as hydrochloric acid, cleave pepsinogen to pepsin. **Pepsin** digests proteins by cleaving peptide bonds near aromatic amino acids, resulting in short peptide fragments. Because pepsin is activated by the acidic environment, it follows that pepsin is most active at a low pH. This is a unique characteristic among human enzymes, as most human enzymes are most active at physiological pH. Stomach acid also kills most harmful bacteria (with the exception of *Helicobacter pylori*, infection with which is usually asymptomatic but can cause inflammation, ulcers, and even certain gastric cancers). The acidic environment also helps to denature proteins and can break down some intramolecular bonds that hold food together. In addition to HCl, parietal cells secrete **intrinsic factor**, a glycoprotein involved in the proper absorption of vitamin B_{12}.

KEY CONCEPT

The stomach secretes six products:

1. HCl (kills microbes, denatures proteins, and converts pepsinogen into pepsin)
2. Pepsinogen (cleaved in the stomach to pepsin; an enzyme that partially digests proteins)
3. Mucus (protects mucosa)
4. Bicarbonate (protects mucosa)
5. Water (dissolves and dilutes ingested material)
6. Intrinsic factor (required for normal absorption of vitamin B_{12})

The **pyloric glands** contain **G-cells** that secrete gastrin, a peptide hormone. **Gastrin** induces the parietal cells in the stomach to secrete more HCl and signals the stomach to contract, mixing its contents. The digestion of solid food in the stomach results in an acidic, semifluid mixture known as **chyme**. The combined mechanical (the stomach can utilize smooth muscle to churn the mixture) and chemical digestive activities of the stomach result in a significant increase in the surface area of the now unrecognizable food particles, so when the chyme reaches the small intestine, the absorption of nutrients from it can be maximized. There are a few substances that are absorbed directly from the stomach (such as alcohol and aspirin), but the stomach is mainly an organ of digestion.

REAL WORLD

Zollinger–Ellison syndrome is a rare disease resulting from a gastrin-secreting tumor (gastrinoma). Typically, this tumor is found in the pancreas. The excess gastrin leads to excessive HCl production by parietal cells. Not surprisingly, one of the most common signs of Zollinger–Ellison syndrome is the presence of intractable ulcer disease.

Duodenum

The **small intestine** consists of three segments: the duodenum, the jejunum, and the ileum. The small intestine is quite long, up to seven meters. The duodenum is responsible for the majority of chemical digestion and has some minor involvement in absorption. However, most of the absorption in the small intestine takes place in the jejunum and ileum.

Food leaves the stomach through the **pyloric sphincter** and enters the duodenum. The presence of chyme in the duodenum causes the release of brush-border enzymes like *disaccharidases* (*maltase*, *isomaltase*, *lactase*, and *sucrase*) and *peptidases* (including *dipeptidase*). **Brush-border enzymes** are present on the luminal surface of cells lining the duodenum and break down dimers and trimers of biomolecules into absorbable monomers. The duodenum also secretes *enteropeptidase*, which is involved in the activation of other digestive enzymes from the accessory organs of digestion. Finally, it secretes hormones like secretin and cholecystokinin (CCK) into the bloodstream.

The **disaccharidases** digest disaccharides. **Maltase** digests maltose, **isomaltase** digests isomaltose, **lactase** digests lactose, and **sucrase** digests sucrose. Lack of a particular disaccharidase causes an inability to break down the corresponding disaccharide. Then bacteria in the intestines are able to hydrolyze that disaccharide, producing methane gas as a byproduct. In addition, undigested disaccharides can have an osmotic effect, pulling water into the stool and causing diarrhea. This is why people who are lactose intolerant have symptoms of bloating, flatulence, and possibly diarrhea after ingesting dairy products.

Peptidases break down proteins (or peptides, as the name implies). **Aminopeptidase** is a peptidase secreted by glands in the duodenum that removes the N-terminal amino acid from a peptide. **Dipeptidases** cleave the peptide bonds of dipeptides to release free amino acids. Unlike carbohydrates, which must be broken down into monosaccharides for absorption, proteins can be broken down into di- and even tripeptides and can be absorbed across the small intestine wall.

REAL WORLD

Celiac disease results from an immune reaction against gluten, a protein found in grains, especially wheat. In this condition, the immune system develops antibodies against certain components of gluten. These antibodies then cross-react with elements of the small intestine, causing damage to the mucosa. This results in diarrhea and discomfort. Sometimes, this condition also results in malabsorptive syndromes, including the inability to absorb fat and fat-soluble vitamins. Contrary to popular belief, celiac disease and gluten sensitivity are immune conditions, but not true allergies.

Enteropeptidase (formerly called ***enterokinase***) is an enzyme critical for the activation of ***trypsinogen***, a pancreatic protease, to ***trypsin***. Trypsin then initiates an activation cascade, as described later in this chapter. Trypsin can also activate ***procarboxypeptidases A*** and ***B*** to their active forms.

Secretin is a peptide hormone that causes pancreatic enzymes to be released into the duodenum. It also regulates the pH of the digestive tract by reducing HCl secretion from parietal cells and increasing bicarbonate secretion from the pancreas. Secretin is also an **enterogastrone**, a hormone that slows motility through the digestive tract. Slowing of motility allows increased time for digestive enzymes to act on chyme—especially fats.

Finally, **cholecystokinin** (**CCK**) is secreted in response to the entry of chyme (specifically, amino acids and fat in the chyme) into the duodenum. This peptide hormone stimulates the release of both bile and pancreatic juices and also acts in the brain, where it promotes satiety. **Bile** is a complex fluid composed of bile salts, pigments, and cholesterol. **Bile salts** are derived from cholesterol. They are not enzymes and therefore do not directly perform chemical digestion (the enzymatic cleavage of chemical bonds). However, bile salts serve an important role in the mechanical digestion of fats and ultimately facilitate the chemical digestion of lipids. Bile salts have hydrophobic and hydrophilic regions, allowing them to serve as a bridge between aqueous and lipid environments. In fact, bile salts are much like the common soaps and detergents we use to wash our hands, clothes, and dishes. In the small intestine, bile salts **emulsify** fats and cholesterol into smaller droplets. Without bile, fats would spontaneously separate out of the aqueous mixture in the duodenum and would not be accessible to pancreatic lipase, which is water-soluble. These emulsified droplets increase the surface area of the fats, increasing the rate at which lipase can act. After lipase hydrolyzes the ester bonds in triglycerides, the resulting monoglycerides and free fatty acids are incorporated into **micelles**—small transport structures formed by bile salts (see Figure 9.6). A micelle can be thought of as a little hydrophobic "bubble" that can navigate through hydrophilic environments. Micelles facilitate the absorption of lipids by ferrying them to the intestinal lining. Thus, proper fat digestion depends on both bile (for emulsification and transport) and lipase (for chemical breakdown of fats).

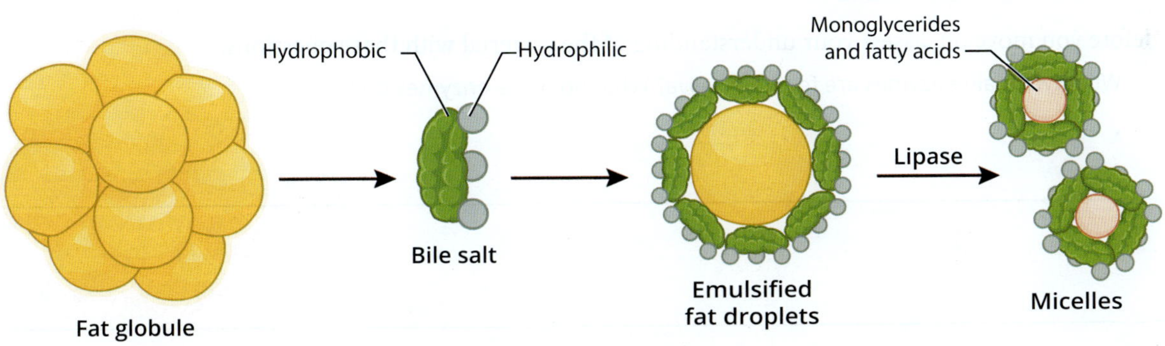

Figure 9.6 Micelle Formation

CCK also promotes the secretion of pancreatic juices into the duodenum, as shown in Figure 9.7. **Pancreatic juices** are a complex mixture of several enzymes in a bicarbonate-rich alkaline solution. This bicarbonate helps to neutralize acidic chyme, as well as provide an ideal working environment for the digestive enzymes, which are most active around pH 8.5. Pancreatic juices contain enzymes that can digest all three types of nutrients: carbohydrates, fats, and proteins. The identities and functions of these enzymes will be discussed in the next section of this chapter.

BRIDGE

The acidic environment of the stomach and basic environment of the duodenum point out the important correlation between pH and enzyme activity. Pepsin is active in the stomach and works best at pH 2. Pancreatic enzymes are active in the duodenum and work best at pH 8.5. pH, temperature, and salinity can all affect enzyme function, as highlighted in Chapter 2 of *MCAT Biochemistry Review*.

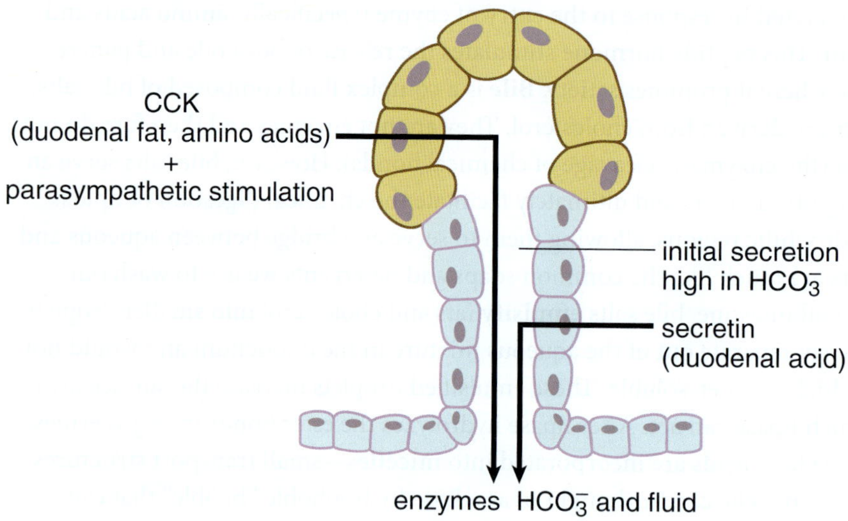

Figure 9.7 Hormonal Control of the Exocrine Pancreas

MCAT CONCEPT CHECK 9.2

Before you move on, assess your understanding of the material with these questions.

1. What two main enzymes are found in saliva? What do these enzymes do?
   -
   -

2. For each of the cell types below, list the major secretions of the cell and the functions of these secretions.

Cell	Secretions	Functions
Mucous cell		
Chief cell		
Parietal cell		
G-cell		

3. For each of the following substances, determine whether it is a digestive enzyme or a hormone and briefly summarize its functions.

Substance	Enzyme or Hormone?	Functions
Sucrase		
Secretin		
Dipeptidase		
Cholecystokinin		
Enteropeptidase		

4. How do bile and pancreatic lipase work together to digest fats?

____

9.3 Accessory Organs of Digestion

LEARNING OBJECTIVES

After Chapter 9.3, you will be able to:

- Recall the pancreatic enzymes and the molecules they help to digest
- Describe the significance and the function of bile, including its production, components, and release
- List the major functions of the liver
- Associate the accessory organs of digestion with their germ layer of origin

Digestion is a complex process that requires the release of enzymes not only from the cells directly lining the alimentary canal, but also from the pancreas, liver, and gallbladder. Collectively, these organs—which all originate as outgrowths of endoderm from the gut tube during development—are called **accessory organs of digestion**.

REAL WORLD

Pancreatitis, or inflammation of the pancreas, is usually caused by gallstones or excessive consumption of alcohol. Regardless of the cause, pancreatitis results from premature activation of pancreatic enzymes and autodigestion of the pancreatic tissue. This is a very painful condition that may result in a long hospital stay and long-term consequences such as diabetes and the reduced digestion of proteins and fats.

Pancreas

The pancreas serves two quite different roles in the body, reflecting its exocrine and endocrine functions. As discussed in Chapter 5 of *MCAT Biology Review*, the endocrine functions of the pancreas include the release of insulin, glucagon, and somatostatin—peptide hormones necessary for the maintenance of proper blood sugar levels. The hormonal function of the pancreas is limited to cells residing in islets of Langerhans scattered throughout the organ. The bulk of the pancreas, however, is made of exocrine cells called **acinar cells** that produce pancreatic juices. As mentioned earlier, pancreatic juices are bicarbonate-rich alkaline secretions containing many digestive enzymes that work on all three classes of biomolecules (sugars, fats, and proteins). ***Pancreatic amylase*** breaks down large polysaccharides into small disaccharides and is therefore responsible for carbohydrate digestion. As shown in Figure 9.8, the pancreatic peptidases (***trypsinogen***, ***chymotrypsinogen***, and ***carboxypeptidases A*** and ***B***) are released in their zymogen form, but once activated are responsible for protein digestion. Enteropeptidase, produced by the duodenum, is the master switch. It converts trypsinogen to trypsin, which can then activate the other zymogens, and also activates procarboxypeptidases A and B. Finally, the pancreas secretes ***pancreatic lipase***, which is capable of breaking down fats into free fatty acids and glycerol.

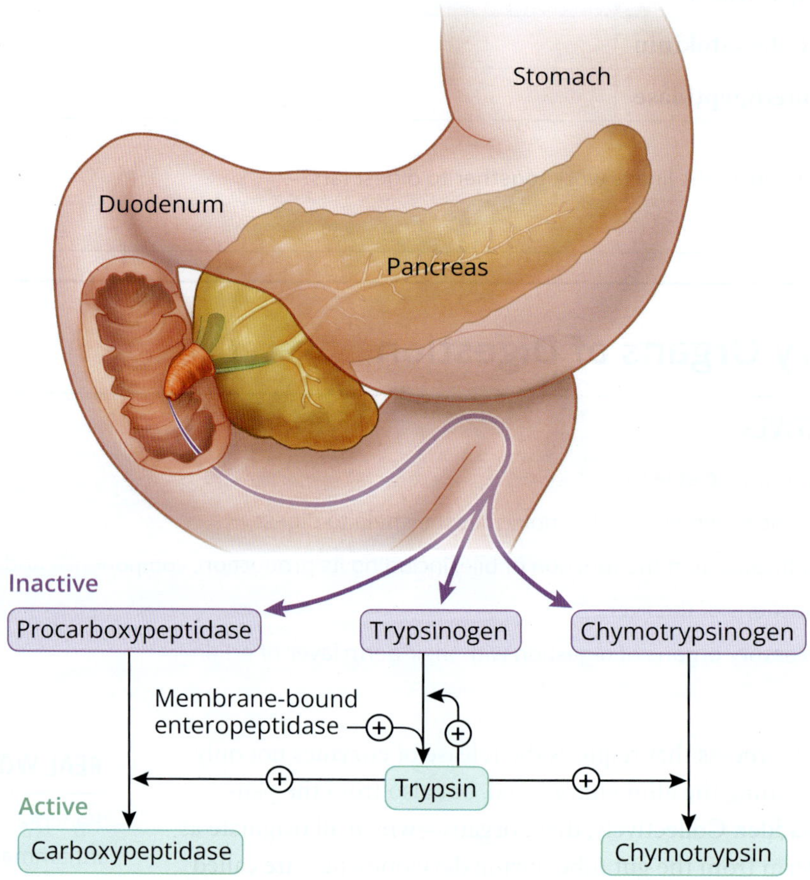

Figure 9.8 Pancreatic Enzyme Activation Cascade

Pancreatic juices are transferred to the duodenum via a duct system that runs along the middle of the pancreas, as shown in Figure 9.9. Like all exocrine cells, acinar cells secrete their products into ducts. These ducts then empty into the duodenum through the **major** and **minor duodenal papillae**.

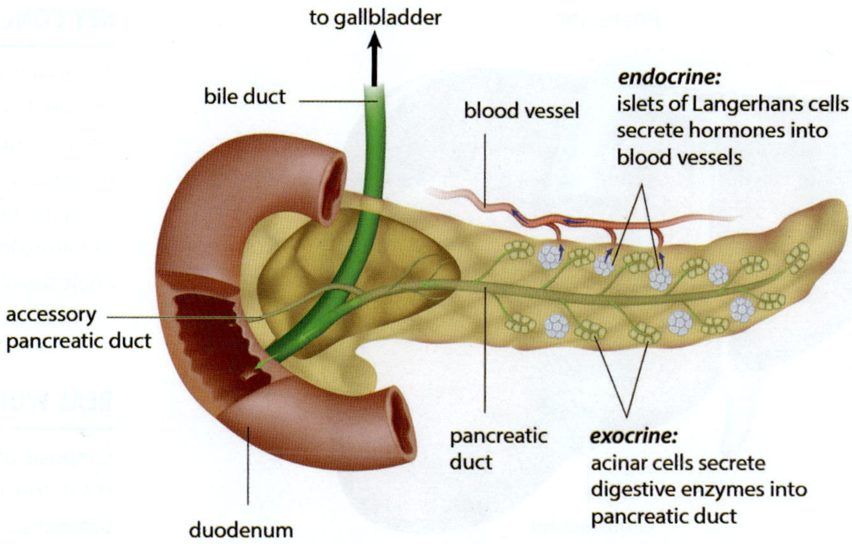

Figure 9.9 Anatomy of the Pancreas

Liver

The **liver** is located in the upper right quadrant of the abdomen and contains two unique structures for communicating with the digestive system. First, **bile ducts** connect the liver with both the gallbladder and small intestine. Bile is produced in the liver and travels down these bile ducts where it may be stored in the gallbladder (the gallbladder's and liver's connection and blood supply is visualized in Figure 9.10) or secreted into the duodenum. The liver also receives all blood draining from the abdominal portion of the digestive tract through the **hepatic portal vein**. This nutrient-rich blood can be processed by the liver before draining into the inferior vena cava on its way to the right side of the heart. For example, the liver takes up excess sugar to create **glycogen**, the storage form of glucose, and stores fats as **triacylglycerols**. The liver can also reverse these processes, producing glucose for the rest of the body through **glycogenolysis** and **gluconeogenesis** and mobilizing fats in **lipoproteins**.

KEY CONCEPT

The functions of the liver include processing and synthesis of nutrients (glycogenesis and glycogenolysis, storage and mobilization of fats, gluconeogenesis), production of urea, detoxification of chemicals, production of bile, and synthesis of albumin and clotting factors.

The liver detoxifies both endogenous compounds (those made in the body) and exogenous compounds (those brought in from the environment). For example, the liver converts ammonia, a toxic waste product of amino acid metabolism, into urea, which can be excreted by the kidneys. The liver also detoxifies and metabolizes alcohol and medications. Some drugs actually require activation by the enzymes of the liver. In addition, some drugs cannot be taken orally because modification of these drugs by the liver renders them inactive.

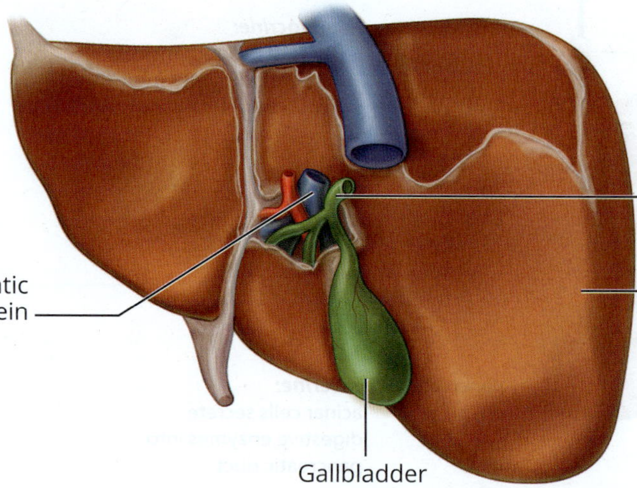

Figure 9.10 The Liver and Gallbladder

Bile production is one of the most significant jobs of the liver *vis-à-vis* the digestive system. As mentioned earlier, bile is composed of bile salts, pigments, and cholesterol. Bile salts are amphipathic molecules that can emulsify fat in the digestive system. The major pigment in bile is **bilirubin**, which is a byproduct of the breakdown of hemoglobin. Bilirubin travels to the liver, where it is **conjugated** to a protein and secreted into the bile for excretion. Bilirubin flows through the digestive system and leaves in waste. Bilirubin is what gives stool its typical brown color. If the liver is unable to process or excrete bilirubin (due to liver damage, excessive red blood cell destruction, or blockage of the bile ducts), **jaundice** or yellowing of the skin may occur.

In addition to bile production, processing of nutrients, and detoxification and drug metabolism, the liver also synthesizes certain proteins necessary for proper body function. These proteins include **albumin**, a protein that maintains plasma oncotic pressure and also serves as a carrier for many drugs and hormones, and **clotting factors** used during blood coagulation.

KEY CONCEPT

The major components of bile are bile salts, which emulsify fats; pigments (especially bilirubin, from the breakdown of hemoglobin); and cholesterol.

REAL WORLD

Cirrhosis of the liver can result from many different processes, including chronic alcohol consumption, hepatitis C infection, autoimmune hepatitis, and fatty liver disease. However, the outcome is the same. Cirrhosis is scarring of the liver, and this scar tissue builds up, creating increased resistance within the portal vein, resulting in portal hypertension. This causes a backup of fluid within the portal system, resulting in swollen veins in the digestive system, especially the esophagus, which may rupture and cause life-threatening bleeding. This often manifests as *hematemesis*, or vomiting of blood. Cirrhosis also causes bleeding disorders because production of clotting factors is disrupted. The inability to properly dispose of ammonia results in increased ammonia in the blood, which affects mentation. Finally, cirrhosis may also cause hepatocellular carcinoma, or cancer of the hepatocytes.

Gallbladder

The **gallbladder** is located just beneath the liver and both stores and concentrates bile. Upon release of CCK, the gallbladder contracts and pushes bile out into the **biliary tree**. The bile duct system merges with the pancreatic duct, as shown in Figure 9.9 earlier, before emptying into the duodenum.

The gallbladder is a common site of cholesterol or bilirubin stone formation. This painful condition causes inflammation of the gallbladder. The stones may also travel into the bile ducts and get stuck in the biliary tree. In some cases, stones can get caught just before entering the duodenum, resulting in blockage of not only the biliary tree, but the pancreatic duct as well, causing pancreatitis.

The functions of the various digestive enzymes (and bile) are summarized in Table 9.2.

BRIDGE

Stone formation is nothing more than precipitation of a solid once its concentration has reached the K_{sp} of the compound. This is particularly common in the gallbladder because bile is concentrated there. Solubility and K_{sp} are discussed in Chapter 9 of *MCAT General Chemistry Review*.

Nutrient	Enzyme	Site of Production	Site of Function	Function
Carbohydrates	Salivary amylase (ptyalin)	Salivary glands	Mouth	Hydrolyzes starch to maltose and dextrins
	Pancreatic amylase	Pancreas (acinar cells)	Duodenum	Hydrolyzes starch to maltose and dextrins
	Maltase	Intestinal glands	Duodenum	Hydrolyzes maltose to two glucose molecules
	Isomaltase	Intestinal glands	Duodenum	Hydrolyzes isomaltose to two glucose molecules
	Sucrase	Intestinal glands	Duodenum	Hydrolyzes sucrose to glucose and fructose
	Lactase	Intestinal glands	Duodenum	Hydrolyzes lactose to glucose and galactose
Proteins	Pepsin(ogen)	Gastric glands (chief cells)	Stomach	Hydrolyzes specific peptide bonds; activated by HCl
	Trypsin(ogen)	Pancreas (acinar cells)	Duodenum	Hydrolyzes specific peptide bonds; converts chymotrypsinogen to chymotrypsin; activated by enteropeptidase
	Chymotrypsin (ogen)	Pancreas (acinar cells)	Duodenum	Hydrolyzes specific peptide bonds; activated by trypsin
	(Pro)carboxy peptidases A and B	Pancreas (acinar cells)	Duodenum	Hydrolyzes terminal peptide bond at carboxy end; indirectly activated by enteropeptidase via trypsin
	Aminopeptidase	Intestinal glands	Duodenum	Hydrolyzes terminal peptide bond at amino end
	Dipeptidases	Intestinal glands	Duodenum	Hydrolyzes pairs of amino acids
	Enteropeptidase	Intestinal glands	Duodenum	Converts trypsinogen to trypsin and procarboxypeptidases A and B to carboxypeptidases A and B
Lipids	Bile*	Liver (stored in gallbladder)	Duodenum	Emulsifies fat
	Lipase	Pancreas (acinar cells)	Duodenum	Hydrolyzes lipids

*Note: Bile is not an enzyme, but is involved in mechanical digestion of fats.

Table 9.2 Digestive Enzymes

A summary of the digestion of each major class of biomolecules is provided in Figure 9.11.

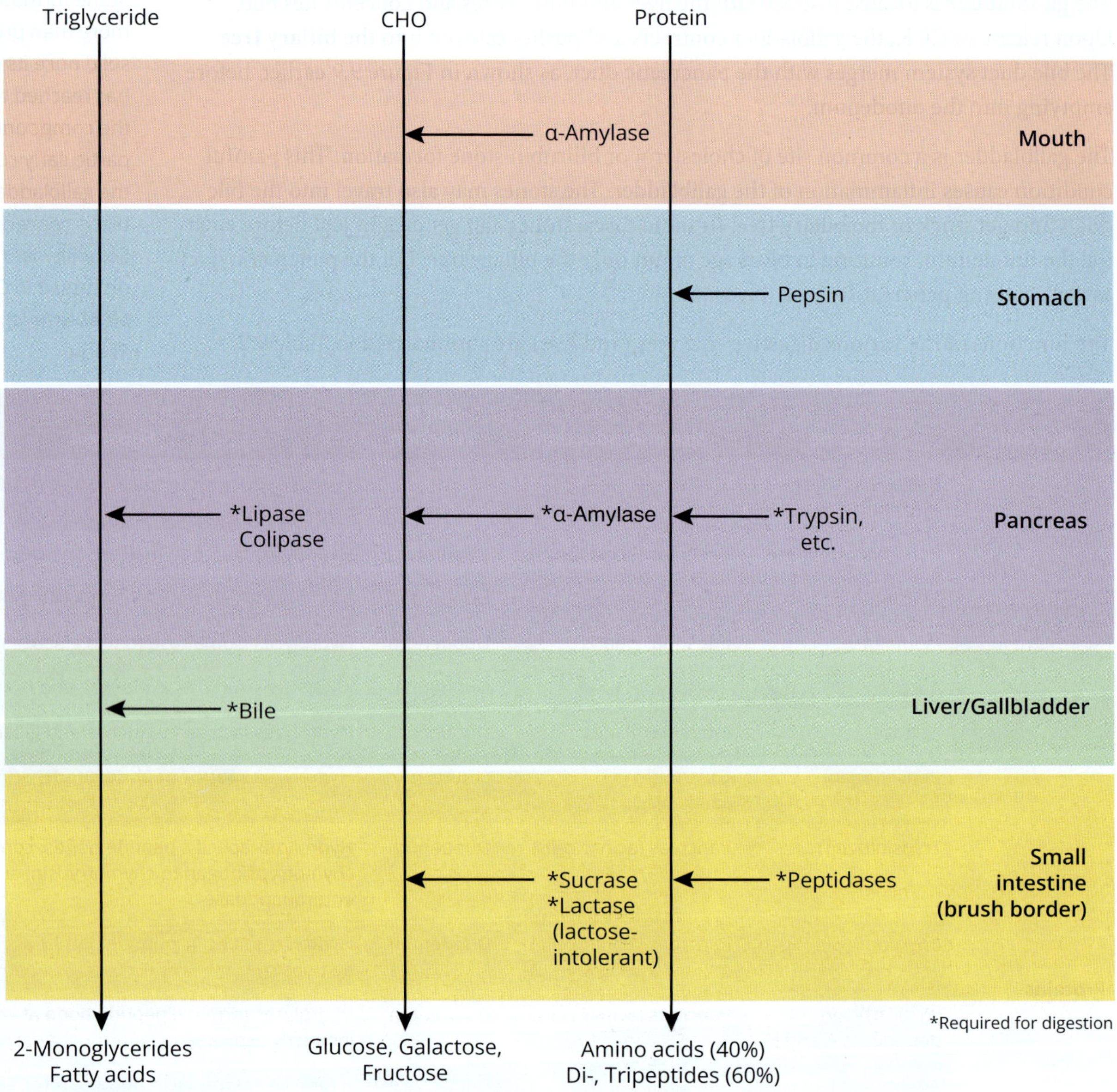

Figure 9.11 Summary of Digestive Processes

MCAT CONCEPT CHECK 9.3

Before you move on, assess your understanding of the material with these questions.

1. List at least one pancreatic enzyme that digests each of the three major classes of biomolecules:
   - Carbohydrates:
   - Proteins:
   - Fats:
2. What are the main components of bile?
3. Where is bile synthesized? Where is bile stored? Where does bile carry out its digestive function?
   - Synthesized:
   - Stored:
   - Carries out function:
4. List at least four functions of the liver:
   -
   -
   -
   -
5. The accessory organs of digestion originate from which primary germ layer?

9.4 Absorption and Defecation

LEARNING OBJECTIVES

After Chapter 9.4, you will be able to:

- Recall the four fat-soluble vitamins
- Order the three sections of the small intestine and the three sections of the large intestine
- Predict the portions of the gut impacted by a disease when given a digestive symptom, such as watery stool
- Identify the biomolecules typically absorbed into each vessel of the villus:

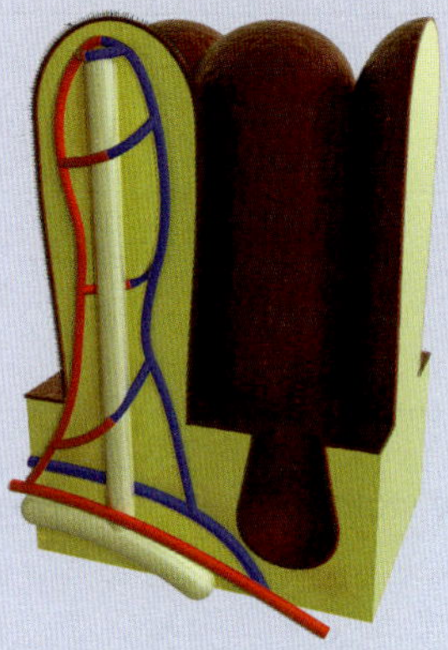

Absorption of nutrients primarily occurs in the small intestine, especially in the jejunum and ileum. The large intestine largely absorbs water.

Jejunum and Ileum

The small intestine consists of three segments: the duodenum, the jejunum, and the ileum. As discussed previously, the **duodenum** is primarily involved in digestion. The **jejunum** and **ileum** are involved in the absorption of nutrients. The small intestine is lined with **villi**, which are small, finger-like projections from the epithelial lining, as shown in Figure 9.12. Each villus has many **microvilli**, drastically increasing the surface area available for absorption. In addition, at the middle of each villus there is a capillary bed for the absorption of water-soluble nutrients and a **lacteal**, a lymphatic channel that takes up fats for transport into the lymphatic system.

MNEMONIC

Segments of the small intestine: **D**ow **J**ones **I**ndustrial

- **D**uodenum
- **J**ejunum
- **I**leum

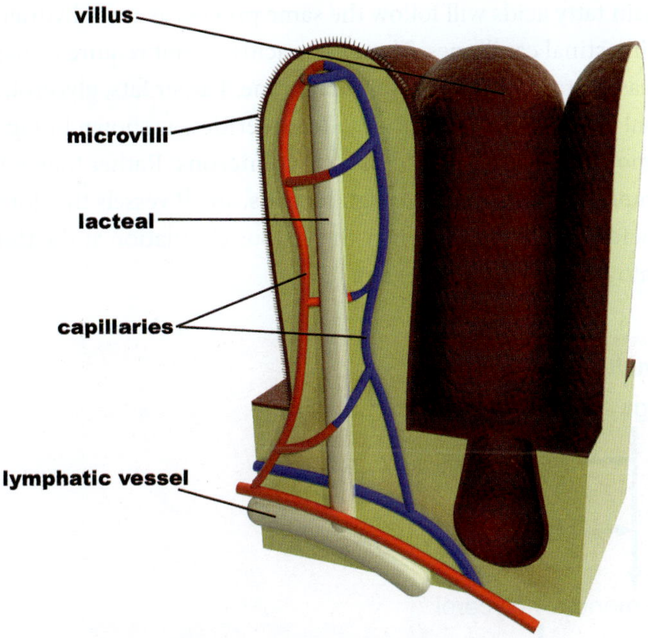

Figure 9.12 Structure of a Villus

Simple sugars, such as glucose, fructose, and galactose, and amino acids are absorbed by secondary active transport and facilitated diffusion into the epithelial cells lining the small intestine, as shown in Figure 9.13. Then, these substances move across the epithelial cell membrane into the intestinal capillaries. Blood is constantly passing by the epithelial cells, carrying the carbohydrate and amino acid molecules away. This new incoming blood maintains a lower concentration of monosaccharides and amino acids than inside the epithelial cells. This sustained concentration gradient always allows for the intake of those energy containing molecules, which can be seen in Figure 9.13. Thus, simple carbohydrates and amino acids diffuse from the epithelial cells into the capillaries. The absorbed molecules then go to the liver via the hepatic portal circulation.

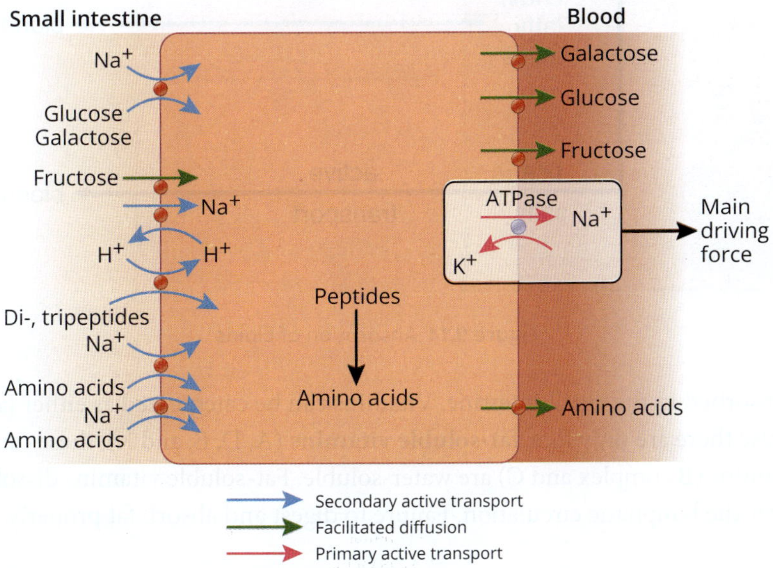

Figure 9.13 Absorption of Carbohydrates and Amino Acids in the Small Intestine

What about fats? Short-chain fatty acids will follow the same process as carbohydrates and amino acids by diffusing directly into the intestinal capillaries. These fatty acids do not require transporters because they are nonpolar, so they can easily traverse the cellular membrane. Larger fats, glycerol, and cholesterol move separately into the intestinal cells but then reform into triglycerides, as shown in Figure 9.14. The triglycerides and esterified cholesterol molecules are packaged into **chylomicrons**. Rather than entering the bloodstream, chylomicrons enter the lymphatic circulation through **lacteals**, small vessels that form the beginning of the lymphatic system. These lacteals converge and enter the venous circulation at the **thoracic duct** in the base of the neck, which empties into the left subclavian vein.

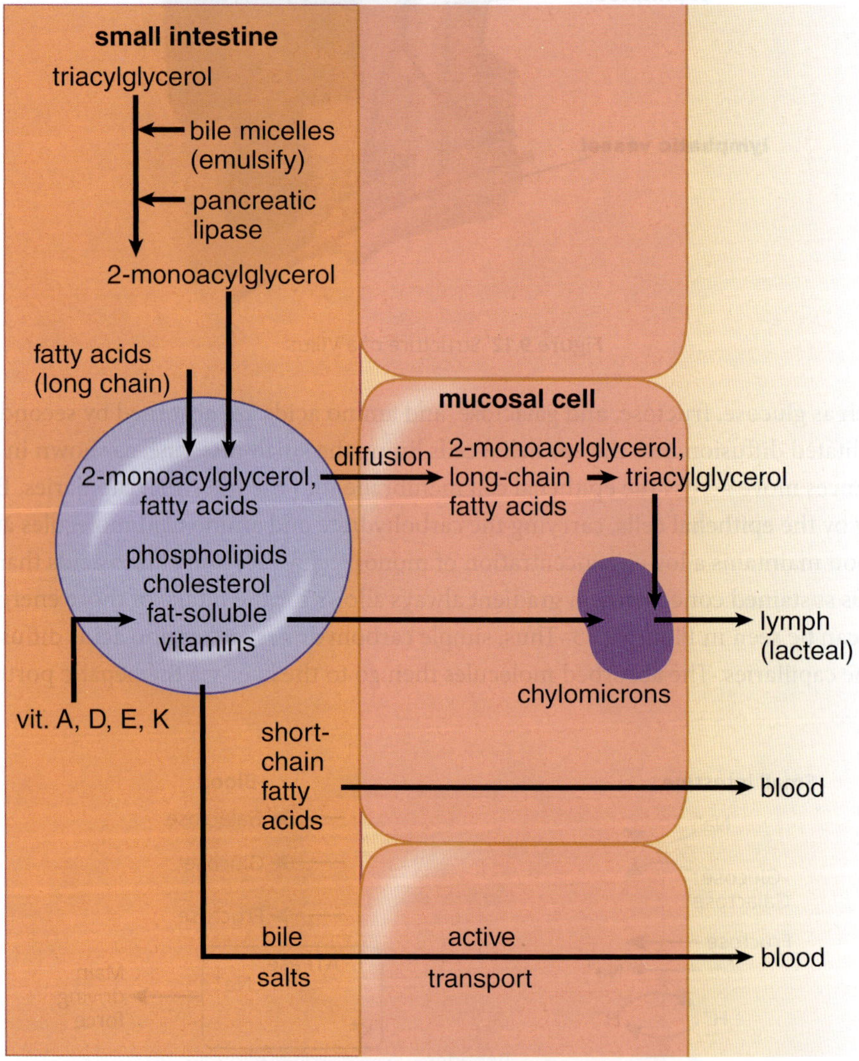

Figure 9.14 Absorption of Lipids

Vitamins are also absorbed in the small intestine. Vitamins can be categorized as either fat-soluble or water-soluble. Because there are only four **fat-soluble vitamins** (A, D, E, and K), these can be easily memorized. All other vitamins (B complex and C) are water-soluble. Fat-soluble vitamins dissolve directly into chylomicrons to enter the lymphatic circulation. Failure to digest and absorb fat properly, which can be due to pathologies in the liver, gallbladder, pancreas, or small intestine, may lead to deficiencies of fat-soluble vitamins. The **water-soluble vitamins** are taken up, along with water, amino acids, and carbohydrates, across the endothelial cells of the small intestine, passing directly into the plasma.

In addition to fats, carbohydrates, amino acids, and vitamins, the small intestine also absorbs water. Much of the water in chyme is actually the result of secretions. On average, a person may consume up to two liters of fluid per day, but secretions into the upper gastrointestinal tract may total up to seven liters of fluid per day. In order to maintain proper fluid levels within the body, much of this fluid must be reabsorbed by osmosis. As solutes are absorbed into the bloodstream, water is drawn with them, eventually reaching the capillaries. Water passes not only **transcellularly** (across the cell membrane), but also **paracellularly** (squeezing between cells) to reach the blood.

Large Intestine

The final part of the gastrointestinal tract is the **large intestine**. It is primarily involved in water absorption. The large intestine has a larger diameter but shorter length than the small intestine. It is divided into three major sections: the cecum, the colon, and the rectum. The **cecum** is simply an outpocketing that accepts fluid exiting the small intestine through the **ileocecal valve** and is the site of attachment of the **appendix**. The appendix is a small finger-like projection that was once thought to be **vestigial**. Recent evidence, however, suggests that it may have a role in warding off certain bacterial infections and repopulating the large intestine with normal flora after episodes of diarrhea. Inflammation of the appendix (appendicitis) is a surgical emergency; in fact, it is the most common reason for an unscheduled surgery in the United States.

The **colon** itself is divided into the ascending, transverse, descending, and sigmoid colons (see Figure 9.15). Its main function is to absorb water and salts (such as sodium chloride) from the undigested material left over from the small intestine. The small intestine actually absorbs much more water than the colon, so the colon primarily concentrates the remaining material to form **feces**. There is a balance to this concentration function because too little or too much water absorption can cause diarrhea or constipation, respectively.

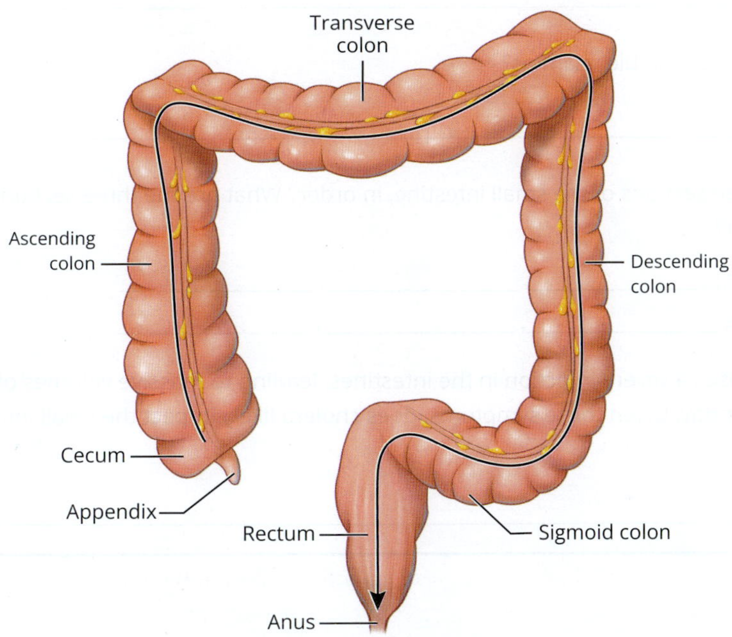

Figure 9.15 The Large Intestine

Finally, the rectum serves as a storage site for feces, which consists of indigestible material (for example, fiber), water, bacteria (*E. coli* and others), and certain digestive secretions that are not reabsorbed (enzymes and some bile). The **anus** is the opening through which wastes are eliminated and consists of two sphincters: the **internal** and **external anal sphincters**. The external sphincter is under voluntary control (somatic), but the internal sphincter is under involuntary control (autonomic).

The large intestine—and even the small intestine—is home to many different species of bacteria. In fact, 30 percent of the dry matter in stool consists of bacteria. Most of these bacteria are anaerobes, but the cecum is also home to many aerobic bacteria. The presence of bacteria in the colon represents a symbiotic relationship: the bacteria are provided with a steady source of food, and the byproducts produced by the bacteria are beneficial to humans. For example, bacteria in the gut produce vitamin K, which is essential for the production of clotting factors, and biotin (vitamin B_7), which is a coenzyme for many metabolic enzymes.

BRIDGE

Note the similarity between the muscles that control voiding of urine and feces. In both cases, there is an internal sphincter under autonomic control (internal urethral sphincter and internal anal sphincter) and an external sphincter under somatic control (external urethral sphincter and external anal sphincter). Urination is discussed in Chapter 10 of *MCAT Biology Review*.

MCAT CONCEPT CHECK 9.4

Before you move on, assess your understanding of the material with these questions.

1. What are the two circulatory vessels in a villus? What biomolecules are absorbed into each?
   - ____________________
   - ____________________
2. What are the four fat-soluble vitamins?

   ____
3. What are the three sections of the small intestine, in order? What are the three sections of the large intestine, in order?
   - Small intestine: ________, ________, ________
   - Large intestine: ________, ________, ________
4. *Vibrio cholera* causes a severe infection in the intestines, leading to massive volumes of watery diarrhea—up to 20 liters per day. Given these symptoms, does cholera likely impact the small intestine or the large intestine?

   ____

Conclusion

In this chapter, we have reviewed a lot of information about the digestive system that we can use to our advantage on Test Day. We began with an overview of the anatomy, keeping in mind that the system is designed to carry out extracellular digestion. Considering that all our foodstuffs are made up of fats, proteins, and carbohydrates, these compounds have to be broken down to their simplest molecular forms before they can be absorbed and distributed to the tissues and cells of the body. As we moved through the gastrointestinal tract, we discussed whether each organ was a site of absorption, digestion, or both. We spent a good bit of time discussing each of the enzymes involved in digestion and their specific purposes. While digestion occurs primarily in the oral cavity, stomach, and duodenum, absorption occurs primarily in the jejunum and ileum, where the method of transport into the circulatory system is slightly different depending on the compound. Finally, we discussed the three segments of the large intestine and their roles in water and salt absorption, as well as the temporary storage of waste products. Although the amount of information about the digestive system may seem overwhelming, the underlying concepts are relatively straightforward, and a systematic approach (such as charts, tables, or flashcards) will help you manage this content.

In the end, the digestive system's main purpose is to break down energy-containing compounds and get them into the circulation so they can be used by the rest of the body. Equally important are the systems the body has for getting rid of compounds from the blood. Buildup of waste products like ammonia, urea, potassium, and hydrogen ions can lead to serious pathology. For instance, hyperammonemia (buildup of ammonia in the blood) can lead to severe, permanent neurological damage. Hyperkalemia (buildup of potassium in the blood) can quickly cause a fatal heart attack. Temperature regulation is similarly important; both hyperthermia and hypothermia can lead to organ dysfunction and, ultimately, death. In the next chapter, we turn our attention to these regulatory systems: the renal system and the skin.

GO ONLINE

You've reviewed the content, now test your knowledge and critical thinking skills by completing a test-like passage set in your online resources!

CONCEPT SUMMARY

Anatomy of the Digestive System

- **Intracellular digestion** involves the oxidation of glucose and fatty acids to make energy. **Extracellular digestion** occurs in the lumen of the **alimentary canal**.
  - **Mechanical digestion** is the physical breakdown of large food particles into smaller food particles.
  - **Chemical digestion** is the enzymatic cleavage of chemical bonds, such as the peptide bonds of proteins or the glycosidic bonds of starches.
- The pathway of the digestive tract is: oral cavity → pharynx → esophagus → stomach → small intestine → large intestine → rectum
- The **accessory organs of digestion** are the salivary glands, pancreas, liver, and gallbladder.
- The **enteric nervous system** is in the wall of the alimentary canal and controls peristalsis. Its activity is upregulated by the parasympathetic nervous system and downregulated by the sympathetic nervous system.

Ingestion and Digestion

- Multiple hormones regulate feeding behavior, including antidiuretic hormone (ADH or vasopressin) and aldosterone, which promote thirst; glucagon and ghrelin, which promote hunger; and leptin and cholecystokinin, which promote satiety.
- In the **oral cavity**, **mastication** starts the mechanical digestion of food, while **salivary amylase** and **lipase** start the chemical digestion of food. Food is formed into a **bolus** and swallowed.
- The **pharynx** connects the mouth and posterior nasal cavity to the esophagus.
- The **esophagus** propels food to the stomach using peristalsis. Food enters the stomach through the **lower esophageal (cardiac) sphincter**.
- The stomach has four parts: **fundus**, **body**, **antrum**, and **pylorus**. The stomach has a **lesser** and **greater curvature** and is thrown into folds called **rugae**. Numerous secretory cells line the stomach.
  - **Mucous cells** produce bicarbonate-rich mucus to protect the stomach.
  - **Chief cells** secrete **pepsinogen**, a protease activated by the acidic environment of the stomach.
  - **Parietal cells** secrete hydrochloric acid and **intrinsic factor**, which is needed for vitamin B_{12} absorption.
  - **G-cells** secrete **gastrin**, a peptide hormone that increases HCl secretion and gastric motility.

- After mechanical and chemical digestion in the stomach, the food particles are now called **chyme**. Food passes into the duodenum through the **pyloric sphincter**.
- The **duodenum** is the first part of the small intestine and is primarily involved in chemical digestion.
  - **Disaccharidases** are brush-border enzymes that break down maltose, isomaltose, lactose, and sucrose into monosaccharides.
  - Brush-border **peptidases** include **aminopeptidase** and **dipeptidases**.
  - **Enteropeptidase** activates trypsinogen and procarboxypeptidases, initiating an activation cascade.
  - **Secretin** stimulates the release of pancreatic juices into the digestive tract and slows motility.
  - **Cholecystokinin** stimulates bile release from the gallbladder, release of pancreatic juices, and satiety.

Accessory Organs of Digestion

- **Acinar cells** in the pancreas produce pancreatic juices that contain bicarbonate, **pancreatic amylase**, pancreatic peptidases (**trypsinogen**, **chymotrypsinogen**, **carboxypeptidases A** and **B**), and **pancreatic lipase**.
- The **liver** synthesizes **bile**, which can be stored in the gallbladder or secreted into the duodenum directly.
  - Bile emulsifies fats, making them soluble and increasing their surface area.
  - The main components of bile are **bile salts**, pigments (especially **bilirubin** from the breakdown of hemoglobin), and cholesterol.
- The liver also processes nutrients (through glycogenesis and glycogenolysis, storage and mobilization of fats, and gluconeogenesis), produces urea, detoxifies chemicals, activates or inactivates medications, produces bile, and synthesizes albumin and clotting factors.
- The **gallbladder** stores and concentrates bile.

Absorption and Defecation

- The **jejunum** and **ileum** of the small intestine are primarily involved in absorption.
  - The small intestine is lined with **villi**, which are covered with **microvilli**, increasing the surface area available for absorption.
  - Villi contain a capillary bed and a **lacteal**, a vessel of the lymphatic system.
  - Water-soluble compounds, such as monosaccharides, amino acids, water-soluble vitamins, small fatty acids, and water, enter the capillary bed.
  - Fat-soluble compounds, such as fats, cholesterol, and fat-soluble vitamins, enter the lacteal.
- The **large intestine** absorbs water and salts, forming semisolid feces.
  - The **cecum** is an outpocketing that accepts fluid from the small intestine through the **ileocecal valve** and is the site of attachment of the **appendix**.
  - The **colon** is divided into ascending, transverse, descending, and sigmoid portions.
  - The **rectum** stores feces, which are then excreted through the **anus**.
  - Gut bacteria produce vitamin K and biotin (vitamin B_7).

ANSWERS TO CONCEPT CHECKS

9.1

1. Mechanical digestion, such as chewing, physically breaks down food into smaller pieces. Chemical digestion involves hydrolysis of bonds and breakdown of food into smaller biomolecules.
2. Oral cavity (mouth) → pharynx → esophagus → stomach → small intestine → large intestine → rectum → anus
3. The parasympathetic nervous system increases secretions from all of the glands of the digestive system and promotes peristalsis. The sympathetic nervous system slows peristalsis.

9.2

1. Saliva contains salivary amylase (ptyalin), which digests starch into smaller sugars (maltose and dextrin); and lipase, which digests fats.
2.

Cell	Secretions	Functions
Mucous cell	Mucus	Protects lining of stomach, increases pH (bicarbonate)
Chief cell	Pepsinogen	Digests proteins, activated by H^+
Parietal cell	HCl, intrinsic factor	HCl: decreases pH, kills microbes, denatures proteins, carries out some chemical digestion; intrinsic factor: absorption of vitamin B_{12}
G-cell	Gastrin	Increases HCl production, increases gastric motility

3.

Substance	Enzyme or Hormone?	Functions
Sucrase	Enzyme	Brush-border enzyme; breaks down sucrose into monosaccharides
Secretin	Hormone	Increases pancreatic secretions, especially bicarbonate; reduces HCl secretion; decreases motility
Dipeptidase	Enzyme	Brush-border enzyme; breaks down dipeptides into free amino acids
Cholecystokinin	Hormone	Recruits secretions from gallbladder and pancreas; promotes satiety
Enteropeptidase	Enzyme	Activates trypsinogen, which initiates an activation cascade

4. Bile accomplishes mechanical digestion of fats, emulsifying them and increasing their surface area. Pancreatic lipase accomplishes chemical digestion of fats, breaking their ester bonds.

9.3

1. Carbohydrates: pancreatic amylase; proteins: trypsin, chymotrypsin, carboxypeptidases A and B; fats: pancreatic lipase
2. Bile is composed of bile salts (amphipathic molecules derived from cholesterol that emulsify fats), pigments (especially bilirubin from the breakdown of hemoglobin), and cholesterol.
3. Bile is synthesized in the liver, stored in the gallbladder, and serves its function in the duodenum.
4. The liver processes nutrients (through glycogenesis and glycogenolysis, storage and mobilization of fats, and gluconeogenesis), produces urea, detoxifies chemicals, activates or inactivates medications, produces bile, and synthesizes albumin and clotting factors.
5. As outgrowths of the gut tube, the accessory organs of digestion arise from embryonic endoderm.

9.4

1. The two circulatory vessels are capillaries and lacteals. The capillary absorbs water-soluble nutrients like monosaccharides, amino acids, short-chain fatty acids, water-soluble vitamins, and water itself. The lacteal absorbs fat-soluble nutrients, like fats, cholesterol, and fat-soluble vitamins.
2. The fat-soluble vitamins are A, D, E, and K.
3. The small intestine consists of the duodenum, jejunum, and ileum. The large intestine consists of the cecum, colon, and rectum.
4. While the large intestine's main function is to absorb water, the small intestine actually absorbs a much larger volume of water. Thus, massive volumes of watery diarrhea are more likely to arise from infections in the small intestine than in the large intestine.

SCIENCE MASTERY ASSESSMENT EXPLANATIONS

1. **B**

Chief cells secrete pepsinogen, a protease secreted as a zymogen that is activated by the acidic environment of the stomach. G-cells secrete gastrin, parietal cells secrete hydrochloric acid and intrinsic factor, and mucous cells secrete alkaline mucus, eliminating the other answer choices.

2. **B**

The small intestine is divided into three sections: the duodenum, the jejunum, and the ileum. The cecum is part of the large intestine, making **(B)** the correct answer.

3. **B**

Aminopeptidase is a brush-border peptidase secreted by the cells lining the duodenum; it does not require enteropeptidase for activation. Both trypsinogen and procarboxypeptidases A and B are activated by enteropeptidase, eliminating **(A)** and **(D)**. Once activated, trypsin can activate chymotrypsinogen; if trypsinogen cannot be activated, then chymotrypsinogen will not be activated either, eliminating **(C)**.

4. **D**

Lipase is involved in the digestion of fats, but its function is not to emulsify fats—this is the job of bile. Rather, lipase chemically digests fats in the duodenum, allowing them to be brought into duodenal cells and packaged into chylomicrons. The other associations given here are all correct.

5. **C**

Protein digestion begins in the stomach, where pepsin (secreted as pepsinogen) hydrolyzes specific peptide bonds. Protein digestion continues in the small intestine as trypsin (secreted as trypsinogen), chymotrypsin (secreted as chymotrypsinogen), carboxypeptidases A and B (secreted as procarboxypeptidases A and B), aminopeptidase, and dipeptidases hydrolyze specific parts of the peptide. No protein digestion occurs in the mouth or large intestine.

6. **A**

Sucrase is a brush-border enzyme found on duodenal cells and is not secreted by the salivary glands. This enzyme hydrolyzes sucrose (a disaccharide) to form glucose and fructose (monosaccharides). The other associations are all correct.

7. **B**

The question is basically asking us to identify the structure that lies between the stomach and the small intestine. This is the pyloric sphincter; the presentation given in the question is a classic example of what is called pyloric stenosis, in which the pyloric sphincter is thickened and cannot relax to permit chyme through. The cardiac sphincter, **(A)**, lies between the esophagus and the stomach. The ileocecal valve, **(C)**, lies between the ileum of the small intestine and the cecum of the large intestine. The internal anal sphincter, **(D)**, lies at the end of the rectum.

8. **B**

The parasympathetic nervous system has many roles in the digestive system. It promotes motility of the gut tube and secretion from glands. Therefore, blocking the parasympathetic nervous system would likely result in dry mouth (from reduced secretion of saliva), slow gastric emptying (from decreased peristalsis), and decreased gastric acid production (from reduced HCl secretion from the parietal cells in the gastric glands), eliminating **(A)**, **(C)**, and **(D)**. **(B)** is the correct answer because we would expect constipation in such an individual, not diarrhea: slowed motility through the colon would lead to increased water reabsorption, making the feces too firm and causing constipation.

9. **B**

The first graph shows maximal activity at a very acidic pH, implying that this is an enzyme acting in the stomach. The second graph shows maximal activity around pH 8.5, implying that this is an enzyme acting in the duodenum. The only choice that matches the first graph with a stomach enzyme (pepsin) and the second with a duodenal enzyme (carboxypeptidase B) is **(B)**.

10. **C**

Elevated bilirubin implies a blockage to bile flow, increased production of bilirubin (from massive hemoglobin release), or an inability of the liver to produce bile. If the bile duct were occluded, as in **(A)**, then bile would not be able to flow into the digestive tract and would build up, increasing bilirubin levels in the blood. If many red blood cells were lysed, as in **(B)**, then bilirubin levels would rise in accordance with the increased hemoglobin release. If liver failure occurred, as in **(D)**, then the liver would be unable to produce bile, and bilirubin would again build up. **(C)** refers to a pathology in the stomach—the key word given here is rugae, which are the folds in the stomach wall. Lack of gastric function would have no effect on bilirubin levels, making this the correct choice.

11. **A**

Chylomicrons contain triacylglycerols, cholesteryl esters, and fat-soluble vitamins and are secreted by intestinal cells into lacteals. Amino acids, fat-soluble vitamins (like vitamins A and E), and cholesterol are all absorbed in the small intestine.

12. **B**

The cleavage of a fat described in this question stem refers to the breakdown of triacylglycerides, which is a hydrolysis reaction in which water is added across the ester linkage of the fatty acids to the glycerol backbone, breaking these bonds. For this reason, chemical digestion, **(B)**, is correct. Note that, the location of this reaction occurs in the lumen of a digestive organ, so this reaction could also be classified as an extracellular reaction. This observation is important because it eliminates **(C)**.

13. **A**

While the capillaries from the intestine come together to form the portal vein, which drains to the liver, the lacteals come together to form the thoracic duct, which drains directly into the left subclavian vein. Therefore, fat-soluble compounds do not pass through the liver before reaching the right side of the heart. Only **(A)**, vitamin D, is fat-soluble.

14. **C**

Ghrelin promotes a sensation of hunger, increasing feeding behavior. Both leptin and cholecystokinin promote satiety, decreasing feeding behavior—eliminating **(A)** and **(B)**. Gastrin increases acid production and gastric motility, but does not have any significant relationship with feeding behavior, eliminating **(D)**.

15. **D**

The liver serves many functions, including carrying out metabolic processes (glycogenesis and glycogenolysis, fat storage, and gluconeogenesis), detoxification or activation of medications, and synthesis of bile. Germane to this question are the roles of converting ammonia into urea through the urea cycle and synthesis of proteins, including albumin and clotting factors. A patient with liver failure would thus not be able to convert ammonia into urea and would have high concentrations of ammonia and low concentrations of urea in the blood, eliminating **(A)** and **(C)**. With decreased synthetic activity, both albumin and clotting factor concentrations would be low, eliminating **(B)** and making **(D)** the correct answer.

GO ONLINE

Consult your online resources for additional practice.

SHARED CONCEPTS

Biochemistry Chapter 2
Enzymes

Biochemistry Chapter 9
Carbohydrate Metabolism I

Biochemistry Chapter 11
Lipid and Amino Acid Metabolism

Biology Chapter 5
The Endocrine System

Biology Chapter 7
The Cardiovascular System

Biology Chapter 8
The Immune System

SCIENCE MASTERY ASSESSMENT

Every pre-med knows this feeling: there is so much content I have to know for the MCAT! How do I know what to do first or what's important?

While the high-yield badges throughout this book will help you identify the most important topics, this Science Mastery Assessment is another tool in your MCAT prep arsenal. This quiz (which can also be taken in your online resources) and the guidance below will help ensure that you are spending the appropriate amount of time on this chapter based on your personal strengths and weaknesses. Don't worry though—skipping something now does not mean you'll never study it. Later on in your prep, as you complete full-length tests, you'll uncover specific pieces of content that you need to review and can come back to these chapters as appropriate.

How to Use This Assessment

If you answer 0–7 questions correctly:

Spend about 1 hour to read this chapter in full and take limited notes throughout. Follow up by reviewing **all** quiz questions to ensure that you now understand how to solve each one.

If you answer 8–11 questions correctly:

Spend 20–40 minutes reviewing the quiz questions. Beginning with the questions you missed, read and take notes on the corresponding subchapters. For questions you answered correctly, ensure your thinking matches that of the explanation and you understand why each choice was correct or incorrect.

If you answer 12–15 questions correctly:

Spend less than 20 minutes reviewing all questions from the quiz. If you missed any, then include a quick read-through of the corresponding subchapters, or even just the relevant content within a subchapter, as part of your question review. For questions you answered correctly, ensure your thinking matches that of the explanation and review the Concept Summary at the end of the chapter.

1. Which of the following would most likely be filtered through the glomerulus into Bowman's space?
   - **A.** Erythrocytes
   - **B.** Monosaccharides
   - **C.** Platelets
   - **D.** Proteins

2. In which of the following segments of the nephron is sodium NOT actively transported out of the nephron?
   - **A.** Proximal convoluted tubule
   - **B.** Thin portion of the ascending limb of the loop of Henle
   - **C.** Distal convoluted tubule
   - **D.** Thick portion of the ascending limb of the loop of Henle

3. Which region of the kidney has the lowest solute concentration under normal physiological circumstances?
   - **A.** Cortex
   - **B.** Outer medulla
   - **C.** Inner medulla
   - **D.** Renal pelvis

4. Which of the following sequences correctly shows the passage of blood through the vessels of the kidney?
   - **A.** Renal artery → afferent arterioles → glomerulus → efferent arterioles → vasa recta → renal vein
   - **B.** Afferent arterioles → renal artery → glomerulus → vasa recta → renal vein → efferent arterioles
   - **C.** Glomerulus → renal artery → afferent arterioles → efferent arterioles → renal vein → vasa recta
   - **D.** Renal vein → efferent arterioles → glomerulus → afferent arterioles → vasa recta → renal artery

5. Which of the following statements is FALSE?
   - **A.** ADH increases water reabsorption in the kidney.
   - **B.** Aldosterone indirectly increases water reabsorption in the kidney.
   - **C.** ADH acts directly on the proximal convoluted tubule.
   - **D.** Aldosterone stimulates reabsorption of sodium from the collecting duct.

6. In the nephron, amino acids enter the vasa recta via the process of:
   - **A.** filtration.
   - **B.** secretion.
   - **C.** excretion.
   - **D.** reabsorption.

7. On a very cold day, a person waits for over an hour at the bus stop. Which of the following structures helps the person's body set and maintain a normal temperature?
   - **A.** Hypothalamus
   - **B.** Kidneys
   - **C.** Posterior pituitary
   - **D.** Brainstem

8. Glucose reabsorption in the nephron occurs in the:
   - **A.** loop of Henle.
   - **B.** distal convoluted tubule.
   - **C.** proximal convoluted tubule.
   - **D.** collecting duct.

9. Under normal physiological circumstances, the primary function of the nephron is to create urine that is:
   - **A.** hypertonic to the blood.
   - **B.** hypotonic to the blood.
   - **C.** isotonic to the filtrate.
   - **D.** hypotonic to the vasa recta.

10. Diabetic nephropathy is commonly detected by finding protein in the urine of a patient. In such a disease, where is the likely defect in the nephron?
    - **A.** Glomerulus
    - **B.** Proximal convoluted tubule
    - **C.** Loop of Henle
    - **D.** Collecting duct

11. A laceration cuts down into a layer of loose connective tissue in the skin. Which layer of the skin is this?
    - **A.** Stratum corneum
    - **B.** Stratum lucidum
    - **C.** Papillary layer
    - **D.** Reticular layer

12. When the pH of the blood is high, which substance is likely to be excreted in larger quantities in the urine?

A. Urea
B. Ammonia
C. Hydrogen ions
D. Bicarbonate ions

13. In which layer of the skin can the stem cells of keratinocytes be found?

A. Stratum lucidum
B. Stratum granulosum
C. Stratum basale
D. Stratum corneum

14. A drug is used that prevents the conversion of angiotensin I to angiotensin II. What is a likely effect of this drug?

A. Increased sodium reabsorption
B. Increased potassium reabsorption
C. Increased blood pressure
D. Increased blood pH

15. Sarin is a potent organophosphate that can be used in chemical warfare. As an inhibitor of acetylcholinesterase, sarin causes excessive buildup of acetylcholine in all synapses where it is the neurotransmitter. Which of the following symptoms would most likely be seen in an individual with sarin poisoning?

A. Increased urination and increased sweating
B. Increased urination and decreased sweating
C. Decreased urination and increased sweating
D. Decreased urination and decreased sweating

Answer Key

1. **B** (See section 10.1)
2. **B** (See section 10.1)
3. **A** (See section 10.1)
4. **A** (See section 10.1)
5. **C** (See section 10.1)
6. **D** (See section 10.1)
7. **A** (See section 10.2)
8. **C** (See section 10.1)
9. **A** (See section 10.1)
10. **A** (See section 10.1)
11. **C** (See section 10.2)
12. **D** (See section 10.1)
13. **C** (See section 10.2)
14. **B** (See section 10.1)
15. **A** (See section 10.1)

The relevant section of the chapter to review for each question is given in parentheses after the correct answer. Detailed explanations can be found at the end of the chapter.

CHAPTER 10

HOMEOSTASIS

In This Chapter

CHAPTER PROFILE

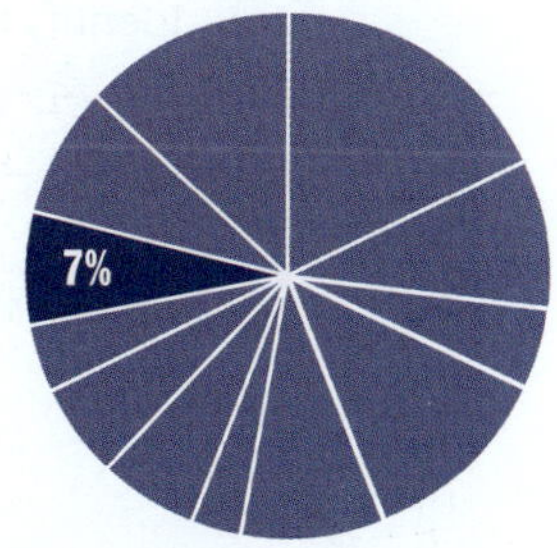

The content in this chapter should be relevant to about 7% of all questions about biology on the MCAT.

This chapter covers material from the following AAMC content category:

3B: Structure and integrative functions of the main organ systems

Introduction

Have a headache? Take an ibuprofen. Backache? Works for that, too. Ibuprofen, which has been around for over 50 years, is a relatively inexpensive, over-the-counter, nonsteroidal anti-inflammatory drug (NSAID). Ibuprofen is known as an analgesic, or pain reliever. When used in moderation, ibuprofen carries relatively little risk. However, taking multiple doses for many years can profoundly affect the kidneys. Years of analgesic use (usually as self-therapy) can lead to kidney failure, known as analgesic nephropathy. If untreated, kidney failure is universally fatal.

If kidney failure is detected, however, dialysis (or a kidney transplant) could save an individual's life. How does dialysis save a patient with kidney failure? Dialyzing fluid has many of the same solutes as blood, in strategic concentrations, and it is kept separate from blood by a semipermeable membrane. As blood is filtered through the dialysis machine, fluid and solutes diffuse down their concentration gradients, limited only by size (as determined by the membrane). The dialysis machine therefore performs filtration to purify the blood and excrete wastes, a crucial function that the kidneys would normally perform.

In this chapter, we'll learn more about filtration, as well as reabsorption and secretion. These processes are collectively responsible for osmoregulation. Osmoregulation is just one mechanism the body uses to maintain homeostasis in its fluids and tissues. We'll also discuss the skin, which plays a significant role in temperature homeostasis (thermoregulation).

10.1 The Excretory System High Yield

LEARNING OBJECTIVES

After Chapter 10.1, you will be able to:

- List the structures of the secretory pathway
- Order the vessels in the renal vascular pathway
- Identify the nervous system components used to control the detrusor muscle
- Describe the processes by which components of the kidney are able to exchange solutes between the filtrate and the blood
- Identify the function(s) of each segment of the nephron:

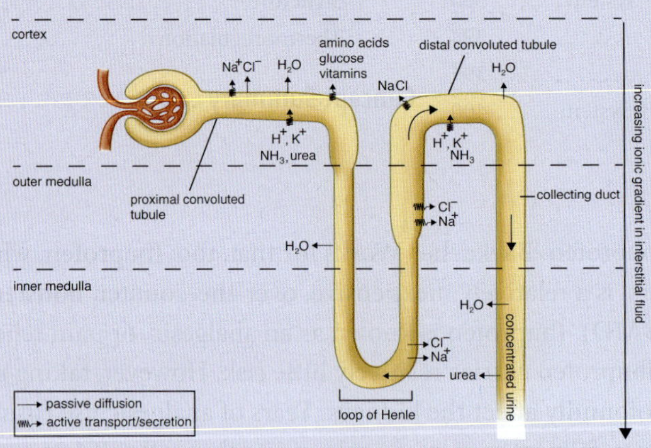

The **excretory system** serves many functions, including the regulation of blood pressure, blood osmolarity, acid–base balance, and removal of nitrogenous wastes. The kidneys play an essential role in these functions.

Anatomy of the Excretory System

The excretory system consists of the kidneys, ureters, bladder, and urethra, as shown in Figure 10.1. The kidneys are two bean-shaped structures located behind the digestive organs at the level of the bottom rib. The functional unit of the kidney is the nephron; each kidney has approximately 1 million nephrons. All of the nephrons eventually empty into the renal pelvis, which narrows to form the ureter. Urine travels through the ureter to the bladder. From the bladder, urine is transported through the urethra to exit the body.

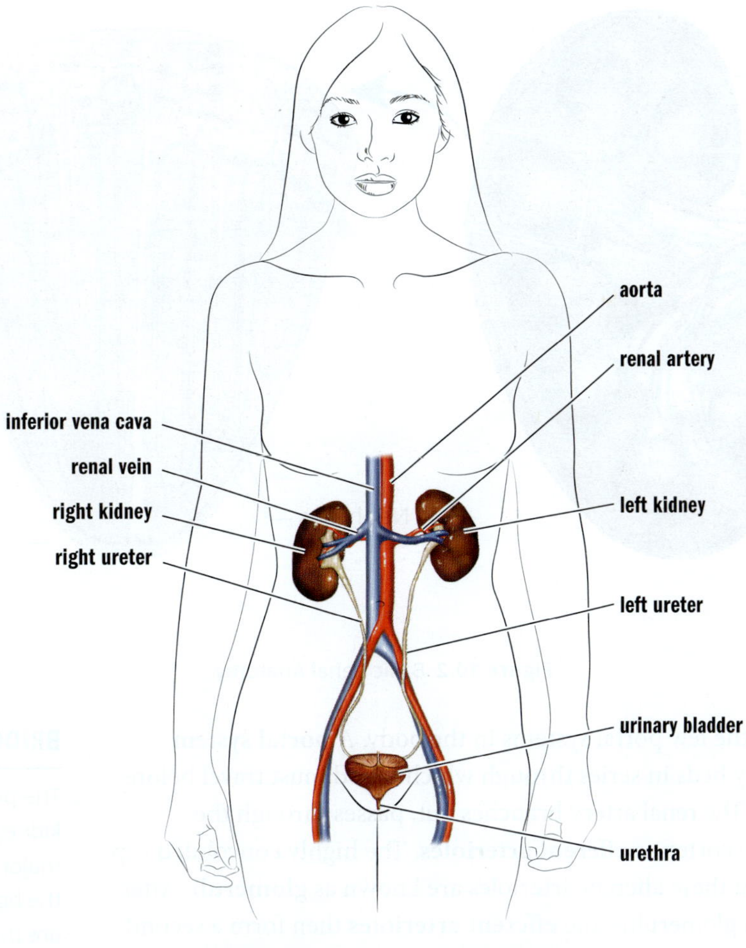

Figure 10.1 The Excretory System
Once it leaves the kidneys, urine moves through the ureters to be stored in the urinary bladder until it is excreted through the urethra.

Kidney Structure

Each kidney is subdivided into a cortex and a medulla, as shown in Figure 10.2. The **cortex** is the kidney's outermost layer, while the **medulla** of the kidney sits within the cortex. Each kidney also has a renal **hilum**, which is a deep slit in the center of its medial surface. The widest part of the ureter, the **renal pelvis**, spans almost the entire width of the renal hilum. The **renal artery**, **renal vein**, and **ureter** enter and exit through the renal hilum.

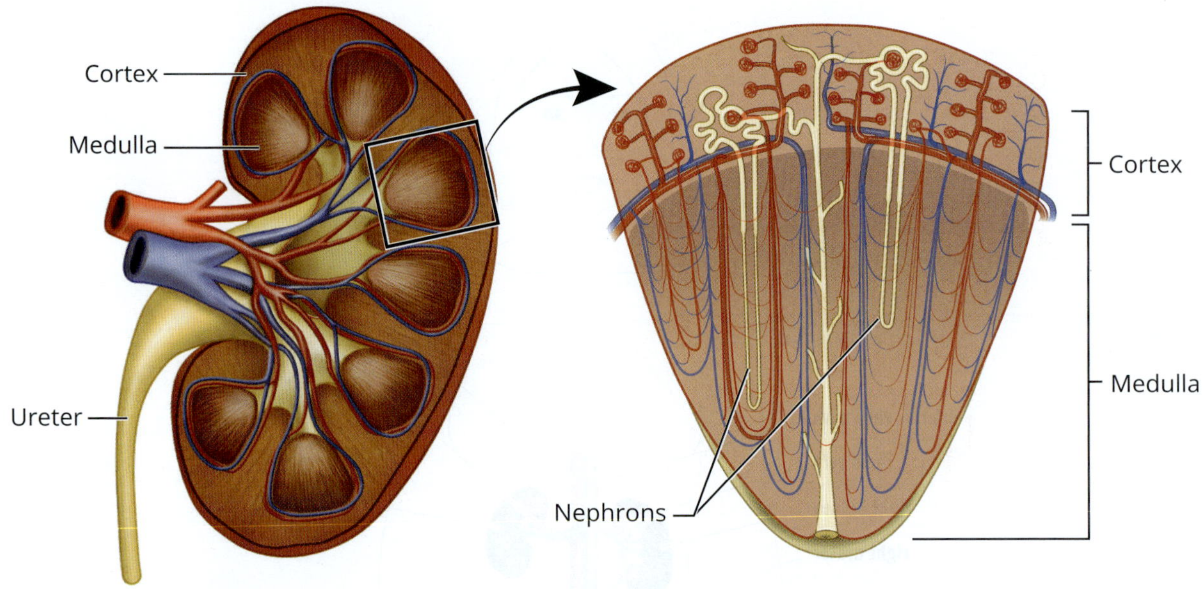

Figure 10.2 Basic Renal Anatomy

The kidney has one of the few portal systems in the body. A **portal system** consists of two capillary beds in series through which blood must travel before returning to the heart. The renal artery branches out, passes through the medulla, and enters the cortex as **afferent arterioles**. The highly convoluted capillary tufts derived from these afferent arterioles are known as **glomeruli**. After blood passes through a glomerulus, the **efferent arterioles** then form a second capillary bed. These capillaries surround the loop of Henle and are known as **vasa recta**. The renal vascular system is shown in Figure 10.3.

Also visible in Figure 10.3 is the structure of the nephron. Around the glomerulus is a cup-like structure known as **Bowman's capsule**. Bowman's capsule leads to a long tubule with many distinct areas; in order, these are the proximal convoluted tubule, descending and ascending limbs of the Loop of Henle, distal convoluted tubule, and collecting duct. The kidney's ability to excrete waste is intricately tied to the specific placement of these structures and their physiology.

BRIDGE

The portal system in the kidney is one of three major portal systems in the body. The other two are the hypophyseal portal system, which connects the hypothalamus and the anterior pituitary (discussed in Chapter 5 of *MCAT Biology Review*), and the hepatic portal system, which connects the gut tube and the liver (discussed in Chapter 9 of *MCAT Biology Review*). In each case, blood passes through two capillary beds before returning to the heart.

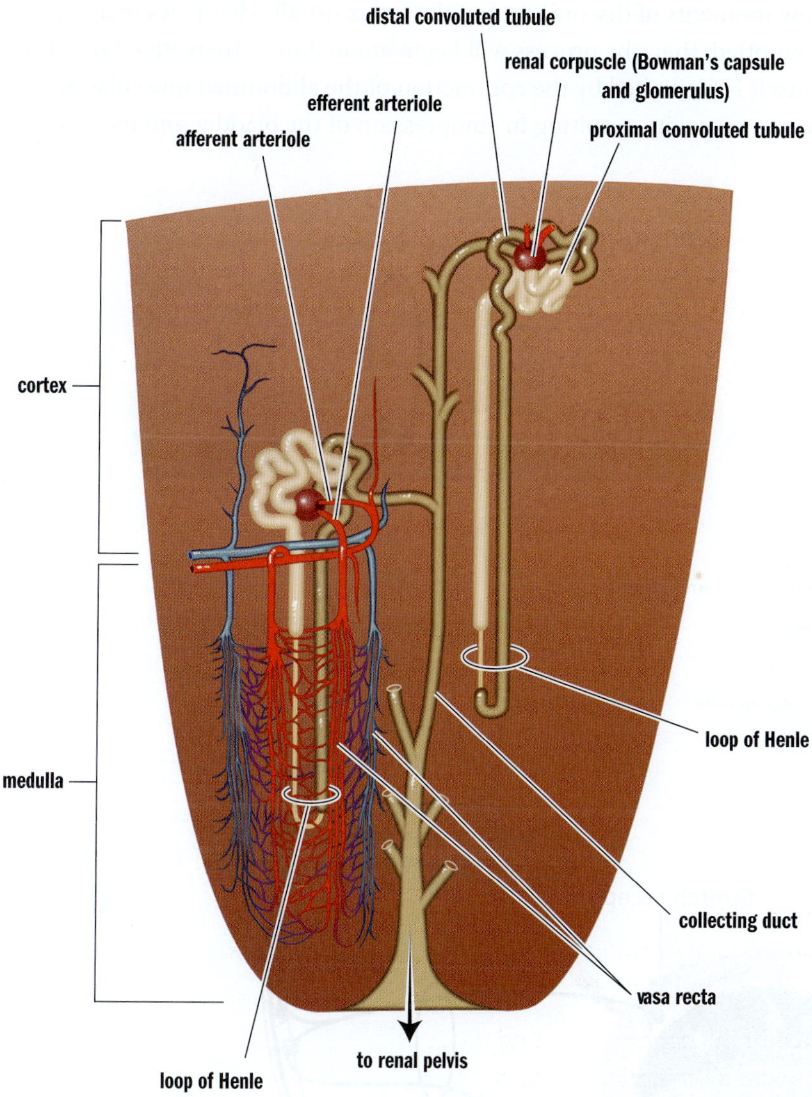

Figure 10.3 Microanatomy of the Renal Vascular System and the Nephron

BRIDGE

Our discussion of neurons in Chapter 4 of *MCAT Biology Review* used some of the same terms as those that describe the organization of blood vessels in the kidney. Afferent neurons carry sensory information toward the central nervous system much as afferent arterioles carry blood toward the glomeruli. Efferent neurons relay signals away from the central nervous system just as efferent arterioles carry blood away from the glomerulus.

Bladder Structure

The ureters from the kidneys empty the filtered fluid into the bladder, which is a hollow cavity. The wall of the bladder is made up of several layers, including **transitional epithlium (urothelium)**, which contains cells that change shape in response to stetching to allow for bladder elasticity. The bladder also has a muscular lining known as the **detrusor muscle**. Parasympathetic activity causes the detrusor muscle to contract. However, in order to leave the body, urine must pass through two sphincters—the internal and external urethral sphincters. The **internal urethral sphincter**, consisting of smooth muscle, is contracted in its normal state. Because the internal sphincter is made of smooth muscle, it is under involuntary control. The **external urethral sphincter** consists of skeletal muscle and is under voluntary control. When the bladder is full, stretch receptors convey to the nervous system that the bladder requires emptying. This causes parasympathetic neurons to fire, and the detrusor muscle contracts. This contraction also causes the internal sphincter to relax. This reflex is known as the **micturition reflex** and is shown in Figure 10.4. The next step is up to the individual. The person can choose to relax the external sphincter to urinate, or can maintain the tone of the external sphincter to prevent urination. This can cause a few moments of discomfort, but the reflex usually dissipates in a few minutes. However, if the bladder is not emptied, then the process will begin anew shortly thereafter. Once the external sphincter is relaxed, urination itself is facilitated by the contraction of the abdominal musculature, which increases pressure within the abdominal cavity, resulting in compression of the bladder and increased urine flow rate.

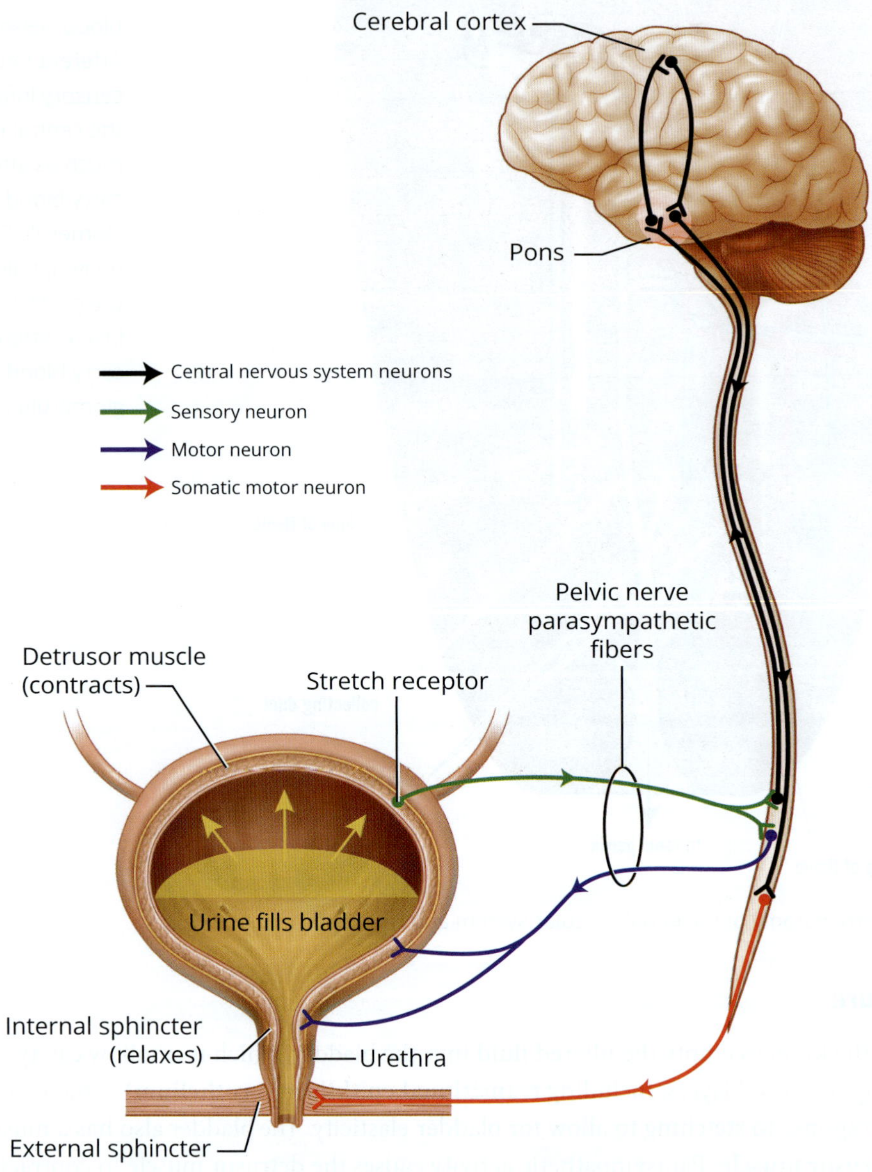

Figure 10.4 The Micturition Reflex

Osmoregulation

The kidney filters the blood to form urine. The composition and quantity of urine is determined by the present state of the body. For example, if blood volume is low and blood osmolarity is high, then it is most beneficial to the body to maximally retain water. This results in low-volume, highly concentrated urine. Likewise, a patient receiving large amounts of intravenous fluids is likely to produce a larger volume of less concentrated urine. Thus, the primary job of the kidneys is to regulate blood volume and osmolarity. In order to do this, kidney function may be divided into three different processes: filtration, secretion, and reabsorption.

Filtration

The nephron's first function is **filtration**. In the kidneys, approximately 20 percent of the blood that passes through the glomerulus is filtered as fluid into Bowman's space. The collected fluid is known as the **filtrate**. The movement of fluid into Bowman's space is governed by **Starling forces**, which account for the pressure differentials in both hydrostatic and oncotic pressures between the blood and Bowman's space, as shown in Figure 10.5. The hydrostatic pressure in the glomerulus is significantly higher than that in Bowman's space, which causes fluid to move into the nephron. On the other hand, the osmolarity of blood is higher than that of Bowman's space, resulting in pressure opposing the movement of fluid into the nephron. However, the hydrostatic pressure is much larger than the oncotic pressure, so the net flow is still from blood into the nephron.

BRIDGE

Like the electromotive force discussed in Chapter 6 of *MCAT Physics and Math Review*, Starling *forces* are really a misnomer. Rather than forces, it is a pressure differential that causes the net movement of fluid from the glomerulus to Bowman's space. Pressure is discussed in Chapter 4 of *MCAT Physics and Math Review.*

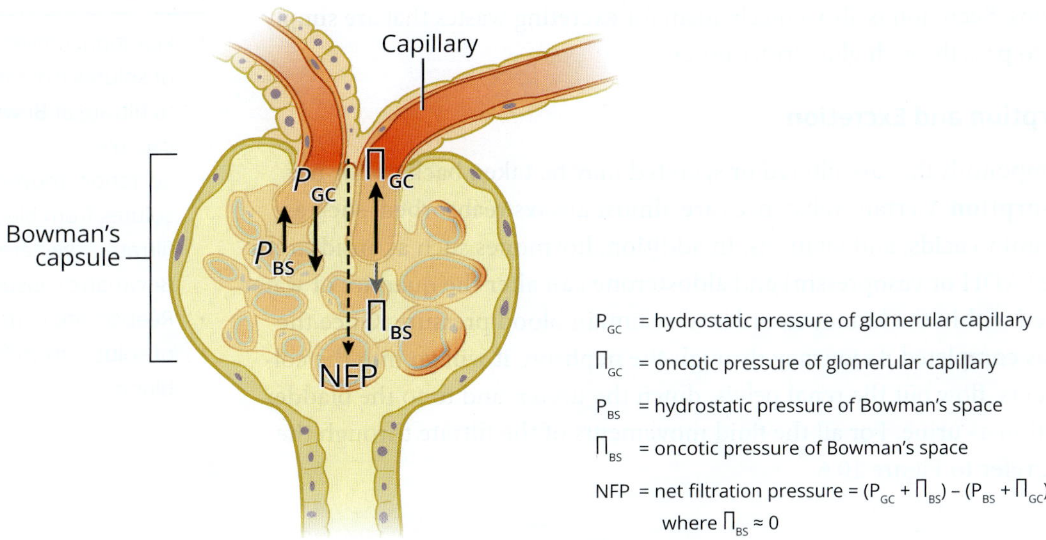

Figure 10.5 Starling Forces
The relative hydrostatic and oncotic pressure gradients determine the direction and rate of filtration.

Under most circumstances, fluid will flow from the glomerulus into Bowman's space. However, various pathologies can cause derangements of this flow. Consider what might happen if the ureter was obstructed by a kidney stone. An obstruction would result in a buildup of urine behind the stone. Eventually, enough fluid will build up and cause distention of the renal pelvis and the nephrons. What will happen to filtration in this case? The hydrostatic pressure in Bowman's space would increase to the point that filtration could no longer occur because there would be excessive pressure opposing movement of fluid into the nephron.

The filtrate is similar in composition to blood but does not contain cells or proteins due to the filter's ability to select based on size. In other words, molecules or cells that are larger than glomerular pores will remain in the blood. As described earlier, the blood remaining in the glomerulus then travels into the efferent arterioles, which empty into the vasa recta. The filtrate is isotonic to blood so that neither the capsule nor the capillaries swell. Our kidneys filter about 180 liters per day, which is approximately 36 times our blood volume. This means that the entire volume of a person's blood is filtered about every 40 minutes. This hyperfiltration by both kidneys is why people can donate a kidney and still function.

Secretion

In addition to filtering blood, the nephrons are able to **secrete** salts, acids, bases, and urea directly into the tubule by either active or passive transport. The quantity and identity of the substances secreted into the nephron are directly related to the needs of the body at that time. For example, a diet heavy in meat results in the intake of large amounts of protein, which contains a significant amount of nitrogen. Ammonia (NH_3) is a byproduct of the metabolism of nitrogen-containing compounds and, as a base, can disturb the pH of blood and cells. The liver converts the ammonia to **urea**, a neutral compound, which travels to the kidney and is secreted into the nephron for excretion in the urine. The kidneys are capable of eliminating ions or other substances when present in relative excess in the blood, such as potassium cations, hydrogen ions, or metabolites of medications. Secretion is also a mechanism for excreting wastes that are simply too large to pass through glomerular pores.

Reabsorption and Excretion

Some compounds that are filtered or secreted may be taken back up for use via **reabsorption**. Certain substances are almost always reabsorbed, such as glucose, amino acids, and vitamins. In addition, hormones such as antidiuretic hormone (ADH or vasopressin) and aldosterone can alter the quantity of water reabsorbed within the kidney in order to maintain blood pressure. Once the filtrate has completed its journey through the nephron, it will go into the collecting ducts, flow out the renal pelvis, down the ureter, and to to the bladder for excretion as urine. For all the fluid movements of the filtrate through the nephron, refer to Figure 10.6.

KEY CONCEPT

Imagine that the glomerulus is like a sieve or colander. Small molecules dissolved in the blood will pass through the tiny pores (such as glucose, which is later reabsorbed), whereas large molecules such as proteins and blood cells will not. If blood cells or proteins are found in the urine, this indicates a health problem at the level of the glomerulus.

KEY CONCEPT

- Filtration: movement of solutes from blood to filtrate at Bowman's capsule
- Secretion: movement of solutes from blood to filtrate anywhere besides Bowman's capsule
- Reabsorption: movement of solutes from filtrate to blood

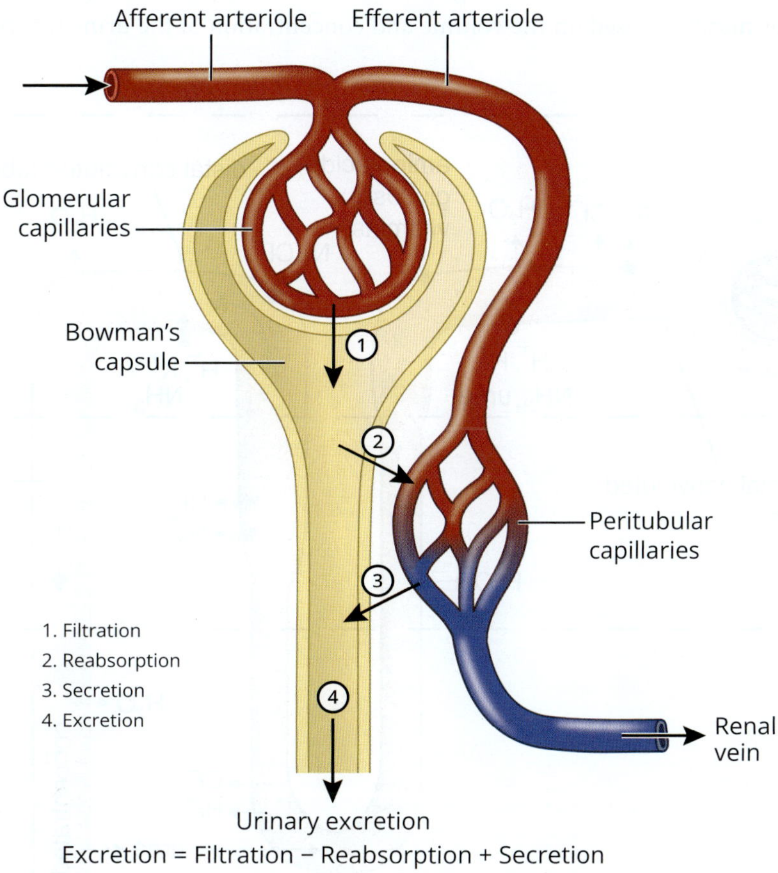

Figure 10.6 Renal Mechanisms for Moving Material

Nephron Function

The kidney uses mechanisms such as filtration, secretion, and reabsorption to produce urine and to regulate the blood volume and osmolarity. However, the function of the nephron isn't quite that simple. In fact, renal physiology is often considered one of the most difficult topics covered in medical school.

In order to simplify this topic, it is important to understand that the kidney has two main goals: keep what the body needs and lose what it doesn't, and concentrate the urine to conserve water. The kidney allows the human body to reabsorb certain materials for reuse, while also selectively eliminating waste. For example, glucose and amino acids are not usually present in the urine because the kidney is able to reabsorb these substances for later use. On the contrary, waste products like hydrogen and potassium ions, ammonia, and urea remain in the filtrate and are excreted. Finally, water is reabsorbed in large quantities in order to maintain blood pressure and adequate hydration.

KEY CONCEPT

Anything that makes it into the filtrate and that is not reabsorbed will be lost from the body in the urine.

In order to understand this complex organ, we will study the nephron piece-by-piece, discussing exactly what is occurring in each segment. Follow along with the nephron diagram shown in Figure 10.7. As a theme, note that segments that are horizontal in the diagram (Bowman's capsule, the proximal convoluted tubule, and the distal convoluted tubule) are primarily focused on the *identity* of the particles in the urine (*keep what the body needs and lose what it doesn't*). In contrast, the segments that are vertical in the diagram (the loop of Henle and collecting duct) are primarily focused on the volume and concentration of the urine (*concentrate the urine to conserve water*).

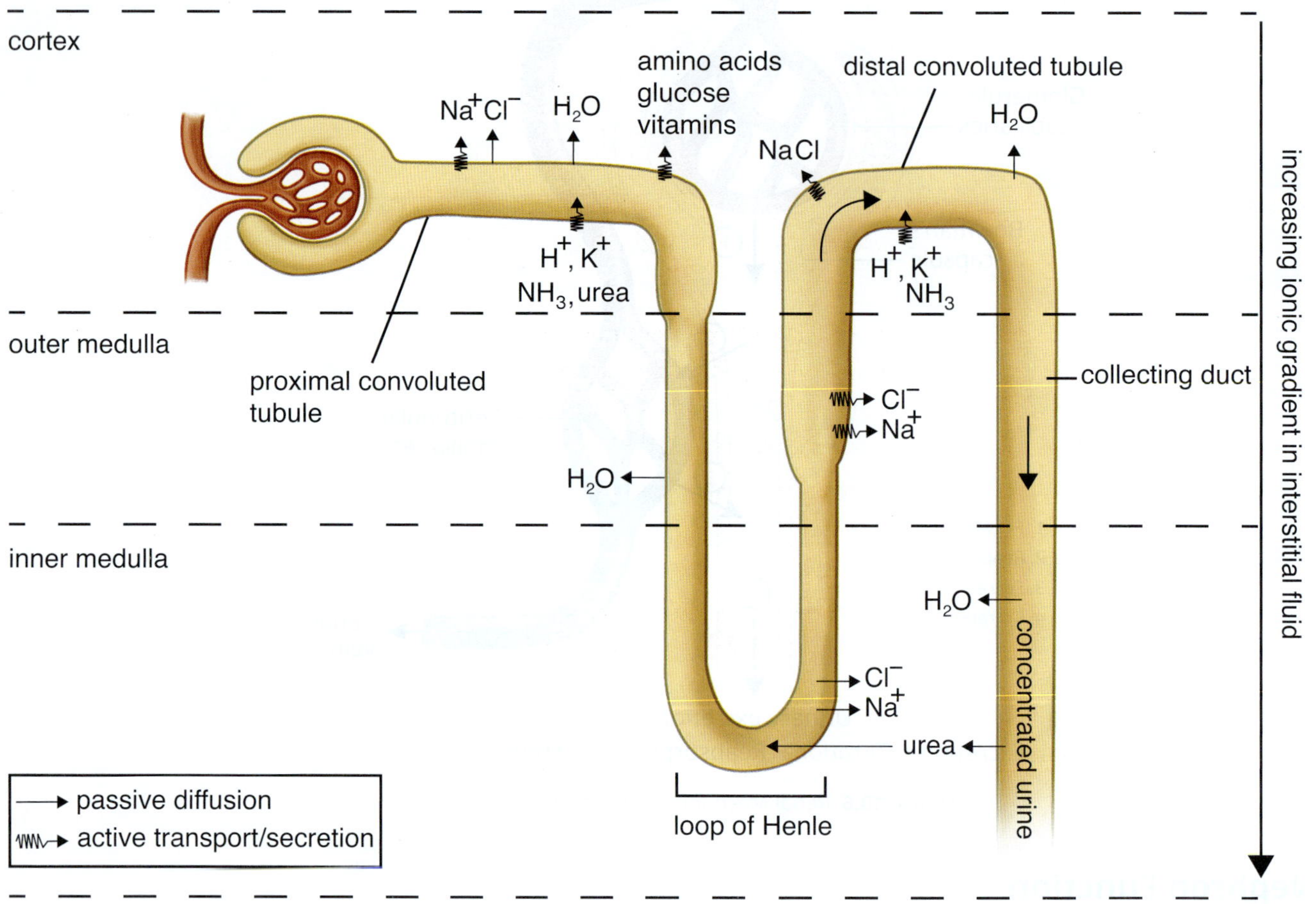

Figure 10.7 Reabsorption and Secretion in the Nephron

Proximal Convoluted Tubule

The filtrate first enters the **proximal convoluted tubule** (**PCT**). In this region, amino acids, glucose, water-soluble vitamins, and the majority of salts are reabsorbed along with water. Almost 70 percent of filtered sodium will be reabsorbed here, but the filtrate remains isotonic to the interstitium, as other solutes and a large volume of water are also reabsorbed. Solutes that enter the **interstitium**—the connective tissue surrounding the nephron—are picked up by the vasa recta to be returned to the bloodstream for reuse within the body. The PCT is also the site of secretion for a number of waste products, including hydrogen ions, potassium ions, ammonia, and urea.

MNEMONIC

Major waste products excreted in the urine: **Dump the HUNK**

- **H^+**
- **U**rea
- **N**H_3
- **K**$^+$

Loop of Henle

Filtrate from the proximal convoluted tubule then enters the **descending limb of the loop of Henle**, which dives deep into the medulla before turning around to become the **ascending limb of the loop of Henle**. The descending limb is permeable only to water, and the medulla has an ever-increasing osmolarity as the descending limb travels deeper into it. Think for a moment how this would affect the flow of water. As the descending limb traverses deeper into the medulla, the increasing interstitial concentration favors the outflow of water from the descending limb, which is reabsorbed into the vasa recta.

The kidney is capable of altering the osmolarity of the interstitium. This creates a gradient that, coupled with selective permeability of the nephron, allows maximal reabsorption and conservation of water. In the normal physiological state, the osmolarity in the cortex is approximately the same as that of the blood and remains at that level. Deeper in the medulla, the osmolarity in the interstitium can range from isotonic with blood (when trying to excrete water) to four times as concentrated (when trying to conserve water). If the concentration is the same in the tubule and in the interstitium, there is no driving force (gradient), and the water will be lost in urine. If the interstitium is more concentrated, then water will move out of the tubule, into the interstitium, and eventually back into the blood.

Together, the vasa recta and nephron create a **countercurrent multiplier system** (shown in Figure 10.8). This means that the flow of filtrate through the loop of Henle is in the opposite direction from the flow of blood through the vasa recta. If the two flowed in the same direction, they would quickly reach equilibrium and the kidney would be unable to reabsorb as much water. By making the two flow in opposite directions, the filtrate is constantly being exposed to hypertonic blood, which allows maximal reabsorption of water.

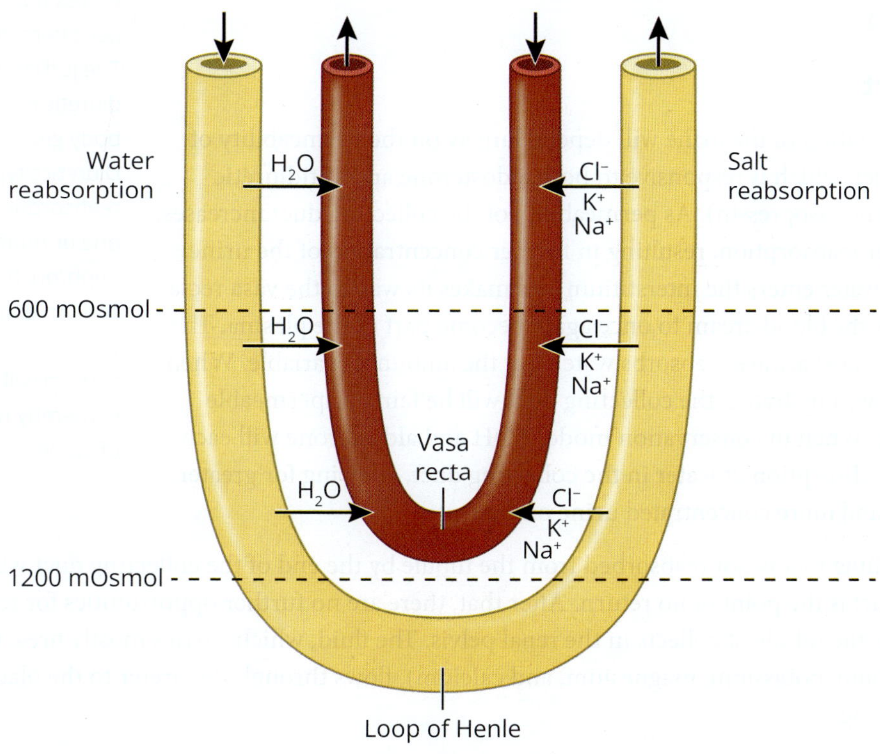

Figure 10.8 The Countercurrent Multiplier System

As the descending limb transitions to become the ascending limb of the loop of Henle, a change in permeability occurs. The ascending limb is only permeable to salts and is impermeable to water. So while the descending limb maximizes water reabsorption by taking advantage of increasing medullary osmolarity, the ascending limb maximizes salt reabsorption by taking advantage of *decreasing* medullary osmolarity.

At the transition from the inner to outer medulla, the loop of Henle becomes thicker in what is termed the **diluting segment**. This is not because the lumen within the tube has enlarged, but because the cells lining the tube are larger. These cells contain large amounts of mitochondria, which allow the reabsorption of sodium and chloride by active transport. Indeed, because so much salt is reabsorbed while water is stuck in the nephron, the filtrate actually becomes hypotonic compared to the interstitium. While we tend to focus on the concentrating abilities of the nephron, this segment (coupled with the countercurrent multiplier system) is noteworthy because it can produce urine that is more dilute than the blood. This is important during periods of *overhydration* and provides a mechanism for eliminating excess water.

At the beginning of the loop of Henle, the filtrate is isotonic to the interstitium. Thus, from the beginning of the loop of Henle to the end, there is a slight degree of dilution. Far more important, however, is the fact that the volume of the filtrate has been significantly reduced, demonstrating a net reabsorption of a large volume of water.

Distal Convoluted Tubule

Next, the filtrate enters the **distal convoluted tubule** (**DCT**). The DCT responds to aldosterone, which promotes sodium reabsorption. Because sodium ions are osmotically active particles, water will follow the sodium, concentrating the urine and decreasing its volume. The DCT is also a site of waste product secretion, like the PCT.

Collecting Duct

The final concentration of the urine will depend largely on the permeability of the collecting duct, which is responsive to both aldosterone and antidiuretic hormone (ADH or vasopressin). As permeability of the collecting duct increases, so too does water reabsorption, resulting in further concentration of the urine. The reabsorbed water enters the interstitium and makes its way to the vasa recta, where it reenters the bloodstream to once again become part of the plasma. The collecting duct almost always reabsorbs water, but the amount is variable. When the body is very well hydrated, the collecting duct will be fairly impermeable to salt and water. When in conservation mode, ADH and aldosterone will each act to increase reabsorption of water in the collecting duct, allowing for greater water retention and more concentrated urine output.

REAL WORLD

In certain conditions, such as congestive heart failure, the body accumulates excess fluid in the lungs or peripheral tissues (edema). The judicious use of a diuretic drug can help the body get rid of excess fluid. Diuretics typically inhibit the reabsorption of sodium in one or more regions of the nephron, thereby increasing sodium excretion. As an osmotically active particle, sodium will pull water with it, thereby relieving the body of some of its excess fluid.

Ultimately, anything that is not reabsorbed from the tubule by the end of the collecting duct will be excreted; the collecting duct is the point of no return. After that, there are no further opportunities for reabsorption. As the filtrate leaves the tubule, it collects in the renal pelvis. The fluid, which carries mostly urea, uric acid, and excess ions (sodium, potassium, magnesium, and calcium), flows through the ureter to the bladder where it is stored until voiding.

Functions of the Excretory System

The kidneys use osmolarity gradients and selective permeability to filter, secrete, and reabsorb materials in the process of making urine. However, these processes have larger implications for the human body as a whole. The selective elimination of water and solutes allows the kidneys, in conjunction with the endocrine, cardiovascular, and respiratory systems, to control blood pressure, blood osmolarity, and acid–base balance.

Blood Pressure

In Chapter 5 of *MCAT Biology Review*, we discussed two hormones that are very important for the maintenance of proper blood pressure: aldosterone and antidiuretic hormone (ADH or vasopressin).

Aldosterone is a steroid hormone that is secreted by the adrenal cortex in response to decreased blood pressure. Decreased blood pressure stimulates the release of **renin** from **juxtaglomerular cells** in the kidney. Renin then cleaves **angiotensinogen**, a liver protein, to form **angiotensin I**. This peptide is then metabolized by **angiotensin-converting enzyme** in the lungs to form **angiotensin II**, which promotes the release of aldosterone from the adrenal cortex.

Aldosterone works by altering the ability of the distal convoluted tubule and collecting duct to reabsorb sodium. Remember that water does not move on its own, but rather travels down its osmolarity gradient. Thus, if we reabsorb more sodium, water will flow with it. This reabsorption of isotonic fluid has the net effect of increasing blood volume and therefore blood pressure. Aldosterone will also increase potassium and hydrogen ion excretion.

Antidiuretic hormone (**ADH**, also known as **vasopressin**) is a peptide hormone synthesized by the hypothalamus and released by the posterior pituitary in response to high blood osmolarity (see Figure 10.9). It directly alters the permeability of the collecting duct, allowing more water to be reabsorbed by increasing the number of aquaporins on the cells lining the collecting duct. Increased concentration in the interstitium (hypertonic to the filtrate) will then cause the reabsorption of water from the tubule. Alcohol and caffeine both inhibit ADH release and lead to the frequent excretion of dilute urine.

REAL WORLD

Aldosterone increases blood pressure by increasing the reabsorption of sodium. In medicine, we exploit this characteristic by using drugs that actually block angiotensin-converting enzyme or the angiotensin II receptor. In Chapter 5 of *MCAT Biology Review*, we mentioned the ACE inhibitors, which mostly end with *–pril*. The angiotensin II receptor blockers mostly end with *–sartan* (*losartan*, *valsartan*, *irbesartan*). Blocking this receptor limits aldosterone release, which limits salt and water reabsorption, and therefore results in lowered blood pressure.

KEY CONCEPT

ADH only governs water reabsorption and thus results in a lower blood osmolarity. Aldosterone causes both salt and water reabsorption and does not change blood osmolarity.

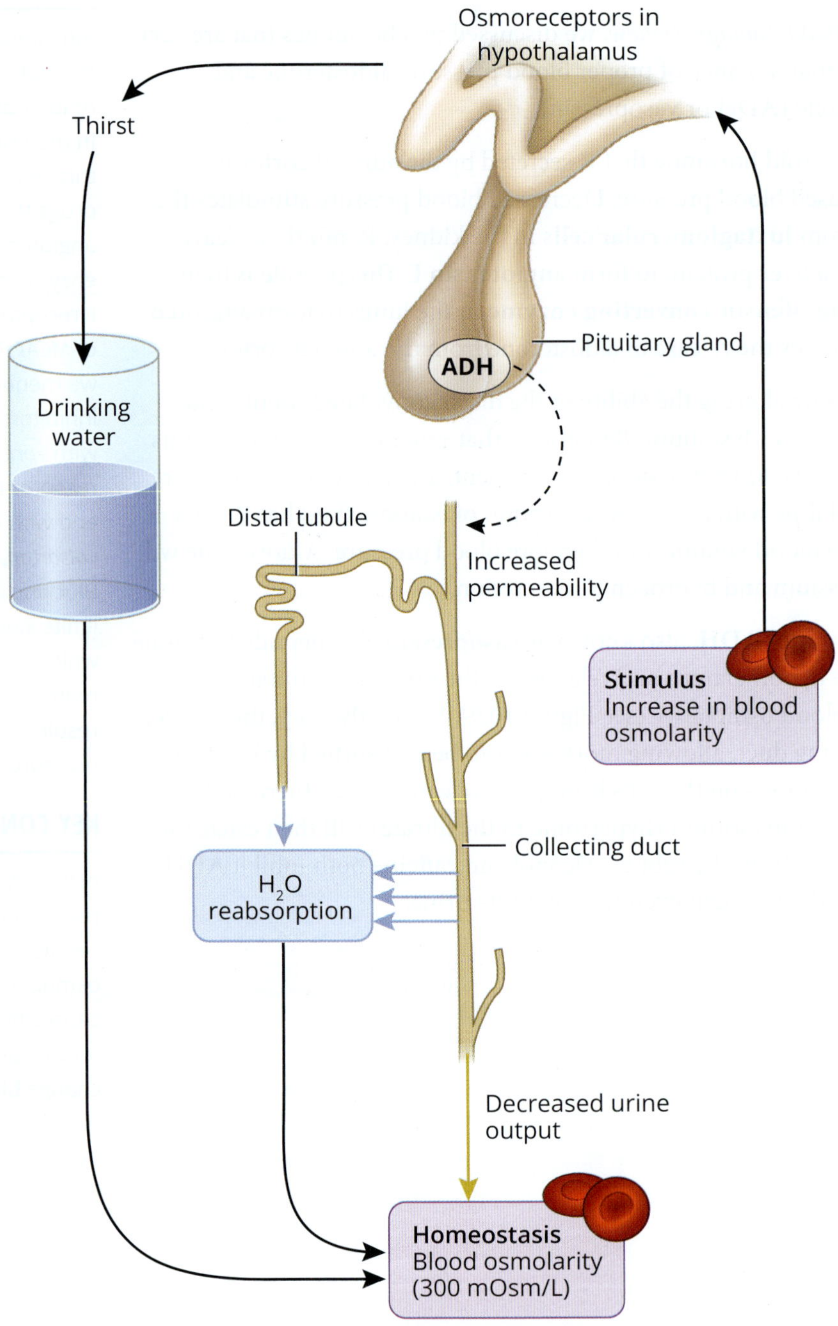

Figure 10.9 Mechanism of Antidiuretic Hormone (ADH)

In addition to the kidneys, the cardiovascular system also regulates blood pressure, specifically by vasoconstricting or vasodilating in order to maintain blood pressure. Constriction of the afferent arteriole will lead to a lower pressure of blood reaching the glomeruli, which are adjacent to the juxtaglomerular cells. Therefore, this vasoconstriction will secondarily lead to renin release, which will also help raise blood pressure.

Osmoregulation

The osmolarity of the blood must be tightly controlled to ensure correct oncotic pressures within the vasculature. A note on terminology: **osmotic pressure** is the "sucking" pressure that draws water into the vasculature caused by all dissolved particles. **Oncotic pressure**, on the other hand, is the osmotic pressure that is attributable to dissolved proteins specifically. Blood osmolarity is usually maintained at approximately 290 milliosmoles (mOsm) per liter. As described earlier, the kidneys control osmolarity by modulating the reabsorption of water and by filtering and secreting dissolved particles. When blood osmolarity is low, excess water will be excreted, while solutes will be reabsorbed in higher concentrations. In contrast, when blood osmolarity is high, water reabsorption increases and solute excretion increases.

Acid–Base Balance

The **bicarbonate buffer system** is the major regulator of blood pH. Remind yourself of the buffer equation:

$$CO_2\,(g) + H_2O\,(l) \leftrightharpoons H_2CO_3\,(aq) \leftrightharpoons H^+\,(aq) + HCO_3^-\,(aq)$$

In Chapter 6 of *MCAT Biology Review*, we talked about how the respiratory system can contribute to acid–base balance by increasing or decreasing the respiratory rate. If the blood pH is too low, then increasing the respiratory rate blows off more CO_2 and favors the conversion of H^+ and HCO_3^- to water and carbon dioxide, increasing the pH. If the blood pH is too high, then decreasing the respiratory rate causes the opposite effects. The respiratory system can react to derangements of pH quickly. What can the excretory system do to contribute? The kidneys are able to selectively increase or decrease the secretion of hydrogen ions and bicarbonate. When blood pH is too low, the kidneys excrete more hydrogen ions and increase reabsorption of bicarbonate, resulting in a higher pH. Likewise, when blood pH is too high, the kidneys can excrete more bicarbonate and increase the reabsorption of hydrogen ions. This is slower than the respiratory response, but it is a highly effective way for the body to maintain acid–base balance. The specific renal responses to acidosis and alkalosis are summarized in Table 10.1.

	Hydrogen Ion		Bicarbonate Ion		
Condition	**Effect**	**Nephron segment involved**	**Effect**	**Nephron segment involved**	**Net Result**
Low pH (acidosis)	Increased secretion	Proximal tubule and collecting duct	Increased reabsorption	Proximal tubule	Net H^+ excretion, net HCO_3^- conservation
High pH (alkalosis)	Decreased secretion	Collecting duct	Increased secretion	Collecting duct	Net HCO_3^- excretion, net H^+ conservation

Table 10.1 Kidney Responses to Acidosis and Alkalosis

BIOLOGY GUIDED EXAMPLE WITH EXPERT THINKING

Carbonic anhydrases are a group of zinc metalloenzymes that catalyze the reversible hydration of carbon dioxide into carbonic acid, which in solution rapidly dissociates into bicarbonate and a proton. The second isoform, carbonic anhydrase II (CAII) is soluble and is expressed in most tissues including red blood cells, osteoclasts, and the kidney. CAII physically and functionally interacts with aquaporin-1 (AQP1) to increase permeability of AQP1 to water. AQP1 is expressed in the lumen facing and the interstitium facing membranes of the proximal tubule, as well as the thin descending limb (TDL) of the loop of Henle. Our observation that CAII augments water flux through AQP1 led us to posit that CAII may contribute to water reabsorption and consequently to urinary concentrating ability. To test this hypothesis, we examined water homeostasis in CAII-deficient (CAII def) mice. These mice were found to be polydipsic (high water intake) and polyuric (high urine volume). Analysis of the osmolarity of the urine is seen in Figure 1. We also measured the following properties in the interstitium of the renal cortex, inner strip of the outer medulla (ISOM), which lies between the cortex and the medulla, and the inner medulla (IM): osmolarity (Figure 2) and sodium ion concentration (Figure 3).
*Represents $p < 0.05$

CA = enzyme that catalyzes CO_2 into bicarbonate ion

CAII isoform is expressed in most tissues

CAII interacts with AQP1 → more water reabsorption

APQ1 is found in the proximal convoluted tubule and descending limb of loop of Henle

Hypothesis: CAII helps with water resorption and concentrating urine

Knocked out CAII in mice, looked at water homeostasis

CAII-def mice drank lots of water, had high volume of urine

Fig 1: urine osmolarity

Looked at three different kidney areas: cortex, between cortex and medulla, and medulla

Fig 2: osmolarity in three kidney regions

Fig 3: sodium ion concentration in three kidney regions

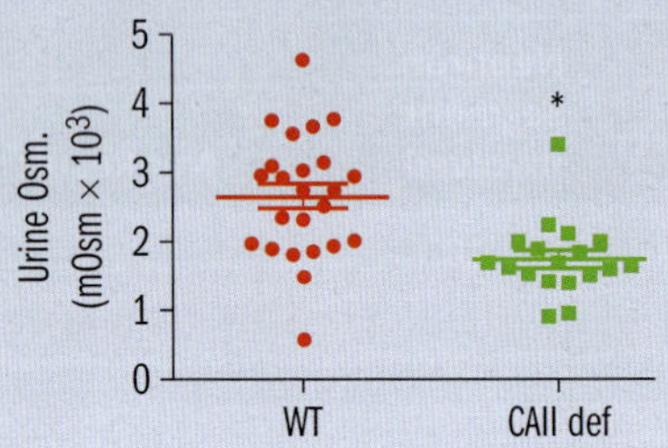

Figure 1

IV: wild-type or CAII-def mice

DV: urine osmolarity

Trend: CAII-def mice have significantly lower urine osmolarity

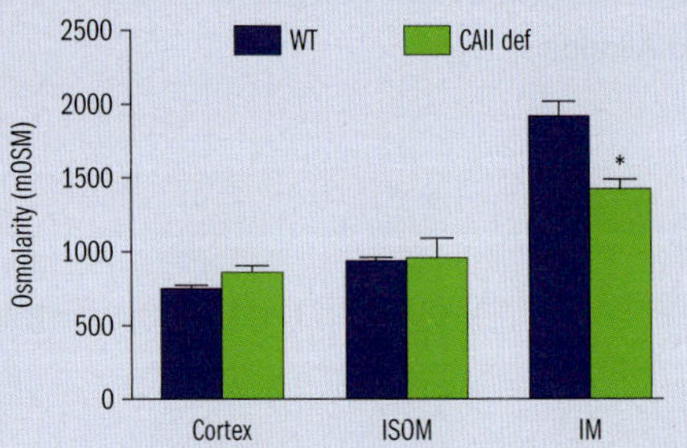

Figure 2

IV: region of kidney, type of mice (WT or CAII-def)

DV: interstitium osmolarity

Trend: inner medulla of kidney interstitium has significantly lower osmolarity in CAII-def mice compared to WT

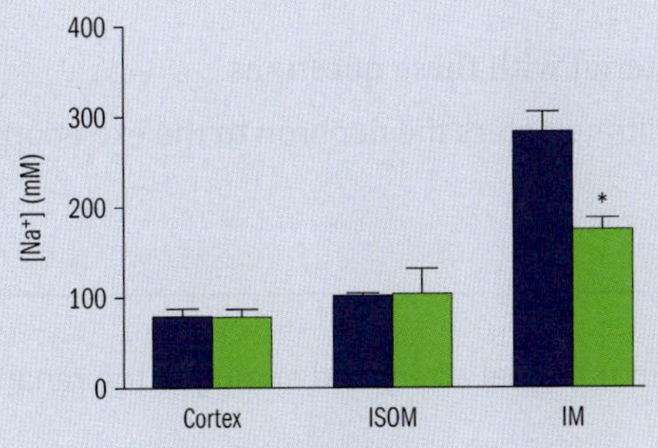

Figure 3

IV: region of kidney, type of mice (WT or CAII-def)

DV: interstitium sodium concentration

Trend: inner medulla of kidney interstitium has significantly lower sodium concentration in CAII-def mice compared to WT

Adapted from Krishnan, D., Pan, W., Beggs, M. R., Trepiccione, F., Chambrey, R., Eladari, D., Cordat, E., Dimke, H., ... Alexander, R. T. (2018). Deficiency of carbonic anhydrase II results in a urinary concentrating defect. *Frontiers in Physiology* 8, 1108. doi:10.3389/fphys.2017.01108.

According to the data, lack of CAII has the greatest impact on which portion of the nephron?

Since the question is asking us to use the data to pinpoint a specific area of the nephron being affected, it's important to understand the experimental setup and the results, and to be prepared to use our outside content knowledge. The researcher's goal is to better understand the role CAII plays in water resorption through its interaction with AQP1. We should know from our content background that aquaporin (AQP) is a water-specific membrane channel found in many parts of the nephron, and AQP availability on the membrane allows for movement of water from the filtrate back into the body. We're also given some information about CAII—it's the enzyme responsible for creating bicarbonate ions, and we're told it interacts with AQP1 to increase water permeability.

In creating mice with deficient CAII, the researchers are looking for a change in the osmolarity of the urine and the kidney. We're told in paragraph 2 that the CAII-deficient mice have a high urine volume and high water intake, supporting the hypothesis that the mice are not reabsorbing enough water, but instead are excreting it as urine. Figure 1 also supports this conclusion by showing that urine is more dilute in CAII-deficient mice than in wild-type (controls). However, this data doesn't answer the question of where specifically in the nephron lack of CAII is having the greatest impact. Figures 2 and 3 both have information about specific parts of the kidney, which is where our answer is going to come from. Recall that cortex refers to the outer region of the organ, while medulla refers to the inner part. We're given an additional area called the ISOM, which is the boundary between the cortex and medulla. We can see from those two figures that the osmolarity of the interstitium in the inner medulla (IM) is significantly lower than in normal mice, indicating that the part of the nephron existing in the inner medulla is the problem area. Paragraph 1 states that AQP1 is found in the proximal tubule and the thin descending limb of the loop of Henle. The proximal tubule would be in the outer part of the kidney in the cortex, and the thin descending limb would go deep into the kidney, moving into the inner medulla, making the descending limb the part of the nephron that is being most affected. While this satisfies the requirements of the question, this brings up another issue: why does less water being reabsorbed into the interstitium result in less osmolarity? Shouldn't the expected result be a higher osmolarity? This ultimately comes down to how the nephron works as a whole to concentrate your urine. Lack of water being reabsorbed by the thin descending limb will result in a decrease of ions being passively reabsorbed in the ascending limb, giving us that drop in osmolarity.

Using the results of the data, we can conclude that the CAII-deficient mice are being most impacted by the reduced efficacy of AQP1 in the thin descending limb of the loop of Henle.

MCAT CONCEPT CHECK 10.1

Before you move on, assess your understanding of the material with these questions.

1. List the structures in the excretory pathway, from where filtrate enters the nephron to the excretion of urine from the body.

____

2. List the vessels in the renal vascular pathway, starting from the renal artery and ending at the renal vein.

____

3. What arm of the nervous system is responsible for contraction of the detrusor muscle?

____

4. What are the three processes by which solutes are exchanged between the filtrate and the blood? What happens in each process?
   - ____
   - ____
   - ____

5. For each segment of the nephron listed below, what are its major functions?
   - Bowman's capsule: ____
   - Proximal convoluted tubule: ____
   - Descending limb of the loop of Henle: ____
   - Ascending limb of the loop of Henle: ____
   - Distal convoluted tubule: ____
   - Collecting duct: ____

10.2 Skin

LEARNING OBJECTIVES

After Chapter 10.2, you will be able to:

- Recall the predominant cell type in the epidermis
- Order the layers of the epidermis and dermis
- Describe the mechanisms the body uses to regulate temperature using the integument

By both weight and size, the **skin** (**integument**) is the largest organ in our bodies. It makes up about 16 percent of total body weight, on average. Skin is one of the major components of nonspecific immune defense, protecting us from exposure to the elements and invasion by pathogens.

Structure

The skin has several layers. Starting from the deepest layer and working outward, these layers are the **hypodermis** (**subcutaneous** layer), **dermis**, and **epidermis**, as shown in Figure 10.10. Skin is derived from the ectoderm.

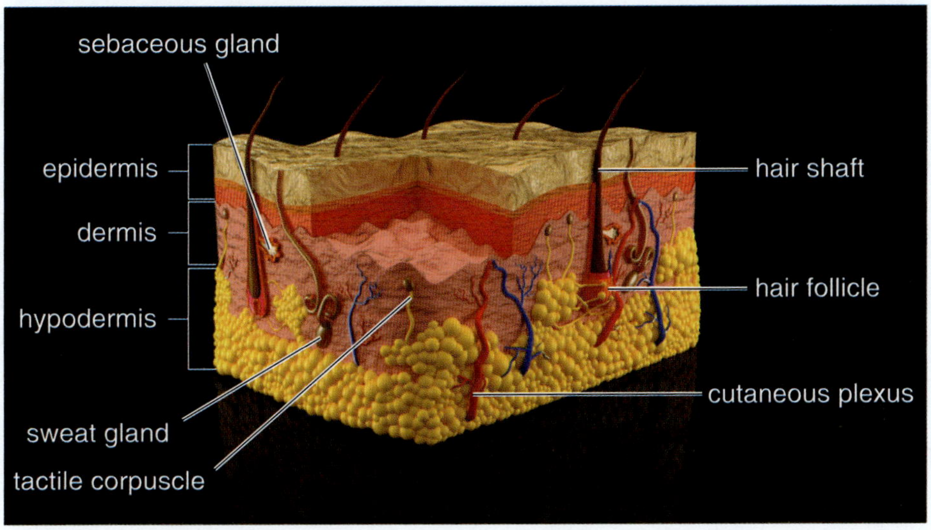

Figure 10.10 Anatomy of the Skin and Subcutaneous Tissue

The Epidermis

The **epidermis** is also subdivided into layers called **strata**. From the deepest layer outward, these are the stratum basale, stratum spinosum, stratum granulosum, stratum lucidum, and stratum corneum, as shown in Figure 10.11. The **stratum basale** contains stem cells and is responsible for proliferation of **keratinocytes**, the predominant cells of the skin, that produce **keratin**. In the **stratum spinosum**, these cells become connected to each other; this layer is also the site of Langerhans cells, described below. In the **stratum granulosum**, the keratinocytes die and lose their nuclei. The **stratum lucidum** is only present in thick, hairless skin, such as the skin on the sole of the foot or the palms, and is nearly transparent. Finally, the **stratum corneum** contains up to several dozen layers of flattened keratinocytes, forming a barrier that prevents invasion by pathogens and that helps to prevent loss of fluids and salt. Hair projects above the skin, and there are openings for sweat and sebaceous glands.

MNEMONIC

Layers of the skin (superficial to deep): **C**ome, **L**et's **G**et **S**un **B**urned

- Stratum **c**orneum
- Stratum **l**ucidum
- Stratum **g**ranulosum
- Stratum **s**pinosum
- Stratum **b**asale

REAL WORLD

People who have albinism suffer from a genetic metabolic disorder characterized by the inability to synthesize melanin. Typically, albinism is inherited in an autosomal recessive fashion. As would be expected, patients with albinism are extremely sensitive to the harmful effects of the sun. Depigmentation can also occur in vitiligo, an autoimmune disorder in which melanocytes are killed by the individual's immune system.

BRIDGE

Evaporation is an endothermic process and, thus, substances absorb energy from the surroundings to undergo this phase change. Further, the presence of dissolved solutes in sweat increases the boiling point of sweat slightly in comparison to pure water; this allows the absorption of even more heat energy. Boiling point elevation is a colligative property that is discussed in Chapter 9 of *MCAT General Chemistry Review*.

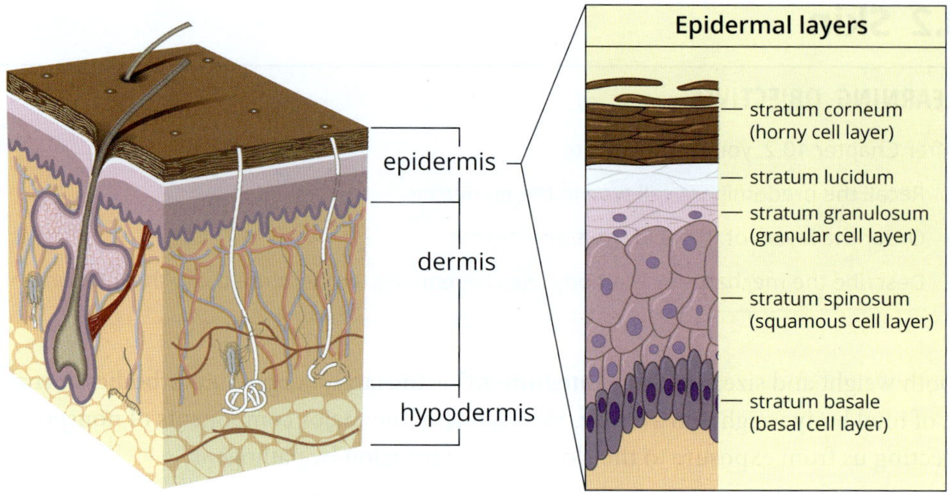

Figure 10.11 Layers of the Epidermis

Other Cells of the Epidermis

In the epidermis, the main cells are keratinocytes. Keratin, mentioned above, is resistant to damage and provides protection against injury, water, and pathogens. **Calluses** form from excessive keratin deposition in areas of repeated strain due to friction; they provide protection to avoid damage in the future. **Fingernails** and **hair** are also formed from keratin and are produced by specialized cells in the skin.

Melanocytes are a cell type derived from neural crest cells and found in the stratum basale. These cells produce **melanin**, a pigment that serves to protect the skin from DNA damage caused by ultraviolet radiation. Once produced, the pigment is transferred to the keratinocytes. All humans have comparable numbers of melanocytes; skin color is caused by varying levels of activity of the melanocytes. More active melanocytes result in darker skin tones. Upon exposure to ultraviolet radiation, melanocytes increase activity, resulting in a darker skin color.

Langerhans cells are actually special macrophages that reside within the stratum spinosum. These cells are capable of presenting antigens to T-cells in order to activate the immune system.

The Dermis

The dermis also consists of multiple layers. The upper layer (right below the epidermis) is the **papillary layer**, which consists of loose connective tissue. Below the papillary layer is the denser **reticular layer**. Sweat glands, blood vessels, and hair follicles originate in the dermis.

Most sensory receptors are also located in the dermis. **Merkel cells (discs)**, for example, are sensory receptors present at the epidermal–dermal junction. These cells are connected to sensory neurons and are responsible for deep pressure and texture sensation within the skin. Other sensory organs in the skin include free nerve endings, which respond to pain; **Meissner's corpuscles**, which respond to light touch; **Ruffini endings**, which respond to stretch; and **Pacinian corpuscles**, which respond to deep pressure and vibration. These receptors are illustrated in Figure 10.12.

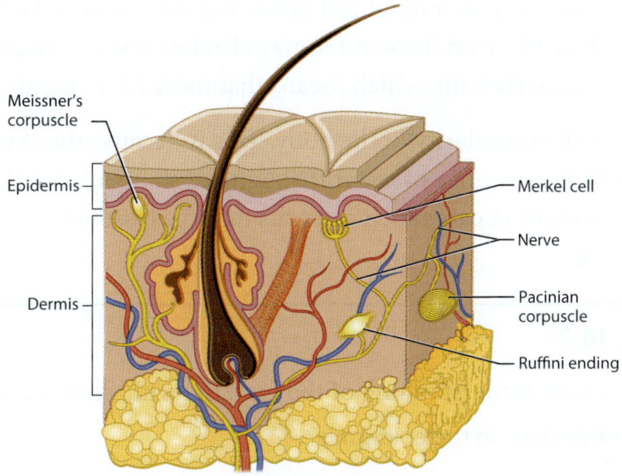

Figure 10.12 Sensory Structures of the Dermis

The Hypodermis

Finally, the **hypodermis** is a layer of connective tissue that connects the epithelium to the rest of the body. This layer contains loose connective tissue known as **areolar tissue**. Areolar tissue plays an important role in allowing for nutrient and waste exchange.

Thermoregulation

We have already mentioned that the skin protects us from the elements and microbes. It also has other functions, including ultraviolet protection (via melanin) and transduction of sensory information from the outside world. In this section, we look at another function of the skin: thermoregulation.

Thermoregulation is achieved by sweating, piloerection, vasodilation, and vasoconstriction. **Sweating** is an excellent cooling mechanism that is controlled by the autonomic nervous system. When body temperature rises above the set point determined by the hypothalamus, thermoregulation processes must occur in order to rid the body of heat. Postganglionic sympathetic neurons that utilize acetylcholine innervate sweat glands and promote the secretion of water with certain ions onto the skin. Heat is then absorbed from the body as the water molecules undergo a phase change to evaporate. The production of sweat itself is not the main mechanism of cooling; it is the evaporation of water from the skin which absorbs body heat. At the same time, arteriolar vasodilation occurs to maximize heat loss. This brings a large quantity of blood to the skin, which accelerates the evaporation of sweat by maximizing the heat energy available for the liquid–gas phase change.

In cold conditions, **arrector pili** muscles contract, causing the hairs of the skin to stand up on end (**piloerection**). This helps to trap a layer of heated air near the skin. It is important to note that the extent of this ability's efficacy is determined by how much hair an organism has. For most humans, the erector pili muscles result in what is widely referred to as goosebumps. In addition, the arterioles that feed the capillaries of the skin constrict, limiting the quantity of blood reaching the skin. Skeletal muscle may also begin to contract rapidly, causing shivering. **Shivering** requires a sizeable amount of ATP; however, a significant portion of the energy from ATP is converted into thermal energy. In addition

BRIDGE

The neurons that innervate sweat glands are actually very unusual. Unlike all other postganglionic sympathetic neurons, these neurons are cholinergic—not noradrenergic (that is, they release acetylcholine, not norepinephrine). All preganglionic neurons in the autonomic nervous system and postganglionic neurons in the parasympathetic nervous system are cholinergic as well. These neurons are discussed in Chapter 4 of *MCAT Biology Review*.

to these mechanisms, humans possess a layer of fat just below the skin. This fat helps to insulate the body. In addition to this fat, which is called **white fat**, **brown fat** may also be present, especially in infants. Brown fat has a much less efficient electron transport chain, which means that more heat energy is released as fuel is burned.

The skin also helps to maintain the osmolarity of the body. This is because the skin is relatively impermeable to water. This prevents not only the entrance of water through the skin, but also the loss of water from the tissues. This becomes very important in cases such as burns or large losses of skin as dehydration of the tissues becomes a real threat to survival.

MCAT CONCEPT CHECK 10.2

Before you move on, assess your understanding of the material with these questions.

1. What is the predominant cell type in the epidermis?

___

2. What are the layers of the epidermis, from superficial to deep?

   -
   -
   -
   -
   -

3. What are the layers of the dermis, from superficial to deep?

   -
   -

4. What are some mechanisms the body uses to cool itself? What are some mechanisms the body uses to retain heat?

   - Cooling:
   - Retaining heat:

Conclusion

Two main organ systems were discussed in this chapter: the excretory system and the skin. Both of these systems play an essential role in homeostasis. However, this chapter also demonstrated a very MCAT-worthy concept: no system works alone. Multiple systems participate in homeostasis. While the kidneys are the major players in salt, water, and acid–base balance, their function depends on the endocrine system, circulatory system, and respiratory system. While the skin is an important immune organ in and of itself, its function as a thermoregulatory organ is dependent on the nervous system—and it also sends sensory signals *to* the nervous system. As you move on to the last organ system in the next chapter—the musculoskeletal system—notice how each system interacts with other systems in order to produce a fully functioning organism. The MCAT is far more focused on how you conceptualize the big picture, and not on how many details you memorize. As you study, focus on understanding these systems and how each system influences the rest of the body.

▶ GO ONLINE

You've reviewed the content, now test your knowledge and critical thinking skills by completing a test-like passage set in your online resources!

CONCEPT SUMMARY

The Excretory System

- The **excretory system** serves many functions, including the regulation of blood pressure, blood osmolarity, acid–base balance, and removal of nitrogenous wastes.
- The **kidney** produces urine, which flows into the **ureter** at the **renal pelvis**. Urine is then collected in the **bladder** until it is excreted through the **urethra**.
- The kidney contains a cortex and a medulla. Each kidney has a **hilum**, which contains a renal artery, renal vein, and ureter.
- The kidney contains a **portal system** with two capillary beds in series.
  - Blood from the renal artery flows into **afferent arterioles**, which form **glomeruli** in Bowman's capsule (the first capillary bed).
  - Blood then flows through the **efferent arteriole** to the **vasa recta** (the second capillary bed), which surround the nephron, before leaving the kidney through the renal vein.
- The bladder has a muscular lining known as the **detrusor muscle**, which is under parasympathetic control. It also has two muscular sphincters.
  - The **internal urethral sphincter** consists of smooth muscle and is under involuntary (parasympathetic) control.
  - The **external urethral sphincter** consists of skeletal muscle and is under voluntary control.
- The kidney participates in solute movement through three processes:
  - **Filtration** is the movement of solutes from blood to filtrate at Bowman's capsule. The direction and rate of filtration is determined by **Starling forces**, which account for the hydrostatic and oncotic pressure differentials between the glomerulus and Bowman's space.
  - **Secretion** is the movement of solutes from blood to filtrate anywhere other than Bowman's capsule.
  - **Reabsorption** is the movement of solutes from filtrate to blood.
- Each segment of the nephron has a specific function.
  - The **proximal convoluted tubule** (**PCT**) is the site of bulk reabsorption of glucose, amino acids, soluble vitamins, salt, and water. It is also the site of secretion for hydrogen ions, potassium ions, ammonia, and urea.
  - The **descending limb of the loop of Henle** is permeable to water but not salt; therefore, as the filtrate moves into the more osmotically concentrated renal medulla, water is reabsorbed from the filtrate. The vasa recta and nephron flow in opposite directions, creating a **countercurrent multiplier system** that allows maximal reabsorption of water.
  - The **ascending limb of the loop of Henle** is permeable to salt but not water; therefore, salt is reabsorbed both passively and actively. The **diluting segment** is in the outer medulla; because salt is actively reabsorbed in this site, the filtrate actually becomes hypotonic compared to the blood.
  - The **distal convoluted tubule** (**DCT**) is responsive to aldosterone and is a site of salt reabsorption and waste product excretion, like the PCT.
  - The **collecting duct** is responsive to both aldosterone and antidiuretic hormone and has variable permeability, which allows reabsorption of the right amount of water depending on the body's needs.

- The kidney is under hormonal control. When blood pressure (and volume) are low, two different hormonal systems are activated.
  - **Aldosterone** is a steroid hormone regulated by the renin–angiotensin–aldosterone system that increases sodium reabsorption in the distal convoluted tubule and collecting duct, thereby increasing water reabsorption. This results in an increased blood volume (and pressure), but no change in blood osmolarity.
  - **Antidiuretic hormone** (**ADH** or **vasopressin**) is a peptide hormone synthesized by the hypothalamus and released by the posterior pituitary. Its release is stimulated not only by low blood volume but also by high blood osmolarity. It increases the permeability of the collecting duct to water, increasing water reabsorption. This results in an increased blood volume (and pressure) and a decreased blood osmolarity.
- The kidney can regulate pH by selective reabsorption or secretion of bicarbonate or hydrogen ions.

Skin

- The skin acts as a barrier, protecting us from the elements and invasion by pathogens.
- The skin is composed of three major layers: the **hypodermis** (**subcutaneous** layer), **dermis**, and **epidermis**.
  - The epidermis is composed of five layers: the **stratum basale**, **stratum spinosum**, **stratum granulosum**, **stratum lucidum**, and **stratum corneum**. The stratum basale contains stem cells that proliferate to form keratinocytes. Keratinocyte nuclei are lost in the stratum granulosum, and many thin layers form in the stratum corneum.
  - **Melanocytes** produce **melanin**, which protects the skin from DNA damage caused by ultraviolet radiation; melanin is passed to keratinocytes.
  - **Langerhans cells** are special macrophages that serve as antigen-presenting cells in the skin.
  - The dermis is composed of two layers: the **papillary layer** and the **reticular layer**.
  - Many sensory cells are located in the dermis, including **Merkel cells** (deep pressure and texture), free nerve endings (pain), **Meissner's corpuscles** (light touch), **Ruffini endings** (stretch), and **Pacinian corpuscles** (deep pressure and vibration).
  - The hypodermis contains fat and connective tissue and connects the skin to the rest of the body.
- The skin is important for thermoregulation, or the maintenance of a constant internal temperature.
  - Cooling mechanisms include **sweating**, which draws heat from the body through evaporation of water from sweat, and vasodilation. Sweat glands are innervated by postganglionic cholinergic sympathetic neurons.
  - Warming mechanisms include: piloerection, in which arrector pili muscles contract, causing hairs to stand on end (trapping a layer of warmed air around the skin); vasoconstriction; shivering; and insulation provided by fat.
- The skin also prevents dehydration and salt loss from the body.

ANSWERS TO CONCEPT CHECKS

10.1

1. Bowman's space → proximal convoluted tubule → descending limb of the loop of Henle → ascending limb of the loop of Henle → distal convoluted tubule → collecting duct → renal pelvis → ureter → bladder → urethra
2. Renal artery → afferent arteriole → glomerulus → efferent arteriole → vasa recta → renal vein
3. The parasympathetic nervous system causes contraction of the detrusor muscle.
4. Filtration is the movement of solutes from blood into filtrate at Bowman's capsule. Secretion is the movement of solutes from blood into filtrate anywhere besides Bowman's capsule. Reabsorption is the movement of solutes from filtrate into blood.
5. Bowman's capsule is the site of filtration, through which water, ions, amino acids, vitamins, and glucose pass (essentially everything besides cells and proteins). The proximal convoluted tubule controls solute identity, reabsorbing vitamins, amino acids, and glucose, while secreting potassium and hydrogen ions, ammonia, and urea. The descending limb of the loop of Henle is important for water reabsorption, and uses the medullary concentration gradient. The ascending limb of the loop of Henle is important for salt reabsorption and dilution of the urine in the diluting segment. The distal convoluted tubule, like the PCT, is important for solute identity by reabsorbing salts while secreting potassium and hydrogen ions, ammonia, and urea. The collecting duct is important for urine concentration; its variable permeability allows water to be reabsorbed based on the needs of the body.

10.2

1. Keratinocytes are the primary cells of the epidermis.
2. Stratum corneum, stratum lucidum, stratum granulosum, stratum spinosum, stratum basale
3. The papillary layer and the reticular layer
4. The body can cool itself through sweating and vasodilation. The body can warm itself through vasoconstriction, piloerection, and shivering.

SCIENCE MASTERY ASSESSMENT EXPLANATIONS

1. **B**

The glomerulus functions like a sieve; small molecules dissolved in the fluid will pass through the glomerulus, including glucose, which is later reabsorbed. Large molecules, such as proteins, and cells, such as erythrocytes and platelets, will not be able to pass through the glomerular filter.

2. **B**

Sodium is actively transported out of the nephron in the proximal and distal convoluted tubules, where the concentration of sodium outside of the nephron is higher than inside; thus, energy is required to transport the sodium molecules against their concentration gradient, eliminating **(A)** and **(C)**. In the inner medulla, however, sodium and other ions (such as chloride) diffuse passively down their concentration gradients at the thin ascending limb of the loop of Henle, making **(B)** the correct answer. The thick ascending limb of the loop of Henle is thick because its cells contain many mitochondria—which produce the ATP needed for active transport of sodium and chloride out of the filtrate, eliminating **(D)**.

3. **A**

The region of the kidney that has the lowest solute concentration is the cortex, where the proximal convoluted tubule and a part of the distal convoluted tubule are found. The solute concentration increases as one descends into the medulla, and concentrated urine can be found in the renal pelvis.

4. **A**

Blood enters the kidney through the renal artery, which divides into many afferent arterioles that run through the medulla and into the cortex. Each afferent arteriole branches into a convoluted network of capillaries called a glomerulus. Rather than converging directly into a vein, the capillaries converge into an efferent arteriole, which divides into a fine capillary network known as the vasa recta. The vasa recta capillaries envelop the nephron tubule, where they reabsorb various ions, and then converge into the renal vein. The arrangement of tandem capillary beds is known as a portal system.

5. **C**

All of the answer choices describe ADH or aldosterone. These two hormones ultimately act to increase water reabsorption in the kidney; their respective mechanisms of action, however, are different. ADH increases water reabsorption by increasing the permeability of the collecting duct to water, whereas aldosterone stimulates reabsorption of sodium from the distal convoluted tubule and collecting duct. Using this knowledge, we can now evaluate the answer choices. **(C)** is the correct answer because ADH does not act on the proximal convoluted tubule, but rather on the collecting duct.

6. **D**

Essential substances, such as glucose, salts, amino acids, and water, are reabsorbed from the filtrate and returned to the blood in the vasa recta. In general, reabsorption refers to the movement of solutes from the filtrate back into the blood.

7. **A**

The hypothalamus functions as a thermostat that regulates body temperature. When it's cold outside, nervous stimulation to the blood vessels in the skin is increased, causing the vessels to constrict. This constriction diminishes blood flow to the skin surface and prevents heat loss. Sweat glands are turned off to prevent heat loss through evaporation. Skeletal muscles are stimulated to shiver (rapidly contract), which increases the metabolic rate and produces heat. The hypothalamus is also involved in other processes, including the release of endocrine hormones, regulation of appetite, and circadian rhythms.

8. **C**

The filtrate enters Bowman's capsule and then flows into the proximal convoluted tubule, where virtually all glucose, amino acids, and other important organic molecules are reabsorbed via active transport.

9. **A**

The kidneys function to eliminate wastes such as urea, while reabsorbing various important substances such as glucose and amino acids for reuse by the body. Generation of a solute concentration gradient from the cortex to the medulla allows a considerable amount of water to be reabsorbed. Excretion of concentrated urine serves to limit water losses from the body and helps to preserve blood volume. Thus, the primary function of the nephron is to create urine that is hypertonic to the blood, making **(A)** the correct answer and eliminating **(B)** and **(D)**. Water should be reabsorbed from the filtrate, so urine should be hypertonic to the filtrate, eliminating **(C)**.

10. **A**

The glomerulus is the most likely location of pathology if large proteins are detected in the urine. This is because large proteins should not be able to pass through the filter of the glomerulus in the first place. Once large proteins are in the filtrate, no other nephron structure can reabsorb them. Thus, the only likely source of protein in the urine is glomerular pathology.

11. **C**

The layer of the skin that is predominantly loose connective tissue is the papillary layer of the dermis. The stratum corneum and stratum lucidum, **(A)** and **(B)**, contain dead keratinocytes, while the reticular layer, **(D)**, consists of dense connective tissue.

12. **D**

When the pH of the blood is high, this indicates that the blood is alkalemic. In order to correct the pH of the blood, the kidney will increase the excretion of a base, namely bicarbonate. Excretion of urea would have little effect on the pH, eliminating **(A)**. While ammonia is a base, it is quite toxic and is generally converted into urea before excretion, eliminating **(B)**. Excretion of hydrogen ions would exacerbate the alkalemia, eliminating **(C)**.

13. **C**

The stratum basale contains the stem cells that proliferate to form keratinocytes, which then ascend through the other layers of skin until they are shed from the stratum corneum.

14. **B**

Normally, angiotensin II causes secretion of aldosterone from the adrenal cortex. Aldosterone serves to increase reabsorption of sodium, while promoting excretion of potassium and hydrogen ions. Thus, blocking the release of aldosterone should result in decreased reabsorption of sodium, while decreasing excretion of potassium and hydrogen ions. This eliminates **(A)** and **(D)** and makes **(B)** the correct answer. In the absence of aldosterone, less sodium reabsorption will occur, leading to less water reabsorption, eliminating **(C)**.

15. **A**

An excess of acetylcholine will lead to activation of all parasympathetic neurons, preganglionic sympathetic neurons, and the postganglionic sympathetic neurons that innervate sweat glands. Because the parasympathetic nervous system causes contraction of the bladder, one would expect increased urination. The increased activation of sweat glands would lead to increased sweating as well.

GO ONLINE

Consult your online resources for additional practice.

SHARED CONCEPTS

Behavioral Sciences Chapter 2
Sensation and Perception

Biochemistry Chapter 8
Biological Membranes

Biology Chapter 6
The Respiratory System

Biology Chapter 7
The Cardiovascular System

Biology Chapter 8
The Immune System

General Chemistry Chapter 9
Solutions

CHAPTER 11

THE MUSCULOSKELETAL SYSTEM

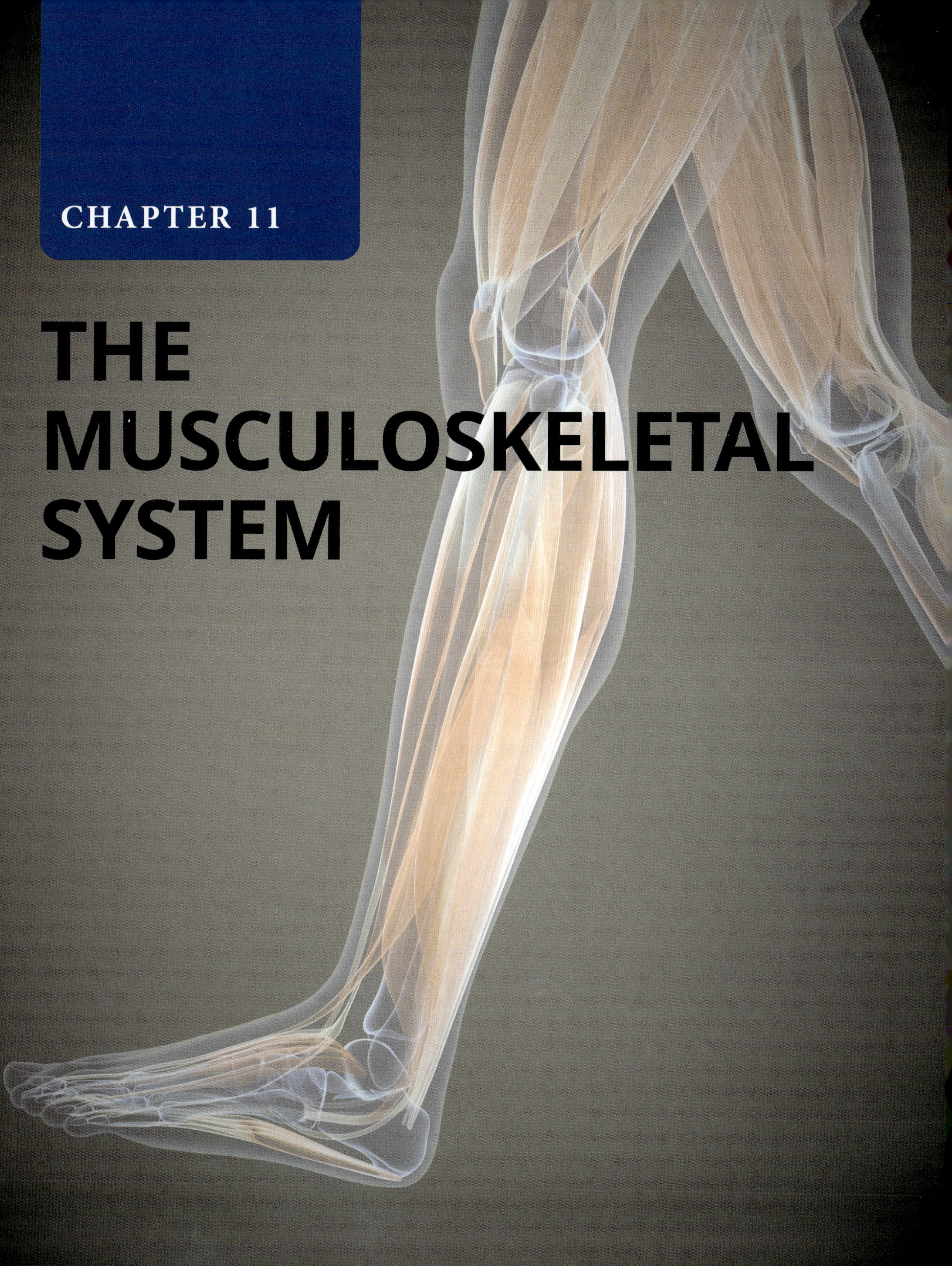

SCIENCE MASTERY ASSESSMENT

Every pre-med knows this feeling: there is so much content I have to know for the MCAT! How do I know what to do first or what's important?

While the high-yield badges throughout this book will help you identify the most important topics, this Science Mastery Assessment is another tool in your MCAT prep arsenal. This quiz (which can also be taken in your online resources) and the guidance below will help ensure that you are spending the appropriate amount of time on this chapter based on your personal strengths and weaknesses. Don't worry though—skipping something now does not mean you'll never study it. Later on in your prep, as you complete full-length tests, you'll uncover specific pieces of content that you need to review and can come back to these chapters as appropriate.

How to Use This Assessment

If you answer 0–7 questions correctly:

Spend about 1 hour to read this chapter in full and take limited notes throughout. Follow up by reviewing **all** quiz questions to ensure that you now understand how to solve each one.

If you answer 8–11 questions correctly:

Spend 20–40 minutes reviewing the quiz questions. Beginning with the questions you missed, read and take notes on the corresponding subchapters. For questions you answered correctly, ensure your thinking matches that of the explanation and you understand why each choice was correct or incorrect.

If you answer 12–15 questions correctly:

Spend less than 20 minutes reviewing all questions from the quiz. If you missed any, then include a quick read-through of the corresponding subchapters, or even just the relevant content within a subchapter, as part of your question review. For questions you answered correctly, ensure your thinking matches that of the explanation and review the Concept Summary at the end of the chapter.

Questions 1, 2, and 3 are based on the following diagram:

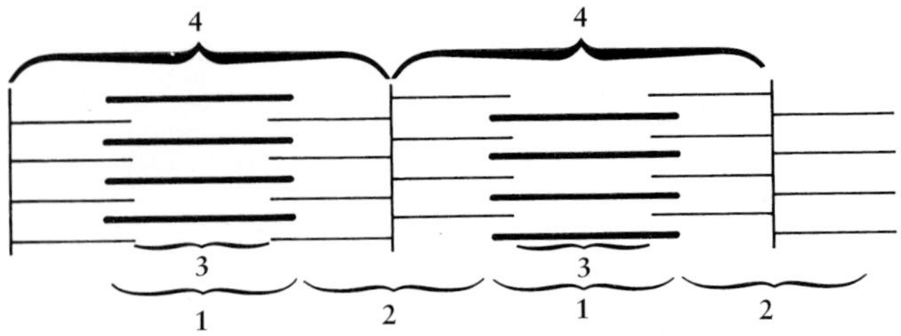

1. During muscle contraction, which of the following regions decrease(s) in length?

A. 1 only
B. 1 and 2 only
C. 3 and 4 only
D. 2, 3, and 4 only

2. Region 1 refers to:

A. the thick filaments only.
B. the thin filaments only.
C. the A-band.
D. the I-band.

3. Which region represents one sarcomere?

A. 1
B. 2
C. 3
D. 4

4. With which of the following molecules does Ca^{2+} bind after its release from the sarcoplasmic reticulum to regulate muscle contraction?

A. Myosin
B. Actin
C. Troponin
D. Tropomyosin

5. Which of the following cells is correctly coupled with its definition?

A. Osteoblasts—bone cells involved in the secretion of bone matrix
B. Osteoclasts—immature bone cells
C. Osteocytes—polynucleated cells actively involved in bone resorption
D. Chondrocytes—undifferentiated bone marrow cells

6. An X-ray of the right femur in a child shows that it is shorter than the opposite femur, and below the average length for a child of this age. Which region of the bone is most likely to have caused this abnormality?

A. Diaphysis
B. Metaphysis
C. Epiphysis
D. Periosteum

7. Which of the following INCORRECTLY pairs a type of muscle fiber with a characteristic of that fiber?

A. Red fibers—rich in mitochondria
B. Red fibers—high levels of myoglobin
C. White fibers—fast-twitching
D. White fibers—predominantly use aerobic respiration

8. When the knee moves back and forth during walking, what prevents the surfaces of the leg bones from rubbing against each other?

A. Articular cartilage
B. Epiphyses
C. Synovial fluid
D. Smooth muscle

9. Which type(s) of muscle is/are always multinucleated?

I. Cardiac muscle
II. Skeletal muscle
III. Smooth muscle

A. I only
B. II only
C. III only
D. I and II only

10. Which type(s) of muscle has/have myogenic activity?
  I. Cardiac muscle
  II. Skeletal muscle
  III. Smooth muscle

  A. I only
  B. II only
  C. III only
  D. I and III only

11. Red bone marrow is involved in erythrocyte formation. In contrast, yellow bone marrow:
  A. is involved in leukocyte formation.
  B. is responsible for drainage of lymph.
  C. causes the formation of spicules.
  D. contains predominantly adipose tissue.

12. Which of the following statements regarding the periosteum is INCORRECT?
  A. The periosteum serves as a site of attachment of bone to muscle.
  B. Cells of the periosteum may differentiate into osteoblasts.
  C. The periosteum is a fibrous sheath that surrounds long bones.
  D. The periosteum secretes fluid into the joint cavity.

13. Which of the following bones is NOT a part of the appendicular skeleton?
  A. The triquetrum, one of the carpal bones
  B. The calcaneus, which forms the heel
  C. The ischium, one of the fused pelvic bones
  D. The sternum, or breastbone

14. To facilitate the process of birth, an infant's head is somewhat flexible. This flexibility is due in part to the two fontanelles, which are soft spots of connective tissue in the infant's skull. With time, the fontanelles will close through a process known as:
  A. endochondral ossification.
  B. intramembranous ossification.
  C. bone resorption.
  D. longitudinal growth.

15. A young patient presents to the emergency room with a broken hip. The patient denies any recent history of trauma to the joint. Blood tests reveal a calcium concentration of 11.5 $\frac{mg}{dL}$ (normal: 8.4–10.2). Which tissue is likely responsible for these findings?
  A. Thyroid
  B. Cartilage
  C. Parathyroid
  D. Smooth muscle

Answer Key

1. **D** (See section 11.1)
2. **C** (See section 11.1)
3. **D** (See section 11.1)
4. **C** (See section 11.1)
5. **A** (See section 11.2)
6. **C** (See section 11.2)
7. **D** (See section 11.1)
8. **A** (See section 11.2)
9. **B** (See section 11.1)
10. **D** (See section 11.1)
11. **D** (See section 11.2)
12. **D** (See section 11.2)
13. **D** (See section 11.2)
14. **B** (See section 11.2)
15. **C** (See section 11.2)

The relevant section of the chapter to review for each question is given in parentheses after the correct answer. Detailed explanations can be found at the end of the chapter.

CHAPTER 11

THE MUSCULOSKELETAL SYSTEM

In This Chapter

CHAPTER PROFILE

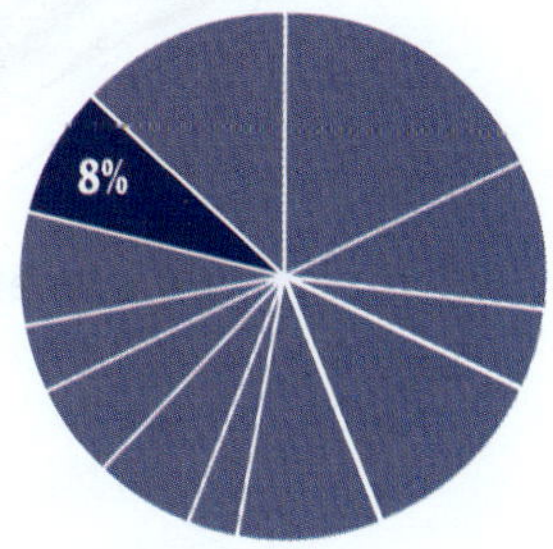

The content in this chapter should be relevant to about 8% of all questions about biology on the MCAT.

This chapter covers material from the following AAMC content category:

3B: Structure and integrative functions of the main organ systems

Introduction

Large disasters or traumatic events like wars or earthquakes can deeply affect the health of populations, which also has an impact on the practice of medicine, sometimes leading to the discovery of new medical conditions. During World War II, Nazi Germany bombed London for 57 consecutive days during the beginning of what came to be known as the *Blitzkrieg*, or an eight-month "lightning war." Victims of the Blitz, as it is known in London, included those afflicted with a specific set of symptoms: pain and swelling with accompanying effects of depleted blood volume (shock, weakness, low blood pressure, and decreased urine output). Less obvious was acute kidney failure, which could lead quickly to death if left untreated.

What caused the Blitz victims to suffer from these symptoms? Extreme physical trauma to muscles—namely, compression—destroys skeletal muscle tissue. This condition is called *rhabdomyolysis* (*rhabdo–* refers to striation, *myo–* to muscle, and *–lysis* to breakdown) and its mechanism is shown in Figure 11.1. The products of skeletal muscle destruction, some of which are toxic, circulate in the blood until they are filtered out. *Creatine kinase* is one of these products; in fact, rhabdomyolysis is diagnosed with a creatine kinase level five times the normal upper limit. Myoglobin is another. Much like hemoglobin, myoglobin uses heme to carry oxygen; however, it is not housed within a red blood cell, and it only possesses one heme group. Thus, an erythrocyte-free urine sample that tests positive for heme points compellingly toward rhabdomyolysis. Myoglobin oxygen reserves are just one of the specialized features of muscles, as we will see in this chapter.

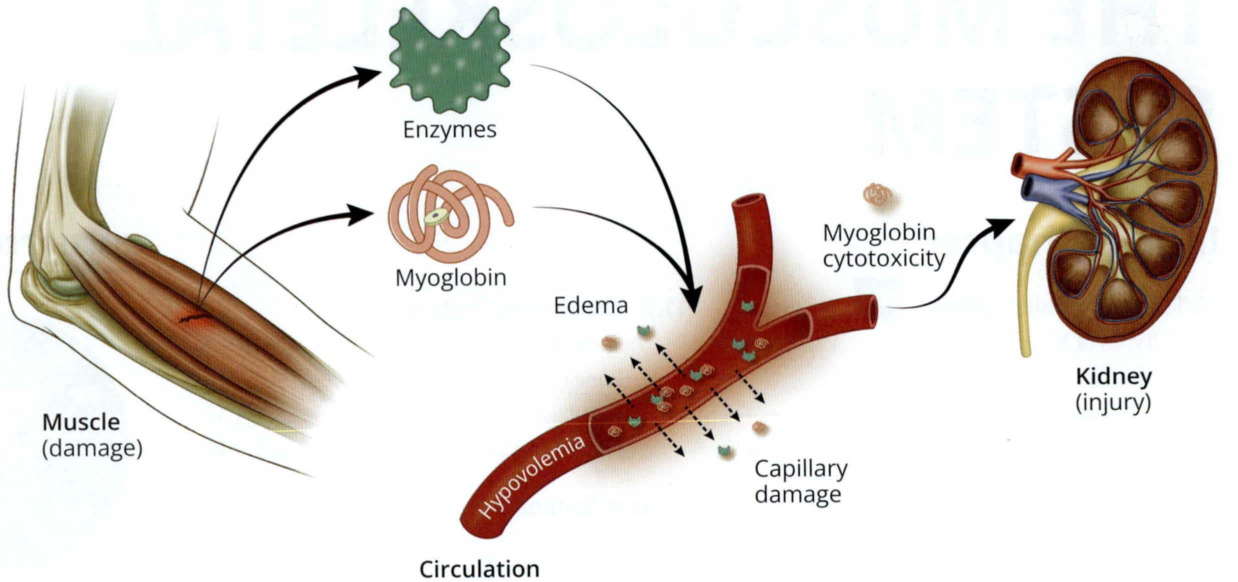

Figure 11.1 Rhabdomyolysis

Skeletal muscles are only able to exert an effect on the body by moving bony structures around joints. Further, skeletal muscle isn't the only form of muscle in the body; smooth muscle plays roles in the cardiovascular, respiratory, reproductive, and digestive systems, and cardiac muscle comprises the contractile tissue of the heart. Bones are more than simply a support structure, however; they also provide protection to internal organs, serve as a storage reserve of calcium and other minerals, and are the site of hematopoiesis. In this chapter, we'll explore the biology of all of these tissues, completing our tour of systems anatomy and physiology.

11.1 The Muscular System High Yield

LEARNING OBJECTIVES

After Chapter 11.1, you will be able to:

- Categorize muscles as skeletal, smooth, or cardiac based on their innervation and structure
- Order the series of events in muscular contraction
- Explain the relationship between ATP binding and muscular contraction
- Recall the meaning of the terms summation, simple twitch, and tetanus
- Identify the zones and bands within a sarcomere and predict their length changes during contraction:

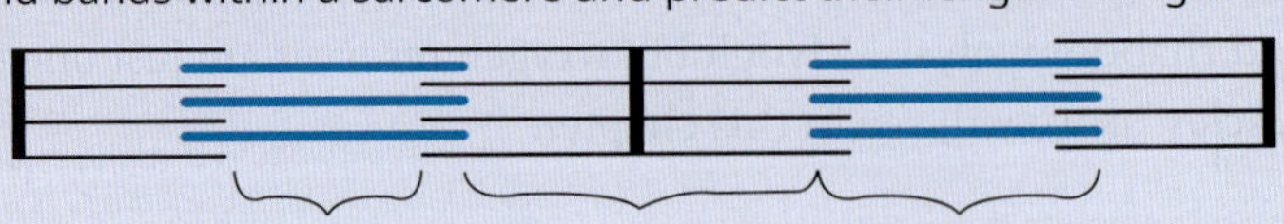

The muscular system is composed of not only skeletal muscle, but also smooth muscle and cardiac muscle. Skeletal muscle is essential for supporting the body and facilitating movement. The contraction of skeletal muscle also compresses venous structures and helps propel blood through the low-pressure venous system toward the heart, as well as lymph through the lymphatic system. Rapid muscle contraction also leads to shivering, which is important in thermoregulation. Smooth muscle is responsible for involuntary movement, such as the rhythmic contractions of smooth muscle in the digestive system called peristalsis. Smooth muscle also aids in the regulation of blood pressure by constricting and relaxing the vasculature. Cardiac muscle is a special type of muscle that is able to maintain rhythmic contraction of the heart without nervous system input. In this section, we will discuss each type of muscle as well as the physiology of muscles.

Types of Muscle

Muscle can be divided into the three different subtypes: skeletal muscle, smooth muscle, and cardiac muscle (Figure 11.2). Each muscle type performs specific functions, although they share some similarities. All muscle is capable of contraction, which relies on calcium ions. All muscle is innervated, although—as we will see—the part of the nervous system that innervates the muscle and the ability of the muscle to contract without nervous input varies from type to type.

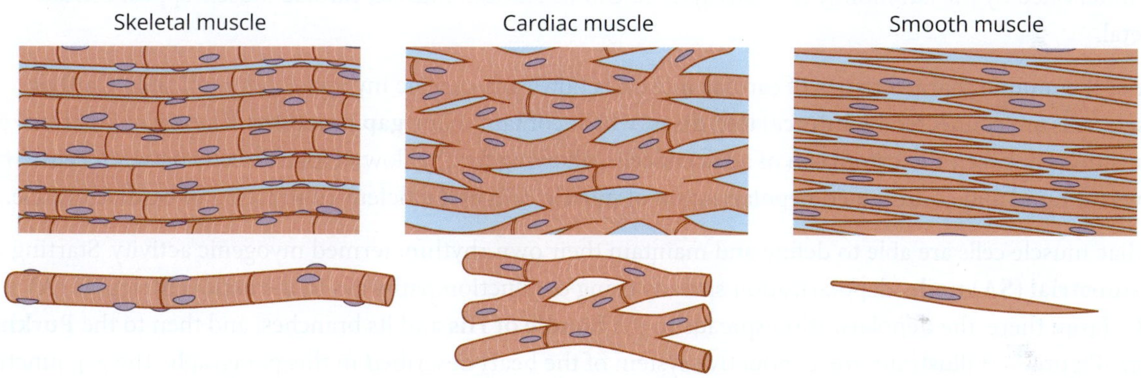

Figure 11.2 The Three Muscle Types

Skeletal Muscle

Skeletal muscle is responsible for voluntary movement and is therefore innervated by the somatic nervous system. Due to the arrangement of actin and myosin into repeating units called **sarcomeres**, it appears striped or **striated** when viewed microscopically. Skeletal muscle is multinucleated because it is formed as individual muscle cells fuse into long rods during development.

There are multiple different types of fibers within skeletal muscle. **Red fibers**, also known as **slow-twitch fibers**, have high myoglobin content and primarily derive their energy aerobically. **Myoglobin** is an oxygen carrier that uses iron in a heme group to bind oxygen, imparting a red color. Red fibers also contain many mitochondria to carry out oxidative phosphorylation. **White fibers**, also known as **fast-twitch fibers**, contain much less myoglobin. Because there is less myoglobin, and therefore less iron, the color is lighter. These two types of fibers can be mixed in muscles. Muscles that contract slowly, but that can sustain activity (such as the muscles that support posture), contain a predominance of red fibers. Muscles that contract rapidly, but fatigue quickly, contain mostly white fibers.

REAL WORLD

Poultry provides a great example of the difference between red and white fibers. Most muscles of support, such as the thigh, are considered dark meat and contain a high concentration of red fibers. The pectoral muscles (breast meat), used by some poultry for only short bursts of flight, are considered white meat and have a high concentration of white fibers.

Smooth Muscle

Smooth muscle is responsible for involuntary action. Thus, smooth muscle is controlled by the autonomic nervous system. It is found in the respiratory tree, digestive tract, bladder, uterus, blood vessel walls, and many other locations. Smooth muscle cells have a single nucleus located in the center of the cell. Just like skeletal muscle, smooth muscle cells contain actin and myosin, but the fibers are not as regularly organized at a macroscopic level, so striations cannot be seen. The fibers are instead organized in sporadic, diagonal directions. Compared to skeletal muscle, smooth muscle is capable of more sustained contractions; a constant state of low-level contraction, as may be seen in the blood vessels, is called **tonus**. Smooth muscle can actually contract without nervous system input in what is known as **myogenic activity**. In this case, the muscle cells contract directly in response to stretch or other stimuli.

MCAT EXPERTISE

The MCAT loves to test the fact that both smooth and cardiac muscle exhibit myogenic activity. These muscle cells will respond to nervous input, but do not require external signals to undergo contraction.

Cardiac Muscle

Cardiac muscle has characteristics of both smooth and skeletal muscle types. Cardiac muscle is primarily uninucleated, but cells may contain two nuclei. Like smooth muscle, cardiac muscle contraction is involuntary and innervated by the autonomic nervous system. Unlike smooth muscle, cardiac muscle appears striated like skeletal.

One of the unique characteristics of cardiac muscle is how each cardiac myocyte communicates. Cardiac muscle cells are connected by **intercalated discs**, which contain many **gap junctions**. These gap junctions are connections between the cytoplasm of adjacent cells, allowing for the flow of ions directly between cells. This allows for rapid and coordinated depolarization of muscle cells and efficient contraction of cardiac muscle.

Cardiac muscle cells are able to define and maintain their own rhythm, termed myogenic activity. Starting at the **sinoatrial (SA) node**, depolarization spreads using conduction pathways to the **atrioventricular (AV) node**. From there, the depolarization spreads to the **bundle of His** and its branches, and then to the **Purkinje fibers**. Figure 11.3 illustrates the conductive system of the heart described in this paragraph. The gap junctions allow for progressive depolarizations to spread via ion flow across the gap junctions between cells.

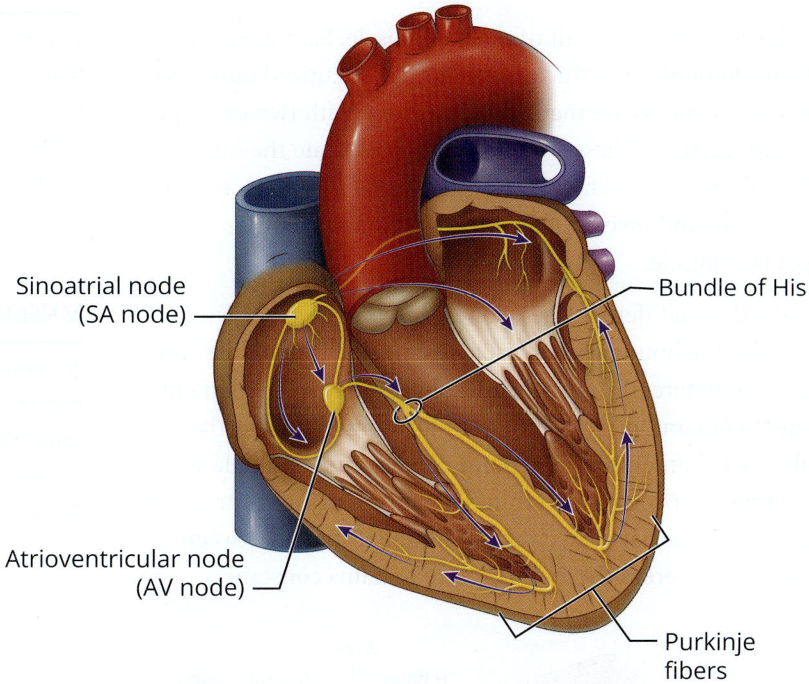

Figure 11.3 The Conductive System of the Heart

The nervous and endocrine systems also play a role in the regulation of cardiac muscle contraction. The vagus nerve provides parasympathetic outflow to the heart and slows the heart rate. Norepinephrine from sympathetic neurons or epinephrine from the adrenal medulla binds to adrenergic receptors in the heart, causing an increased heart rate and greater contractility. One of the ways epinephrine does this is by increasing intracellular calcium levels within cardiac myocytes. Ultimately, cardiac contraction—like that of all types of muscle—relies on calcium.

The main characteristics of each muscle type are summarized in Table 11.1.

Skeletal Muscle	Cardiac Muscle	Smooth Muscle
Striated	Striated	Nonstriated
Voluntary	Involuntary	Involuntary
Somatic innervation	Autonomic innervation	Autonomic innervation
Many nuclei per cell	1–2 nuclei per cell	1 nucleus per cell
Ca^{2+} required for contraction	Ca^{2+} required for contraction	Ca^{2+} required for contraction

Table 11.1 Types of Muscle

Microscopic Structure of Skeletal Muscle

Each type of muscle has a specific microscopic structure. However, the MCAT tends to focus on the contractile elements and microscopic structure of skeletal muscle. In order to accurately answer those questions on Test Day, let's take a moment to discuss skeletal muscle in detail.

The Sarcomere

The **sarcomere** is the basic contractile unit of skeletal muscle. Sarcomeres are made of **thick** and **thin filaments**. The thick filaments are organized bundles of **myosin**, whereas the thin filaments are made of **actin** along with two other proteins: **troponin** and **tropomyosin**. These proteins help to regulate the interaction between the actin and myosin filaments. Another protein, **titin**, acts as a spring and anchors the actin and myosin filaments together, preventing excessive stretching of the muscle.

Each sarcomere is divided into different lines, zones, and bands, as shown in Figure 11.4. **Z-lines** define the boundaries of each sarcomere. The **M-line** runs down the center of the sarcomere, through the middle of the myosin filaments. The **I-band** is the region containing exclusively thin filaments, whereas the **H-zone** contains only thick filaments. The **A-band** contains the thick filaments in their entirety, including any overlap with thin filaments. During contraction, the H-zone, I-band, the distance between Z-lines, and the distance between M-lines all become smaller, whereas the A-band's size remains constant.

MNEMONIC

To remember which filament is associated with **t**roponin and **t**ropomyosin, remember that ac**t**in has a **T** in it.

MNEMONIC

To remember which is the thin and thick filament, remember **acthin: actin** filaments are **thin** (while myosin filaments are thick).

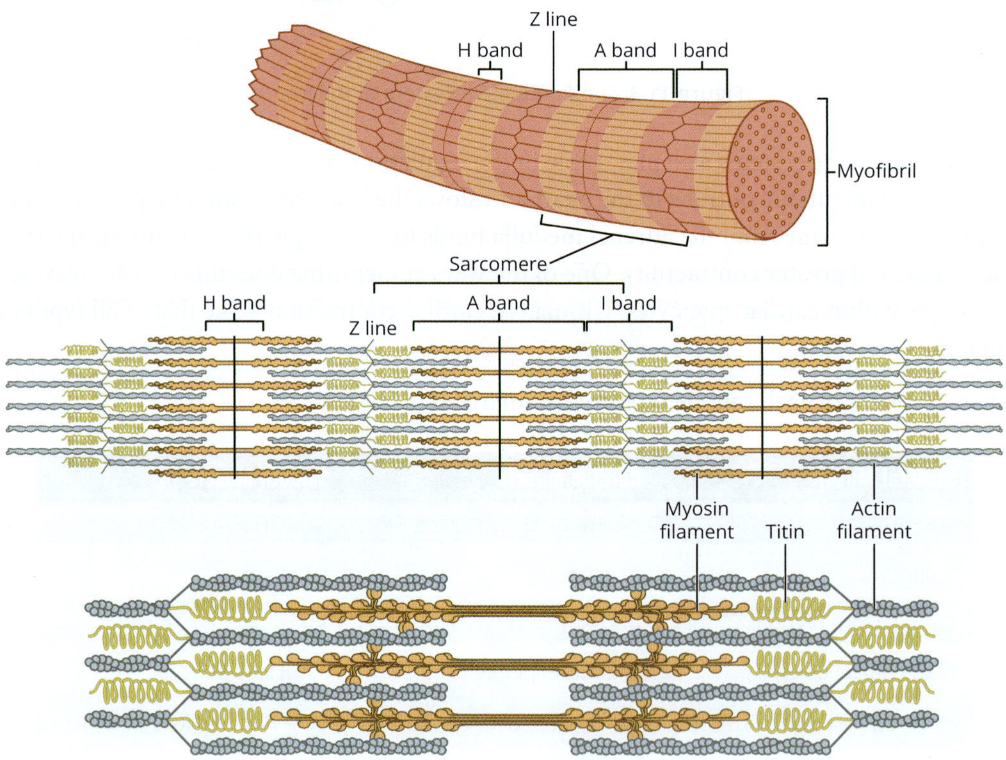

Figure 11.4 The Sarcomere
Sarcomeres are the functional units of striated muscle.

Gross Structure of Myocytes

Sarcomeres are attached end-to-end to form **myofibrils**. Myofibrils are surrounded by a covering known as the **sarcoplasmic reticulum** (**SR**), a modified endoplasmic reticulum that contains a high concentration of Ca^{2+} ions. The **sarcoplasm** is a modified cytoplasm located just outside the sarcoplasmic reticulum. The cell membrane of a myocyte is known as the **sarcolemma**. The sarcolemma is capable of propagating an action potential and can distribute the action potential to all sarcomeres in a muscle using a system of **transverse tubules** (**T-tubules**) that are oriented perpendicularly to the myofibrils, as shown in Figure 11.5. Each **myocyte**, or muscle cell, contains many myofibrils arranged in parallel and can also be called a **muscle fiber**. The nuclei, of which there are many, are usually found at the periphery of the cell. Finally, many myocytes in parallel form a muscle.

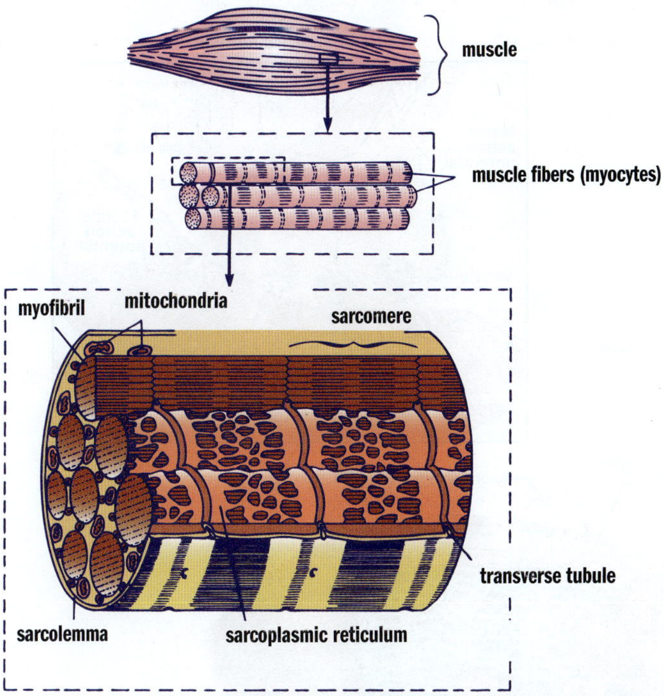

Figure 11.5 Architecture of Skeletal Muscle
A muscle is composed of parallel myocytes (muscle fibers), which are composed of parallel myofibrils.

MNEMONIC

Parts of the sarcomere:

- **Z—Z** is the end of the alphabet, and the end of the sarcomere
- **M—M**iddle of the **m**yosin filaments
- **I—I** is a **thin** letter (**thin** filaments only)
- **H—H** is a **thick** letter (**thick** filaments only)
- **A—A**ll of the thick filament, whether or not it is overlapping

KEY CONCEPT

The sarcoplasmic reticulum is just a fancy name for the specialized endoplasmic reticulum in muscle cells.

KEY CONCEPT

A myofibril is an arrangement of many sarcomeres in series. A muscle fiber (or myocyte, or muscle cell) contains many myofibrils within it, arranged in parallel. A muscle is made up of parallel muscle fibers. These names are very similar; pay careful attention to terminology when reading about muscle structure!

Muscle Contraction

Contraction of muscle requires a series of coordinated steps that are repeated to induce further shortening. This process depends on both ATP and calcium.

Initiation

Contraction starts at the **neuromuscular junction**, where the nervous system communicates with muscles via **motor (efferent) neurons**. This signal travels down the neuron until it reaches the **nerve terminal (synaptic bouton)**, where acetylcholine is released into the synapse. In the case of the neuromuscular junction, as seen in Figure 11.6, the *motor end plate* is a specialized postsynaptic membrane that receives the signal from the innervating axon terminal. Acetylcholine binds to receptors on the sarcolemma, causing depolarization. Each nerve terminal controls a group of myocytes; together, the nerve terminal and its myocytes constitute a **motor unit**.

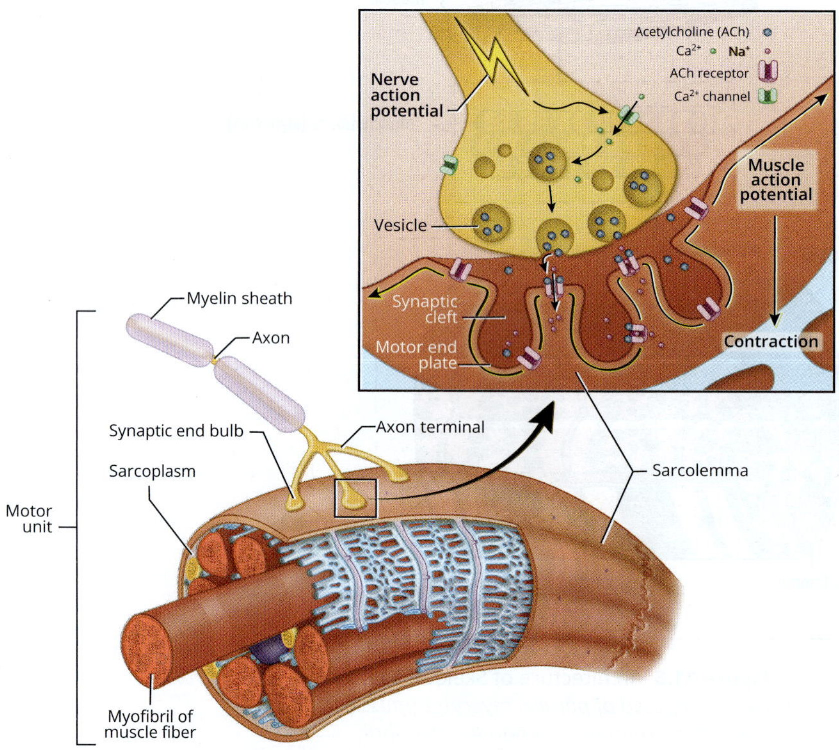

Figure 11.6 Neuromuscular Junction

Depolarization triggers an action potential, which spreads down the sarcolemma to the T-tubules. The action potential travels down the T-tubules into the muscle tissues to the sarcoplasmic reticulum. When the action potential reaches the sarcoplasmic reticulum, Ca^{2+} is ultimately released. The calcium ions bind to a regulatory subunit in troponin, triggering a change in the confirmation of tropomyosin, to which troponin is bound. This change exposes the **myosin-binding sites** on the actin thin filament, as shown in Figure 11.7.

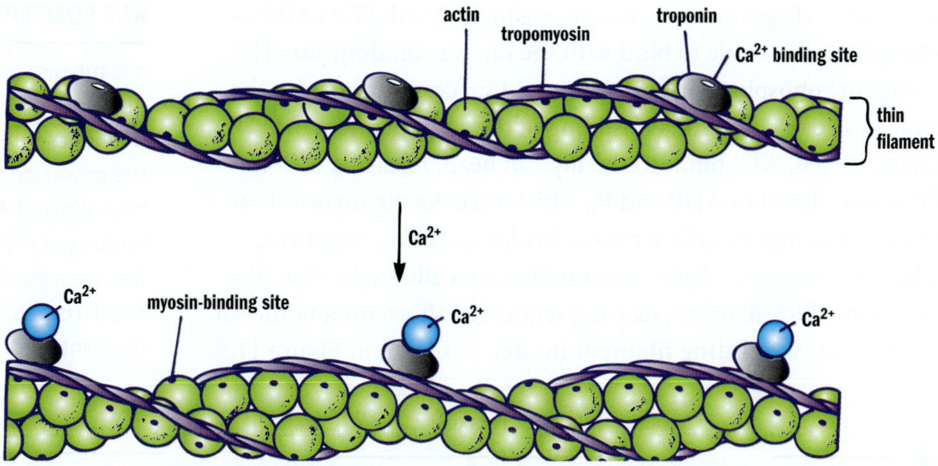

Figure 11.7 Regulation of Contraction with Calcium
Calcium binds to troponin, leading to a conformational change in tropomyosin, which exposes the myosin-binding sites of actin.

Shortening of the Sarcomere

The free globular heads of the myosin molecules move toward and bind with the exposed sites on actin. The newly formed actin–myosin cross bridges then allow myosin to pull on actin, which draws the thin filaments toward the M-line, resulting in shortening of the sarcomere. The actin–myosin cross-bridge cycle is illustrated in Figure 11.8.

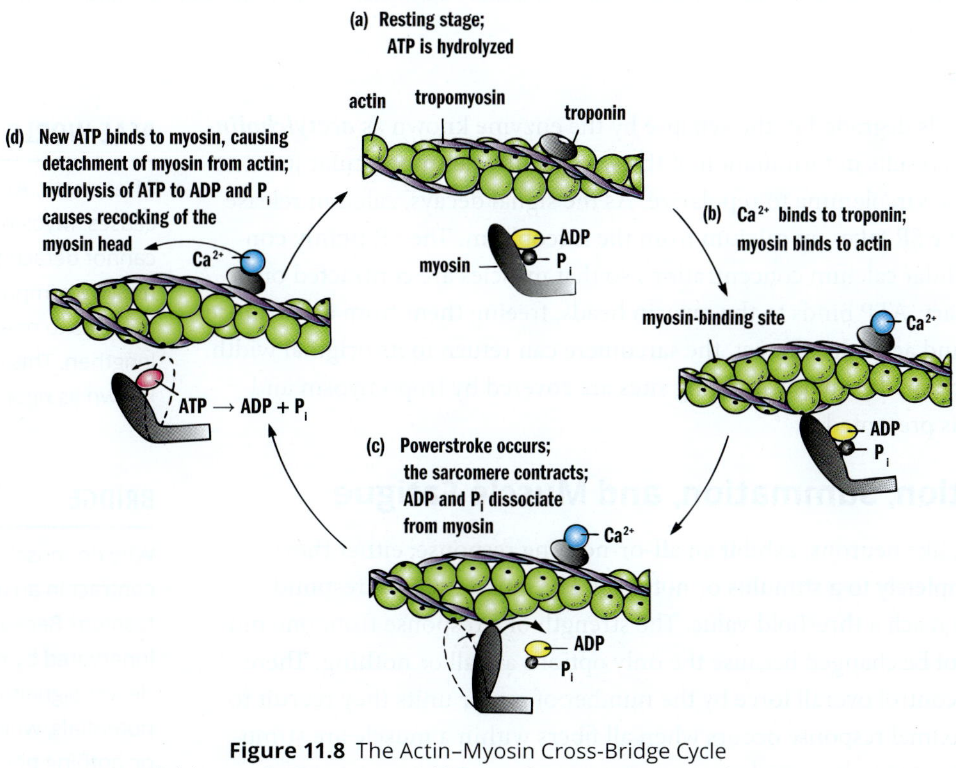

Figure 11.8 The Actin–Myosin Cross-Bridge Cycle
Calcium and ATP are essential for muscle contraction and relaxation.

Starting at the top of the diagram, myosin carrying hydrolyzed ATP (ADP and an inorganic phosphate, P_i) is able to bind with the myosin-binding site. The release of the inorganic phosphate and ADP in rapid succession provides the energy for the powerstroke and results in sliding of the actin filament over the myosin filament. Then, ATP binds to the myosin head, releasing it from actin. This ATP is hydrolyzed to ADP and P_i, which **recocks** the myosin head so that it is in position to initiate another cross-bridge cycle. The repetitive binding and releasing of myosin heads on actin filaments allows the thin filament to slide along the thick filament, causing sequential shortening of the sarcomere. This is known as the **sliding filament model**, as shown in Figure 11.9.

KEY CONCEPT

It is the dissociation of ADP and P_i from myosin that is responsible for the powerstroke, not the hydrolysis of ATP. The binding of ATP is required for releasing the myosin head from the actin filament.

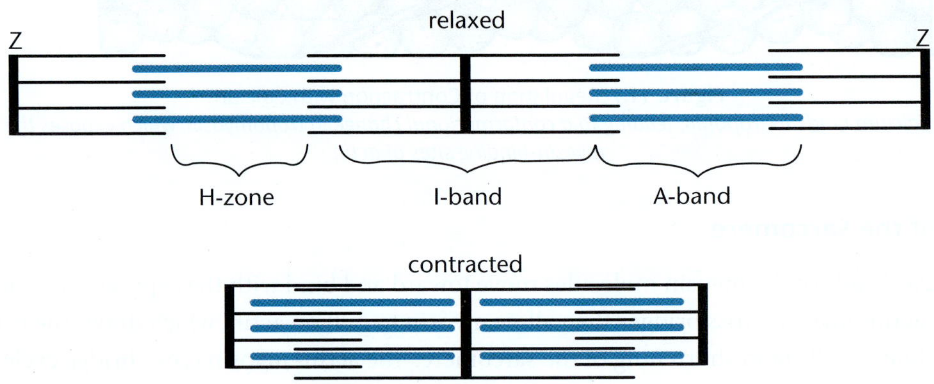

Figure 11.9 Sarcomere Contraction
When a sarcomere contracts, both the H-zone and I-band shorten, while the A-band is unchanged.

Relaxation

Acetylcholine is degraded in the synapse by the enzyme known as ***acetylcholinesterase***. This results in termination of the signal at the neuromuscular junction and allows the sarcolemma to repolarize. As the signal decays, calcium release ceases, and the SR takes up calcium from the sarcoplasm. The SR tightly controls intracellular calcium concentrations so that muscles are contracted only when necessary. ATP binds to the myosin heads, freeing them from actin. Once the myosin and actin disconnect, the sarcomere can return to its original width. Without calcium, the myosin-binding sites are covered by tropomyosin and contraction is prevented.

REAL WORLD

After death, ATP production ceases. Myosin heads cannot detach from actin, making it impossible for muscles to relax and lengthen. This condition is known as rigor mortis.

Stimulation, Summation, and Muscle Fatigue

Muscle cells, like neurons, exhibit an all-or-nothing response; either they respond completely to a stimulus or not at all. For muscle cells to respond, stimuli must reach a threshold value. The strength of a response from one muscle cell cannot be changed because the only options are all or nothing. Therefore, nerves control overall force by the number of motor units they recruit to respond. Maximal response occurs when all fibers within a muscle are stimulated to contract simultaneously.

BRIDGE

Why do muscle fibers contract in an all-or-nothing fashion? Because they are innervated by neurons that deliver signals using action potentials, which are all-or-nothing phenomena as well. Action potentials are discussed in Chapter 4 of *MCAT Biology Review*.

Simple Twitch

A simple twitch is the response of a single muscle fiber to a brief stimulus at or above threshold, as shown in Figure 11.10(a). It consists of a latent period, contraction period, and relaxation period. The **latent period** is the time between reaching threshold and the onset of contraction. It is during this time that the action potential spreads along the muscle and allows for calcium to be released from the sarcoplasmic reticulum. The muscle then contracts, and, assuming calcium is cleared from the sarcoplasm, it then relaxes.

Summation and Tetanus

If a muscle fiber is exposed to frequent and prolonged stimulation, it will have insufficient time to relax. The contractions will combine, become stronger and more prolonged. This is known as **frequency summation**, as shown in Figure 11.10(b). If the contractions become so frequent that the muscle is unable to relax at all, this is known as **tetanus**. Prolonged tetanus will result in muscle fatigue, explained below. Note that tetanus (the disease) includes tetanus (the physiological phenomenon) as one of its primary clinical features, but that tetanic physiology also occurs under normal circumstances with multiple simple twitches in succession.

REAL WORLD

The disease *tetanus* is caused by a bacterium called *Clostridium tetani* that releases the toxin *tetanospasmin*. Tetanospasmin blocks the release of GABA from the neurons that *inhibit* motor neurons, making the motor neurons overexcitable. This leads to constant contraction of muscles, which can be so strong as to fracture bones. Tetanus can usually be prevented after exposure by administration of a tetanus immunoglobulin.

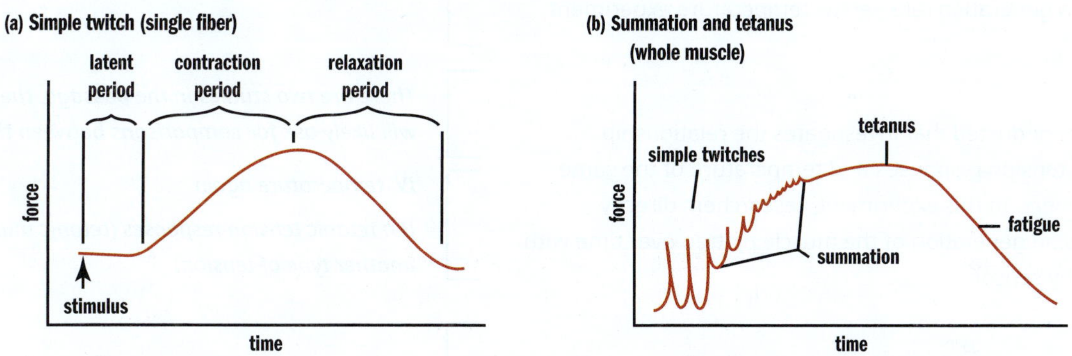

Figure 11.10 Force of Muscle Contraction Due to a Simple Twitch and Tetanus
(a) A simple twitch contraction; (b) Summation of frequent simple twitches can lead to tetanus.

BIOLOGY GUIDED EXAMPLE WITH EXPERT THINKING

Study 1

Previous research has shown muscle tension generation is influenced by temperature of the muscle fibers. To further establish the connection between how temperature interacts with muscle tension generation, researchers measured the rate of tension rise at various temperatures. More specifically, researchers established change in the rate of tension rise is different at high temperatures (25°C to 35°C) and low temperatures (20°C to 10°C).

IV: temperature

DV: muscle tension generation

Experiment is trying to test the connection between temperature and tension

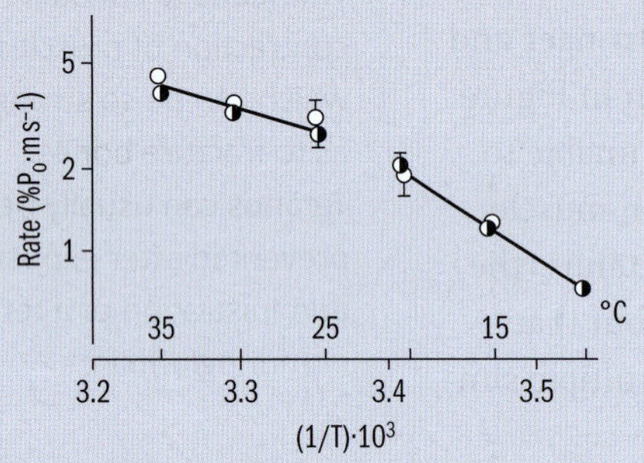

Figure 1 Tension generation rate versus temperature experiment results.

Trend: Tension generation rate is lower and the slope of the line is more steep at lower temperatures

Study 2

Another study is conducted that investigates the relationship between tetanic tension responses and temperature of the same type of muscle fibers. In this experiment, researchers directly observe the tension generation of the muscle plotted over time with electromyography sensor.

There are two studies in the passage, the MCAT will likely ask for comparisons between the two

IV: temperature again

DV: tetanic tension responses (tetanic must be another type of tension)

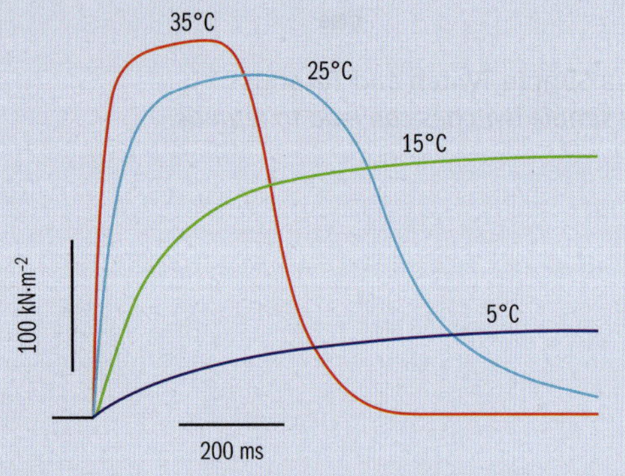

Figure 2 Tetanic tension responses obtained from one intact fiber bundle at four different temperatures, using suitable stimulation frequencies and duration.

Trend: as temperature decreases, the curve flattens out (i.e., change in tension remains low)

Adapted from Ranatunga K. W. (2018). Temperature effects on force and actin–myosin interaction in muscle: a look back on some experimental findings. *International Journal of Molecular Sciences*, 19(5), 1538. doi:10.3390/ijms19051538.

Does Study 2's data conflict with Study 1's data?

This question asks us whether two sets of data conflict with one another. To analyze this relationship, we need to draw the proper conclusions from each data set, and see how these two data sets are related. Conflict is when one data set reveals a relationship that is either not validated by similar data sets, or directly contradicted by similar data sets.

To start, we'll want to make sure we can understand each data set separately. The first study seeks to investigate how temperature affects the rate of tension generation by the muscle tissues. The results of this experiment are displayed as a line graph. One of the first things to look at when analyzing any figure are axes labels and their corresponding units. On the y-axis, we see the rate of tension rise. So, a higher value on that axis means the muscle can generate tension faster, or in other words, have a higher rate. For the x-axis, things are a bit more confusing. The axis displays temperature, but in two ways. Technically, it is the reciprocal of temperature, but fortunately for us the graph is also labeled with the corresponding real temperature location. Because of the reciprocal, higher temperatures are found closer to the left, and temperature decreases going toward the right. Besides this complication, the graph shows a pretty straightforward relationship. At higher temperatures (close to physiological temperature), the rate of tension rise is high, with the drop in rate from 35°C to 25°C being relatively minor. At lower temperatures, the rate of tension rise is much lower, and the change in rate as temperature decreases is more dramatic.

Study 2 examined a similar relationship between temperature and muscle tension. Here the graph shows a more visual representation of how the tension is generated in those muscles. From the shape of the curve, it appears that the measurement is for one stimulation, as the tension rises once and quickly tapers off. From the graph, we can make some quick observations. At higher temperatures, the max tension generated is higher, as well as the time required to reach peak tension. When temperature is lowered, muscle tension generation drops significantly.

To evaluate whether Study 2's data conflicts with Study 1's data, we need to compare and assess how the two data sets are related. Both of these graphs have temperature as the independent variable, so we must look at what each data set demonstrates with that change in temperature. Study 1 shows a rise in rate of tension. While Study 2 does not report rate of tension rise explicitly, it does show tension over time, which is essentially rate! At 35°C and 25°C, the slope of tension increase is sharp, meaning that the rate of tension increase is high. At lower temperature, the slope is more gentle, and tension generation takes significantly longer. This means that Study 2 corroborates Study 1's data in that higher temperature is correlated with a higher rate, while lower temperature is correlated with lower rate.

What about the *change* in rate? How is that visualized? Study 1 shows that change in the rate of tension rise at high temperature is more mild than the change in rate at lower temperatures. From Study 2's graph, we can see that from 35°C to 25°C, the change in the slope (and therefore rate) of the tension is rather small. However, the change in slope between 15°C and 5°C is much more dramatic. Since we know that the slope represents the rate of tension rise, the change in slope must represent the change in rate.

Thus, Study 2 does not conflict with Study 1. In fact, the two studies corroborate each other!

Oxygen Debt and Muscle Fatigue

Muscles require ATP to function. Slow-twitch (red) muscle fibers have high levels of mitochondria and thus use oxidative phosphorylation to make ATP. However, this means that high concentrations of oxygen are required to generate the large amounts of ATP muscle cells need. There are two supplemental energy reserves in muscle. **Creatine phosphate** is created by transferring a phosphate group from ATP to creatine during times of rest. This reaction can then be reversed at the onset of intense physical activity to quickly generate ATP from the rapidly growing supply of ADP:

$$\text{creatine} + \text{ATP} \rightleftharpoons \text{creatine phosphate} + \text{ADP}$$

Muscle also contains myoglobin, which binds oxygen with high affinity. As exercising muscles run out of oxygen, they use myoglobin reserves to keep aerobic metabolism going. Fast-twitch (white) muscle fibers have fewer mitochondria and must rely on glycolysis and fermentation to make ATP under most circumstances. When a person exercises, heart rate and respiratory rate increase in order to move more oxygen to actively respiring muscles. The oxyhemoglobin dissociation curve undergoes a right shift in the presence of increased carbon dioxide concentration, increased hydrogen ion concentration (decreased pH), and increased temperature. However, even with these adaptations, muscle use can quickly overwhelm the ability of the body to deliver oxygen. Then, even red muscle fibers must switch to anaerobic metabolism and produce lactic acid, at which point the muscle begins to fatigue. The difference between the amount of oxygen needed by the muscles and the actual amount present is called the **oxygen debt**. After the cessation of strenuous exercise, the body must metabolize all of the lactic acid it has produced. Most lactic acid is converted back into pyruvate, which can enter the citric acid cycle via the Cori cycle (Figure 11.11). This process requires oxygen, and the amount of oxygen required to recover from strenuous exercise is equal to the oxygen debt.

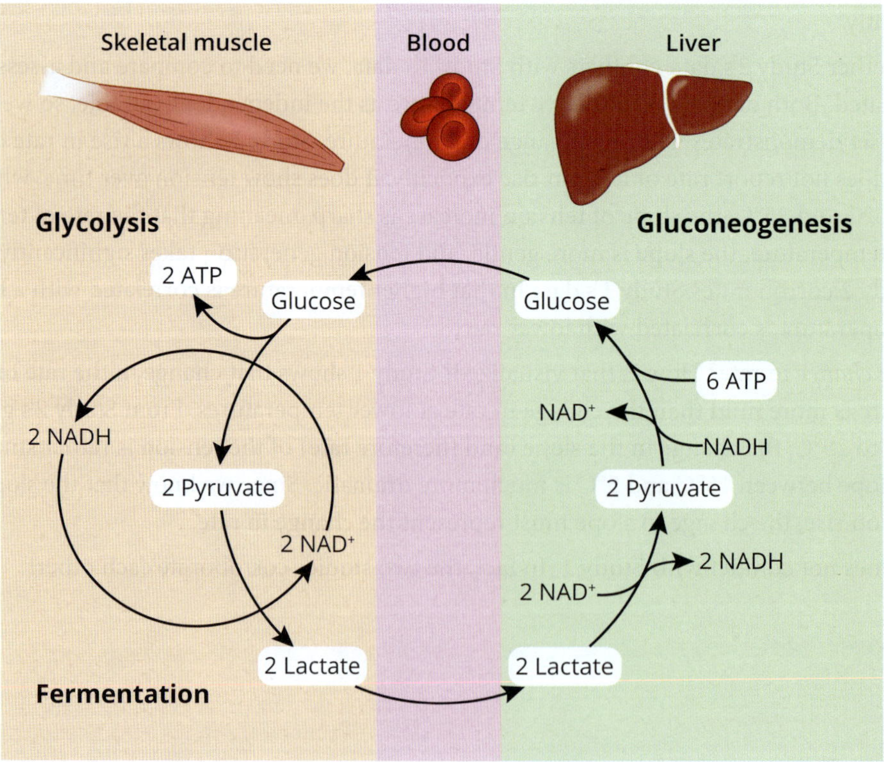

Figure 11.11 The Cori Cycle

MCAT CONCEPT CHECK 11.1

Before you move on, assess your understanding of the material with these questions.

1. What type(s) of muscle (skeletal, smooth, or cardiac) does each of the following describe? (Note: Circle the correct response(s) next to each item.)

• Striated:	Skeletal	Smooth	Cardiac
• Always uninucleated:	Skeletal	Smooth	Cardiac
• Always polynucleated:	Skeletal	Smooth	Cardiac
• Voluntary:	Skeletal	Smooth	Cardiac
• Innervated by the autonomic nervous system:	Skeletal	Smooth	Cardiac
• Exhibits myogenic activity:	Skeletal	Smooth	Cardiac

2. Which zone or band in the sarcomere does NOT change its length during muscle contraction? Why?

____

3. What are the events that initiate muscle contraction, in order? Start with neurotransmitter release and trace the pathway to the point where myosin binds with actin.

____

4. What role does the binding of ATP to the myosin head play in the cross-bridge cycle? What about the dissociation of ADP and inorganic phosphate from the myosin head?

    • Binding of ATP:

____

    • Dissociation of ADP and inorganic phosphate:

____

5. What is tetanus (the physiological phenomenon, not the disease)?

____

11.2 The Skeletal System

LEARNING OBJECTIVES

After Chapter 11.2, you will be able to:

- Distinguish between compact and spongy bone
- Identify the three structural parts of a bone and their relative contributions to growth
- Recall the major chemical component of bone
- Describe the function(s) of osteoblasts, osteoclasts, and chondrocytes
- Name the substance that lubricates movable joints and where it is produced

There are two types of skeletons: exoskeletons and endoskeletons. **Exoskeletons** encase whole organisms and are usually found in arthropods, such as crustaceans and insects. Vertebrates, including humans, have **endoskeletons**. Endoskeletons are internal, but are not able to protect the soft tissue structures as well as exoskeletons. However, exoskeletons must be shed and regrown to accommodate growth. Endoskeletons are much better able to accommodate the growth of a larger organism.

Skeletal Structure

The components of our skeletal system are divided into axial and appendicular skeletons (see Figure 11.13 below). The **axial skeleton** consists of the skull, vertebral column, rib cage, and hyoid bone (a small bone in the anterior neck used for swallowing); it provides the basic central framework for the body. The **appendicular skeleton** consists of the bones of the limbs (humerus, radius and ulna, carpals, metacarpals, and phalanges in the upper limb; and femur, tibia and fibula, tarsals, metatarsals, and phalanges in the lower limb); the pectoral girdle (scapula and clavicle); and pelvis. Both skeleton types are covered by other structures (muscle, connective tissue, and vasculature). The structure of the skeleton is shown in Figure 11.12, with many of the bones labeled.

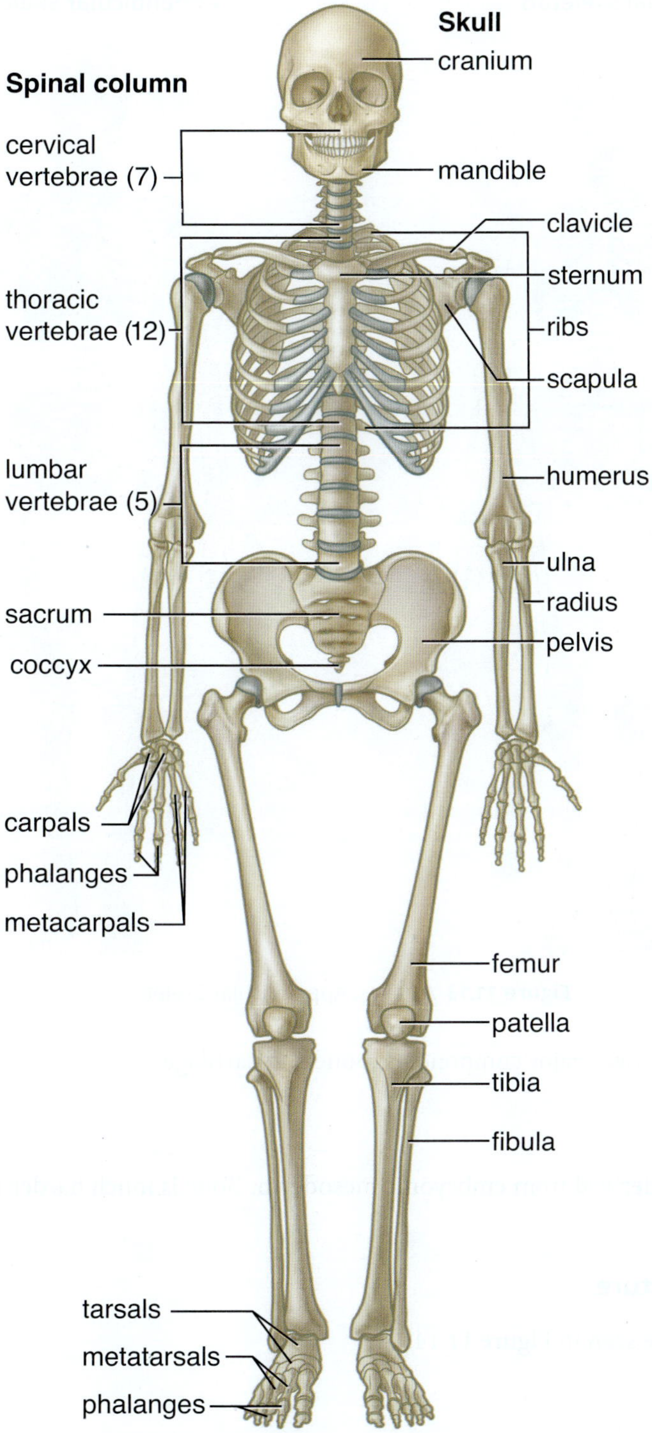

Figure 11.12 Anatomy of the Human Skeleton

REAL WORLD

An adult human has 206 bones. Over 100 of these are in the hands and feet.

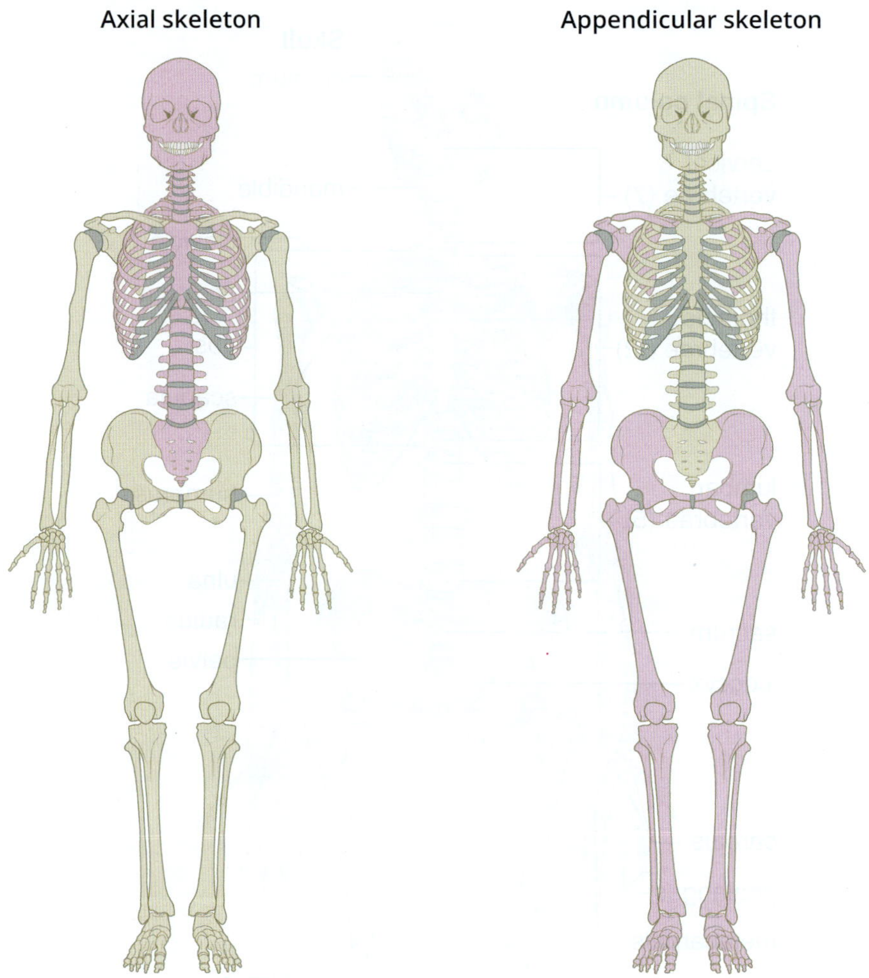

Figure 11.13 Axial vs. Appendicular Skeleton

The skeleton is created from two major components: bone and cartilage.

Bone Composition

Bone is a connective tissue derived from embryonic mesoderm. Bone is much harder than cartilage, but is relatively lightweight.

Macroscopic Bone Structure

The structure of bone can be seen in Figure 11.14.

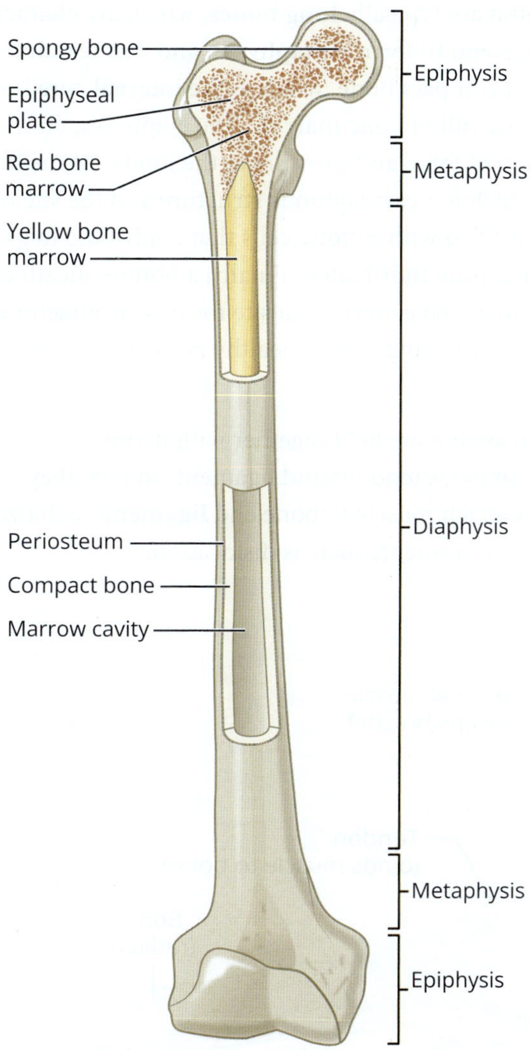

Figure 11.14 Anatomy of a Long Bone (Humerus)

Bone's characteristic strength comes specifically from **compact bone**. It lives up to its name, as it is both dense and strong. The other type of bone structure is **spongy** or **cancellous** bone. The lattice structure of spongy bone is visible under microscopy and consists of bony spicules (points) known as **trabeculae**. The cavities between trabeculae are filled with **bone marrow**, which may be either red or yellow. **Red marrow** is typically concentrated in flat bones and the ends of long bones and is filled with hematopoietic stem cells, which are responsible for the generation of all the cells in our blood; **yellow marrow** is typically housed in the shaft of long bones and is composed primarily of fat, so it is relatively inactive. As people age, more of their red bone marrow will convert into yellow marrow. However, there are certain situations that may facilitate yellow marrow reverting back to red marrow (such as anemia).

Bones in the appendicular skeleton are typically **long bones**, which are characterized by cylindrical shafts called **diaphyses** that swell at each end to form **metaphyses**, and that terminate in **epiphyses**. The outermost portions of bone are composed of compact bone, whereas the internal core is made of spongy bone. Long bone diaphyses and metaphyses are full of bone marrow. The epiphyses, on the other hand, use their spongy cores for more effective dispersion of force and pressure at the joints. At the internal edge of the epiphysis is an **epiphyseal (growth) plate**, which is a cartilaginous structure and the site of longitudinal growth. Prior to adulthood, the epiphyseal plate is filled with mitotic cells that contribute to growth; during puberty, these epiphyseal plates close and vertical growth is halted. Finally, a fibrous sheath called the **periosteum** surrounds the long bone to protect it as well as serve as a site for muscle attachment. Some periosteal cells are capable of differentiating into bone-forming cells; a healthy periosteum is necessary for bone growth and repair.

Structures in the musculoskeletal system are held together with dense connective tissue. Figure 11.15 compares tendons and ligaments in how they are utilized in the body. **Tendons** attach muscle to bone and **ligaments** stabilize and protect joints from damaging movements such as dislocation.

BRIDGE

The root *lig–* comes from Latin, where it means to "to tie; bind." Think of *DNA ligase*, discussed in Chapter 6 of *MCAT Biochemistry Review*. Think of ligands in complex ions, discussed in Chapter 9 of *MCAT General Chemistry Review*. In this case, ligaments tie bones to each other to stabilize joints.

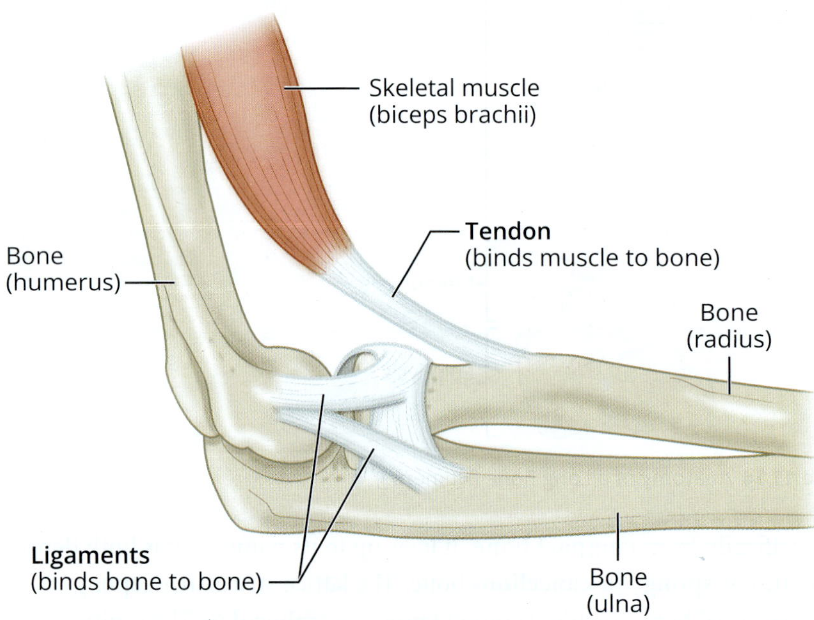

Figure 11.15 Tendons vs. Ligaments

Microscopic Bone Structure

The strength of compact bone comes from the **bone matrix**, which has both organic and inorganic components. The organic components include collagen, glycoproteins, and other peptides. The inorganic components include calcium, phosphate, and hydroxide ions, which harden together to form **hydroxyapatite** crystals ($Ca_{10}(PO_4)_6(OH)_2$). Minerals such as sodium, magnesium, and potassium are also stored in bone.

Strong bones require uniform distribution of organic and inorganic materials. The bony matrix is ordered into structural units known as **osteons** or **Haversian systems**, as shown in Figure 11.16. Each of these osteons contains concentric circles of bony matrix called **lamellae** surrounding a central microscopic channel. Longitudinal channels (those with an axis parallel to the bone) are known as **Haversian canals**, while transverse channels (those with an axis perpendicular to the bone) are known as **Volkmann's canals**. These canals contain the blood vessels, nerve fibers, and lymph vessels that maintain the health of the bone. Between the lamellar rings are small spaces called **lacunae**, which house mature bone cells known as **osteocytes**. The lacunae are interconnected by tiny channels called **canaliculi** that allow for the exchange of nutrients and wastes between osteocytes and the Haversian and Volkmann's canals.

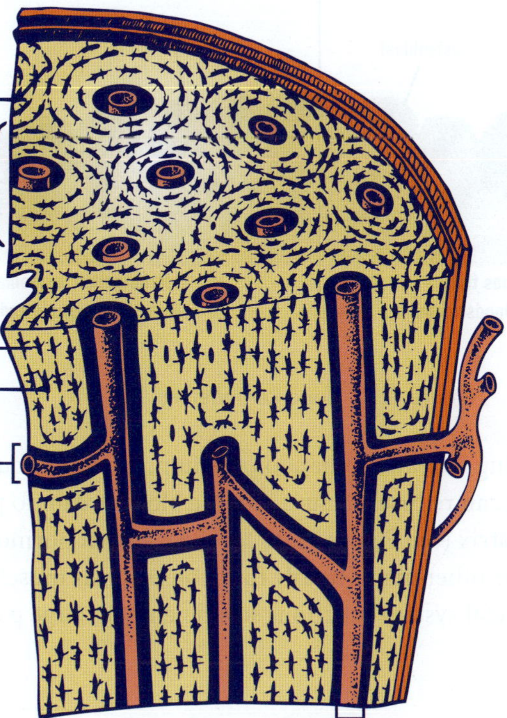

Figure 11.16 Bone Matrix
Cross-sectional and longitudinal views highlighting Haversian systems

KEY CONCEPT

Bone appears to be rigid and static, but it is actually quite dynamic. It is both vascular and innervated, which is why it hurts so much to break a bone. In addition, bone remains in a vigorous equilibrium between construction and destruction, known as bone remodeling.

Bone Remodeling

Two cell types are largely responsible for building and maintaining strong bones: osteoblasts and osteoclasts. **Osteoblasts** build bone, whereas **osteoclasts**, polynucleated resident macrophages of bone, resorb it. These processes together contribute to the constant turnover of bone, as shown in Figure 11.17. During bone formation, essential ingredients such as calcium and phosphate are obtained from the blood. During bone resorption, these ions are released back into the bloodstream. Bone remodeling occurs in response to stress, and bone actually remodels in such a way as to accommodate the repetitive stresses faced by the body. Endocrine hormones may also affect bone metabolism. **Parathyroid hormone**, a peptide hormone released by the parathyroid glands in response to low blood calcium, promotes resorption of bone, increasing the concentration of calcium and phosphate in the blood. **Vitamin D**, which is activated by parathyroid hormone, also promotes the

REAL WORLD

Osteoporosis is the most common bone disease in the United States. It is thought to be the result of increased osteoclast resorption and some concomitant slowing of bone formation, both of which lead to loss of bone mass. Estrogen is believed to help prevent osteoporosis by stimulating osteoblast activity.

resorption of bone. This may seem counterintuitive at first—isn't vitamin D used to promote bone growth? Indeed, the resorption of bone in response to vitamin D actually encourages the growth of new, stronger bone, thus overcompensating for the effect of resorbing bone in the first place. Finally, **calcitonin**, a peptide hormone released by the parafollicular cells of the thyroid in response to high blood calcium, promotes bone formation, lowering blood calcium levels.

MNEMONIC

Osteo**b**lasts **b**uild bone.
Osteo**c**lasts **c**hew bone.

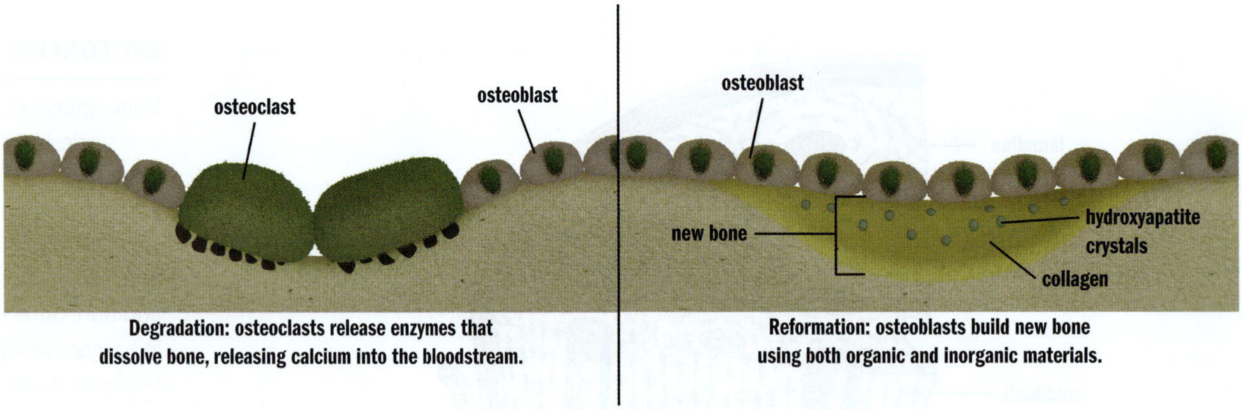

Figure 11.17 Bone Remodeling

As stated, bone structure and remodeling is heavily reliant on calcium, the most abundant mineral in the body. This process of bone remodeling can release calcium into the bloodstream to perform other functions aside from forming the strong bone matrix (see Figure 11.18 for the role that hormones play in regulating this process). Calcium is responsible for other major bodily functions such as muscle contractions and neurotransmitter release. The musculoskeletal system functions so efficiently in large part due to the versatility of calcium.

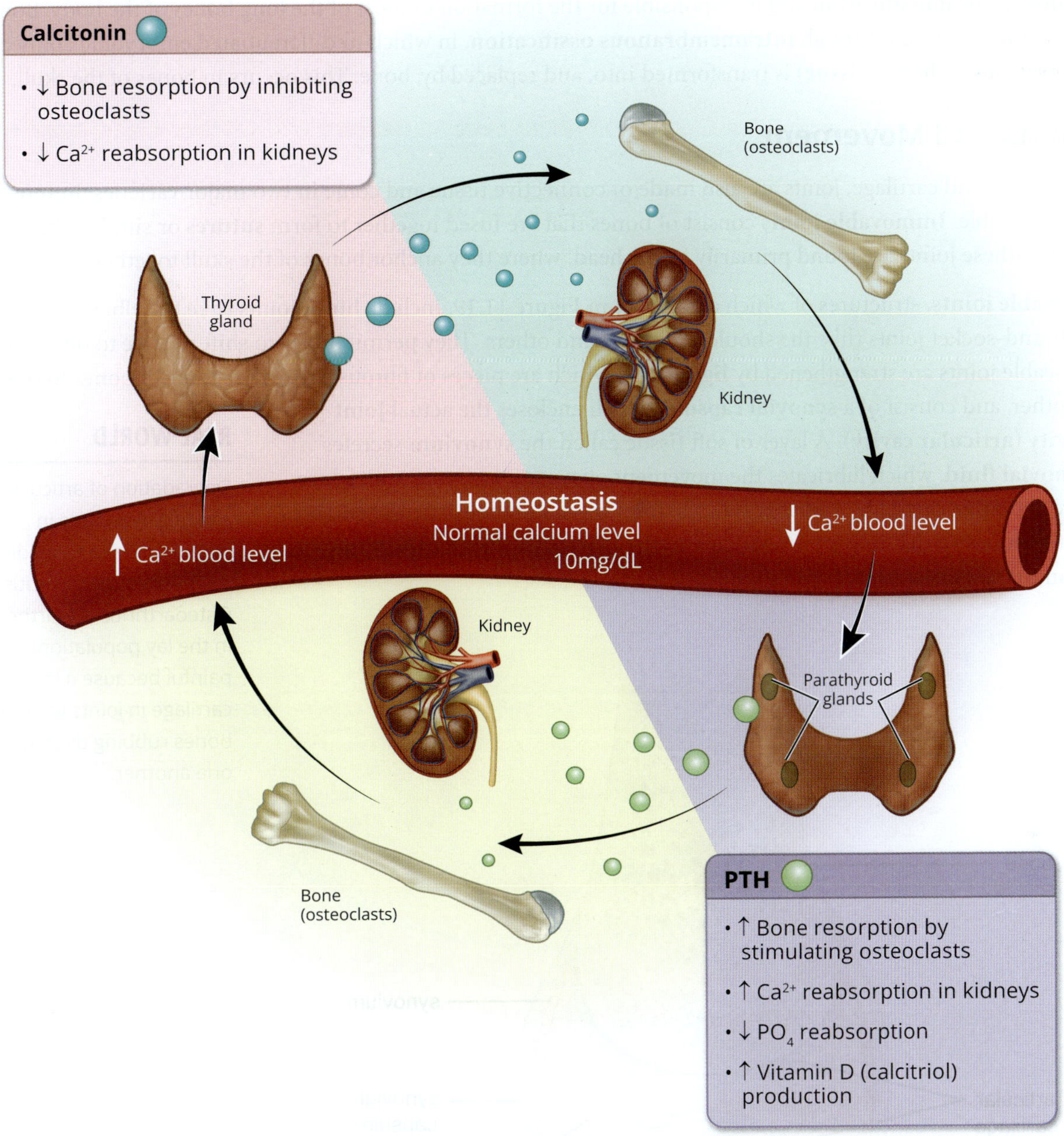

Figure 11.18 The Homeostatic Functions of Calcitonin and Parathyroid Hormone

Cartilage

Cartilage is softer and more flexible than bone. Cartilage consists of a firm but elastic matrix called **chondrin** that is secreted by cells called **chondrocytes**. Fetal skeletons are mostly made up of cartilage. This is advantageous because fetuses must grow and develop in a confined environment and then must traverse the birth canal. Adults have cartilage only in body parts that need a little extra flexibility or cushioning (external ear, nose, walls of the larynx and trachea, intervertebral discs, and joints). Cartilage also differs from bone in that it is avascular (without blood and lymphatic vessels) and is not innervated.

Most of the bones of the body are created by the hardening of cartilage into bone. This process is known as **endochondral ossification** and is responsible for the formation of most of the long bones of the body. Bones may also be formed through **intramembranous ossification**, in which undifferentiated embryonic connective tissue (**mesenchymal tissue**) is transformed into, and replaced by, bone. This occurs in bones of the skull.

Joints and Movement

Like bone and cartilage, joints are also made of connective tissue and come in two major varieties: immovable and movable. **Immovable joints** consist of bones that are fused together to form **sutures** or similar fibrous joints. These joints are found primarily in the head, where they anchor bones of the skull together.

Movable joints, structures of which are shown in Figure 11.19, include hinge joints (like the elbow or knee), ball-and-socket joints (like the shoulder or hip), and others. They permit bones to shift relative to one another. Movable joints are strengthened by **ligaments**, which are pieces of fibrous tissue that connect bones to one another, and consist of a **synovial capsule**, which encloses the actual **joint cavity** (**articular cavity**). A layer of soft tissue called the **synovium** secretes **synovial fluid**, which lubricates the movement of structures in the joint space. The **articular cartilage** contributes to the joint by coating the articular surfaces of the bones so that impact is restricted to the lubricated joint cartilage, rather than to the bones.

REAL WORLD

Degradation of articular cartilage (cartilage in joints) can lead to medical issues like osteoarthritis. Osteoarthritis (or "arthritis" in the lay population) is painful because a lack of cartilage in joints leads to bones rubbing directly on one another.

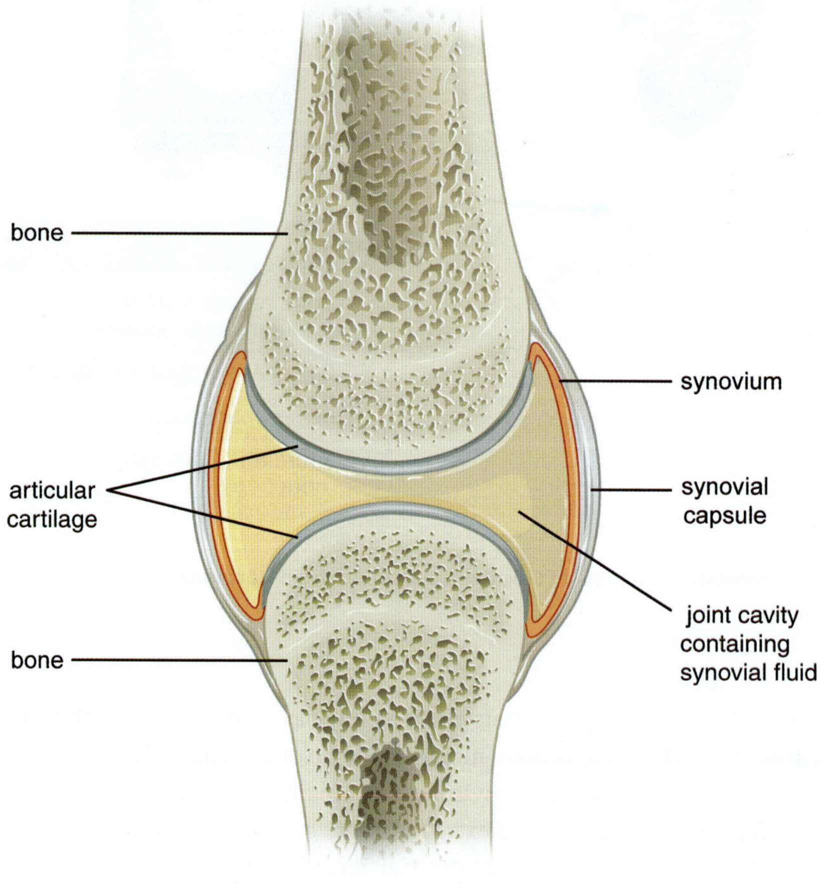

Figure 11.19 Structures in a Movable Joint

When a muscle is attached to two bones, its contraction will cause one of the bones to move. The end of the muscle with a larger attachment to bone (usually the proximal connection) is called the **origin**. The end with the smaller attachment to bone (usually the distal connection) is called the **insertion**. Often, our muscles work in **antagonistic pairs**; one relaxes while the other contracts. Such is the case in the arm, where the biceps brachii and triceps brachii work antagonistically, as shown in Figure 11.20. When the biceps contracts and the triceps relaxes, the elbow is flexed; when the triceps contracts and the biceps relaxes, the elbow is extended. Muscles can also be **synergistic**—working together to accomplish the same function.

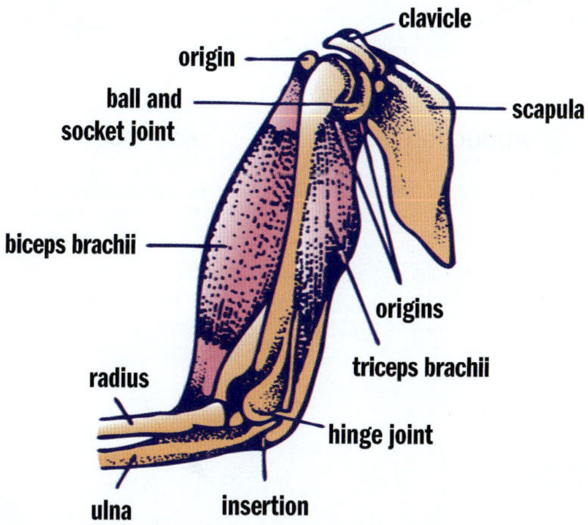

Figure 11.20 Antagonistic Muscle Pairs
The biceps brachii and triceps brachii are an example of a muscle pair that works antagonistically; the contraction of one causes the other to elongate.

Muscles may also be classified by the types of movements they coordinate (Figure 11.21). A **flexor** muscle decreases the angle across a joint (for the hip, one flexor is the iliopsoa); an **extensor** increases or straightens this angle (for the hip, one extensor is the gluteus maximus). An **abductor** moves a part of the body away from the midline (like the deltoid); an **adductor** moves a part of the body toward the midline (like the pectoralis major). **Medial** and **lateral rotation** describe motions that occur in limbs; a medial rotator rotates the axis of the limb toward the midline (like the subscapularis), whereas a lateral rotator rotates the axis of the limb away from the midline (like the infraspinatus).

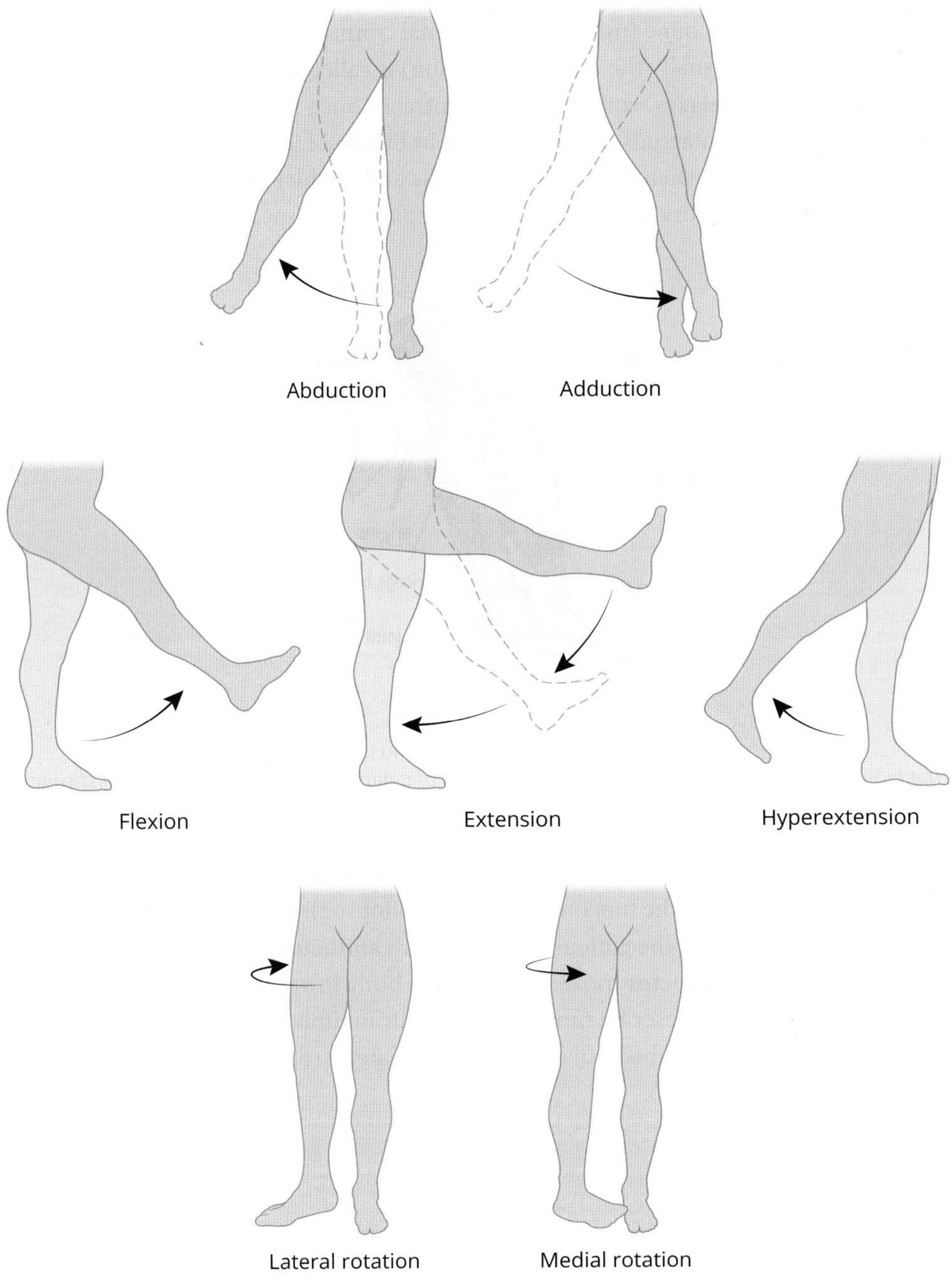

Figure 11.21 Muscle Movement Types

MCAT CONCEPT CHECK 11.2

Before you move on, assess your understanding of the material with these questions.

1. What is the difference between compact and spongy bone?
   - Compact bone:

   - Spongy bone:

   ---

2. What are the three structural parts of a bone? Which part contributes most to linear growth?

---

3. What chemical forms most of the inorganic component of bone?

---

4. What are the functions of osteoblasts, osteoclasts, and chondrocytes?
   - Osteoblast:

   - Osteoclast:

   - Chondrocyte:

   ---

5. What liquid provides the lubrication for movable joints? What tissue produces it?

Conclusion

One concept that has been emphasized throughout the past eight chapters on anatomy and physiology is the notion that organ systems work together in order to achieve a desired effect. The musculoskeletal system is no different. Usually, we think of the musculoskeletal system as being responsible for movement, but to limit the musculoskeletal system to that function would be shortsighted. The bones are reservoirs of calcium and other minerals that can be released through hormonal signaling. They protect the internal organs and provide support for the body. Muscle tissue not only moves these bones, but pumps blood through the body and is key to the function of a number of other systems, including respiration, digestion, blood pressure and vascular tone, and reproduction and childbirth. As you review anatomy and physiology and master the fundamentals of each organ system, be sure to pay special attention to how each organ system interacts with the others. While the MCAT expects you to understand each individual organ system, it will also challenge you by asking you to think critically about how one system impacts another. By spending some time in your studies looking at these interactions, you will be one step ahead on Test Day.

In our final chapter of *MCAT Biology Review*, we will switch gears and look at the transfer of information from generation to generation. This picks up on a discussion from the first three chapters of the book in which we explored the organization of cells and their genetic material, reproduction, and embryogenesis and development. In the next chapter, we'll describe classical (Mendelian) inheritance and conclude with a note on how the gene pool can change over time with the topic of evolution.

GO ONLINE

You've reviewed the content, now test your knowledge and critical thinking skills by completing a test-like passage set in your online resources!

CONCEPT SUMMARY

The Muscular System

- There are three main types of muscle: skeletal muscle, smooth muscle, and cardiac muscle.
  - **Skeletal muscle** is involved in support and movement, propulsion of blood in the venous system, and thermoregulation. It appears **striated**, is under voluntary (somatic) control, is polynucleated, and can be divided into **red (slow-twitch) fibers** that carry out oxidative phosphorylation and **white (fast-twitch) fibers** that rely on anaerobic metabolism.
  - **Smooth muscle** is in the respiratory, reproductive, cardiovascular, and digestive systems. It appears nonstriated, is under involuntary (autonomic) control, and is uninucleated. It can display **myogenic activity**, or contraction without neural input.
  - **Cardiac muscle** comprises the contractile tissue of the heart. It appears striated, is under involuntary (autonomic) control, and is uninucleated (sometimes binucleated). It can also display myogenic activity. Cells are connected with **intercalated discs** that contain **gap junctions**.
- The **sarcomere** is the basic contractile unit of striated muscle.
  - Sarcomeres are made of thick (**myosin**) and thin (**actin**) filaments.
  - **Troponin** and **tropomyosin** are found on the thin filament and regulate actin–myosin interactions.
- The sarcomere can be divided into different lines, zones, and bands.
  - The boundaries of each sarcomere are defined by **Z-lines**.
  - The **M-line** is located in the middle of the sarcomere.
  - The **I-band** contains only thin filaments.
  - The **H-zone** consists of only thick filaments.
  - The **A-band** contains the thick filaments in their entirety. It is the only part of the sarcomere that maintains a constant size during contraction.
- Sarcomeres attach end-to-end to become **myofibrils**, and each **myocyte** (muscle cell or **muscle fiber**) contains many myofibrils.
  - Myofibrils are surrounded by the **sarcoplasmic reticulum**, a calcium-containing modified endoplasmic reticulum, and the cell membrane of a myocyte is known as the **sarcolemma**.
  - A system of **T-tubules** is connected to the sarcolemma and oriented perpendicularly to the myofibrils, allowing the action potential to reach all parts of the muscle.
- Muscle contraction begins at the **neuromuscular junction**, where the motor neuron releases acetylcholine that binds to receptors on the sarcolemma, causing depolarization.
  - This depolarization spreads down the sarcolemma to the T-tubules, triggering the release of calcium ions.
  - Calcium binds to troponin, causing a shift in tropomyosin and exposure of the myosin-binding sites on the actin thin filament.
  - Shortening of the sarcomere occurs as myosin heads bind to the exposed sites on actin, forming cross bridges and pulling the actin filament along the thick filament, which results in contraction. This is known as the **sliding filament model**.
  - The muscle relaxes when acetylcholine is degraded by acetylcholinesterase, terminating the signal and allowing calcium to be brought back into the SR. ATP binds to the myosin head, allowing it to release from actin.

- Muscle cells exhibit an all-or-nothing response called a **simple twitch**.
  - Addition of multiple simple twitches before the muscle has an opportunity to fully relax is called **frequency summation**.
  - Simple twitches that occur so frequently as to not let the muscle relax at all can lead to **tetanus**, a more prolonged and stronger contraction.
- Muscle cells have additional energy reserves to reduce **oxygen debt** (the difference between the amount of oxygen needed and the amount present) and forestall fatigue.
  - **Creatine phosphate** can transfer a phosphate group to ADP, forming ATP.
  - **Myoglobin** is a heme-containing protein that is a muscular oxygen reserve.

The Skeletal System

- Internal skeletons (like those in humans) are called **endoskeletons**; external skeletons (like those in arthropods) are called **exoskeletons**.
- The human skeletal system can be divided into axial and appendicular skeletons.
  - The **axial skeleton** consists of structures in the midline such as the skull, vertebral column, rib cage, and hyoid bone.
  - The **appendicular skeleton** consists of the bones of the limbs, the pectoral girdle, and the pelvis.
- Bone is derived from embryonic mesoderm and includes both compact and spongy (cancellous) types.
  - **Compact bone** provides strength and is dense.
  - **Spongy** or **cancellous bone** has a lattice-like structure consisting of bony spicules known as **trabeculae**. The cavities are filled with bone marrow.
  - Long bones contain shafts called **diaphyses** that flare to form **metaphyses** and terminate in **epiphyses**. The epiphysis contains an **epiphyseal (growth) plate** that causes linear growth of the bone.
  - Bone is surrounded by a layer of connective tissue called **periosteum**.
  - Bones are attached to **muscles** by tendons and to each other by **ligaments**.
- **Bone matrix** has both organic components, like collagen, glycoproteins, and other peptides; and inorganic components, like **hydroxyapatite**.
  - Bone is organized into concentric rings called **lamellae** around a central **Haversian** or **Volkmann's canal**. This structural unit is called an **osteon** or **Haversian system**.
  - Between lamellar rings are **lacunae**, where osteocytes reside, which are connected with **canaliculi** to allow for nutrient and waste transfer.
- Bone remodeling is carried out by osteoblasts and osteoclasts. **Osteoblasts** build bone, while **osteoclasts** resorb bone.
  - **Parathyroid hormone** increases resorption of bone, increasing calcium and phosphate concentrations in the blood.
  - **Vitamin D** also increases resorption of bone, leading to increased turnover and, subsequently, the production of stronger bone.
  - **Calcitonin** increases bone formation, decreasing calcium concentrations in the blood.

- Cartilage is a firm, elastic material secreted by **chondrocytes**. Its matrix is called **chondrin**.
    - Cartilage is usually found in areas that require more flexibility or cushioning.
    - Cartilage is avascular and is not innervated.
- In fetal life, bone forms from cartilage through **endochondral ossification**. Some bones, especially those of the skull, form directly from undifferentiated tissue (**mesenchyme**) in **intramembranous ossification**.
- Joints may be classified as immovable or movable.
    - **Immovable joints** are fused together to form sutures or similar fibrous joints.
    - **Movable joints** are usually strengthened by ligaments and contain a **synovial capsule**.
    - **Synovial fluid**, secreted by the **synovium**, aids in motion by lubricating the joint.
    - Each bone in the joint is coated with **articular cartilage** to aid in movement and provide cushioning.
- Muscles that serve opposite functions come in **antagonistic pairs**; when one muscle contracts, the other lengthens.

ANSWERS TO CONCEPT CHECKS

11.1

1. Skeletal and cardiac muscle are striated. Smooth muscle is always uninucleated. Skeletal muscle is always polynucleated. Skeletal muscle is voluntary. Smooth and cardiac muscle are innervated by the autonomic nervous system. Smooth and cardiac muscle exhibit myogenic activity.
2. The A-band does not change length during muscle contraction because it is the entire length of the myosin filament. The filaments do not change length, but rather slide over each other; thus, the A-band should remain a constant length during contraction.
3. Release of acetylcholine from motor neuron → activation of acetylcholine receptors in sarcolemma → depolarization of sarcolemma → spreading of signal using T-tubules → release of calcium from sarcoplasmic reticulum (SR) → binding of calcium to troponin → conformational shift in tropomyosin → exposure of myosin-binding sites → myosin binds to actin
4. ATP binding allows the myosin filament to disconnect from actin. Dissociation of ADP and inorganic phosphate from myosin causes the powerstroke.
5. Tetanus is the summation of multiple simple twitches that occur too quickly for the muscle to relax. This leads to a stronger and more prolonged contraction of the muscle.

11.2

1. Compact bone is dense and is used for its strength; it forms most of the outer layers of a bone. Spongy (cancellous) bone has many spaces between bony spicules called trabeculae and is the site of marrow production. It is found in the interior core of the bone and also helps distribute forces or pressures on the bone.
2. The three parts of a bone are the diaphysis, metaphysis, and epiphysis. Growth plates are found in epiphyses and contribute to linear growth.
3. Most inorganic bone is composed of hydroxyapatite crystals.
4. Osteoblasts build bone. Osteoclasts "chew" bone (break it down). Chondrocytes form cartilage.
5. Synovial fluid, produced by the synovium, lubricates movable joints.

SCIENCE MASTERY ASSESSMENT EXPLANATIONS

1. **D**

We are given a diagram of a sarcomere and asked to determine which regions shorten during muscle contraction. All bands and zones of the sarcomere shorten during contraction except the A-band, which is the full length of the thick filaments. In this diagram, that is region 1. Thus, the remaining regions all shorten, making **(D)** the correct answer. Region 2 represents the I-band, region 3 represents the H-zone, and region 4 is the length of the sarcomere between Z-lines.

2. **C**

Region 1 contains both thick and thin filaments overlapping each other. This region refers to the A-band and is measured from one end of the thick filaments to the other. This is also the only portion of the sarcomere that does not change length during muscle contraction.

3. **D**

The sarcomere is the contractile unit in striated muscle cells. One sarcomere is represented by the area between the two vertical lines, referred to as the Z-lines. In addition, the Z-lines anchor the thin filaments. In the diagram, a sarcomere is therefore defined by region 4.

4. **C**

Calcium is released from the sarcoplasmic reticulum into the sarcoplasm. It binds the troponin molecules on the thin filaments, causing the strands of tropomyosin to shift, thereby exposing the myosin-binding sites on the thin filaments.

5. **A**

Let's quickly define each one of the four cells discussed in the answer choices. Osteoblasts are bone cells involved in the secretion of bone matrix, as **(A)** states. Osteoclasts are large, polynucleated cells involved in bone resorption. Osteocytes are mature bone cells that eventually become surrounded by their matrix; their primary role is bone maintenance. Finally, chondrocytes are cells that secrete chondrin, an elastic matrix that makes up cartilage.

6. **C**

This question is essentially asking where longitudinal growth occurs in bones. The most likely site of abnormalities in this child's femur is the epiphyseal plate, a disc of cartilaginous cells at the internal border of the epiphysis, because the epiphyseal plate is the site of longitudinal growth. Damage to the epiphysis (with or without metaphysis involvement) can imply damage to the epiphyseal plate.

7. **D**

Red fibers are slow-twitching fibers that have high levels of myoglobin and many mitochondria. They derive their energy from aerobic respiration and are capable of sustained vigorous activity. This eliminates **(A)** and **(B)**. White fibers, on the other hand, are fast-twitching fibers and contain lower levels of myoglobin and fewer mitochondria. Because of their composition, they derive more of their energy anaerobically and fatigue more easily. This eliminates **(C)** and makes **(D)** the correct answer.

8. **A**

The articular surfaces of the bones are covered with a layer of smooth articular cartilage. The epiphysis is a portion of the bone itself, eliminating **(B)**. Synovial fluid lubricates the movement in the joint space, but does not stop the bones from contacting one another; this is the job of articular cartilage, eliminating **(C)**. There is no appreciable function for smooth muscle in the joint space, eliminating **(D)**.

9. **B**

The only type of muscle that is always multinucleated is skeletal muscle, making **(B)** the correct answer. Cardiac muscle may contain one or two centrally located nuclei, so Statement I is incorrect. Smooth muscle, on the other hand, always has only one centrally located nucleus.

10. **D**

Myogenic activity refers to the ability of a muscle to contract without nervous stimulation, such as in response to other stimuli like stretching. Smooth and cardiac muscle both possess myogenic activity.

11. **D**

Yellow marrow is largely inactive and is infiltrated by adipose tissue, making **(D)** the correct answer.

12. **D**

The periosteum, a fibrous sheath that surrounds long bones, is the site of attachment to muscle tissue. Some periosteum cells are capable of differentiating into bone-forming cells called osteoblasts. This eliminates **(A)**, **(B)**, and **(C)**. It is the synovium that secretes fluid into the joint cavity (joint space), not the periosteum, making **(D)** the correct answer.

13. **D**

The axial skeleton includes the skull, vertebral column, rib cage, and hyoid bone. The sternum is a point of attachment of the rib cage and is thus a part of the axial, not appendicular, skeleton. The limb bones, pectoral girdle, and pelvis are all part of the appendicular skeleton.

14. **B**

Bones form in one of two ways: endochondral ossification and intramembranous ossification. Endochondral ossification is the replacement of cartilage with bone and occurs mostly in long bones, eliminating **(A)**. Intramembranous ossification is the formation of bone from undifferentiated connective tissue cells (mesenchyme) and occurs mostly in the skull, making **(B)** the correct answer. Bone resorption is the breakdown of bone, not its formation, eliminating **(C)**. Longitudinal growth occurs in long bones and is responsible for increasing height over time, but does not play a role in fontanelle ossification, eliminating **(D)**.

15. **C**

An unprovoked fracture of the hip is not a normal finding in a person who is younger. Given that the patient has a high calcium level, it is likely that the patient has an increased level of bone resorption that is causing the bones to be more fragile. Parathyroid hormone causes calcium release from bones. If this patient had an overactive parathyroid gland—or even cancer in this gland—then it is likely that calcium could still be resorbed from the bones even though blood calcium levels are already high.

GO ONLINE

Consult your online resources for additional practice.

SHARED CONCEPTS

Biology Chapter 4
The Nervous System

Biology Chapter 5
The Endocrine System

Biology Chapter 6
The Respiratory System

Biology Chapter 7
The Cardiovascular System

General Chemistry Chapter 9
Solutions

Physics and Math Chapter 1
Kinematics and Dynamics

CHAPTER 12

GENETICS AND EVOLUTION

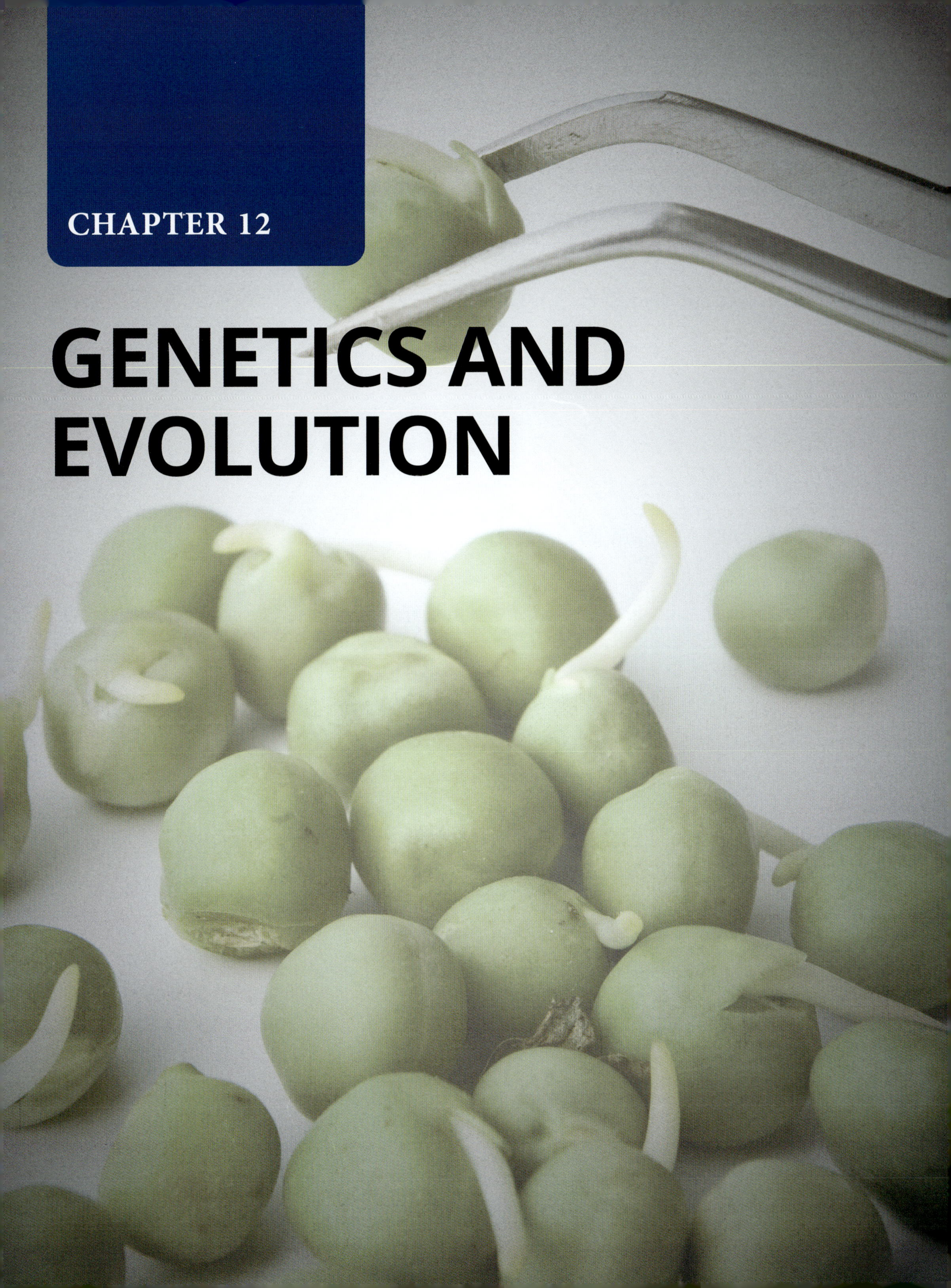

SCIENCE MASTERY ASSESSMENT

Every pre-med knows this feeling: there is so much content I have to know for the MCAT! How do I know what to do first or what's important?

While the high-yield badges throughout this book will help you identify the most important topics, this Science Mastery Assessment is another tool in your MCAT prep arsenal. This quiz (which can also be taken in your online resources) and the guidance below will help ensure that you are spending the appropriate amount of time on this chapter based on your personal strengths and weaknesses. Don't worry though—skipping something now does not mean you'll never study it. Later on in your prep, as you complete full-length tests, you'll uncover specific pieces of content that you need to review and can come back to these chapters as appropriate.

How to Use This Assessment

If you answer 0–7 questions correctly:

Spend about 1 hour to read this chapter in full and take limited notes throughout. Follow up by reviewing **all** quiz questions to ensure that you now understand how to solve each one.

If you answer 8–11 questions correctly:

Spend 20–40 minutes reviewing the quiz questions. Beginning with the questions you missed, read and take notes on the corresponding subchapters. For questions you answered correctly, ensure your thinking matches that of the explanation and you understand why each choice was correct or incorrect.

If you answer 12–15 questions correctly:

Spend less than 20 minutes reviewing all questions from the quiz. If you missed any, then include a quick read-through of the corresponding subchapters, or even just the relevant content within a subchapter, as part of your question review. For questions you answered correctly, ensure your thinking matches that of the explanation and review the Concept Summary at the end of the chapter.

1. What is the gene order of linked genes M, N, O, and P, given the following recombination frequencies?

MN: 6%	NO: 18%
MO: 12%	NP: 1%
MP: 5%	OP: 17%

A. MOPN
B. NPMO
C. ONPM
D. PNMO

2. Suppose that in a mammalian species, the allele for black hair (B) is dominant to the allele for brown hair (b), and the allele for curly hair (C) is dominant to the allele for straight hair (c). When an organism of unknown genotype is crossed against one with straight, brown hair, the phenotypic ratio is as follows:

I. 25% curly black hair
II. 25% straight black hair
III. 25% curly brown hair
IV. 25% straight brown hair

What is the genotype of the unknown parent?

A. BbCC
B. bbCc
C. Bbcc
D. BbCc

3. If a genotypical male who has hemophilia (X_hY) is crossed with a genotypical female carrier of both color blindness and hemophilia (X_cX_h), what is the probability that a genotypically female child would be born without either condition?

A. 0%
B. 25%
C. 50%
D. 100%

4. If a test cross on a species of plant reveals the appearance of a recessive phenotype in the offspring, what must be true of the phenotypically dominant parent?

A. It must be genotypically heterozygous.
B. It must be genotypically homozygous.
C. It could be either genotypically heterozygous or homozygous.
D. It must have the same genotype as the test cross control parent.

5. Which of the following definitions is FALSE?

A. Penetrance—the percentage of individuals in the population carrying the allele who actually express the phenotype associated with it
B. Expressivity—the percentage of individuals in the population carrying the allele who do not express the phenotype associated with it
C. Incomplete dominance—occurs when the phenotype of the heterozygote is an intermediate of the phenotypes of the homozygotes
D. Codominance—occurs when multiple alleles exist for a given gene and more than one of them is dominant

6. In a species of plant, a homozygous red flower (RR) is crossed with a homozygous yellow flower (rr). If the F_1 generation is self-crossed and the F_2 generation has a phenotypic ratio of red:orange:yellow of 1:2:1, which characteristic accounts for these results?

A. Codominance
B. Incomplete dominance
C. Penetrance
D. Expressivity

7. Which of the following statements is INCORRECT regarding inheritance of traits according to the modern synthesis model?

A. A mutation due to excessive amounts of ultraviolet light occurs in an unfertilized egg; this will affect the child who is born from that egg.
B. The muscular strength gained by a weight lifter over a lifetime is inherited by the weight lifter's children.
C. A green-feathered bird that survived all of the predators in the forest will pass on the green feather genes to its offspring.
D. A flower with a tasty nectar eaten by a butterfly is more likely to pass on its genes through the pollen spread by the butterfly than a flower with less desirable nectar.

8. Which of the following statements is FALSE based on Darwin's theory of natural selection?
   A. Natural selection is the driving force for evolution.
   B. Favorable genetic variations become more and more common in individuals throughout their lives.
   C. Natural selection can drive organisms living in groups to ultimately become distinct species.
   D. Fitness is measured by reproductive success.

9. Which of the following is NOT a necessary condition for Hardy–Weinberg equilibrium?
   A. Large population size
   B. No mutations
   C. Monogamous mating partners
   D. No migration into or out of the population

10. As the climate became colder during the Ice Age, a particular species of mammal evolved a thicker layer of fur. What kind of selection occurred in this population?
    A. Stabilizing selection
    B. Directional selection
    C. Disruptive selection
    D. Speciation selection

11. At what point are two populations descended from the same ancestral stock considered to be separate species?
    A. When they can no longer produce viable, fertile offspring
    B. When they look significantly different from each other
    C. When they can interbreed successfully and produce offspring
    D. When their habitats are separated by a significantly large distance so that they cannot meet

12. In a nonevolving population, there are two alleles, R and r, which code for the same trait. The frequency of R is 30 percent. What are the frequencies of all the possible genotypes?
    A. 49% RR, 42% Rr, 9% rr
    B. 30% RR, 21% Rr, 49% rr
    C. 0.09% RR, 0.42% Rr, 0.49% rr
    D. 9% RR, 42% Rr, 49% rr

13. In a particular Hardy–Weinberg population, there are only two eye colors: brown and blue. Of the population, 36% have blue eyes, the recessive trait. What percentage of the population is heterozygous?
    A. 24%
    B. 48%
    C. 60%
    D. 64%

14. Tay-Sachs disease is an autosomal recessive disorder characterized by defective hexosaminidase A. Proteomic analysis of a cell affected by this condition revealed a shortened protein with an abnormal amino acid sequence at the C-terminus. Based on this information, which mutation is mostly likely?
    A. Silent mutation
    B. Missense mutation
    C. Nonsense mutation
    D. Frameshift mutation

15. A child is born with a number of rare phenotypic features and genetic testing is performed. The child is determined to have partial trisomy 21, with three copies of some segments of DNA from chromosome 21, and partial monosomy 4, with only one copy of some segments of DNA from chromosome 4. Which of the following mutations could have occurred in one of the parental gametes during development to explain both findings?
    A. Deletion
    B. Insertion
    C. Translocation
    D. Inversion

Answer Key

1. **B** (See section 12.3)
2. **D** (See section 12.3)
3. **C** (See section 12.3)
4. **A** (See section 12.3)
5. **B** (See section 12.1)
6. **B** (See section 12.1)
7. **B** (See section 12.1)
8. **B** (See section 12.4)
9. **C** (See section 12.3)
10. **B** (See section 12.4)
11. **A** (See section 12.4)
12. **D** (See section 12.3)
13. **B** (See section 12.3)
14. **D** (See section 12.2)
15. **C** (See section 12.2)

The relevant section of the chapter to review for each question is given in parentheses after the correct answer. Detailed explanations can be found at the end of the chapter.

CHAPTER 12

GENETICS AND EVOLUTION

In This Chapter

CHAPTER PROFILE

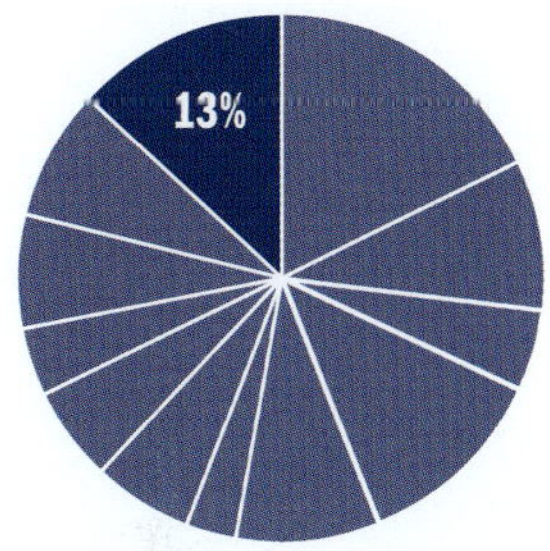

The content in this chapter should be relevant to about 13% of all questions about biology on the MCAT.

This chapter covers material from the following AAMC content category:

1C: Transmission of heritable information from generation to generation and the processes that increase genetic diversity

Introduction

For generations, European royal families practiced what is known as royal intermarriage. For purposes of establishing or continuing political alliances, maintaining bloodline purity, or smoothing out diplomatic relations, marriages between royal families were arranged, resulting in such an interweaving of bloodlines that eventually much of European royalty was—and still is—genetically related.

Such marriage unions led to rather severe restrictions on the gene pool, or all the alleles represented in the royal family lines, by limiting **gene flow** artificially. Offspring of parents who were also related to each other through blood lineage (consanguinity) came to have greater similarities in their genotypes, and certain alleles became so frequent that their phenotypic expression became almost a hallmark of royal descent. The House of Habsburg, which ruled a number of European kingdoms from the 11th century until the late 18th century, was perhaps the most infamous for its inbreeding practices. Members of this royal family bore the unmistakable mark of their restricted genes through a jaw malformation that even came to be known as the *Habsburg lip*. Medically termed *prognathism* (Greek: "forward jaw"), the condition is a misalignment of the mandible and maxilla. The Habsburg family portraits present individuals with prominent, forward-thrusting lower jaws and chins characteristic of mandibular prognathism. The genetic condition has more than just aesthetic implications; it can lead to serious disfigurement and disability. Charles II of Spain suffered from the worst case of the Habsburg lip on record—his lower teeth protruded so much farther than his upper teeth that he was not able to chew his food. Figure 12.1 is a portrait of Charles II from his time.

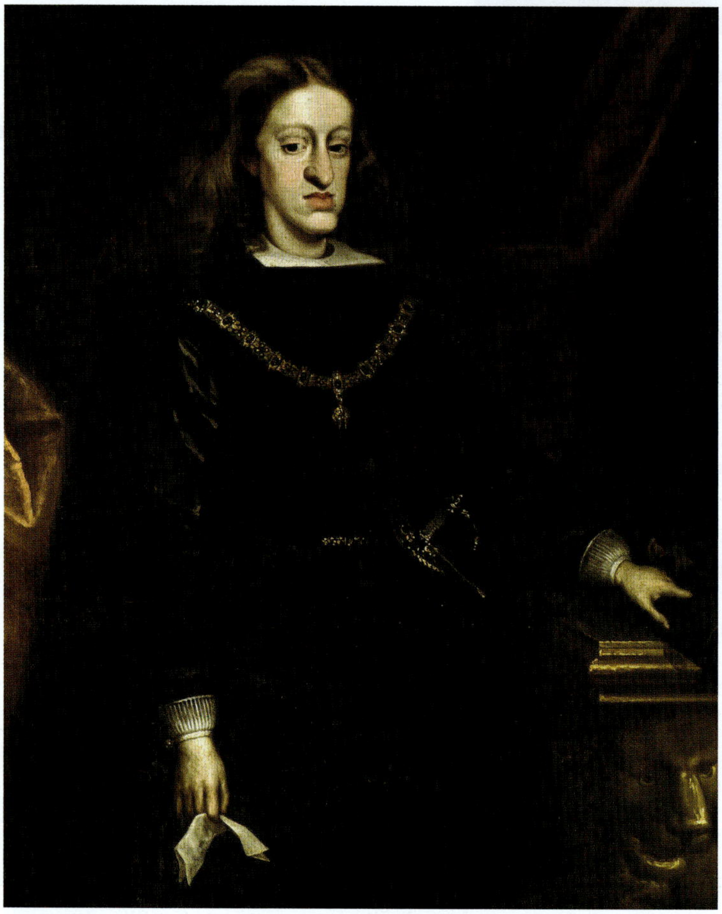

Figure 12.1 The Habsburg Lip
This is a portrait of King Charles II of Spain.

In this chapter, we will explore the concepts of classical genetics, which were originally described in the mid-1800s. Consider this chapter in tandem with the discussions of molecular genetics in Chapters 6 and 7 of *MCAT Biochemistry Review*. Then, we will explore the changes in the gene pool that occur over time with a discussion of evolution. We'll also quantify the genetics of populations that are *not* undergoing evolution with the Hardy–Weinberg principle.

12.1 Fundamental Concepts of Genetics High Yield

LEARNING OBJECTIVES

After Chapter 12.1, you will be able to:

- Recall what traits make alleles dominant or recessive
- Differentiate between homozygous, heterozygous, and hemizygous genotypes
- Compare and contrast complete dominance, codominance, and incomplete dominance
- Explain the difference between penetrance and expressivity
- Connect Mendel's laws with the phase of meiosis to which they are most closely correlated

The physical and biochemical characteristics of every living organism are determined by **genes**, which are DNA sequences that code for heritable traits that can be passed from one generation to the next. Taken together, all genes (as well as a large supply of noncoding DNA) are organized into **chromosomes** to ensure that genetic material is passed easily to daughter cells during mitosis and meiosis. Each gene may have alternative forms called **alleles**. We've already explored the ABO blood antigens as an example of three alleles for the same gene (I^A, I^B, and i). The genetic combination possessed by an individual is known as a **genotype**, and the manifestation of a given genotype as an observable trait is known as a **phenotype**.

BRIDGE

Blood type A individuals carry the A antigen on their erythrocytes and have circulating anti-B antibodies. Blood type B individuals carry the B antigen on their erythrocytes and have circulating anti-A antibodies. Those with type AB have both antigens and neither antibody; those with type O have neither antigen and both antibodies. That makes type O individuals universal donors and type AB individuals universal recipients. Blood typing is discussed in Chapter 7 of *MCAT Biology Review* and shown again here in Figure 12.2.

Human beings typically possess two copies of each chromosome, called **homologues**, with the exception of the sex chromosomes of genotypical males, who have one X chromosome and one Y chromosome. Each gene has a particular **locus**, or location on a specific chromosome. The normal locus of a particular gene is consistent among human beings—a gene can be described by its location. Because each chromosome is part of a homologous pair, a person will inherit two alleles for all genes (again, except for male sex chromosomes). Alleles can be categorized based on their expression. If only one copy of an allele is needed to express a given phenotype, the allele is said to be **dominant** and is usually represented with a capital letter. If two copies are needed, the allele is said to be **recessive** and is usually represented with a lowercase letter. The terms dominant and recessive refer to how the alleles would affect the phenotype when paired with each other. If both alleles are the same for a given gene, the individual is said to have a **homozygous** genotype. If the alleles are different, the individual has a **heterozygous** genotype. A **hemizygous** genotype describes a situation in which only one allele is present for a given gene, as is the case for parts of the X chromosome in genotypical males.

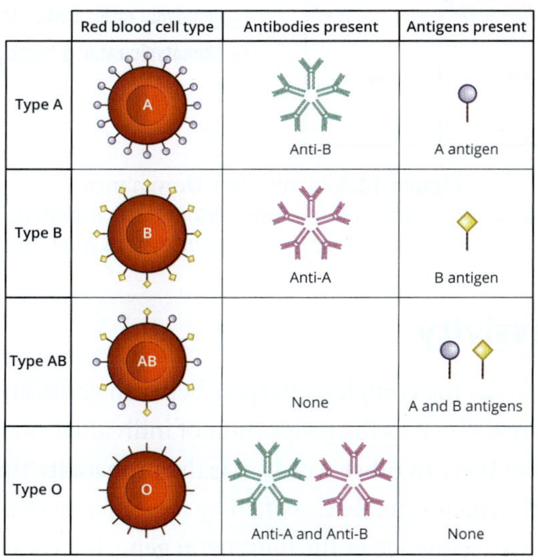

Figure 12.2 Blood Types

Patterns of Dominance

When only one dominant and one recessive allele exist for a given gene, there is said to be **complete dominance**. In this case, the presence of one dominant allele will mask the recessive allele, if present. When more than one dominant allele exists for a given gene, there is **codominance**. For example, a person with one allele for the A blood antigen and one allele for the B blood antigen will express both antigens simultaneously. Finally, **incomplete dominance** occurs when a heterozygote expresses a phenotype that is intermediate between the two homozygous genotypes. A classic example of incomplete dominance is the mating of certain flowers, in which a red flower crossed with a white flower results in pink flowers, as shown in Figure 12.3.

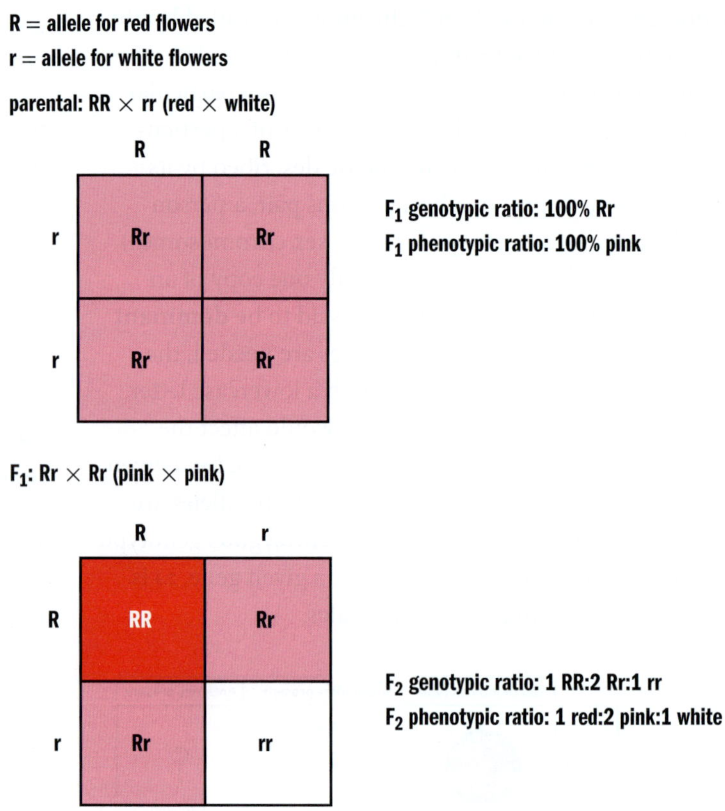

Figure 12.3 Incomplete Dominance
Snapdragons display incomplete dominance, in which neither allele is dominant and the heterozygous phenotype is a mixture of the two homozygous phenotypes.

Penetrance and Expressivity

Penetrance and expressivity both reveal the complex interplay between genes and the environment (Figure 12.4). **Penetrance** is a population measure defined as the proportion of individuals in the population carrying the allele who actually express the phenotype. In other words, it is the probability that, given a particular genotype, a person will express the phenotype. Alleles can be classified by their degree of penetrance; Huntington's disease, caused by an expansion of a repetitive sequence in the *huntingtin* gene, is a classic example. Individuals with more than 40 sequence repeats have **full penetrance**—100 percent of individuals with this allele show symptoms of Huntington's disease. Individuals with fewer sequence repeats show **high penetrance**, wherein most (but not all) of those with the allele show symptoms of the disease. With fewer sequence repeats, the gene comes to have **reduced penetrance**, **low penetrance**, or even **nonpenetrance**.

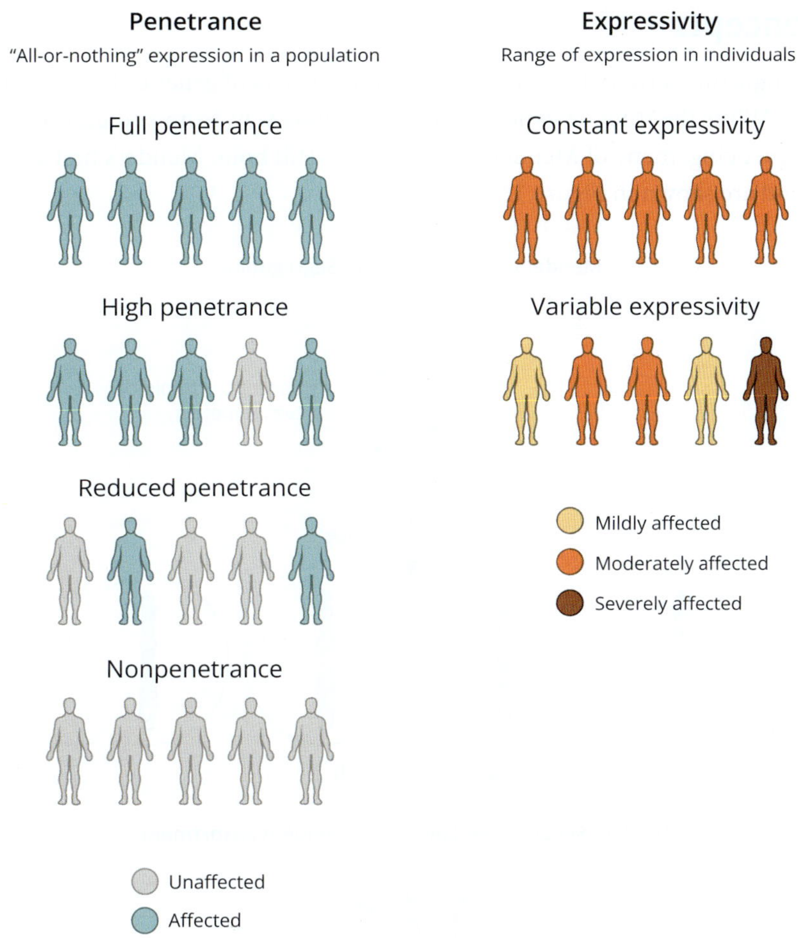

Figure 12.4 Penetrance vs. Expressivity

A related but distinct concept is **expressivity**, which is defined as varying phenotypes despite identical genotypes. If expressivity is **constant**, then all individuals with a given genotype express the same phenotype. However, if expressivity is **variable**, then individuals with the same genotype may have different phenotypes. Whereas penetrance is a population parameter (what percentage of individuals with a given genotype express the phenotype?), expressivity reflects the gray area in expression and is more commonly considered at the individual level. For example, the disease *neurofibromatosis type II* is an autosomal dominant disease that results from a mutation of the gene *NF2* (*merlin*). Interestingly, a range of phenotypes is associated with carrying the defective allele. Many patients have debilitating tumors of the vestibulocochlear nerve, which is needed for hearing and balance. Some have cataracts, while others have tumors in the skin called neuromas; still others have spinal lesions. A small proportion of the population is nonpenetrant. Nonpenetrant refers to a situation in which an individual possesses the genotype for a specific phenotype but fails to express the expected characteristics in a significant way. The disease shows variable expressivity because presentations range from no clinical effect to severe disability.

KEY CONCEPT

- **Penetrance**—the proportion of the population with a given genotype who actually express the phenotype
- **Expressivity**—the different manifestations of the same genotype across the population

Mendelian Concepts

Gregor Mendel, an Augustinian friar, developed several of the tenets of genetics in the 1860s based on his work with pea plants. While the study of genetics has come a long way, from pedigree analysis to DNA probes to whole-genome sequencing, many of Mendel's original ideas still hold. Mendel's first and second laws are among those ideas and are shown in Figure 12.5.

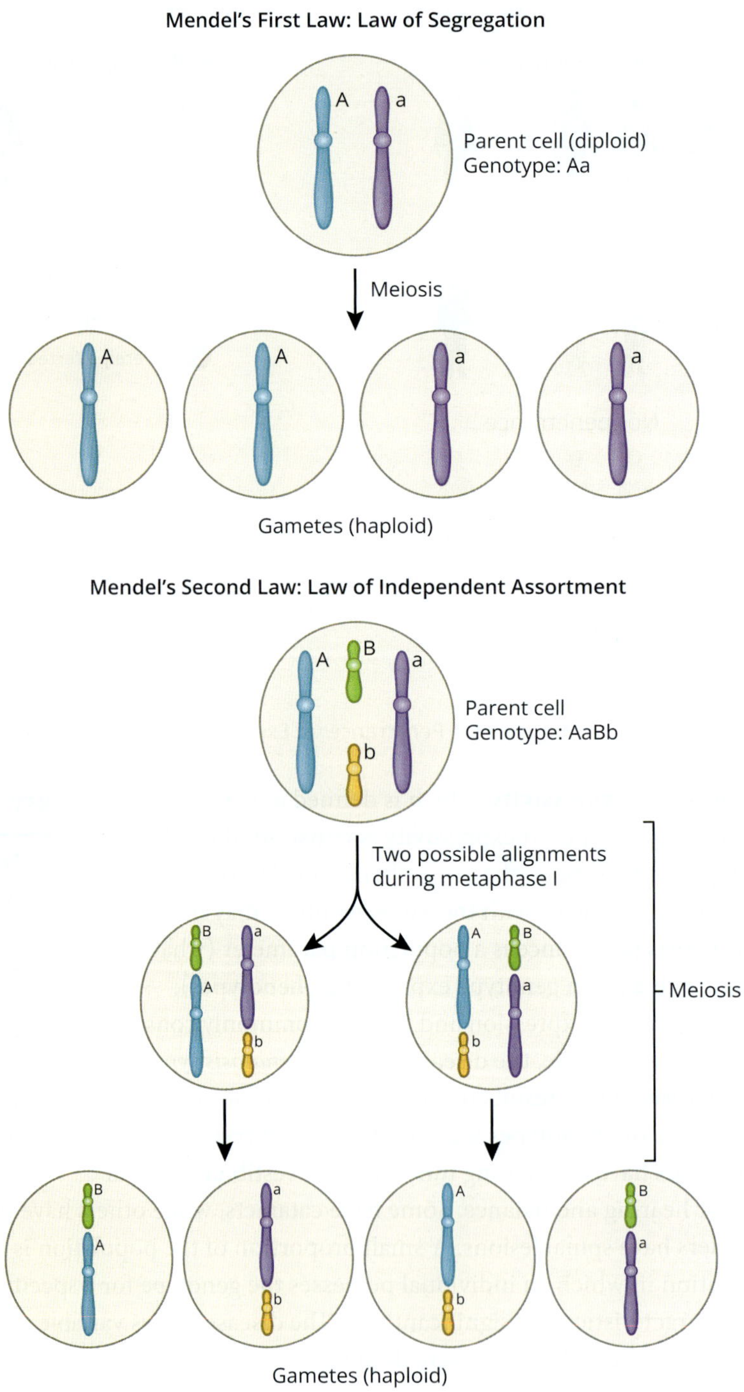

Figure 12.5 Mendel's Two Laws

Mendel's First Law: Law of Segregation

There are four basic tenets of the modern interpretation of **Mendel's first law** (**of segregation**), some which have already been discussed:

- Genes exist in alternative forms (alleles).
- An organism has two alleles for each gene—one inherited from each parent.
- The two alleles segregate during meiosis, resulting in gametes that carry only one allele for any inherited trait.
- If two alleles of an organism are different, only one will be fully expressed and the other will be silent. The expressed allele is said to be dominant, while the silent allele is recessive. (Keep in mind that codominance and incomplete dominance are exceptions to this rule.)

The key cellular correlate to draw here is the separation of homologous chromosomes during anaphase I of meiosis. By separating—segregating—these chromosomes into different cells, each gamete carries only one allele for any given trait.

Mendel's Second Law: Law of Independent Assortment

Mendel's second law (**of independent assortment**) states that the inheritance of one gene does not affect the inheritance of another gene. Remember from Chapter 2 of *MCAT Biology Review* that spermatogonia and oogonia undergo genome replication before meiosis I. The daughter DNA strand is held to the parent strand at the **centromere**. Together, these DNA strands are known as **sister chromatids**. During prophase I of meiosis, homologous chromosomes pair up to form **tetrads**, which derive their name from the four chromatids involved (two chromatids in each of two homologous chromosomes). Small segments of genetic material are swapped between chromatids in homologous chromosomes (**crossing over**), resulting in novel combinations of alleles that were not present in the original chromosomes (**recombination**). This contributes to genetic diversity by shuffling alleles on the same chromosome, while Mendel's second law of independent assortment describes the random segregation of entire homologous chromosomes into gametes.

Mendel's second law has been complicated by the discovery of linked genes. We will discuss nonindependent assortment and linkage later in this chapter in the section on analytical approaches in genetics.

Both segregation of homologous chromosomes and independent assortment of alleles increase the genetic diversity of gametes and, subsequently, the genetic diversity of offspring. This has been demonstrated to improve the ability of a species to evolve and adapt to environmental stresses.

KEY CONCEPT

Segregation of chromosomes and independent assortment of alleles allow for greater genetic diversity in the offspring.

DNA as Genetic Material

While Mendel noticed there were certain patterns of inheritance, what he did not know was that DNA was the genetic material transferred to offspring and that genes were made of DNA. In fact, the scientific community rejected Mendel's initial papers on inheritance. It wasn't until the early 1900s that his work was rediscovered. In the early to mid-1900s, it was largely believed that protein was the heritable material. In the mid-1900s, there were three experiments conducted that largely pointed to DNA's role in genetic inheritance.

In the 1920s, Frederick Griffith was a scientist working for the British government, studying *Streptococcus pneumoniae*, a bacteria that causes pneumonia. Two strains of *S. pneumoniae* were identified: a virulent (disease-causing) strain and a nonvirulent strain. In successive trials, Griffith exposed mice to these strains of bacteria under different conditions and observed whether the mice lived or died, as shown in Figure 12.6. The virulent *S. pneumonia* has a smooth capsule that helps the bacterium evade the immune system and cause disease. He injected this strain into mice, which resulted in death of the mice. Naturally, if the virulent bacteria were killed prior to injection, no disease resulted. Likewise, exposure of the mice to the nonvirulent strain, which has a rough capsule, did not cause disease. However, when both dead virulent bacteria and live nonvirulent bacteria were injected into the mouse, the mouse died and live bacteria with smooth capsules could be found in the mice. He theorized that the live, nonvirulent bacteria must have acquired the ability to form smooth capsules from the dead virulent bacteria. This was known as the *transforming principle*.

BRIDGE

The transforming principle described in Griffith's experiment is the same as bacterial transformation discussed in Chapter 1 of *MCAT Biology Review*. Remember that transformation is one of three main ways bacteria increase genetic variability; the other two are conjugation and transduction.

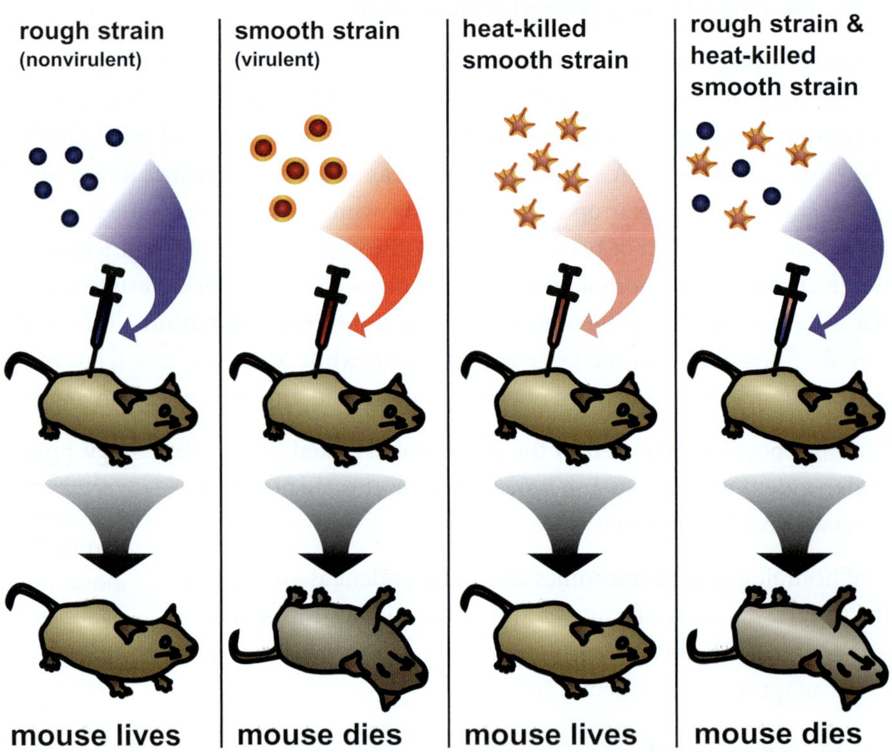

Figure 12.6 The Griffith Experiment

Researchers at the Rockefeller Institute confirmed the transformation principle. Three American scientists—Oswald Avery, Colin MacLeod, and Maclyn McCarty—were attempting to identify the exact material underlying the transformation principle. These scientists purified a very large quantity of heat-killed virulent *S. pneumoniae* bacteria and separated the subcellular components of the bacteria into different extracts. It was noted that the addition of one particular extract to nonvirulent *S. pneumoniae* transformed the bacteria and enabled them to kill the mouse when injected. When this substance was treated with enzymes known to degrade DNA, the bacteria were not transformed and the mice lived. However, when the substance was treated with enzymes known to degrade proteins, the bacteria were still transformed and the mice died. Thus, the group concluded that the transforming substance must be DNA.

In 1952 (one year before the description of the Watson–Crick model), Alfred Hershey and Martha Chase worked to confirm the idea that DNA could independently carry genetic information via the process depicted in Figure 12.7. These scientists created bacteriophages with radiolabeled DNA and protein. One group of bacteriophages contained radiolabeled sulfur, which is found in protein but not in DNA. Another group contained radiolabeled phosphorus, which is found in DNA but not in protein. Each of these bacteriophages was permitted to infect a group of nonlabeled bacteria. Recall from Chapter 1 of *MCAT Biology Review* that when bacteriophages infect a bacterium, they inject their genetic material into the cell and leave their capsid outside. After the phages and bacteria were incubated, the sample was centrifuged to separate the material that remained outside the cell from the bacterial cells themselves. It was determined that while no radiolabeled sulfur (protein) entered the cells, radiolabeled phosphorus (DNA) had. It was known that viruses must enter a cell to cause disease and replicate, so this experiment once again helped confirm that DNA was the heritable genetic material.

BRIDGE

Radiolabeling sulfur was an appropriate choice to tag proteins in the Hershey–Chase experiment. Recall from Chapter 1 of *MCAT Biochemistry Review* that two amino acids—cysteine and methionine—contain sulfur in their R group, while no nucleotides contain any sulfur.

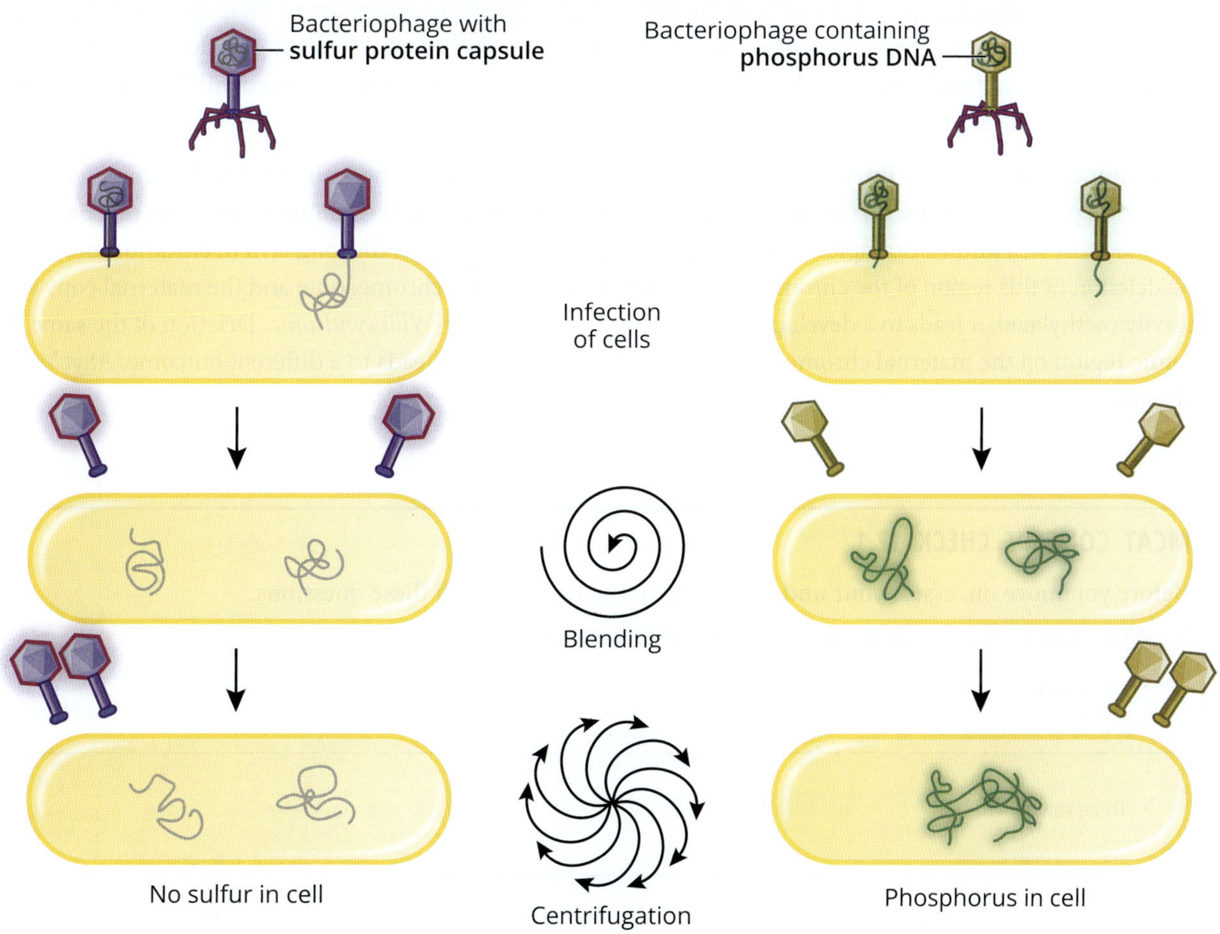

Figure 12.7 The Hershey-Chase Experiment

Epigenetics

Epigenetics is a general term for changes in DNA that do not involve an alteration to the nucleotide sequence. The prefix *epi–* is Greek for "over" or "above," so the name suggests regulatory mechanisms that are in addition to the traditional features of inheritance. Epigenetic modifications can include the covalent attachment of different chemical groups to nucleotides and histone proteins, including but not limited to methylation or acetylation. These modifications can be temporary and function to increase or decrease the expression of specific genes. In general, modifications like methylation of DNA promoter regions tends to decrease the expression of specific genes, whereas modifications of lysines and/or arginines on histones have variable effects on the expression of genes.

Because almost all cells in the body contain the same genetic code, epigenetics allows cells to undergo differentiation, where different cells are able to express certain genes while silencing others. One prominent example of this is X-inactivation in cells that have two X chromosomes, in which one of the two X chromosomes is transcriptionally silenced via methylation; the inactive X chromosome is called a **Barr body**.

BRIDGE

Methylation of DNA is commonly used for transcriptional regulation. Recall from Chapter 7 of the *MCAT Biochemistry Review* that the addition of methyl groups to adenine and cytosine is linked to gene silencing.

Epigenetic changes can have significant clinical impact. Hypermethylation of tumor suppressor genes and hypomethylation of oncogenes have been implicated in some forms of cancer. Furthermore, studies have shown that epigenetic changes can be a mechanism by which organisms' responses to their changing environment can be passed down to their progeny. Indeed, the Överkalix study found that the grandchildren of those who had experienced food scarcity had different health outcomes compared to the grandchildren of those who had not experienced famine.

Another important concept is **imprinting**, an epigenetic process in which gene expression is determined by the contributing parent. There are certain genes that are differentially methylated when inherited from one parent; one of the most well known examples of imprinting comes from a region on the long arm of chromosome 15. If the deletion of this region of the chromosome occurs on the paternal chromosome and the maternal copy is heavily methylated, it leads to a developmental disorder called *Prader-Willi syndrome*. Deletion of the same genomic region on the maternal chromosome and paternal methylation leads to a different outcome, *Angelman syndrome*.

MCAT CONCEPT CHECK 12.1

Before you move on, assess your understanding of the material with these questions.

1. What does it mean for an allele to be dominant? Recessive?
   - Dominant:

   ____

   - Recessive:

   ____

2. What does it mean for a genotype to be homozygous? Heterozygous? Hemizygous?
    - Homozygous:

    ____

    - Heterozygous:

    ____

    - Hemizygous:

    ____

3. What is the difference between complete dominance, codominance, and incomplete dominance?
    - Complete dominance:

    ____

    - Codominance:

    ____

    - Incomplete dominance:

    ____

4. What is the difference between penetrance and expressivity?
    - Penetrance:

    ____

    - Expressivity:

    ____

5. With which phase of meiosis does each of Mendel's laws most closely correlate?
    - Mendel's first law:

    ____

    - Mendel's second law:

    ____

12.2 Changes in the Gene Pool

LEARNING OBJECTIVES

After Chapter 12.2, you will be able to:

- Identify the three main types of point mutations and the genetic changes they are associated with
- Recall the two main types of frameshift mutation
- Explain why genetic leakage would increase within the last century
- Describe the relationship between genetic drift, small population, and the founder effect
- Identify the main types of chromosomal mutation and the impact they have at the chromosomal level:

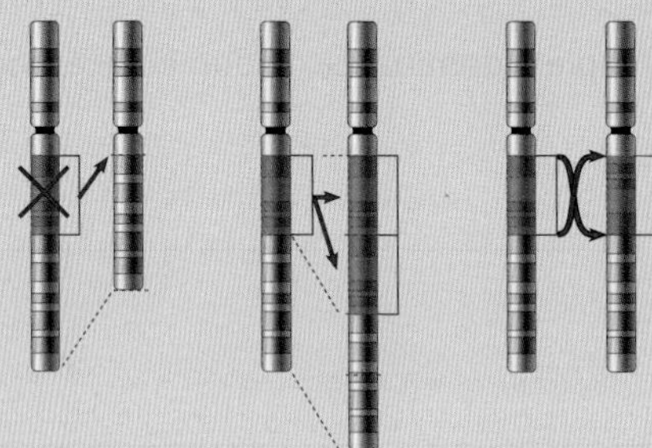

All of the alleles that exist within a species are known as the **gene pool**. When mutations or genetic leakage occur, new genes are introduced into the gene pool. Genetic variability is essential for the survival of a species because it allows it to evolve to adapt to changing environmental stresses. Certain traits may be more desirable than others and confer a selective advantage that allows for an individual to produce more viable, fertile offspring. In this section, we will consider genetic diversity and mutations, leakage, and genetic drift, which cause changes to the alleles or their frequency in the gene pool.

Mutations

A **mutation** is a change in DNA sequence, and it results in a mutant allele. Mutant alleles can be contrasted with their **wild-type** counterparts, which are alleles that are considered "normal" or "natural" and are ubiquitous in the study population. New mutations may be introduced in a variety of ways. Ionizing radiation, such as ultraviolet rays from the sun, and chemical exposures can damage DNA; substances that can cause mutations are called **mutagens**. *DNA polymerase* is subject to making mistakes during DNA replication, albeit at a very low rate; proofreading mechanisms help prevent mutations from occurring through this mechanism. Elements known as **transposons** can insert and remove themselves from the genome. If a transposon inserts in the middle of a coding sequence, the mutation will disrupt the gene.

Flawed proteins can arise in other ways without an underlying change in DNA sequence. Incorrect pairing of nucleotides during transcription or translation, or a tRNA molecule charged with the incorrect amino acid for its anticodon, can result in derangements of the normal amino acid sequence.

The major types of nucleotide-level mutations are discussed in great detail in Chapter 7 of *MCAT Biochemistry Review*, so we offer just a brief overview here of each type.

Nucleotide-Level Mutations

Many mutations occur at the level of a single nucleotide (or a very small number of nucleotides). These mutations are shown in Figure 12.8 and are summarized below.

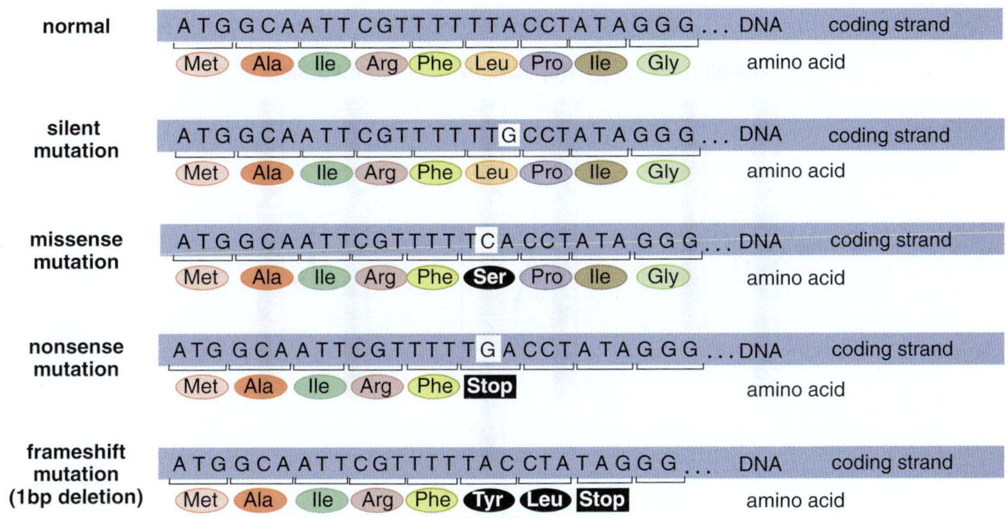

Figure 12.8 Common Nucleotide-Level Mutations

Point mutations occur when one nucleotide in DNA (A, C, T, or G) is swapped for another. These can be subcategorized as silent, missense, or nonsense mutations:

- **Silent mutations** occur when the change in nucleotide has no effect on the final protein synthesized from the gene. This most commonly occurs when the changed nucleotide is transcribed to be the third nucleotide in a codon because there is **degeneracy** (**wobble**) in the genetic code.
- **Missense mutations** occur when the change in nucleotide results in substituting one amino acid for another in the final protein.
- **Nonsense mutations** occur when the change in nucleotide results in substituting a **stop codon** for an amino acid in the final protein.

Frameshift mutations occur when nucleotides are inserted into or deleted from the genome. Because mRNA transcribed from DNA is always read in three-letter sequences called **codons**, insertion or deletion of nucleotides can shift the **reading frame**, usually resulting in either changes in the amino acid sequence or premature truncation of the protein (due to the generation of a nonsense mutation). These can be subcategorized as **insertion** or **deletion mutations**.

Chromosomal Mutations

Chromosomal mutations are larger-scale mutations in which large segments of DNA are affected, as demonstrated in Figure 12.9 and summarized below.

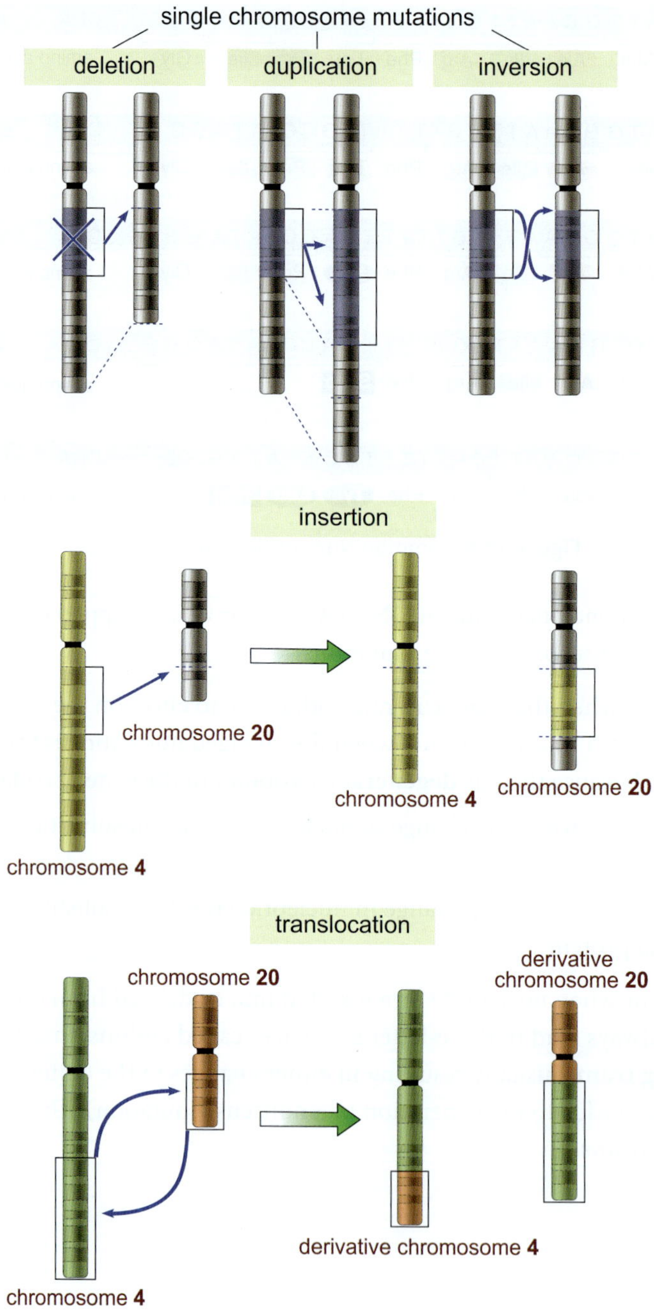

Figure 12.9 Common Chromosomal Mutations

- **Deletion mutations** occur when a large segment of DNA is lost from a chromosome. Small deletion mutations are considered frameshift mutations, as described previously.
- **Duplication mutations** occur when a segment of DNA is copied multiple times in the genome.
- **Inversion mutations** occur when a segment of DNA is reversed within the chromosome.
- **Insertion mutations** occur when a segment of DNA is moved from one chromosome to another. Small insertion mutations (including those where the inserted DNA is not from another chromosome) are considered frameshift mutations, as described previously.
- **Translocation mutations** occur when a segment of DNA from one chromosome is swapped with a segment of DNA from another chromosome.

Consequences of Mutations

Mutations can have many different consequences. Some mutations can be **advantageous**, conferring a positive selective advantage that may allow the organism to produce fitter offspring. For example, sickle cell disease is a single nucleotide mutation that causes sickled hemoglobin. While the disease itself is detrimental to life, heterozygotes for sickle cell disease usually have minor symptoms, if any, and have natural resistance to malaria because their red blood cells have a slightly shorter lifespan—just short enough that the parasitic *Plasmodium* species that causes malaria cannot reproduce in them. Thus, heterozygotes for sickle cell disease have a selective advantage because they are less likely to die from malaria. This advantage is more common in African regions with high malaria prevalence, as can be seen in maps such as Figure 12.10.

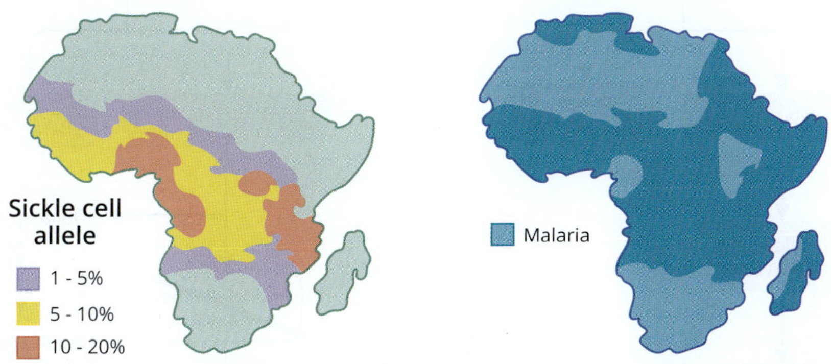

Figure 12.10 Geographical Correlation between Prevalence of Malaria and Prevalence of Sickle Cell Alleles

On the other hand, some mutations can be detrimental or **deleterious**. For example, *xeroderma pigmentosum* (XP) is an inherited defect in the nucleotide excision repair mechanism. In patients with XP, DNA that has been damaged by ultraviolet radiation cannot be repaired appropriately. Ultraviolet radiation can introduce cancer-causing mutations; since they lack a repair mechanism, patients with XP are frequently diagnosed with malignancies, especially of the skin.

One important class of deleterious mutations is known as **inborn errors of metabolism**. These are deficiencies in genes required for metabolism. Children born with these deficient genes often require very early intervention in order to prevent permanent damage from the buildup of metabolites in various pathways. For example, in *phenylketonuria* (PKU), the enzyme *phenylalanine hydrolase*, which completes the metabolism of the amino acid phenylalanine, is defective (see Figure 12.11). In the absence of this enzyme, toxic metabolites of phenylalanine accumulate, causing seizures, impairment of cerebral function, and learning disabilities, as well as a musty odor to bodily secretions. However, if the disease is discovered shortly after birth, then dietary phenylalanine can be eliminated by avoiding foods like meat, eggs, dairy products, and soft drinks. Diet change is the first line of defense for the individual, but there are treatments that can be administered to aid in metabolizing any remaining phenylalanine.

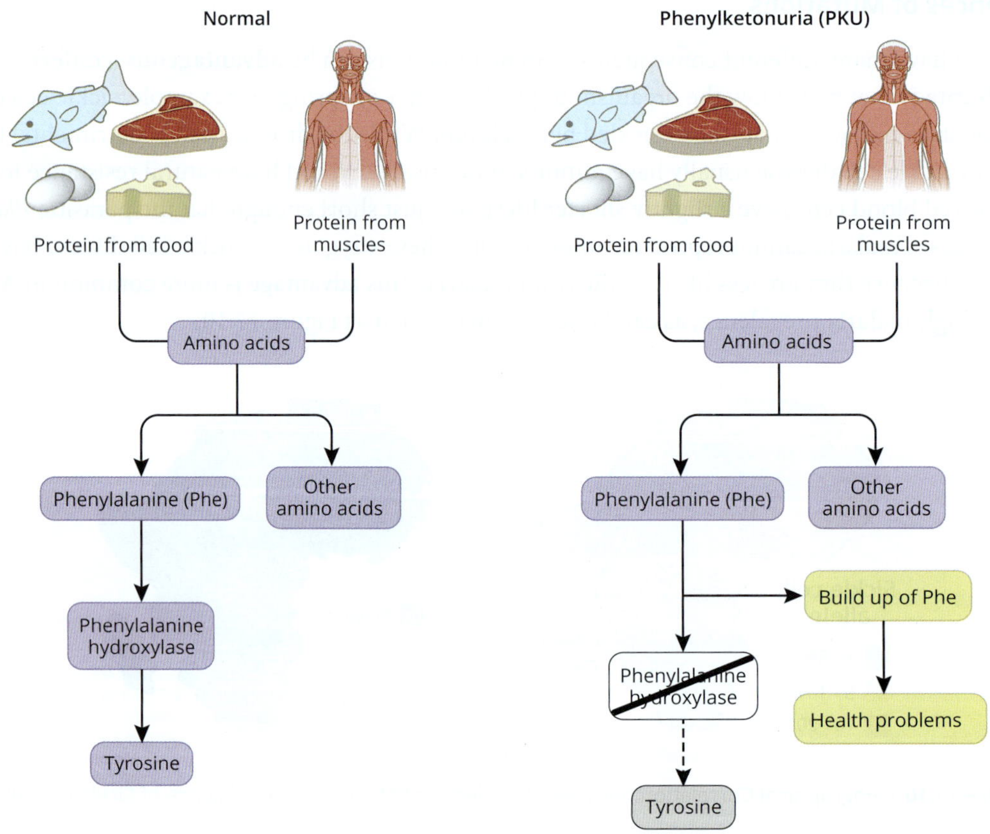

Figure 12.11 Phenylketonuria (PKU) Pathway

Leakage

Genetic **leakage** is a flow of genes between species. In some cases, individuals from different (but closely related) species can mate to produce **hybrid** offspring. Many hybrid offspring, such as the mule (hybrid of a male horse and a female donkey), are not able to reproduce because they have odd numbers of chromosomes—horses have 64 chromosomes and donkeys have 62, so mules, with 63 chromosomes, cannot undergo normal homologous pairing in meiosis and cannot form gametes. In some cases, however, a hybrid can reproduce with members of one species or the other, such as the *beefalo* (a cross between cattle and American bison). The hybrid carries genes from both parent species, so this can result in a net flow of genes from one species to the other.

Genetic Drift

Genetic drift refers to changes in the composition of the gene pool due to chance. Genetic drift tends to be more pronounced in small populations. The **founder effect** is a more extreme case of genetic drift in which a small population of a species finds itself in reproductive isolation from other populations as a result of natural barriers, catastrophic events, or other **bottlenecks** that drastically and suddenly reduce the size of the population available for breeding. Both the founder effect and bottlenecks are depicted in Figure 12.12. Because the breeding group is small, **inbreeding**, or mating between two genetically related individuals, may occur in later generations. Inbreeding encourages homozygosity, which increases the prevalence of both homozygous dominant and recessive genotypes. Ultimately, genetic drift, the founder effect, and inbreeding cause a reduction in genetic diversity, which is often the reason why a small population may have increased prevalence of certain traits and diseases. For example, *branched-chain ketoacid dehydrogenase deficiency* (*maple syrup urine disease*), which causes sweet-smelling urine, sweat, and earwax and poor feeding, is especially common in Mennonite communities; this implies a common origin of the mutation, which may have been in a very small original population.

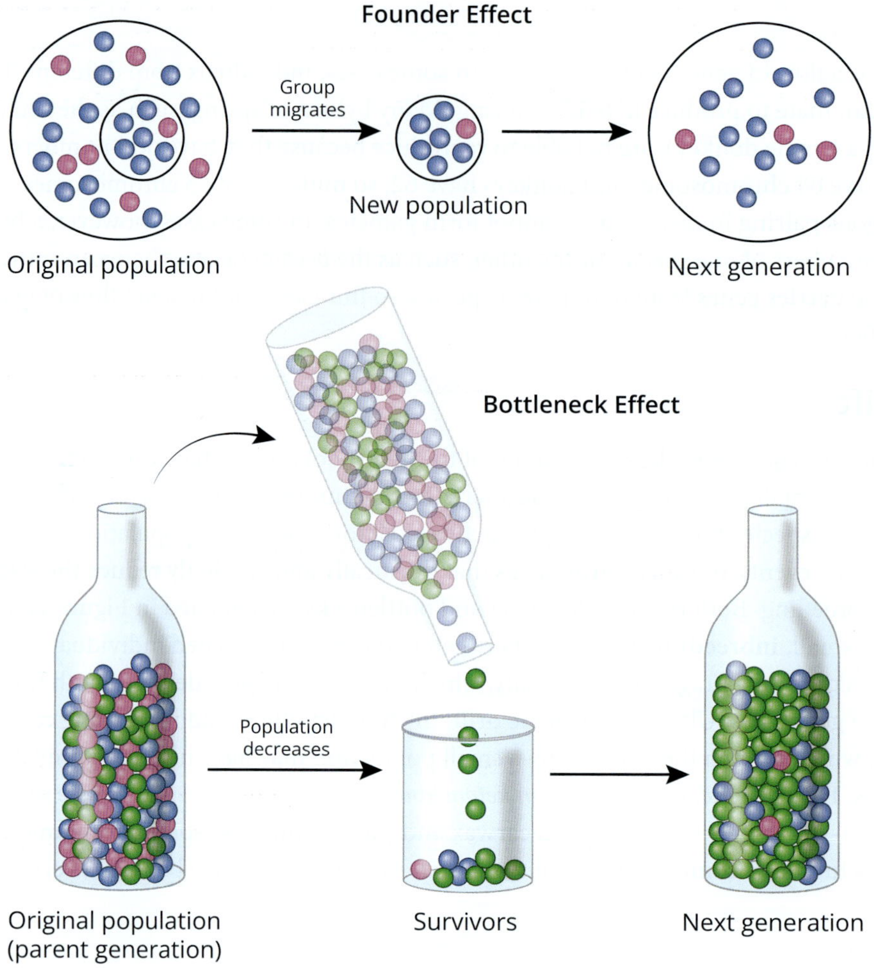

Figure 12.12 The Founder Effect and Bottlenecks

This loss of genetic variation may cause reduced fitness of the population, a condition known as **inbreeding depression**. On the opposite end of the spectrum, **outbreeding** or **outcrossing** is the introduction of unrelated individuals into a breeding group. Theoretically, this could result in increased variation within a gene pool and increased fitness of the population.

MCAT CONCEPT CHECK 12.2

Before you move on, assess your understanding of the material with these questions.

1. What are the three main types of point mutations? What change occurs in each?
   -
   -
   -
2. What are the two main types of frameshift mutations?
   -
   -
3. What are the three main types of chromosomal mutations that do NOT share their name with a type of frameshift mutation? What change occurs in each?
   -
   -
   -
4. Why would genetic leakage in animals be rare prior to the last century?
5. Why is genetic drift more common in small populations? What relationship does this have to the founder effect?

12.3 Analytical Approaches in Genetics

LEARNING OBJECTIVES

After Chapter 12.3, you will be able to:

- Predict the phenotype ratio in the offspring of a cross, such as AaBB × AAbb
- Order genes on a chromosome given their recombination frequencies
- Recall the five criteria of the Hardy–Weinberg principle and the underlying population characteristic each one implies
- Solve calculation problems requiring use of the Hardy–Weinberg equations: $p + q = 1$, and $p^2 + 2pq + q^2 = 1$

Genetics is a field in which a number of **biometric techniques**, or quantitative approaches to biological data, have been developed. These range from pedigrees and the Punnett square to mapping of chromosomes with recombinant frequencies to Hardy–Weinberg equilibrium.

Pedigrees

Pedigree charts are diagrams that show relationships between people within families and indicate the presence or absence of a trait of interest. On the MCAT, only a basic understanding of pedigree charts is required: squares represent biological males, circles represent biological females, empty shapes represent the absence of a trait, and colored-in shapes represent the presence of a trait. Figure 12.13 shows an example of a pedigree chart showing three generations of a family (A, B, and C). In generation A, an unaffected male (A1) and female (A2) had two unaffected children (B1 and B2), while a female with albinism (A3) had two unaffected children (B3 and B4) with an unaffected male (A4). In generation C, two of the three children (C1 and C2) of B2 and B3 also had albinism, while the third female child (C3) was unaffected.

MCAT EXPERTISE

The MCAT will only test a fundamental understanding of how to read pedigree charts. The symbology of pedigree analysis is complex and intricate, and beyond the scope of the MCAT.

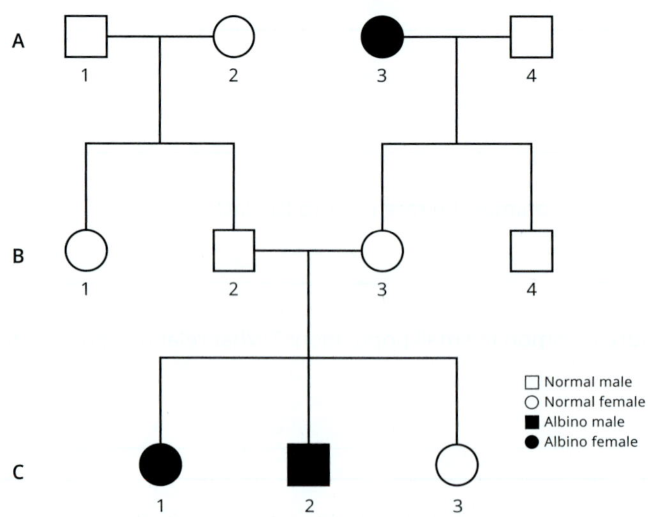

Figure 12.13 Example of a Pedigree Chart
The black square represents a male with albinism, while the black circles represent females with albinism.

Commonly, these types of charts are used to help determine the inheritance pattern of the trait of interest by looking at its inheritance pattern among family generations. The types of inheritance patterns most commonly tested on the MCAT include autosomal dominant, autosomal recessive, X-linked recessive, mitochondrial, and Y-linked.

In an **autosomal dominant** pattern of inheritance, the trait is encoded by a dominant gene on an autosomal chromosome. A tell-tale sign of an autosomal dominant pattern of inheritance is the trait never skips a generation: In other words, an affected child must have at least one affected parent, as demonstrated in Figure 12.14. However, affected parents can have unaffected children if the affected parent is heterozygous and carries one allele that codes for the trait and one allele that does not. Therefore, another indication a pedigree is showing an autosomal dominant pattern of inheritance is two affected parents having an unaffected child.

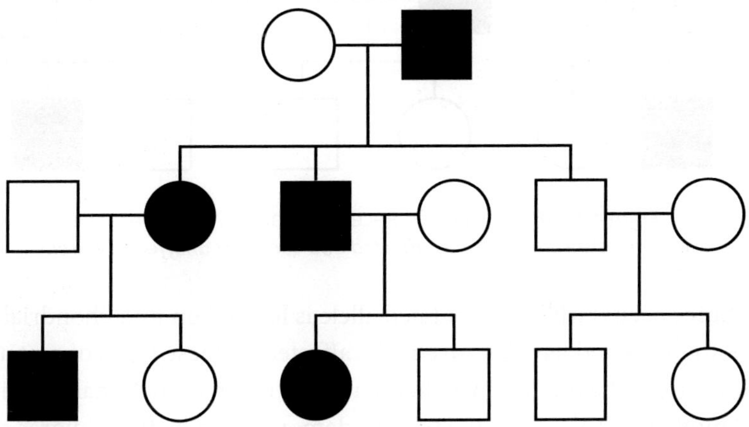

Figure 12.14 An Autosomal Dominant Pattern of Inheritance

In contrast, a pedigree like the ones shown in Figures 12.15 and 12.16, where unaffected individuals have affected children, is indicative of a trait encoded by a recessive allele. In an **autosomal recessive** pattern of inheritance, where the trait is only expressed if an individual has two copies of the recessive allele, both males and females are equally likely to have the trait. Another indication of a recessive trait is when two affected parents only have affected children.

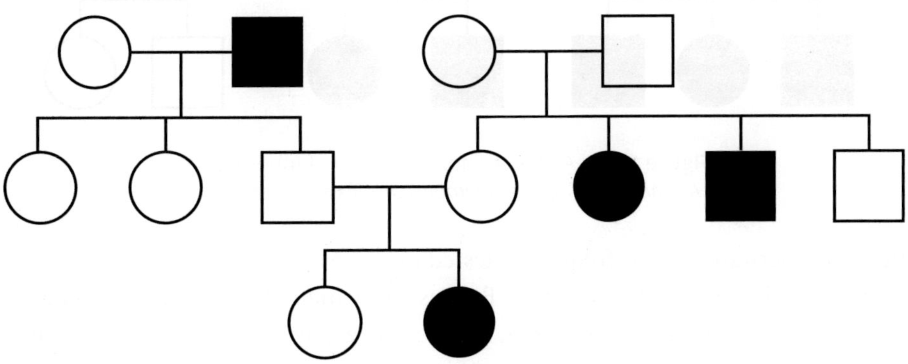

Figure 12.15 An Autosomal Recessive Pattern of Inheritance
Multiple affected members of this family have unaffected parents, suggesting autosomal recessive inheritance.

In an **X-linked recessive** pattern of inheritance, where the trait is encoded by a gene located on the X chromosome, males are disproportionately affected. This is due to the fact that males have only one copy of the X chromosome, while females have two and require both genes to be affected to express the trait. X-linked recessive and autosomal recessive patterns of inheritance can look similar, but there are certain indicators that can favor one inheritance pattern over the other. For example, in X-linked recessive patterns of inheritance, all male children of an affected female will express the trait.

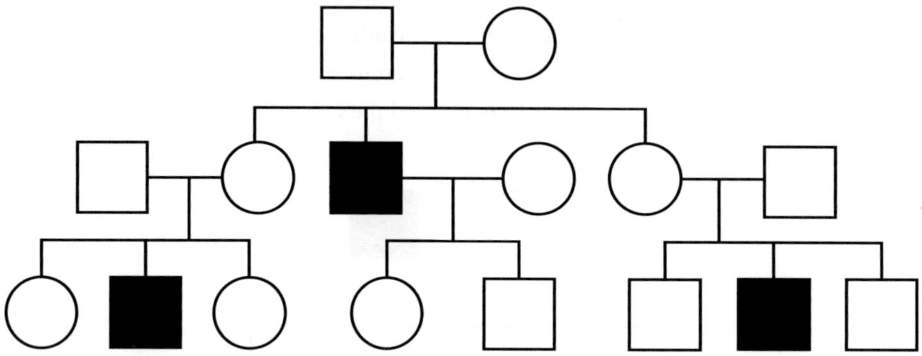

Figure 12.16 An X-Linked Recessive Pattern of Inheritance
Males are disproportionately affected and can have unaffected parents.

Mitochondrial inheritance occurs when the mutated allele is located on mitochondrial DNA rather than nuclear DNA. While both males and females are equally affected by these types of mutations, mitochondrial DNA is only passed down from the mother in a phenomenon known as maternal inheritance. Therefore, all children of an affected mother will also have the trait, as demonstrated by the pedigree shown in Figure 12.17. On the flip side, no child of an affected male and unaffected female will inherit the trait.

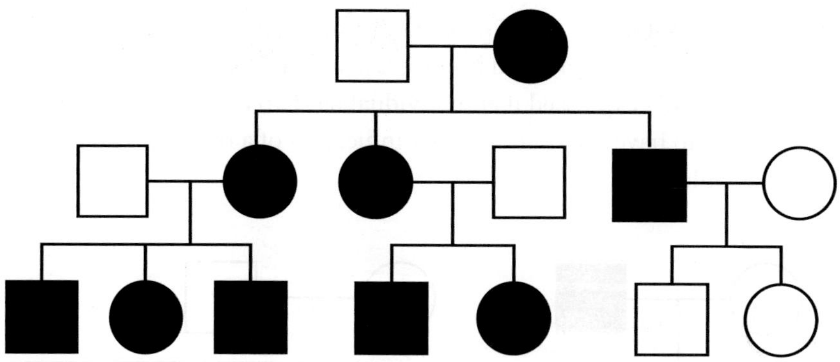

Figure 12.17 A Mitochondrial Pattern of Inheritance
All children of affected females also express the trait.

A **Y-linked** pattern of inheritance is less frequently tested on the MCAT, but refers to an inheritance pattern where a trait is carried on the Y chromosome. Because only males have Y chromosomes, only males are affected and females are unable to pass on the trait. Furthermore, any son of any affected male will also be affected.

Punnett Squares

Punnett squares are diagrams that predict the relative genotypic and phenotypic frequencies that will result from the crossing of two individuals. The alleles of the two parents are arranged on the top and side of the square, with the genotypes of the progeny represented at the intersections of these alleles. The genotypes of the progeny will be the product of the two parental alleles.

Monohybrid Cross

In genetics problems, including those on the MCAT, dominant alleles are assigned capital letters and recessive alleles are assigned lowercase letters. If both copies of the allele are the same, that individual is said to be homozygous; if they are different, the individual is heterozygous.

A cross in which only one trait is being studied is said to be **monohybrid**. The **parent** or **P generation** refers to the individuals being crossed; the offspring are the **filial** or **F generation**. Multiple generations can be denoted F generations by using numeric subscripts. If you think of your grandparents as the P generation, then your parents are in the F_1 generation, and you are in the F_2 generation.

Mendel worked with pea plants that had either purple or white flowers. Before crossing the different plants, each group contained homozygotes; subsequent experimentation revealed that the allele for purple color was dominant (P) and the allele for white color was recessive (p). Thus, crossing a homozygous purple flower with a white flower would be crossing PP with pp, resulting in an F_1 generation that contained 100 percent Pp or heterozygotes, as shown in Figure 12.18. All of the flowers in this generation would be purple because P is a dominant allele.

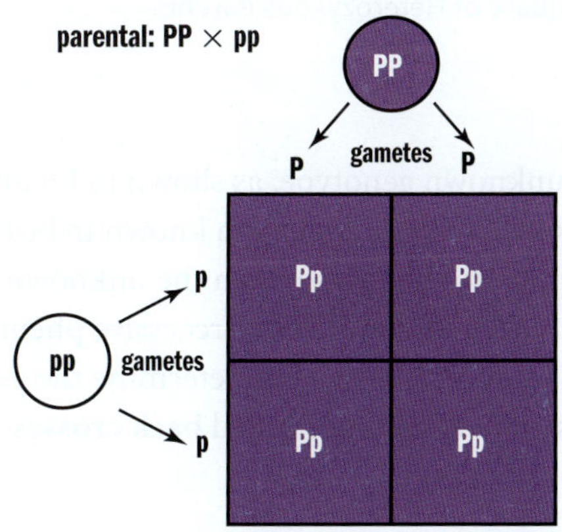

F_1 genotypic ratio: 100% Pp (heterozygous)

F_1 phenotypic ratio: 100% purple

Figure 12.18 Punnett Square of Homozygous Parents

If two members of the F_1 generation were crossed, the resulting offspring in the F_2 generation would be more genotypically and phenotypically diverse than their parents. Crossing two plants with the genotype Pp would result in 25 percent PP, 50 percent Pp, and 25 percent pp offspring, as shown in Figure 12.19. Phenotypically, this would be a 3:1 distribution because both the homozygous dominant and heterozygous dominant offspring would be purple-flowering plants. Thus, crossing two heterozygotes in a case of complete dominance will

KEY CONCEPT

Crossing two heterozygotes for a trait with complete dominance results in a 1:2:1 ratio of genotypes and a 3:1 ratio of phenotypes. Know these ratios cold for Test Day!

result in a 1:2:1 distribution of genotypes (homozygous dominant:heterozygous dominant:homozygous recessive) and a 3:1 distribution of phenotypes (dominant:recessive). These ratios are, of course, theoretical probabilities and will not always hold true—especially in a small population of offspring. Usually, the more offspring parents have, the closer their phenotypic ratios will be to the expected ratios.

MCAT EXPERTISE

The ability to create and read a Punnett square quickly on Test Day is one of the most useful skills for questions involving Mendelian inheritance. Often, an entire passage in the *Biological and Biochemical Foundations of Living Systems* section will be devoted to classical and molecular genetics and will require the use of at least one Punnett square.

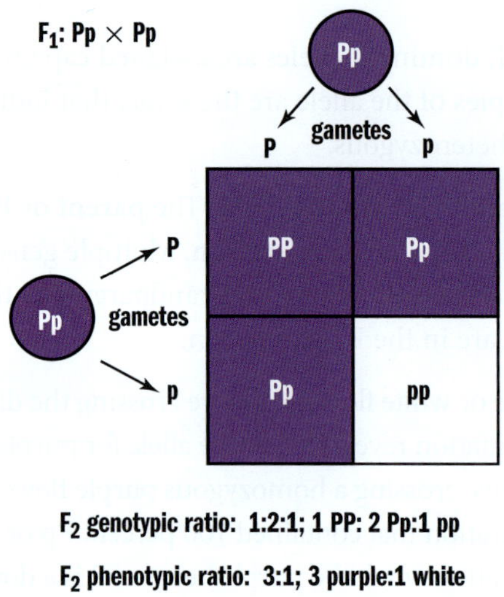

Figure 12.19 Punnett Square of Heterozygous Parents

Test Cross

A **test cross** is used to determine an unknown genotype, as shown in Figure 12.20. In a test cross, the organism with an unknown genotype is crossed with an organism known to be homozygous recessive. If all of the offspring (100 percent) are of the dominant phenotype, then the unknown genotype is likely to be homozygous dominant. If there is a 1:1 distribution of dominant to recessive phenotypes, then the unknown genotype is likely to be heterozygous. Because a test cross is used to determine the genotype of the parent based on the phenotypes of its offspring, test crosses are sometimes called **back crosses**.

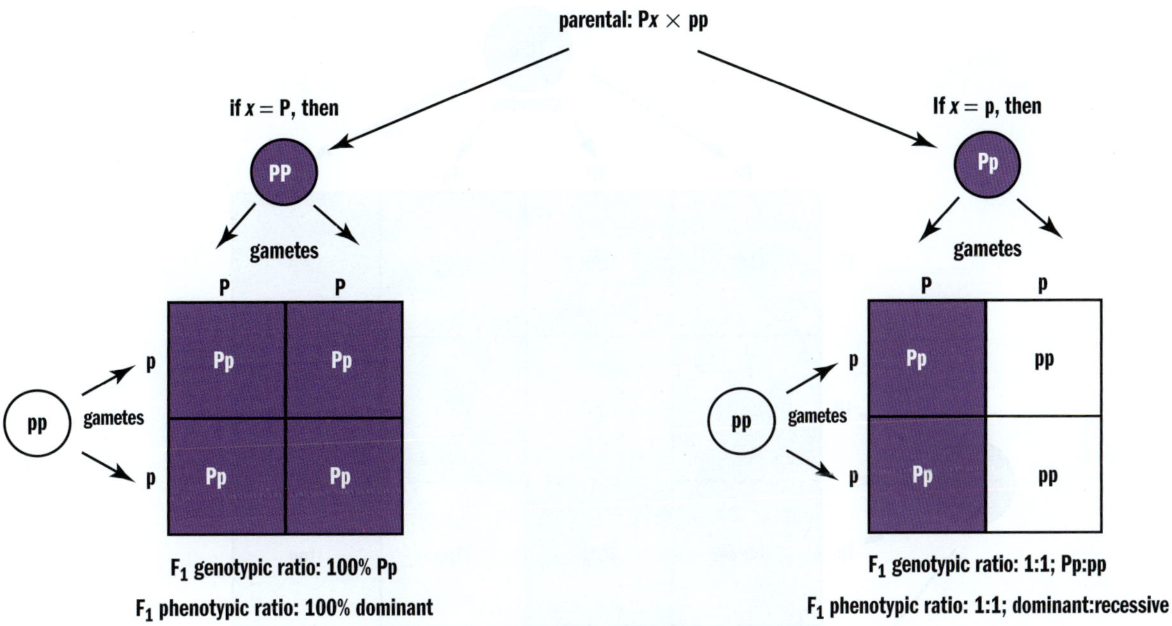

Figure 12.20 Test Cross
An organism with an unknown genotype is crossed with a homozygous recessive organism to identify the unknown genotype using the phenotypes of the resulting offspring.

Dihybrid Cross

We can extend a Punnett square to account for the inheritance of two different genes using a **dihybrid cross**. Remember, according to Mendel's second law (of independent assortment) the inheritance of one gene is independent of the inheritance of the other. This will hold true for **unlinked genes**, although it will be more complicated for linked genes, as described later in this chapter.

If we expand the previous crosses to consider not only flower color, but also plant height, then we can create a 4 × 4 Punnett square as shown in Figure 12.21. Remember that purple is dominant (P) and white is recessive (p); similarly, tall is dominant (T) and short or dwarf is recessive (t). If we cross two plants that are heterozygous for both traits, then the offspring have a phenotypic ratio of 9:3:3:1 (9 tall and purple:3 tall and white:3 dwarf and purple:1 dwarf and white). Note that the 3:1 phenotypic ratio still holds for each trait (12 tall:4 dwarf and 12 purple:4 white), reflecting Mendel's second law.

MCAT EXPERTISE

Just as with the 3:1 phenotypic ratio of a monohybrid cross, it is worth memorizing the 9:3:3:1 distribution for dihybrid crosses between two heterozygotes with complete dominance.

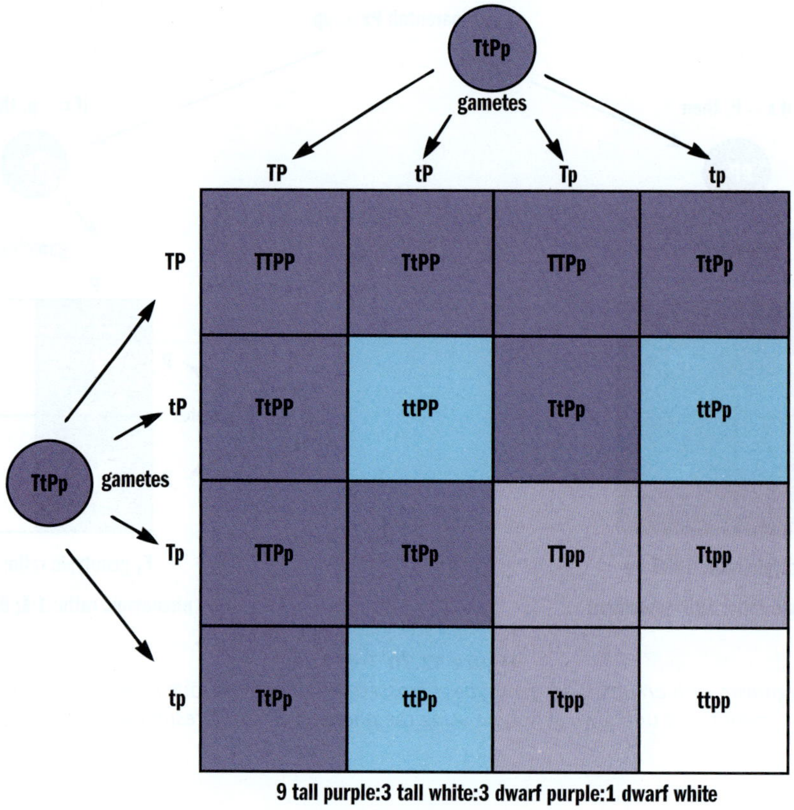

Figure 12.21 Dihybrid Cross

Sex-Linked Crosses

When considering **sex-linked (X-linked) traits**, a slightly different system is used to symbolize the various alleles because genotypical females have two X chromosomes and thus may be homozygous or heterozygous for a condition carried on the X chromosome. Genotypical males have only one X chromosome (and one Y chromosome) and are hemizygous for many genes carried on the X chromosome. This is why sex-linked traits are much more common in genotypical males; having only one recessive allele is sufficient for expression of the recessive phenotype.

When writing genotypes for sex-linked traits, we use X and Y to symbolize normal X and Y chromosomes. An X chromosome carrying a defective allele is commonly given a subscript, such as X_h, to indicate the presence of the disease-carrying allele. Hemophilia is a particularly common example of a sex-linked trait; Punnett squares for a heterozygous (**carrier**) female and both an unaffected (normal) male and affected (hemophiliac) male are shown in Figure 12.22.

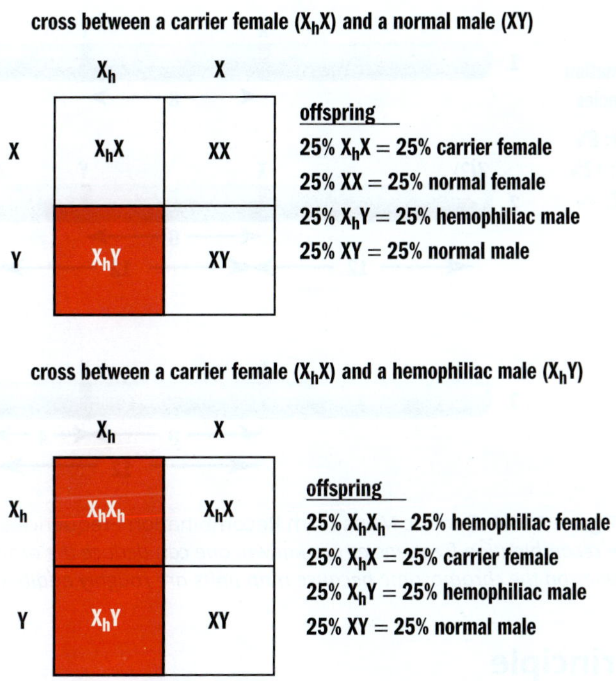

Figure 12.22 Sex-Linked Cross
Unless stated otherwise, assume that all sex-linked traits on the MCAT are X-linked recessive.

KEY CONCEPT

Because an egg necessarily carries an X chromosome, the sperm determines the chromosomal or genotypical sex of a child. It follows that, for genotypical males with a sex-linked trait, genotypically female offspring will either carry the trait or express it, but genotypically male offspring will do neither (unless the X chromosome in the egg contains the affected allele, in which case they will express it).

Gene Mapping

Genes are organized in a linear fashion on chromosomes. As discussed earlier, crossing over during prophase I of meiosis causes alleles to be swapped between homologous chromosomes, supporting Mendel's second law (of independent assortment). However, genes that are located very close together on a chromosome are less likely to be separated from each other during crossing over. In other words, the further apart two genes are, the more likely it is that there will be a point of crossing over, called a **chiasma**, between them. The likelihood that two alleles are separated from each other during crossing over, called the **recombination frequency** (θ), is roughly proportional to the distance between the genes on the chromosome. We can also describe the strength of linkage between genes based on the recombination frequency: tightly linked genes have recombination frequencies close to 0 percent; weakly linked genes have recombination frequencies approaching 50 percent, as expected from independent assortment.

By analyzing recombination frequencies, a **genetic map** representing the relative distance between genes on a chromosome can be constructed. By convention, one **map unit** or **centimorgan** corresponds to a 1 percent chance of recombination occurring between two genes. Thus, if two genes were 25 map units apart, we would expect 25 percent of the total gametes examined to show recombination somewhere between these two genes. Recombination frequencies can be added in a crude approximation to determine the order of genes in the chromosome, as shown in Figure 12.23.

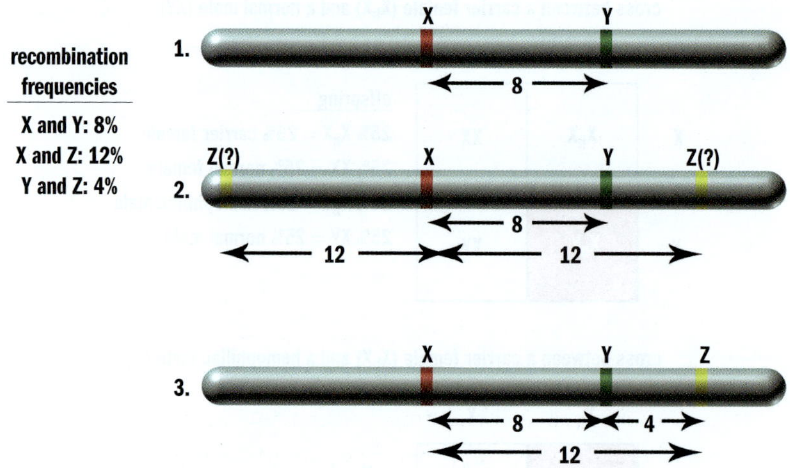

Figure 12.23 Genetic Maps from Recombination Frequencies
If the recombination frequencies are known, one can deduce the order of genes on the chromosome because map units are roughly additive.

Hardy–Weinberg Principle

How often an allele appears in a population is known as its **allele frequency**. For example, if we took a one-cell sample from 50 of Mendel's plants, we could collect 100 copies of alleles for flower color (two from each cell). If 75 of these alleles were the dominant allele, we could say that the allele frequency of P is $75 \div 100 = 0.75$. Note that this does not indicate which flowers contain the allele or if those flowers are homozygous or heterozygous; it only tells us the representation of the allele across all chromosomes in the population. Evolution results from changes in these gene frequencies in reproducing populations over time. However, when the gene frequencies of a population are not changing, the gene pool is stable and evolution is ostensibly *not* occurring. The following five criteria are mandatory for this to be possible:

- The population is very large (no genetic drift).
- There are no mutations that affect the gene pool.
- Mating between individuals in the population is random (no sexual selection).
- There is no migration of individuals into or out of the population.
- The genes in the population are all equally successful at being reproduced.

Provided that all of these conditions are met, the population is said to be in **Hardy–Weinberg equilibrium**, and a pair of equations can be used to predict the allelic and phenotypic frequencies.

Let us define a particular gene as having only two possible alleles, T and t. We will define p to be the frequency of the dominant allele T and q to be the frequency of the recessive allele t. Because there are only these two choices at the same gene locus, $p + q = 1$. That is, the combined allele frequencies of T and t must equal 100 percent. If we square both sides of the equation, we get:

$$(p + q)^2 = 1^2$$

$$p^2 + 2pq + q^2 = 1$$

where p^2 is the frequency of the TT (homozygous dominant) genotype, $2pq$ is the frequency of the Tt (heterozygous dominant) genotype, and q^2 is the frequency of the tt (homozygous recessive) genotype. Note that the sum $p^2 + 2pq$ would represent the frequency of the dominant *phenotype* (both homozygous and heterozygous dominant genotypes).

For Test Day, you should know the two key Hardy–Weinberg equations demonstrated above:

$$p + q = 1$$

$$p^2 + 2pq + q^2 = 1$$

Equation 12.1

Each equation provides us with different information. The first tells us about the frequency of *alleles* in the population, whereas the second provides information about the frequency of *genotypes* and *phenotypes* in the population.

These equations can also be used to demonstrate that evolution is *not* occurring in a population. Assuming that the conditions listed earlier are met, the allele frequencies will remain constant from generation to generation. For example, imagine that we have a population of Mendel's pea plants in which the frequency of the tall allele, T, is 0.80. This value is represented by p. This means that q (the short allele, t) is 0.20 by subtraction. Setting up our F_1 cross for two heterozygotes, we can see the results of such a mating:

	$p = 0.80$ (T = 80%)	$q = 0.20$ (t = 20%)
$p = 0.80$ (T = 80%)	$p^2 = 0.64$ (TT = 64%)	$pq = 0.16$ (Tt = 16%)
$q = 0.20$ (t = 20%)	$pq = 0.16$ (Tt = 16%)	$q^2 = 0.04$ (tt = 4%)

We see that the filial generation contains 64 percent homozygous tall, 32 percent heterozygous tall, and 4 percent homozygous short plants. These are the genotypic frequencies. We can determine the allele frequencies in this generation as follows:

$$\begin{array}{rcl} 64\%\ \text{TT} = 64\%\ \text{T} & \text{and} & 0\%\ \text{t} \\ 32\%\ \text{Tt} = 16\%\ \text{T} & \text{and} & 16\%\ \text{t} \\ 4\%\ \text{tt} = 0\%\ \text{T} & \text{and} & 4\%\ \text{t} \\ \hline \text{allele frequencies} = 80\%\ \text{T} & \text{and} & 20\%\ \text{t} \end{array}$$

Notice that the allele frequencies are unchanged compared to the parent generation. T is still 0.80 and t is still 0.20. Populations in Hardy–Weinberg equilibrium will exhibit this property.

KEY CONCEPT

All you need to know to solve any MCAT Hardy–Weinberg problem is the value of p (or p^2) or q (or q^2). From there, you can calculate everything else using $p + q = 1$ and $p^2 + 2pq + q^2 = 1$.

KEY CONCEPT

The Hardy–Weinberg equations allow you to find two pieces of information: first, the relative frequency of alleles in a population, and second, the frequency of a given genotype or phenotype in the population. Remember that there will be twice as many alleles as individuals in a population because each individual has two autosomal copies of each gene.

MCAT CONCEPT CHECK 12.3

Before you move on, assess your understanding of the material with these questions.

1. For each of the crosses below, what is the phenotypic ratio seen in the offspring?

Cross	Phenotypic Ratio
Bb × Bb	
Aa × aa	
DdEe × ddEE	
$X_qX \times XY$	
$X_rX \times X_rY$	

2. If genes Q and R have a recombination frequency of 2%, genes R and S have a recombination frequency of 6%, genes S and T have a recombination frequency of 23%, and genes Q and T have a recombination frequency of 19%, then what is the order of these four genes in the chromosome?

____

3. All five criteria of the Hardy–Weinberg principle are required to imply what characteristic of the study population?

____

4. Assume that a population is in Hardy–Weinberg equilibrium. If 9% of the population is homozygous dominant, then solve for the following:
   - The frequency of the dominant allele:

   ____

   - The frequency of the recessive allele:

   ____

   - The portion of the population that is heterozygous:

   ____

   - The portion of the population with a homozygous recessive genotype:

   ____

   - The portion of the population with a dominant phenotype:

   ____

12.4 Evolution

LEARNING OBJECTIVES

After Chapter 12.4, you will be able to:

- Describe the key tenets of the major theories of evolution, including punctuated equilibrium, natural selection, inclusive fitness, and the modern synthesis model
- Identify the three patterns of selection and the changes they create in the population phenotype
- Recall the three patterns of evolution between species and the outcome of each
- Recall the biological definition of a species

Evolutionary thought has a relatively short history; the first theories suggesting that new species may arise from older ones were proposed in the 19th century. Significant alterations to these initial theories have been made since then.

Natural Selection

Natural selection, sometimes called *survival of the fittest*, is the theory that certain characteristics or traits possessed by individuals within a species may help those individuals have greater reproductive success, thus passing on those traits to offspring. This theory was originally proposed by Charles Darwin in his 1859 publication *On the Origin of Species*. His theory was built on several basic tenets:

- Organisms produce offspring, few of which survive to reproductive maturity.
- Chance variations within individuals in a population may be heritable. If these variations give an organism even a slight survival advantage, the variation is termed **favorable**.
- Individuals with a greater preponderance of these favorable variations are more likely to survive to reproductive age and produce offspring; the overall result will be an increase in these traits in future generations. This level of reproductive success is termed **fitness**, and an organism's fitness is directly related to the relative genetic contribution of this individual to the next generation.

Darwin's theory was ultimately proven to be correct in many ways—although not completely. In the 20th century, modern genetics led to the development of the currently accepted theory.

Modern Theories

The **modern synthesis model**, sometimes called **neo-Darwinism**, adds knowledge of genetic inheritance and changes in the gene pool to Darwin's original theory. Once scientists showed that inheritance occurs through the passing of genes from parent to child and that genes ultimately change due to mutation or recombination, Darwin's theory was updated to its current form: when mutation or recombination results in a change that is favorable to the organism's reproductive success, that change is more likely to pass on to the next generation. The opposite is also true. This process is termed **differential reproduction**. Over time, those traits passed on by the more successful organisms will become ubiquitous in the gene pool. Because the gene pool changes over time, it is important to note that populations evolve, not individuals.

KEY CONCEPT

Evolution is not equivalent to natural selection. The MCAT likes to test your ability to understand that natural selection is simply a mechanism for evolution. Natural selection is, however, equivalent to *survival of the fittest*.

Also germane to the modernization of Darwin's theory is a shift in scope to focus on inclusive fitness over the fitness of an individual organism. **Inclusive fitness** is a measure of an organism's success in the population, based on the number of offspring, success in supporting offspring, and the ability of the offspring to then support others. Early descriptions of evolutionary success, like those of Darwin, were based solely on the number of viable offspring of an organism. However, contemporary theories take into account the benefits of certain behaviors on the population at large. For example, the existence of altruism could be supported by the observation that close relatives of an individual will share many of the same genes; thus, promoting the reproduction and survival of related or similar individuals can also lead to genetic success. Other species show examples of inclusive fitness by protecting the offspring of the group at large. By endangering themselves to protect the young, these organisms ensure the passing of genes to future generations. Inclusive fitness therefore promotes the idea that altruistic behavior can improve the fitness and success of a species as a whole.

One final theory to consider was proposed as a result of research into the fossil record. Upon examination, it was discovered that little evolution would occur within a lineage of related lifeforms for long periods of time, followed by an explosion in evolutionary change. Niles Eldredge and Stephen Jay Gould proposed the theory of **punctuated equilibrium** to explain this in 1972. In contrast to Darwin's theory, punctuated equilibrium suggests that changes in some species occur in rapid bursts rather than evenly over time.

Modes of Natural Selection

Natural selection may occur as stabilizing selection, directional selection, or disruptive selection, as shown in Figure 12.24.

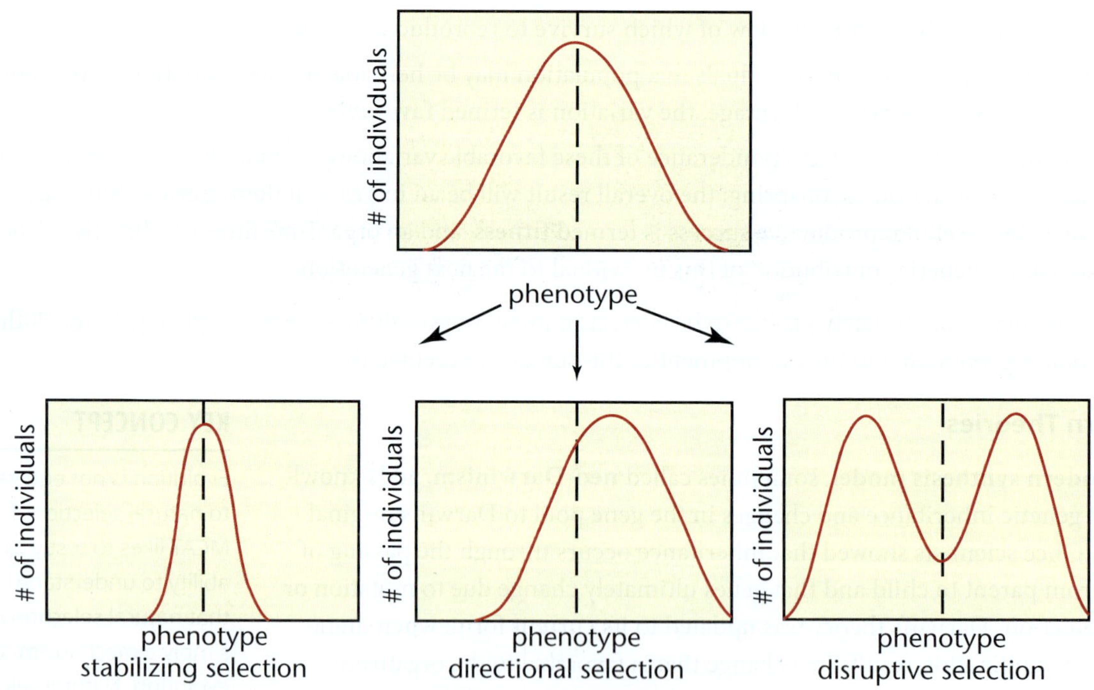

Figure 12.24 Modes of Natural Selection

Stabilizing selection keeps phenotypes within a specific range by selecting against extremes. For instance, human birth weight is maintained within a narrow band by stabilizing selection. Fetuses that weigh too little may not be healthy enough to survive, and fetuses that weigh too much can experience trauma during delivery through the relatively narrow birth canal. In addition, the larger the fetus, the more maternal resources it requires. For all of these reasons, there is a fitness advantage to keeping birth weights within a narrow range.

Adaptive pressure can lead to the emergence and dominance of an initially extreme phenotype through **directional selection**. For example, if we have a heterogeneous plate of bacteria, very few may have resistance to antibiotics. If the plate is then treated with *ampicillin* (an antibiotic), only those colonies that exhibit resistance to this antibiotic will survive. A new standard phenotype emerges as a result of differential survivorship. Natural selection is the history of differential survivorship over time. The emergence of mosquitoes resistant to *dichlorodiphenyltrichloroethane* (DDT), a type of pesticide, is attributed to directional selection.

In **disruptive selection**, two extreme phenotypes are selected over the norm. When Darwin studied finches on the Galapagos Islands, he noted that although there were many species, all the species arguably had a common ancestor, given their similar appearances. However, when he compared beak sizes they were all either large or small, as shown in Figure 12.25. No animals exhibited the intermediate phenotype of medium-size beaks. Darwin hypothesized that the sizes of seeds on the island (the finches' food) led to this effect. Seeds were either quite large or fairly small, requiring a large or small beak, respectively. Thus, if the original ancestor had a medium-size beak, over time the animals with slightly larger or smaller beaks would be selected for. Disruptive selection is facilitated by the existence of **polymorphisms**—naturally occurring differences in form between members of the same population, such as light and dark coloration in the same species of butterfly. **Adaptive radiation** is a related concept that describes the rapid rise of a number of different species from a common ancestor. The benefit of adaptive radiation is that it allows for various species to occupy different niches. A **niche** is a specific environment, including habitat, available resources, and predators, for which a species is specifically adapted. Adaptive radiation is favored by environmental changes or isolation of small groups of the ancestral species.

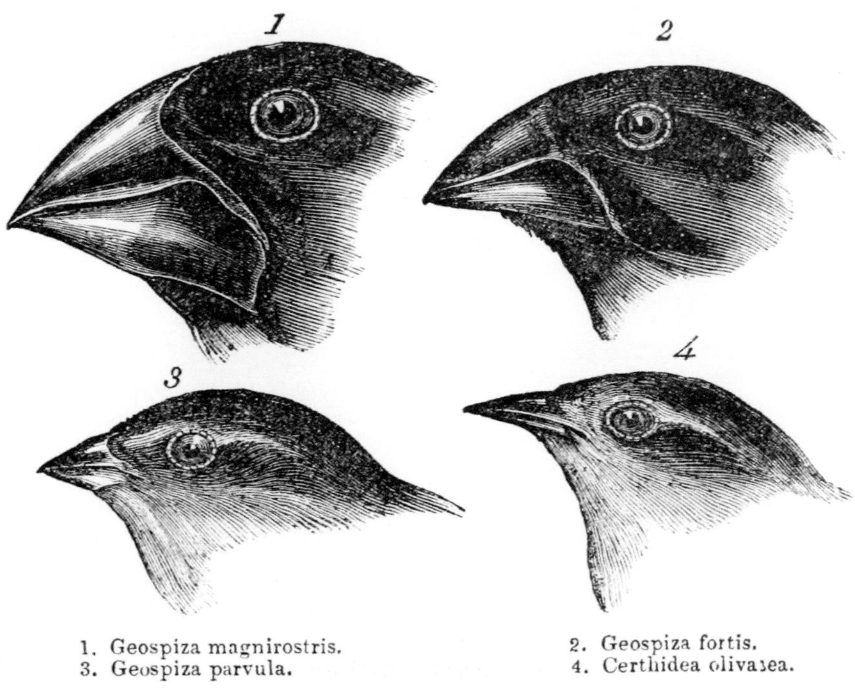

Figure 12.25 Darwin's Finches
Image of Darwin's finches as drawn by John Gould

Speciation

A **species** is defined as the largest group of organisms capable of breeding to form fertile offspring; the formation of a new species through evolution is called **speciation**. If we took two populations from the same species and separated them geographically for a long period of time, different evolutionary pressures would lead to different adaptive changes. If enough time passed, the changes would be sufficient to lead to **isolation**, which means the progeny of these populations could no longer freely interbreed. We would now consider the two groups separate species.

Reproductive isolation may occur either prezygotically or postzygotically. **Prezygotic mechanisms** prevent formation of the zygote completely; **postzygotic mechanisms** allow for gamete fusion but yield either nonviable or sterile offspring. Examples of prezygotic mechanisms include temporal isolation (breeding at different times), ecological isolation (living in different niches within the same territory), behavioral isolation (a lack of attraction between members of the two species due to differences in pheromones, courtship displays, and so on), mechanical isolation (incompatibility of reproductive anatomy), or gametic isolation (intercourse can occur, but fertilization cannot). Postzygotic mechanisms include hybrid inviability (formation of a zygote that cannot develop to term), hybrid sterility (forming hybrid offspring that cannot reproduce), and hybrid breakdown (forming first-generation hybrid offspring that are viable and fertile, but second-generation hybrid offspring that are inviable or infertile). Both prezygotic and postzygotic mechanisms can be observed in Figure 12.26. As described earlier in this chapter, mules are an example of postzygotic hybrid sterility. Although a horse and donkey can produce a viable mule, the mule will be sterile and thus unable to establish a self-perpetuating mule lineage.

Pre-zygotic Isolating Mechanisms		Examples	
Temporal	Mating rythms and patterns are not in sync	Some frogs mate during the summer and some closer to winter	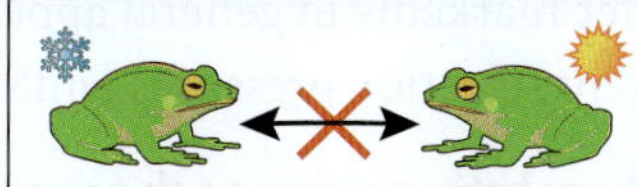
Ecological	The two species no longer occupy the same habitat	Lions and tigers can produce hybrids, but are separated via habitats	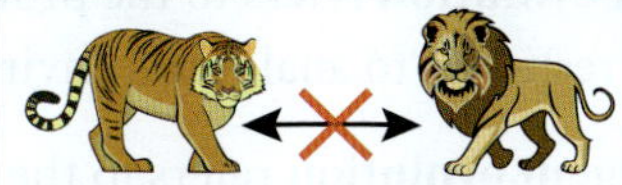
Behavioral	Different species possess different mating behaviors	Two bird species may have different mating calls	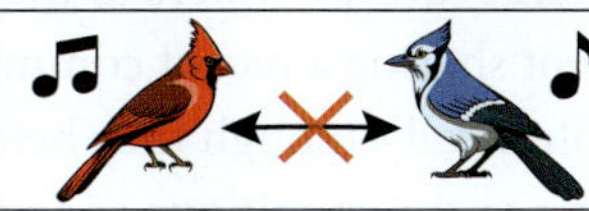
Mechanical	Different species do not mate due to physical differences	Some dog breeds cannot naturally reproduce due to size differences	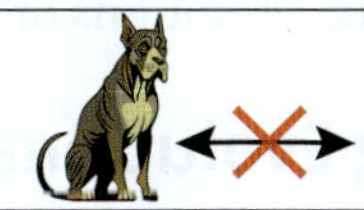
Gametic	Intercourse can occur, but fertilization cannot	Sea urchin egg proteins bind only to same-species sperm	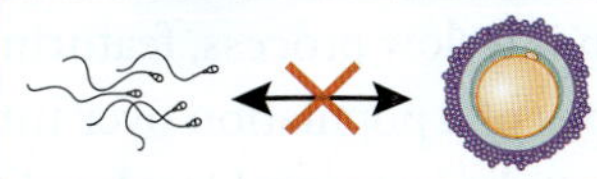

Post-zygotic Isolating Mechanisms		Examples	
Hybrid inviability	Hybrid does not reach reproductive maturity	Hybrid tadpoles do not mature and die before reproducing	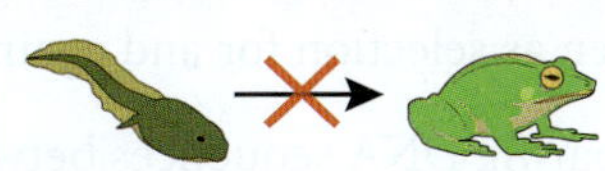
Hybrid sterility	Hybrid cannot produce viable gametes (sterile)	A mule (a cross between horse and donkey) cannot produce functional gametes	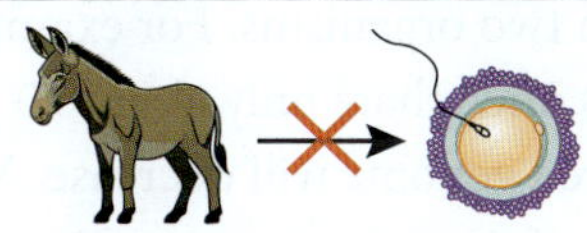
Hybrid breakdown	Second generation hybrids are infertile	Second generation hybrid copepods have reduced fertility	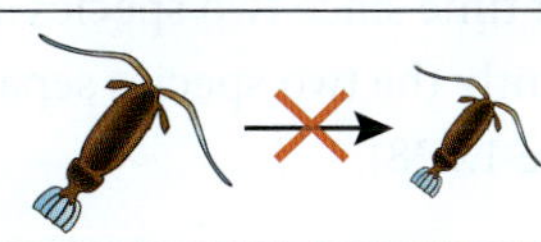

Figure 12.26 Prezygotic and Postzygotic Isolation Mechanisms

Patterns of Evolution

When we look at similarities between two species, we must be careful to determine whether those similarities are due to sharing a common ancestor or sharing a common environment with the same evolutionary pressures. When analyzing species this way, three patterns of evolution emerge: divergent evolution, parallel evolution, and convergent evolution, as shown in Figure 12.27.

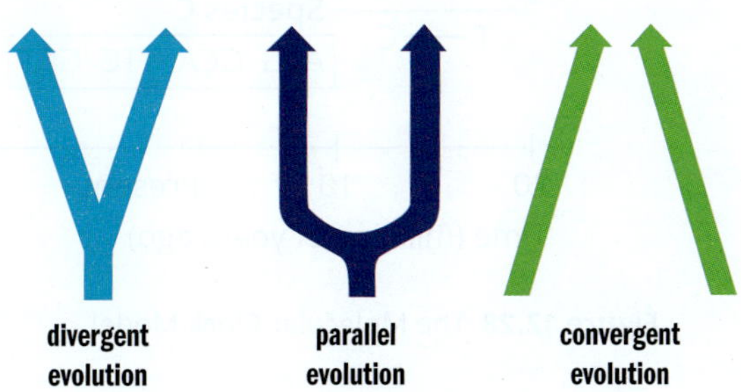

Figure 12.27 Patterns of Evolution

Divergent evolution refers to the independent development of dissimilar characteristics in two or more lineages sharing a common ancestor. For example, seals and cats are both mammals in the order Carnivora, yet they differ markedly in general appearance. These two species live in very different environments and adapted to different selection pressures while evolving.

Parallel evolution refers to the process whereby related species evolve in similar ways for a long period of time in response to analogous environmental selection pressures.

Convergent evolution refers to the independent development of similar characteristics in two or more lineages not sharing a recent common ancestor. For example, fish and dolphins have come to resemble one another physically, though they belong to different classes of vertebrates. They evolved certain similar features in adapting to the conditions of aquatic life.

Measuring Evolutionary Time

Evolution is a slow process, featuring changes in the environment and subsequent changes in genotypes and phenotypes of a population over time. The rate of evolution is measured by the rate of change of a genotype over a period of time and is related to the severity of the evolutionary pressures on the species. In other words, if a species is already perfectly suited to its habitat and there are no changes to the conditions in which it lives, the rate of evolution will be exceedingly slow—although there will still be some small base rate of genetic mutation. On the other hand, if an organism lives in a rapidly changing environment, the rate of evolution will be greater, as selection for and against certain traits will be actively occurring within that population.

By comparing DNA sequences between different species, scientists can quantify the degree of similarity between two organisms. For example, chimpanzees share over 95 percent of their genome with humans, whereas mice share only about 70 percent. As species become more taxonomically distant, the proportion of the shared genome will decrease. Molecular evolutionists correlate the degree of genomic similarity with the amount of time since two species split off from the same common ancestor; the more similar the genomes, the more recently the two species separated from each other. This is sometimes called the **molecular clock model** (see Figure 12.28).

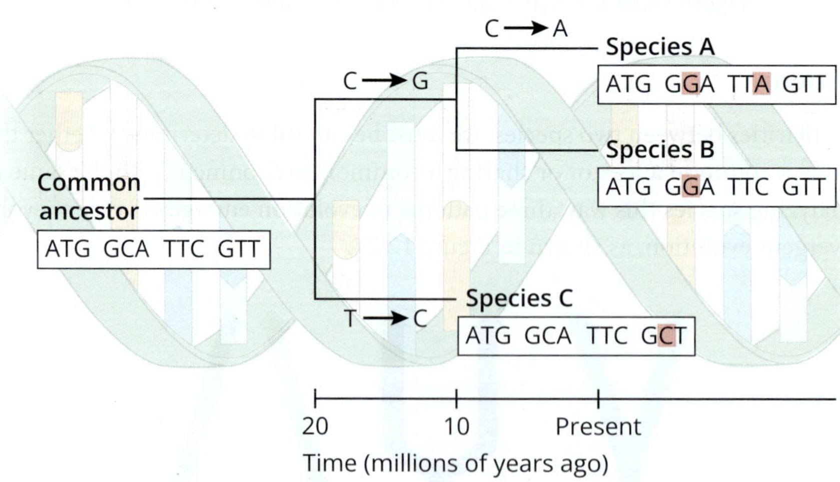

Figure 12.28 The Molecular Clock Model

MCAT CONCEPT CHECK 12.4

Before you move on, assess your understanding of the material with these questions.

1. What are the key tenets of each of the following theories of evolution?
   - Natural selection:

   - Modern synthesis model:

   - Inclusive fitness:

   - Punctuated equilibrium:

   ---

2. What are the three patterns of selection? What changes would each create to the population phenotype?

Pattern of Selection	Change to Population Phenotype

3. What are the three patterns of evolution between species? What is the outcome of each one?

Pattern of Evolution	Outcome

4. What is the biological definition of a species?

BIOLOGY GUIDED EXAMPLE WITH EXPERT THINKING

While the genus *Saccharomyces* is best known for the model and industrial yeast *S. cerevisiae*, it also includes eight closely related additional species.

Saccharomyces has 9 related species

The repeated isolation of *S. cerevisiae* from wine, beer, and other fermented beverages, and the difficulty in finding its truly natural habitats, has led to the common view that this species was a product of domestication. However, the unusual degree of shared physiological characteristics among *Saccharomyces* species along with the recent isolation of *S. cerevisiae* from a natural environment suggests *S. cerevisiae* may be a result of natural evolution.

Issue: Is the formation of S. cervevisiae due to domestication or natural evolution?

In the present work we used a comparative genomics approach and publicly available complete genome sequences of five *Saccharomyces* species to search for proteins exhibiting molecular patterns of evolution. We used the dN/dS ratio [rate of nonsynonymous substitutions per nonsynonymous site (dN)/rate of synonymous substitutions per synonymous site (dS)] of the complete *Saccharomyces* ORFeomes to measure protein divergence and corrected for phylogenetic distance. From this data, we created the phylogenetic tree shown in Figure 1 and searched for genes associated with

There's a lot of technical jargon here, so to rephrase, the key takeaway is that the researchers used comparative genomics to create the phylogenic tree in Figure 1

divergence. Some of the identified genes had been previously associated with adaptation to growth at suboptimal temperatures. This prompted us to examine catabolic fluxes at different temperatures in *Saccharomyces* species with different growth temperature preferences. Figure 1 depicts schematically the phylogenetic relationships of the species in the genus *Saccharomyces* and assigns them to the thermotolerant or cryotolerant groups.

After creating the tree, the researchers saw that optimal growth temperature was a pattern that corresponded to the phylogeny

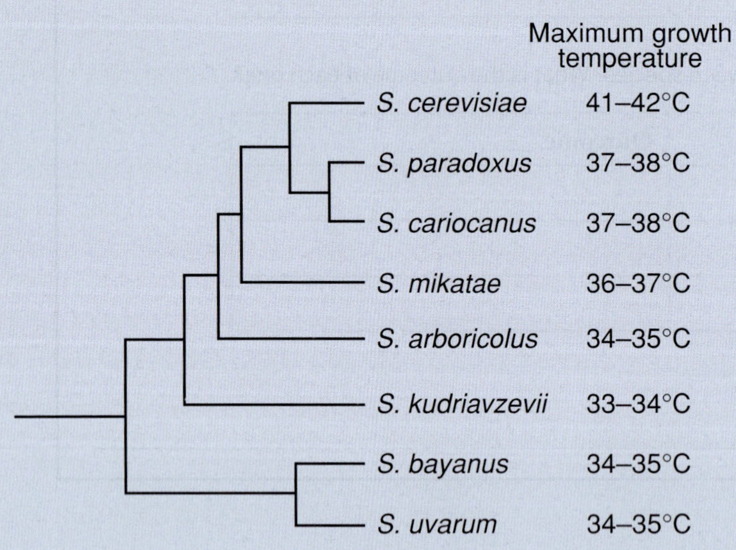

Figure 1

Trend: maximum growth temperature is highest at the top of the tree, and generally descends in order

Adapted from Gonçalves, P., Valério, E., Correia, C., de Almeida, J. M., & Sampaio, J. P. (2011). Evidence for divergent evolution of growth temperature preference in sympatric Saccharomyces species. *PloS One*, 6(6), e20739.

Based on the information provided, could temperature have provided the selective pressure for the divergent evolution of *Saccharomyces* species?

The question is asking us if there is support in the passage and figure for the hypothesis that temperature can explain the divergence of the various *Saccharomyces* species in the phylogenetic tree. Notice the phrasing of the question—it's not asking if we have proof that the evolution was due to temperature selection. This analysis is retrospective, so we would have no way to verify whether or not the relationship between growth and temperature leading up to speciation was causal.

In paragraph 2, the researchers used fairly complex techniques to analyze the genomes of *Saccharomyces* species and arranged them in the phylogenetic tree. We don't need to understand all of the details behind this method. The takeaway is that the phylogeny was generated prior to the analysis of optimal growth temperatures. The researchers then searched for genes associated with divergence and noticed that some of those genes corresponded to adaptations for growth at nonideal temperatures. Finally, an analysis of the optimal growth temperature for the listed *Saccharomyces* species gave us a workable pattern—species that are close together on the tree also have very similar optimal growth temperatures. We know from content background that changes in environment can definitely apply selection pressures strong enough to lead to speciation, or the formation of new species. Recall also that divergent evolution is the development of species with different characteristics despite a shared common ancestor.

Since temperature is an environmental factor, we can say that based on the given information, there is plausible evidence to support that temperature could have provided the selection pressure for divergent evolution of *Saccharomyces* species.

Conclusion

Genetics and the mechanisms of evolution are becoming increasingly important in medicine, as we unintentionally breed strains of highly resistant bacteria. Antibiotic stewardship, or the use of the appropriate antibiotics only as necessary, is very important as the medical community seeks to preserve the effectiveness of antibiotics. In order to understand and apply the concepts of antibiotic stewardship, one must understand that creating environmental pressures leads to directional selection in microorganisms which can increase the frequency of the resistant phenotype. In this chapter, we covered genetics and mutations, as well as evolution. We also gave you some tools to analyze the biometric (statistical) side of genetics through the use of Punnett squares, recombinant frequencies, and the Hardy–Weinberg equations.

It seems fitting to complete this book with a discussion of evolution. You've spent hundreds of pages (and hours!) preparing for the MCAT, learning the basics of cell biology, embryogenesis and development, anatomy and physiology, genetics, and evolution. Our understanding of these topics relies on generations and generations of scientists who came before us, who passed down their knowledge through books, letters, articles, lectures, and—more recently—television, film, and popular media. But science is a field that is constantly evolving itself. At the beginning of medical school, students are often told that no more than 25 percent of what they learn during the first year will remain true by the time they enter practice. We're not sure if this statistic actually holds, but it does speak to the importance of staying on top of the latest research—not only as a medical student, but also as a practitioner. Every day, new discoveries about the human body and the practice of medicine are being made—soon, you'll be one of those making these very discoveries and bringing them to your practice, improving your patients' lives. And at the end of it all, as a provider, an attending physician, or a researcher, you too will pass on your knowledge to future generations of physicians who will also help medical science to evolve and improve. The human body is astoundingly complex. Take a moment to genuinely think about that—*the human body is astoundingly complex*. There's so much more to learn. Medical school and your future awaits!

GO ONLINE

You've reviewed the content, now test your knowledge and critical thinking skills by completing a test-like passage set in your online resources!

CONCEPT SUMMARY

Fundamental Concepts of Genetics

- **Chromosomes** contain **genes** in a linear sequence.
- **Alleles** are alternative forms of a gene.
  - A **dominant** allele requires only one copy to be expressed.
  - A **recessive** allele requires two copies to be expressed.
- A **genotype** is the combination of alleles one has at a given genetic **locus**.
  - Having two of the same allele is termed **homozygous**.
  - Having two different alleles is termed **heterozygous**.
  - Having only one allele is termed **hemizygous** (such as in male sex chromosomes).
  - A **phenotype** is the observable manifestation of a genotype.
- There are different patterns of dominance.
  - **Complete dominance** occurs when the effect of one allele completely masks the effect of another.
  - **Codominance** has more than one dominant allele.
  - **Incomplete dominance** has no dominant alleles; heterozygotes have intermediate phenotypes.
- **Penetrance** is the proportion of a population with a given genotype who express the phenotype.
- **Expressivity** refers to the varying phenotypic manifestations of a given genotype.
- The modern interpretations of Mendel's laws help explain the inheritance of genes from parent to offspring.
  - **Mendel's first law (of segregation)** states that an organism has two alleles for each gene, which segregate during meiosis, resulting in gametes carrying only one allele for a trait.
  - **Mendel's second law (of independent assortment)** states that the inheritance of one allele does not influence the probability of inheriting an allele for a different trait.
- Support for DNA as genetic material came through a number of experiments.
  - The Griffith experiment demonstrated the transforming principle, converting nonvirulent live bacteria into virulent bacteria by exposure to heat-killed virulent bacteria.
  - The Avery–MacLeod–McCarty experiment demonstrated that DNA is the genetic material because degradation of DNA led to a cessation of bacterial transformation.
  - The Hershey–Chase experiment confirmed that DNA is the genetic material because only radiolabeled DNA could be found in bacteriophage-infected bacteria.

Changes in the Gene Pool

- All of the alleles in a given population constitute the **gene pool**.
- **Mutations** are changes in DNA sequence.
- Nucleotide mutations include **point mutations** (the substituting of one nucleotide for another) and **frameshift mutations** (moving the three-letter transcriptional reading frame).
  - A **silent mutation** has no effect on the protein.
  - A **missense mutation** results in the substitution of one amino acid for another.

  - A **nonsense mutation** results in the substitution of a stop codon for an amino acid.
  - **Insertions** and **deletions** result in a shift in the **reading frame**, leading to changes for all downstream amino acids.
- Chromosomal mutations include larger-scale mutations affecting whole segments of DNA.
  - **Deletion mutations** occur when a large segment of DNA is lost.
  - **Duplication mutations** occur when a segment of DNA is copied multiple times.
  - **Inversion mutations** occur when a segment of DNA is reversed.
  - **Insertion mutations** occur when a segment of DNA is moved from one chromosome to another.
  - **Translocation mutations** occur when a segment of DNA is swapped with a segment of DNA from another chromosome.
- Genetic **leakage** is a flow of genes between species through hybrid offspring.
- **Genetic drift** occurs when the composition of the gene pool changes as a result of chance.
- The **founder effect** results from **bottlenecks** that suddenly isolate a small population, leading to **inbreeding** and increased prevalence of certain homozygous genotypes.

Analytical Approaches in Genetics

- **Pedigree charts** track the presence or absence of specific traits among family members, thereby illustrating inheritance patterns.
  - **Autosomal dominant** traits never skip generations and affect males and females equally.
  - **Autosomal recessive** traits also affect males and females equally, but can skip generations; all offspring of two affected parents will be affected.
  - **X-linked recessive** traits can skip generations like autosomal recessive, but disproportionately affect males who have only one X chromosome.
  - **Mitochondrial inheritance** is evident when traits are passed down exclusively through the maternal line: all and only children (both male and female) of affected females are affected.
  - **Y-linked** inheritance is uncommon on the MCAT, but evident when traits only affect males who have Y chromosomes, with all and only sons of affected males also being affected.
- **Punnett squares** visually represent the crossing of gametes from parents to show relative genotypic and phenotypic frequencies.
  - The **parent generation** is represented by P; **filial** (offspring) **generations** are represented by F_1, F_2, and so on in sequence.
  - A **monohybrid cross** accounts for one gene; a **dihybrid cross** accounts for two genes.
  - In **sex-linked crosses**, sex chromosomes are usually used to indicate sex as well as genotype.
- The **recombination frequency** (**θ**) is the likelihood of two alleles being separated during crossing over in meiosis. **Genetic maps** can be made using recombination frequency as the scale in **centimorgans**.
- The **Hardy–Weinberg principle** states that if a population meets certain criteria (aimed at a lack of evolution), then the **allele frequencies** will remain constant (**Hardy–Weinberg equilibrium**).

Evolution

- **Natural selection** states that chance variations exist between individuals and that advantageous variations—those that increase an individual's **fitness** for survival or adaptation to the environment—afford the most opportunities for reproductive success.
- The **modern synthesis model** (**neo-Darwinism**) accounts for mutation and recombination as mechanisms of variation and considers **differential reproduction** to be the mechanism for reproductive success.
- **Inclusive fitness** considers an organism's success to be based on the number of offspring, success in supporting offspring, and the ability of the offspring to then support others; survival of offspring or relatives ensures appearance of genes in subsequent generations.
- **Punctuated equilibrium** considers evolution to be a very slow process with intermittent rapid bursts of evolutionary activity.
- Different types of selection lead to changes in phenotypes.
    - **Stabilizing selection** keeps phenotypes in a narrow range, excluding extremes.
    - **Directional selection** moves the average phenotype toward one extreme.
    - **Disruptive selection** moves the population toward two different phenotypes at the extremes and can lead to **speciation**.
    - **Adaptive radiation** is the rapid emergence of multiple species from a common ancestor, each of which occupies its own ecological **niche**.
- A **species** is the largest group of organisms capable of breeding to form fertile offspring. Species are **reproductively isolated** from each other by **pre-** or **postzygotic mechanisms**.
- Two species can evolve with different relationship patterns.
    - **Divergent evolution** occurs when two species sharing a common ancestor become more different.
    - **Parallel evolution** occurs when two species sharing a common ancestor evolve in similar ways due to analogous selection pressures.
    - **Convergent evolution** occurs when two species not sharing a recent ancestor evolve to become more similar due to analogous selection pressures.
- According to the **molecular clock model**, the degree of difference in the genome between two species is related to the amount of time since the two species broke off from a common ancestor.

ANSWERS TO CONCEPT CHECKS

12.1

1. A dominant allele is one that requires only one copy for expression. A recessive allele requires two copies for expression.
2. A homozygous genotype is one in which the two alleles are the same. A heterozygous genotype is one in which the two alleles are different. A hemizygous genotype is one in which only one allele is present for a given gene (such as parts of the X chromosome in males).
3. Complete dominance occurs when one allele (the dominant one) completely masks the expression of the other (the recessive one). Codominance occurs when a gene has more than one dominant allele, and two different dominant alleles can be expressed simultaneously. Incomplete dominance occurs when a gene has no dominant alleles, and heterozygotes have phenotypes that are intermediate between homozygotes.
4. Penetrance describes the proportion of the population that expresses a phenotype, given a particular genotype. Expressivity describes the differences in expression (severity, location, and so on) of a phenotype in individuals.
5. Mendel's first law (of segregation) most aligns with anaphase I of meiosis. Mendel's second law (of independent assortment) most aligns with prophase I of meiosis.

12.2

1. Silent point mutations occur when one nucleotide is changed for another, but there is no change in the protein coded for by this DNA sequence (due to redundancy in the genetic code). Missense mutations occur when one nucleotide is changed for another, and one amino acid is substituted for another in the final protein. Nonsense mutations occur when one nucleotide is changed for another, and a stop codon substitutes for an amino acid in the final protein.
2. The two types of frameshift mutations are insertion and deletion mutations.
3. Duplication mutations occur when a segment of DNA is copied multiple times in the genome. Inversion mutations occur when a segment of DNA is reversed in the genome. Translocation mutations occur when a segment of DNA from one chromosome is swapped with a segment of DNA from another chromosome.
4. Genetic leakage requires the formation of a hybrid organism that can then mate with members of one or the other parent species. While hybrids existed historically (especially mules), fertile hybrids were certainly rare before a more modern understanding of genetics (and before a commercial, financial, or academic impetus existed to create these organisms).
5. Genetic drift occurs due to chance, so its effects will be more pronounced with a smaller sample size (in smaller populations). The founder effect occurs when a small group is reproductively isolated from the larger population, allowing certain alleles to take on a higher prevalence in the group than in the rest of the population.

12.3

1.

Cross	Phenotypic Ratio
Bb × Bb	3 dominant:1 recessive
Aa × aa	1 dominant:1 recessive
DdEe × ddEE	1 dominant (for D)/dominant (for E): 1 recessive (for D)/dominant (for E)
$\mathbf{X_qX \times XY}$	Female: all unaffected; male: 1 unaffected:1 affected
$\mathbf{X_rX \times X_rY}$	Both male and female: 1 unaffected:1 affected

2. The genes must be in the order SQRT:

$$S \xleftrightarrow{4\%} Q \xleftrightarrow{2\%} R \xleftrightarrow{17\%} T$$

3. The criteria for the Hardy–Weinberg principle all imply that the study population is *not* undergoing evolution; thus, the allele frequencies will remain stable over time.
4. The frequency of the dominant allele (p) is 0.3. The frequency of the recessive allele (q) is 0.7. The fraction of the population with a heterozygous genotype ($2pq$) is $2 \times 0.3 \times 0.7 = 0.42$ (42%). The fraction of the population with a homozygous recessive genotype (q^2) is $(0.7)^2 = 0.49$ (49%). The fraction of the population with a dominant phenotype ($p^2 + 2pq$) is $0.09 + 0.42 = 0.51 = 51\%$.

12.4

1. Natural selection states that certain traits that arise from chance are more favorable for reproductive success in a given environment, and that those traits will be passed on to future generations. The modern synthesis model takes natural selection and explains that selection is for specific alleles, which are passed on to future generations through formation of gametes; the alleles for these favorable traits arise from mutations. Inclusive fitness explains that the reproductive success of an organism is not only due to the number of offspring it creates, but also the ability to care for young (that can then care for others); it explains changes not only at the individual level, but changes based on the survival of the species (and that individual's alleles within the species, including in other related individuals). Punctuated equilibrium states that for some species, little evolution occurs for a long period, which is interrupted by rapid bursts of evolutionary change.

2.

Pattern of Selection	Change to Population Phenotype
Stabilizing	Loss of extremes, maintenance of phenotype in a small window
Directional	Movement toward one extreme or the other
Disruptive	Movement toward both extremes with loss of the norm; speciation may occur

3.

Pattern of Evolution	Outcome
Divergent	Two species with a common ancestor become less similar because of different evolutionary pressures
Parallel	Two species with a common ancestor remain similar because of similar evolutionary pressures
Convergent	Two species with no recent common ancestor become more similar because of similar evolutionary pressures

4. A species is defined as the largest group of organisms capable of breeding to form fertile offspring.

SCIENCE MASTERY ASSESSMENT EXPLANATIONS

1. **B**

This is a gene-mapping problem. Because there is a correlation between the frequency of recombination and the distance between genes on a chromosome, if we are given the frequencies, we can determine gene order. Remember that one map unit equals 1 percent recombination frequency. The easiest way to begin is to determine the two genes that are farthest apart; in this case, N and O recombine with a frequency of 18%, so they are 18 map units apart on the chromosome:

$$N \xleftrightarrow{18\%} O$$

N and P recombine with 1% frequency, and P and O recombine with 17% frequency, so P must be between N and O:

$$N \xleftrightarrow{1\%} P \xleftrightarrow{17\%} O$$

Finally, M and P recombine with 5% frequency, and M and O recombine with 12% frequency, so M must be between P and O:

$$N \xleftrightarrow{1\%} P \xleftrightarrow{5\%} M \xleftrightarrow{12\%} O$$

2. **D**

In this dihybrid problem, a doubly recessive individual is crossed with an individual of unknown genotype; this is known as a test cross. The straight- and brown-haired organism has the genotype bbcc and can thus only produce gametes carrying bc. Looking at the F_1 offspring, there is a 1:1:1:1 phenotypic ratio. The fact that both the dominant and recessive traits are present in the offspring means that the unknown parental genotype must contain both dominant and recessive alleles for each trait. The unknown parental genotype must therefore be BbCc. If you want to double-check the answer, you can work out the Punnett square for the cross BbCc × bbcc:

	BC	Bc	bC	bc
bc	BbCc	Bbcc	bbCc	bbcc
bc	BbCc	Bbcc	bbCc	bbcc
bc	BbCc	Bbcc	bbCc	bbcc
bc	BbCc	Bbcc	bbCc	bbcc
	↓ 25% black curly	↓ 25% black straight	↓ 25% brown curly	↓ 25% brown straight

3. **C**

The female in this example is a carrier of two sex-linked traits; based on the genotype, the affected alleles are found on different X chromosomes. Drawing out a Punnett square, we see that 25% of the offspring will be female hemophiliacs (X_hX_h) and 25% will be female carriers of both alleles (X_cX_h). This question is asking what percentage of females will have a phenotype with no hemophilia or color blindness, which would be half of the females (those who are carriers for both traits).

	X_c	X_h
X_h	X_cX_h	X_hX_h
Y	X_cY	X_hY

offspring
25% female hemophiliac
25% female carrier of both traits (phenotypically normal)
25% male hemophiliac
25% male colorblind

4. **A**

The control parent in a test cross is always recessive. Therefore, if the test parent is phenotypically dominant, yet can provide a recessive allele (as evidenced by the presence of recessive children), then the parent must have both a dominant and recessive allele. Therefore, this test parent must be heterozygous.

5. **B**

The definition given here for expressivity is a much better match for defining penetrance (or, really, one minus the penetrance). Expressivity refers to the variable manifestations of a given genotype as different phenotypes; the degree to which various phenotypes are expressed. All of the other definitions given are accurate.

6. **B**

Some progeny in the second generation are apparently blends of the parental phenotypes. The orange color is the result of the combined effects of the red and yellow alleles. An allele is incompletely dominant if the phenotype of the heterozygotes is an intermediate of the phenotypes of the homozygotes.

7. **B**

To find the correct answer, we have to read each choice and eliminate the ones that fit with the modern-day theories of inheritance, which state that the genes that make an organism most fit for its environment will be passed to offspring. This can be seen in **(C)** and **(D)**, both of which demonstrate that an organism with improved fitness will pass those genes to offspring. **(A)** mentions a gamete being exposed to mutagens; a zygote created from this gamete would contain any mutations that were present in the egg and would be affected by them. Thus, **(B)** must be the correct answer: indeed, acquired characteristics not encoded in the genome should not be passed to offspring according to the modern synthesis model.

8. **B**

Darwin's theory of natural selection argues that chance variations between organisms can help certain organisms survive to reproductive age and produce many offspring, transmitting their variations to the next generation. Thus, natural selection would drive the process of evolution forward, enabling the persistence of characteristics that impart an advantage in the environment, eliminating **(A)**. In Darwin's theory, fitness is measured in terms of reproductive success, as **(D)** states. Through natural selection, organisms may be separated into groups depending on environmental pressures, and these groups can eventually separate to the point of becoming distinct species, eliminating **(C)**. **(B)** is the correct answer because the theory of natural selection applies to a population of organisms, not to a particular individual. As such, favorable genetic variations become more and more common from generation to generation, not during the lifetime of an individual.

9. **C**

Hardy–Weinberg equilibrium exists under certain ideal conditions that, when satisfied, allow one to calculate the gene frequencies within a population. The Hardy–Weinberg equation can be applied only under these five conditions: (1) the population is very large; (2) there are no mutations that affect the gene pool; (3) mating between individuals in the population is random; (4) there is no migration of individuals into or out of the population; (5) the genes in the population are all equally successful at being reproduced. Thus, from the given choices, only **(C)** is false: monogamy is not a necessary condition for Hardy–Weinberg equilibrium.

10. **B**

The situation described in the question stem is an example of directional selection. In directional selection, the phenotypic norm of a particular species shifts toward an extreme to adapt to a selective pressure, such as an increasingly colder environment. Only those individuals with a thicker layer of fur were able to survive during the Ice Age, thus shifting the phenotypic norm.

11. **A**

A species is defined as the largest group of organisms that can interbreed to produce viable, fertile offspring. Therefore, two populations are considered separate species when they can no longer do so.

12. **D**

Let's use the information provided by the question stem to set up our equations. We are told that the frequency of R equals 30%, and as such, $p = 0.30$. The frequency of the recessive gene is $\text{r} = 100\% - 30\% = 70\%$; thus, $q = 0.70$. The frequency of the genotypes, according to the Hardy–Weinberg equilibrium, are given by $p^2 = \text{RR}$, $2pq = \text{Rr}$, and $q^2 = \text{rr}$. Therefore, the frequency of the genotypes are $(0.3)^2 = 0.09 = 9\%$ RR, $2 \times 0.3 \times 0.7 = 0.42 = 42\%$ Rr, and $(0.7)^2 = 0.49 = 49\%$ rr.

13. **B**

Using the information given in the question stem, we can determine that the percentage of the population with blue eyes (genotype bb) $= 36\% = 0.36 = q^2$; therefore, $q = 0.6$. Because this is a Hardy–Weinberg population, we can assume that $p + q = 1$, so $p = 1 - 0.6 = 0.4$. The frequency of heterozygous brown eyes is therefore $2pq = 2 \times 0.4 \times 0.6 = 0.48 = 48\%$.

14. **D**

Frameshift mutations include insertions and deletions of nucleotides that change the triplet reading frame. In such a mutation, the amino acid sequence preceding the mutation is normal, yielding a normal N terminal end. However, the triplet reading frame after the mutation is changed, yielding a drastically different C terminal sequence that often includes a premature stop codon. These factors together support **(D)** as the correct answer. Note that nonsense mutations also introduce premature stop codons. However, **(C)** can be eliminated since a nonsense mutation will create a stop codon directly and will not change the identity of the amino acids before the stop codon.

15. **C**

This scenario—a deletion of some DNA and a duplication of other DNA—would be consistent with a translocation between chromosomes 4 and 21 during development of an egg or sperm. If part of chromosome 21 was swapped with part of chromosome 4, then a gamete resulting from meiosis in this cell would result in a daughter cell with two copies of some of the DNA from 21 and no copies of some of the DNA from 4. Therefore, after fertilization, there would be partial trisomy 21 and partial monosomy 4. While a deletion or insertion could explain one of the findings, it cannot explain both, eliminating **(A)** and **(B)**. An inversion should not lead to partial trisomy or partial monosomy because the DNA is simply reversed, eliminating **(D)**.

GO ONLINE

Consult your online resources for additional practice.

EQUATIONS TO REMEMBER

(12.1) **Hardy–Weinberg equations:**

$$p + q = 1$$

$$p^2 + 2pq + q^2 = 1$$

SHARED CONCEPTS

Behavioral Sciences Chapter 10
Social Thinking

Biochemistry Chapter 6
DNA and Biotechnology

Biochemistry Chapter 7
RNA and the Genetic Code

Biology Chapter 1
The Cell

Physics and Math Chapter 11
Reasoning About the Design and Execution of Research

Physics and Math Chapter 12
Data-Based and Statistical Reasoning

GLOSSARY

Abductor–A muscle that moves a limb away from the center of the body.

Absorption–The process by which substances are taken up into or across tissues.

Acetylcholine–A neurotransmitter found throughout the nervous system (somatic motor neurons, preganglionic parasympathetic and sympathetic nerves, and postganglionic parasympathetic neurons); metabolized by acetylcholinesterase.

Acrosome–The large vesicle at the head of a sperm cell containing enzymes that degrade the ovum cell membrane to allow fertilization.

Actin–A protein found in the cytoskeleton and muscle cells; it is the principal constituent of the thin filaments and microfilaments.

Action potential–An abrupt change in the membrane potential of a nerve or muscle caused by changes in membrane ionic permeability; results in conduction of an impulse in nerves or contraction in muscles.

Active immunity–An immune response (antibody production or cellular immunity) acquired in response to exposure to an antigen.

Active site–Substrate-binding region of an enzyme.

Adaptation–The development of characteristics that enable an organism to survive and reproduce in its habitat.

Adaptive immunity–Highly specific form of immunity that retains chemical memory of each invader encountered and is able to tailor the immune response to the specific pathogen.

Adaptive radiation–The evolutionary process by which one species gives rise to several species, each specialized for different niches.

Adductor–A muscle that moves a limb toward the center of the body.

Adenine–A purine base present in DNA and RNA; it forms hydrogen bonds with thymine and uracil.

Adenosine triphosphate (ATP)–A nucleotide molecule consisting of adenine, ribose, and three phosphate moieties; the outer two phosphates are bound by high-energy bonds.

Adipose–Refers to fatty tissue, fat-storing tissue, or fat within cells.

Aerobic–Refers to a biological process that occurs in the presence of molecular oxygen (O_2) or to organisms that cannot live without molecular oxygen.

Afferent (sensory) neuron–A neuron that picks up impulses from sensory receptors and transmits them toward the central nervous system.

Agranulocyte–Type of leukocyte that does not contain cytoplasmic granules, including lymphocytes and monocytes.

Albumin–Protein synthesized in the liver that maintains the oncotic pressure of the blood and serves as a carrier for many drugs and hormones.

Allantois–One of four embryonic membranes; it contains the growing embryo's waste products.

Allele–Alternative forms of the same gene coding for a particular trait; alleles segregate during meiosis.

Allergy–A type of autoimmunity in which a person's immune system becomes overactivated by common substances in the environment.

Alveolus–Basic functional unit of the lung; a tiny sac specialized for passive gas exchange between the lungs and the blood.

Amino acids–The building blocks of proteins, each containing an amino group, a carboxylic acid group, and a side chain (or R group) attached to the α-carbon.

Amnion–The innermost fluid-filled embryonic membrane; it forms a protective sac surrounding the embryos of birds, reptiles, and mammals.

Amplification–Characteristic of a signaling cascade, in which the binding of a single peptide hormone to a membrane-bound receptor results in a signal that increases in strength through the signaling cascade.

Anaerobic–Refers to a biological process that can occur without oxygen or to organisms that can live without molecular oxygen.

Anaphase–The stage of mitosis or meiosis characterized by the migration of chromatids or homologous chromosomes to opposite poles of the dividing cell.

Androgen–Any male sex hormone, such as testosterone.

Antibiotic–Substance that kills or inhibits the growth of bacteria or fungi (usually by disrupting cell wall assembly or by binding to ribosomes, thus inhibiting protein synthesis).

Antibody–Immune or protective protein whose synthesis is induced by the presence of foreign substances (antigens) in the body;

each antibody binds to a specific antigen in an immune response; also called immunoglobulin.

Antigen–A substance that binds to an antibody; may be foreign or a self-antigen.

Antigen-binding region–Portion of an antibody that is specific for a particular antigen; the area of the antibody to which the antigen binds.

Aortic valve–One of the semilunar valves, separating the left ventricle from the aorta.

Apoptosis–Process by which a cell undergoes programmed cell death in a highly organized manner in response to either external or internal signals.

Appendicular skeleton–Peripheral portion of the skeleton consisting of arms, legs, and pelvic and pectoral girdles.

Archenteron–The central cavity in the gastrula stage of embryological development; it is lined by endoderm and ultimately gives rise to the adult digestive tract.

Areolar tissue–Also called loose connective tissue, this type of tissue is sparse in collagen fibers and is found in the hypodermis, where it allows for nutrient and waste exchange.

Arterioles–Small arterial structures that link the arteries to the capillaries.

Artery–Thick-walled, muscular blood vessel that generally carries blood away from the heart.

Articular cartilage–Cartilaginous coating at the ends of bones that provides a smooth surface for articulation of bones within a joint.

Asexual reproduction–Any reproductive process that does not involve the fusion of gametes (such as budding).

Asters–Star-shaped structures that form around the centrosome during mitosis.

Atrium–One of two paired structures on either side of the heart, into which blood returning from either the body (right atrium) or the lungs (left atrium) flows.

Autocrine–Form of cell–cell communication in which a cell releases a substance that then binds to the membrane of the releasing cell to either inhibit or activate a cellular activity.

Autoimmunity–Inappropriate immune response that targets self-antigens.

Autonomic nervous system–Subdivision of the peripheral nervous system responsible for involuntary activities, which is further subdivided into the parasympathetic and sympathetic nervous systems.

Autosomal dominant–A pattern of inheritance in which the inheritance of one copy of an allele of a gene on an autosomal chromosome is sufficient to result in the expression of a trait.

Autosomal recessive–A pattern of inheritance in which a trait encoded by a gene on an autosomal chromosome is only expressed if an individual has two copies of the allele.

Autosome–Any chromosome other than a sex chromosome.

Axial skeleton–Midline structures of the skeleton including the skull, vertebral column, and rib cage; provides the central framework of the body.

Axon–The long fiber of a neuron; it conducts impulses away from the cell body toward the synapse.

Axon hillock–Transition point between the cell body (soma) and the axon of a neuron; the site of action potential initiation.

Bacillus–Rod-shaped bacterium.

Bacteriophage–A virus that invades bacteria and sometimes uses bacterial RNA and ribosomes to self-replicate.

Barr body–In cells that contain 2 X chromosomes and undergo X-inactivation, the X chromosome that is transcriptionally silenced by methylation.

Basophil–Type of granulocytic leukocyte that largely participates in allergic reactions and local inflammation.

Bile–A solution of salts, pigments, and cholesterol produced by the liver and stored in the gallbladder; it emulsifies large fat droplets when secreted into the small intestine via the bile duct.

Bilirubin–Product of the breakdown of hemoglobin that is modified to a more soluble form in the liver.

Binary fission–A type of asexual reproduction characteristic of prokaryotes in which there is equal nuclear and cytoplasmic division.

Blastocoel–The fluid-filled central cavity of the blastula.

Blastocyst–A mammalian blastula, consisting of the trophoblastic cells and an inner cell mass.

Blastopore–Opening of the archenteron to the external environment in the gastrula stage of embryonic development.

Blastula–The early embryonic stage during which the embryo is a hollow, fluid-filled sphere of undifferentiated cells.

Blastulation–Process by which a solid mass of early embryonic cells, known as the morula, becomes the blastula, a hollow fluid-filled sphere of undifferentiated cells.

Bohr effect–Changes in the affinity of hemoglobin for oxygen caused by changes in the environment; when pH is low (increased concentration of hydrogen ions), the oxyhemoglobin dissociation curve shifts right, indicating a decreased affinity of hemoglobin for oxygen and more efficient off-loading of oxygen from hemoglobin.

Bolus–An initial dose of medication; in the digestive system, chewed food leaving the mouth, traveling through the esophagus, and entering the stomach.

Bone marrow–Central portion of bones, especially long bones, that contains fat and developing blood cells, including erythrocytes, leukocytes, and megakaryocytes.

Bone matrix–Organic and inorganic minerals that provide strength to compact bone; organic components include collagen, glycoproteins, and other peptides; inorganic components include calcium, phosphate, and hydroxide ions (in hydroxyapatite).

Bowman's capsule–The cup-like structure of the nephron; it collects the glomerular filtrate and channels it into the proximal convoluted tubule.

Bronchi–Tube-like passages for air that connect the trachea to the bronchioles.

Bronchioles–Passageways for air that start at the bronchi, dividing into continuously smaller passageways that eventually lead to the alveoli, where gas exchange occurs.

Brush-border enzymes–Group of enzymes present on the luminal surface of cells lining the duodenum that break down larger biomolecules into monomers that are able to be absorbed.

Bundle of His–Part of the conduction system of the heart; it carries impulses from the AV node to the ventricles.

Callus–Area of excessive deposition of keratin in response to repeated strain due to friction.

Canaliculi–Small canals connecting lacunae within the bone matrix with Haversian canals, allowing for the flow of nutrients and wastes.

Capillary–Small, thin-walled blood vessel where gas, nutrient, and waste exchange occurs between blood and tissues.

Capsid–Protein coat surrounding a virus.

Cardiac output–Total blood volume pumped by the left ventricle in one minute, found by multiplying the heart rate by the stroke volume.

Cartilage–A firm, elastic, translucent connective tissue produced by cells called chondrocytes.

Catabolism–The chemical breakdown of complex substances (macromolecules) to yield simpler substances and energy.

Cecum–The first part of the large intestine; accepts material flowing through the ileocecal valve and is the point of attachment of the appendix.

Cell body–Portion of a neuron where the nucleus, endoplasmic reticulum, and ribosomes are located; also known as the soma.

Cell theory–A foundational belief in modern biology that all living things are composed of cells, that the cell is the basic functional unit of life, that all cells arise from preexisting cells, and that DNA is the genetic material.

Cell-mediated immunity–Type of immunity that uses cytotoxic chemicals released from cells to cause death of cells that have been infected by viruses.

Central nervous system (CNS)–The brain and spinal cord.

Centriole–A small organelle in the cytoplasm of animal cells; it organizes the spindle apparatus during mitosis or meiosis.

Centromere–The area of a chromosome where sister chromatids are joined; it is also the point of attachment to the spindle fiber during mitosis and meiosis.

Centrosomes–Paired cylindrical organelles, located in the cytoplasm, that contain the centrioles.

Cerebellum–The section of the mammalian hindbrain that controls muscle coordination and equilibrium.

Cerebral cortex–The outer layer of the forebrain, consisting of grey matter; it is the site of higher cognitive functions in humans.

Cervix–Lower end of the uterus that marks the transition between the vagina and the uterus.

Chemical digestion–Enzymatic cleavage of chemical bonds within foodstuffs, resulting in smaller molecules.

Chemotaxis–Movement of cells toward or away from a chemical within the environment.

Chiasmata–Sites where crossing over occurs between homologous chromosomes during meiosis.

Chief cells–Cells within the stomach that secrete pepsinogen, a zymogen that is converted to its active form, pepsin, by the acidic environment of the stomach.

Cholecystokinin–A peptide hormone released from the small intestine in response to fat and protein that stimulates the gallbladder to release bile and the pancreas to secrete digestive enzymes.

Chondrin–Elastic cartilage matrix substance secreted by chondrocytes.

Chondrocyte–A differentiated cartilage cell that synthesizes the cartilaginous matrix.

Chromatid–Each of the two chromosomal strands formed by DNA replication in the S phase of the cell cycle; held together by the centromere.

Chromosome–A filamentous body found within the nucleus of a eukaryotic cell or nucleoid region of a prokaryotic cell, composed of DNA.

Chylomicron–Soluble lipid molecule that consists of triglycerides and esterified cholesterol molecules; absorbed into lacteals from the digestive tract.

Chyme–Aqueous mixture of food and secretions that leaves the stomach to enter the duodenum.

Cilia–Projection from a cell involved in movement of materials on the outside of the cell.

Ciliated pseudostratified columnar epithelial cells–Cells that contain cilia and appear to be multilayered due to the varying positions of their nuclei, but are actually a single layer of cells. These cells line the bronchi and trachea where they function to catch and remove particulate matter.

Circadian rhythm–A behavioral pattern based on a 24-hour cycle, related to cycling of hormones such as cortisol and melatonin.

Cleavage–A series of mitotic divisions of the zygote immediately following fertilization, resulting in progressively smaller cells with increased nucleus-to-cytoplasm ratios.

Clonal selection–Phenomenon in which only B- or T-cells specific to a particular pathogen are activated.

Coccus–Spherically shaped bacterium.

Codominance–A genetic effect in which the phenotype of a heterozygote is a distinct reflection of both alleles at a particular locus.

Colony forming unit (CFU)–A unit of measurement used to quantify the number of viable bacteria in a sample.

Competence–In the context of transformation, a state in which bacteria can take up extracellular DNA.

Competent–Describes a cell capable of responding to induction signals.

Confocal microscopy–A type of microscopy that increases optical resolution by using a pinhole to block out-of-focus light.

Conjugation–The temporary joining of two organisms via a tube called a pilus, through which genetic material is exchanged; a form of sexual reproduction used by bacteria.

Connective tissue–Animal tissue composed of cells lying in an extracellular proteinaceous network that supports, connects, and surrounds the organs and structures of the body.

Constant region–Portion of an antibody molecule that is not variable and participates in the binding of other immune modulators.

Convergent evolution–The process by which unrelated organisms living in a similar environment develop analogous structures.

Corona radiata–Layer of cells surrounding an oocyte that aids in the development of the ovum.

Corpus albicans–The structure that remains after the corpus luteum degenerates when implantation does not occur.

Corpus luteum–The remnant of the ovarian follicle, which after ovulation continues to secrete progesterone. Its degeneration leads to menstruation; it also maintains the uterine lining during pregnancy.

Cortex–The external layer found in many organs of the body, including the brain, adrenal glands, and kidney.

Cortical reaction–Release of calcium ions by an ovum after fertilization, resulting in the creation of a fertilization membrane, a structure that prevents fertilization of an ovum by multiple sperm cells.

Corticosteroids–Steroid hormones produced in the adrenal cortex, including glucocorticoids (cortisol), mineralocorticoids (aldosterone), and cortical sex hormones.

Crossing over–The exchange of genetic material between homologous chromosomes during meiosis.

Cyclic adenosine monophosphate (cAMP)–An intracellular second messenger in the signaling cascade initiated by a peptide hormone; synthesized from ATP by adenylate cyclase.

Cytokine–Chemical substance that stimulates inflammation and recruits additional immune cells to a specific area.

Cytokinesis–The division and distribution of parent cell cytoplasm to the two daughter cells during mitotic and meiotic cell division.

Cytoplasm–The fluid and solutes within a cell membrane, external to the nucleus and cellular organelles.

Cytotoxic T-cell–T-cell that seeks out infected cells and induces apoptosis in these cells to prevent spread of the pathogen.

Deletion–A type of genetic mutation in which some variable amount of DNA is removed.

Dendrite–The portion of a neuron that receives stimuli and conveys them toward the cell body.

Dermis–The layer of skin cells under the epidermis. Contains sweat glands, hair follicles, fat, and blood vessels.

Determinate cleavage–Rapid mitotic divisions occurring in an embryo that result in cells with predetermined fates; these cells are only capable of differentiating into certain kinds of tissues within an organism.

Determination–Designation of a cell within an embryo as having a particular future function.

Detrusor muscle–The muscular lining of the bladder.

Diaphragm–Thin, muscular structure that divides the thorax from the abdomen and provides the driving force for inhalation.

Diaphysis–Cylindrical shaft of a long bone.

Diastole–The period of relaxation of cardiac muscle during which the atrioventricular valves open and the ventricles fill with blood.

Differentiation–The process by which unspecialized cells become specialized. Involves selective transcription of the genome.

Digestion–The breakdown of macromolecular nutrient material via mechanical and chemical means to simple molecular building blocks; this facilitates absorption.

Diploid–Having two chromosomes of each type per cell; symbolized by $2n$.

Direct hormone–Substance secreted into the bloodstream that causes a change in the physiological activity of cells without requiring an intermediary.

Directional selection–Selective pressures favor the development of an extreme phenotype that provides a selective advantage; this phenotype emerges as the primary phenotype over time.

Disruptive selection–Type of selection in which selective pressures favor extreme phenotypes over the norm.

Divergent evolution–A process of change whereby organisms with a common ancestor evolve dissimilar structures (such as dolphin flippers and human arms).

Dominant–Refers to an allele that requires only one copy for expression.

Ductus arteriosus–Fetal structure that shunts blood from the pulmonary artery to the aorta to bypass the developing lungs.

Ductus venosus–Shunt from the umbilical vein to the inferior vena cava, allowing oxygenated blood returning from the placenta to bypass the liver and enter the systemic circulation.

Duodenum–First segment of the small intestine; the contents of the stomach and the pancreatic and bile ducts empty into it; site of digestion and some absorption.

Ectoderm–Outermost embryonic germ layer; it gives rise to the skin, nervous system, inner ear, lens of the eye, and other structures.

Effector–An organ, muscle, or gland used by an organism to respond to a stimulus.

Efferent (motor) neuron–A neuron that transmits nervous impulses from the central nervous system to an effector.

Embryo–An organism at the early developmental stage; in humans, the term refers to the first eight weeks after fertilization.

Endocrine–A form of cell–cell communication that involves the secretion of hormones into the bloodstream by ductless glands; these hormones then travel to distant locations within the organism to cause a change in cellular activity.

Endoderm–Innermost embryonic germ layer; it later gives rise to the linings of the alimentary canal and of the digestive and respiratory organs.

Endometrium–Uterine lining that is regenerated each month in preparation for implantation of an embryo; absence of an embryo results in sloughing off of the endometrium in a process known as menstruation.

Endoplasmic reticulum–Membrane-bound channels in the cytoplasm that transport proteins and lipids to various parts of the cell.

Endothelium–Lining of blood vessels consisting of endothelial cells.

Enteric nervous system–Collection of neurons within the gastrointestinal tract that governs peristalsis.

Eosinophil–Type of granulocytic leukocyte that largely participates in the immune response against parasites; also involved in the pathogenesis of allergies.

Epidermis–The outermost layer of the skin.

Epididymis–The coiled tube in which sperm gain motility and are stored after production in the testes.

Epigenetics–The study of changes to genes other than alterations to nucleotide sequences.

Epiglottis–The small flap of cartilage that covers the glottis during swallowing, preventing food from entering the larynx.

Epinephrine–A hormone synthesized by the adrenal medulla; it stimulates the fight-or-flight response; also a neurotransmitter in the sympathetic nervous system.

Epiphyseal plate–Cartilaginous structure in the epiphysis where growth occurs.

Epiphysis–Dilated end of a long bone.

Episomes–A specialized subset of plasmids capable of integrating into the genome of bacteria under specific circumstances.

Epithelium–The cellular layer that covers internal and external surfaces of body structures and cavities.

Erythrocyte–Red blood cell; a biconcave, disc-shaped cell that contains hemoglobin and has no nucleus.

Erythropoiesis–The multi-step process of producing mature red blood cells (erythrocytes) from hematopoietic stem cells, primarily occurring within the bone marrow.

Esophagus–Portion of the alimentary canal connecting the pharynx and the stomach.

Eukaryote–A unicellular or multicellular organism composed of cells that contain a membrane-bound nucleus and other membrane-bound organelles.

Evolution–The changes in the gene pool from one generation to the next caused by mutation, nonrandom mating, natural selection, and genetic drift.

Exocrine glands–Glands that release their secretions into ducts (such as the parts of the liver and sweat glands).

Expressivity–Varying expression of disease symptoms despite identical genotypes.

Extensor–A muscle used in the straightening of a limb.

Facultative anaerobes–Prokaryotes that can exist with or without oxygen.

Fertilization–Fusion of two gametes.

Fertilization membrane–Structure created by the cortical reaction after fertilization of an ovum by a sperm cell; prevents fertilization of an ovum by multiple sperm cells.

Fetus–A developing organism that has passed the early developmental stages. In humans, the term refers to an embryo from the ninth week after fertilization until birth.

Fibrin–The insoluble protein that forms the bulk of a blood clot.

Filial generation–Offspring in a genetic cross; may be supplemented with a subscript to show how many generations out from the parents.

Filtration–In the nephron, the process by which blood plasma is forced (under high pressure) out of the glomerulus into Bowman's capsule.

Fitness–Reproductive success of an individual, measured in increased number and survival of offspring.

Flagellum–A microscopic, whip-like filament that functions in the locomotion of sperm cells and some unicellular organisms; composed of microtubules.

Flexor–A muscle used in the bending of a limb.

Fluorescence microscopy–A general term for any type of microscopy that uses fluorescence, or the emission of light by a substance that has absorbed light or other electromagnetic radiation, as a means of visualization.

Follicle–The set of cells surrounding a developing or mature ovum. Secretes nutrients and estrogen and atrophies into the corpus luteum after ovulation.

Foramen ovale–Shunt within the fetal heart between the right and left atria that allows the circulation to largely bypass the developing lungs.

Fragment antigen-binding region (Fab region)–The region of an antibody that contains specific polypeptide sequences that bind to an antigen.

Fragment crystallizable region (Fc region)–The non-antigen-binding region of an antibody, which typically interacts with immune cells such as natural killer cells and macrophages to initiate the complement cascade and other immune pathways.

Gallbladder–Organ below the liver that stores bile; contracts in response to stimulation by cholecystokinin, resulting in release of bile into the biliary system and eventually into the duodenum.

Gamete–Sperm or ovum; a cell that has half the number of chromosomes of a somatic cell (haploid) and can fuse with another gamete to form a zygote.

Ganglion–A mass of neuron cell bodies outside the central nervous system.

Gastrula–The embryonic stage characterized by the presence of ectoderm, mesoderm, and endoderm.

Gene–The basic unit of heredity; a region on a chromosome that codes for a specific product.

Gene flow–The transfer of genetic material from one population to another of the same species through the migration and interbreeding of individuals.

Gene pool–All of the alleles for every gene in every individual in a given population.

Genetic drift–Variations in the gene pool caused by chance.

Genetic map–A diagrammatic representation of a chromosome indicating distance between two genes on a chromosome as determined by recombination frequencies.

Genome–An organism's complete set of chromosomes.

Genotype–The genetic composition of an entire organism or in reference to a particular trait.

Ghrelin–A peptide hormone, often called the "hunger hormone," that is primarily produced by the stomach to stimulate appetite, increase food intake, and promote fat storage.

Glomerulus–The network of capillaries encapsulated by Bowman's capsule. Acts as a filter for blood entering the nephron.

Glottis–The opening to the trachea.

Golgi apparatus–Organelle that plays a role in the packaging and secretion of proteins and other molecules produced intracellularly.

Gonad–Ovary or testis; the reproductive organ in which gametes are produced.

Gram staining–A process of staining bacterial cells such that cells containing large amounts of peptidoglycan within the cell wall are stained purple, while cells with less peptidoglycan within their cell walls appear pink-red after counterstaining.

Granulocyte–Type of leukocyte with cytoplasmic granules that are visible under a microscope, such as neutrophils, basophils, or eosinophils.

Grey matter–Any region in the central nervous system that consists largely of neuron cell bodies, dendrites, and synapses.

Growth factors–Substances that cause induction during embryonic development and ensure the development of the correct structure in the right location.

Haploid–Having only one of each type of chromosome per cell; symbolized by n.

Hardy–Weinberg principle–States that gene ratios and allelic frequencies remain constant through the generations in a non-evolving population.

Haversian canal–Central channel within the osteon (Haversian system) containing blood vessels, nerve fibers, and lymph vessels.

Heavy chain–One of two types of chains, made of peptides, that create an antibody; each antibody consists of two heavy chains and two light chains.

Helper T-cells–Type of T-cell that secretes lymphokines; the specific combination of lymphokines secreted will determine the nature of the immune response; activation of T_h1 cells will result in a cytotoxic response, while a T_h2 response will rely on B-cells.

Hematocrit–Measurement of how much of a blood sample consists of red blood cells, expressed as a percentage.

Hemoglobin–Iron-containing protein found in red blood cells that binds O_2 and transports it throughout the body.

Heterozygous–Having two different alleles for a particular trait.

Hilum–Area of an organ where large vessels or other structures enter or exit; the renal hilum is where the renal artery enters the kidney, the renal vein leaves the kidney, and the ureter exits the kidney to transport urine to the bladder.

Histamine–An inflammatory mediator that causes vasodilation and results in increased movement of fluid and cells out of the blood vessels and into the tissues.

Homeostasis–Maintenance of a stable internal physiological environment in an organism.

Homologous chromosomes–Chromosomes in a diploid cell that carry corresponding genes for the same traits at corresponding loci.

Homozygous–Having two identical alleles for a given trait.

Hormones–Chemical messengers secreted by cells of one part of the body and carried by the bloodstream to cells elsewhere in the body, where they regulate biochemical activity.

Humoral immunity–Form of adaptive immunity that takes place within body fluids, driven by B-cells and antibodies.

Hybrid–The resultant offspring of a cross (mating) either between two different gene types or between two different species.

Hypodermis–Subcutaneous layer beneath the dermis in the skin.

Hypothalamus–The region of the vertebrate forebrain that controls the autonomic nervous system and is the control center for hunger, thirst, body temperature, and other visceral functions; also secretes factors that stimulate or inhibit pituitary secretions.

Ileum–The terminal portion of the small intestine.

Immunohistochemistry–A technique used to label different subcellular components or targets within sample tissues using labeled antibodies.

Imprinting–An epigenetic process in which gene expression is determined by only one parent.

Impulse propagation–Movement of an action potential down an axon, resulting in neurotransmitter release at the synaptic bouton and transmission of the impulse to the target neuron or organ.

Inborn error of metabolism–Genetic mutation that causes a change in an enzyme required for metabolism; early intervention is necessary to prevent the development of life-threatening conditions; some inborn errors of metabolism are ultimately incompatible with life.

Incomplete dominance–A genetic effect in which the phenotype of a heterozygote is a mixture of the two parental phenotypes.

Independent assortment–Unlinked genes within a primary germ cell separate randomly during gametogenesis.

Indeterminate cleavage–Rapid mitotic divisions resulting in cells that are individually capable of becoming complete organisms.

Inducer–A chemical substance passed from an organizing cell to a responsive cell, resulting in differentiation of the responsive cell.

Induction–The initiation of cell differentiation in a developing embryo due to the influence of other cells.

Innate immunity–Form of immunity that is nonspecific and does not require learning.

Integument–The outer layer of the body (skin); provides function for thermoregulation and innate immunity.

Intermediate filament–Collection of fibers that help to maintain the overall integrity of the cytoskeleton.

Interneuron–A neuron that has its cell body and nerve terminals confined to one specific area; often involved in spinal reflexes.

Interphase–The stage between successive nuclear divisions; it is divided into the G_1, S, and G_2 stages; cell growth and DNA replication occur during interphase.

Intracellular digestion–Oxidation of fatty acids and glucose for energy within cells.

Intrapleural space–Fluid-filled potential space between the parietal and visceral pleura that lubricates the two pleural surfaces and allows for a pressure differential between the intrapleural space and the lungs.

Inversion–A chromosomal mutation in which a section of a chromosome breaks off, flips over, and then reattaches in its original spot.

Isolation–Mechanism that prevents genetic exchange between individuals of different species or populations.

Jejunum–The middle portion of the small intestine.

Joint cavity–Space between two bones in a joint; enclosed and maintained by fibrous tissues.

Juxtacrine–A form of cell–cell communication in which a cell releases a substance that binds to receptors on cells directly adjacent to the releasing cell.

Keratin–Protein present in the outermost layer of the skin that is largely responsible for preventing the loss of fluids and salts as well as the entry of foreign substances into the body; also present as an intermediate filament within cells.

Keratinocytes–Cells within the epidermis that produce keratin.

Kidney–Vertebrate organ that regulates water and salt concentration in the blood and is responsible for urine formation.

Kinetochore–A protein structure, located at the centromere, that provides a place for spindle fibers to attach to the chromosome.

Lacteal–Small lymphatic vessel that runs in the center of the villi in the small intestine; site of lipid absorption into the lymphatic system.

Lacunae–Small spaces within the bone matrix where osteocytes reside.

Lamellae–Concentric circles of bony matrix within the Haversian systems of bone.

Langerhans cells–Specialized macrophages that reside within the skin.

Large intestine–Tube-like structure, shorter but wider than the small intestine, largely responsible for resorption of water and the formation of semisolid feces; consists of the cecum, ascending colon, transverse colon, descending colon, sigmoid colon, and rectum.

Larynx–Pathway for air between the pharynx and the trachea. The epiglottis closes to prevent food from entering the larynx.

Latent period–The short interval between the application of a stimulus to a muscle and the contraction of the muscle.

Leakage–Flow of genes between closely related species.

Leptin–A peptide hormone, often called the "satiety hormone," that is produced by fat cells to suppress appetite and increase energy expenditure when the body's energy stores are sufficient.

Leukocytes–White blood cells; can be subdivided into granulocytes and agranulocytes.

Ligament–Connective tissue that joins two bones.

Light chain–One of two types of chains, made of peptides, that create antibodies; each antibody consists of two heavy chains and two light chains.

Light microscopy–A type of microscopy that uses visible light and lenses to magnify an image.

Linkage–Tendency for certain alleles to be inherited together due to proximity on the same chromosome.

Lipase–Enzyme that specifically cleaves the bonds in lipids.

Locus–In genetics, an area or region of a chromosome.

Loop of Henle–The U-shaped section of a mammalian nephron.

Lower esophageal sphincter–Ring-shaped muscular structure that separates the esophagus from the stomach; also known as the cardiac sphincter.

Lumen–The space within a tube or a sac.

Lymph–Clear fluid derived from blood plasma and transported through lymph vessels to the lymphatic ducts, which empty into the circulatory system.

Lymph node–Small, bean-shaped structure that provides a location for antigen presentation and mounting of an attack by the adaptive immune system.

Lymphocyte–A type of white blood cell involved in an organism's specific immune response.

Lysogenic cycle–Bacteriophage infection involving the integration of viral DNA into the bacterial genome without disrupting or destroying the host. The virus may subsequently reemerge and enter a lytic cycle.

Lysosome–A membrane-bound organelle that stores hydrolytic enzymes.

Lytic cycle–Bacteriophage infection involving the destruction (lysis) of the host bacterium.

Macrophage–A phagocytic white blood cell.

Map unit–A unit used to denote a 1 percent recombination frequency between two genes when creating a genetic map; corresponds to one centimorgan.

Mast cell–A granulocyte that releases histamine and causes inflammation.

Mastication–Breaking up of large food particles using the teeth, tongue, and lips; chewing.

Maternal–Of or relating to an individual who is pregnant. (As used in this text, it implies nothing about the gender identity of pregnant individuals.)

Mechanical digestion–Physical breakdown of large food particles into smaller food particles.

Medulla–The internal section of an organ (such as the adrenal glands and the kidney); may generally refer to the medulla oblongata of the mammalian hindbrain.

Medulla oblongata–The part of the brainstem closest to the spinal cord. It controls vital functions, such as breathing and heartbeat.

Megakaryocyte–Precursor cell that gives off platelets.

Meiosis–A process of cell division in which two successive nuclear divisions produce up to four haploid gametes from one diploid germ cell.

Melanin–Skin pigment produced by melanocytes that protects the skin from UV radiation and provides color to skin.

Melanocytes–Melanin-producing cells of the skin.

Memory cell–Lymphocyte of B- or T-cell lineage that remains after an infection is gone in order to recognize the previous invader and rapidly induce a humoral immune response.

Menstruation–The shedding of the uterine lining that occurs every four weeks in phenotypically female individuals who are not presently pregnant but are capable of becoming pregnant.

Mesoderm–The middle embryonic germ layer; it gives rise to the muscular, skeletal, urogenital, and circulatory systems.

Metabolism–The sum of all biochemical reactions that occur in an organism.

Metaphase–The stage of mitosis or meiosis during which single chromosomes or tetrads line up on the central axis of the dividing cell and become attached to spindle fibers.

Microfilaments–Small polymerized rods of actin that participate in muscle contraction, movement of material within the cellular membrane, and amoeboid movement.

Microglia–Phagocytic white blood cells that reside in the central nervous system.

Microtubule–A small, hollow tube composed of two types of protein subunits; serves numerous functions in the cell, such as comprising the internal structures of cilia and flagella and allowing vesicle movement in the cell.

Missense mutation–Type of mutation that results in the substitution of one amino acid for another.

Mitochondria–Membrane-bound cellular organelles in which the reactions of aerobic respiration and ATP synthesis occur.

Mitochondrial inheritance–An inheritance pattern in which the allele of interest is located on mitochondrial DNA, which is only passed down from the mother.

Mitosis–Cellular division that results in the formation of two daughter cells that are genetically identical to each other and to the parent cell.

Mitral valve–The atrioventricular valve separating the left atrium from the left ventricle.

Mixed nerve–Nerve carrying both afferent (sensory) and efferent (motor) fibers.

Monocyte–A white blood cell that transforms into a macrophage or dendritic cell once it enters tissues.

Monohybrid cross–A cross between two members of a species that seeks to study only one trait.

Monosaccharide–A sugar consisting of one monomer (glucose, fructose, or galactose).

Morphogen–Molecule that causes nearby cells to proceed in a specific developmental pathway during embryonic development.

Morula–The solid ball of cells that results from the early stages of cleavage in an embryo.

Mucosa–The type of epithelial tissue that lines moist body cavities; a mucous membrane.

Mucous cells–Type of epithelial cell that secretes mucus.

Multipotent–Stem cell that is able to differentiate into various cells within a particular lineage.

Mutagen–An agent, either chemical or physical, that can cause mutations.

Mutation–A change in DNA sequence.

Myelin–The white, lipid-containing material surrounding the axons of many neurons in the central and peripheral nervous systems.

Myogenic activity–Ability of a muscle cell to contract without input from the nervous system; found in smooth and cardiac muscle types.

Myoglobin–Heme-containing protein that binds molecular oxygen in muscle cells.

Myosin–A protein found in muscle cells that functions in muscle contraction; myosin fibers are also called thick filaments.

Natural selection–An ongoing evolutionary process resulting in changes in gene frequencies, leading to the differential development of phenotypes in a population.

Negative sense–Describes the genome of an RNA virus that contains an RNA sequence that is complementary to the actual transcript for viral protein synthesis.

Nephron–The functional unit of the vertebrate kidney.

Nerve–A bundle of neurons.

Nerve impulse–The self-propagating change in electrical potential across the axon membrane.

Nerve terminal–End of the axon from which neurotransmitter molecules are released; also called a synaptic bouton.

Neural crest cells–Cells that originate at the tip of the neural fold and then migrate outward to form the peripheral nervous system, melanocytes, C-cells of the thyroid, and others.

Neural fold–Group of ectodermal cells that slide together to create a fold, which later becomes the neural tube.

Neural tube–Embryonic hollow tube that subsequently gives rise to the central nervous system.

Neuroglia–Support cells for neurons; responsible for functions such as holding neurons in place, supplying neurons with oxygen and nutrients, insulating neurons from other neurons, destroying pathogens, and removing dead neurons.

Neuron–A cell that conducts electrical impulses; the functional unit of the nervous system.

Neurotransmitter–A chemical agent released into the synaptic cleft by the synaptic bouton of a neuron; binds to receptor sites on postsynaptic neurons or effector membranes to alter activity.

Neutrophil–Type of granulocytic leukocyte that largely participates in the nonspecific immune response against bacteria.

Niche–The specific way of life occupied by a given organism within the environment, including its interactions with other organisms and with the physical environment.

Nodes of Ranvier–Points on a myelinated axon that are not covered by myelin.

Nondisjunction–Failure of homologous chromosomes to separate during meiosis.

Nonsense mutation–A change in nucleotide sequence of DNA that results in a premature stop codon in the mRNA sequence.

Norepinephrine–A hormone synthesized by the adrenal medulla; it stimulates the fight-or-flight response; also, a neurotransmitter in the sympathetic nervous system.

Notochord–A supportive rod running just ventral to the neural tube in vertebrate embryos that induces neurulation.

Nuclear membrane–Double membrane enveloping the nucleus, interrupted periodically by pores; found in eukaryotic cells only; also known as the nuclear envelope.

Nuclear pore–Small hole in the nuclear membrane that allows for two-way exchange of material between the cytoplasm and nucleus.

Nucleoid region–Location in prokaryotic cells where the chromosome is found.

Nucleolus–Dense body visible in a nondividing nucleus; site of ribosomal RNA synthesis.

Nucleus–The eukaryotic membrane-bound organelle that contains the cell's chromosomes; in neuroscience, a collection of cell bodies in the central nervous system.

Oligodendrocyte–Myelin-producing cells in the central nervous system.

Oocyte–An undifferentiated cell that undergoes meiosis to produce an egg cell (ovum).

Oogenesis–Gametogenesis in the ovary leading to the formation of mature ova.

Osmotic pressure–A "sucking" pressure generated by the presence of solutes drawing in water.

Osteoblast–Bone cell responsible for the generation of new bone due to bone remodeling or storage of minerals within the bone matrix.

Osteoclast–Bone cell responsible for the resorption of bone due to bone remodeling or mobilization of minerals from the bone matrix.

Osteocytes–Mature bone cells housed within the bone matrix.

Ovary–The female egg-producing gonad.

Oviduct–The tube leading from the ovary to the uterus; generally, the site of fertilization; also called the fallopian tube.

Ovulation–The release of the mature ovum from the ovarian follicle.

Ovum–The female gamete; egg cell.

Oxygen debt–The amount of oxygen needed to reconvert lactic acid to pyruvate following strenuous exercise; the difference between the amount of oxygen needed by the tissue and the amount of oxygen available.

Pancreas–A gland that secretes digestive enzymes into the duodenum via a duct and synthesizes and secretes the hormones insulin, glucagon, and somatostatin; located between the stomach and the duodenum.

Papillary layer–Upper layer of the dermis, right below the epidermis, that consists of loose connective tissue.

Paracrine–A form of cell–cell communication in which a cell releases a substance into the extracellular fluid and the substance binds to receptors on nearby cells to cause a change in cellular activities.

Parasympathetic nervous system–The subdivision of the autonomic nervous system involved in rest and homeostasis; it is generally antagonistic to the sympathetic nervous system.

Parathyroid glands–Two pairs of glands located on the thyroid that secrete hormones that regulate calcium and phosphorous metabolism.

Parietal cells–Cells within the stomach that are responsible for the secretion of acid into the lumen of the stomach.

Passive immunity–Immunity conferred by the transfer or injection of previously formed antibodies.

Pathogen–An infectious disease-causing agent; includes bacteria, viruses, fungi, parasites, and prions.

Pathogen-associated molecular patterns (PAMPs)–Conserved molecular structures common to broad classes of microbes that are recognized by the innate immune system as a signal of infection.

Pattern recognition receptor–Type of receptor on macrophages and dendritic cells that is able to recognize the nature of the invader (bacteria, virus, or fungi) and release the appropriate cytokines to attract the right immune cells to the area.

Pedigree chart–A diagram that shows relationships between people within families and indicates the presence or absence of a trait of interest.

Penetrance–Percent of individuals with a particular genotype that actually express the associated phenotype.

Peptidase–Enzyme that cleaves peptide bonds.

Periosteum–Fibrous sheath surrounding long bones.

Peripheral nervous system–Includes all neurons outside the central nervous system, including sensory and motor neurons; it is subdivided into the somatic and autonomic nervous systems.

Peristalsis–Rhythmic waves of muscular contraction that move a substance through a tube (most commonly, food through the digestive tract).

Peroxisome–Organelle that contains hydrogen peroxide and participates in the breakdown of very long chain fatty acids.

Pharynx–Pathway for food from the mouth to the esophagus, and for air from the nose and mouth to the larynx.

Phenotype–The physical manifestation of an organism's genotype.

Phospholipid bilayer–A double layer of lipid molecules that forms the fundamental structure of all cell membranes, with hydrophilic heads facing outwards and hydrophobic tails facing inwards.

Pineal gland–Structure within the brain that secretes melatonin, a hormone that aids in the regulation of sleep–wake cycles.

Pituitary–The bilobed endocrine gland that lies just below the hypothalamus; because many of its hormones regulate other endocrine glands, it is known as the "master gland."

Placenta–The structure formed by the wall of the uterus and the chorion of the embryo; contains a network of capillaries through which exchange between maternal and fetal circulation occurs.

Plasma–The fluid component of blood containing dissolved solutes, minus the cells.

Plasma cells–Derived from B-lymphocytes; have the ability to produce and secrete antibodies.

Plasmid–Small circular ring of extrachromosomal DNA found in bacteria.

Platelets–Small, enucleated, disc-shaped shards of blood cells that play an important role in clotting.

Pleura–Connective tissue that surrounds each lung and aids in providing attachment of the lungs to the chest wall; the parietal pleura lies along the chest wall, while the visceral pleura is adherent to the lungs.

Pluripotent–Stem cell that has undergone gastrulation and is able to differentiate into any cell type within the same primary germ layer.

Polar body–A small, nonfunctional haploid cell created during oogenesis.

Population–A group of organisms of the same species living together in a given location.

Portal system–A circuit of blood in which there are two capillary beds in tandem connected by an artery or vein; examples include the hypophyseal, hepatic, and renal portal systems.

Portal vein–A vein that connects two capillary beds in a portal system.

Positive sense–Describes the genome of an RNA virus containing RNA that serves directly as the transcript for viral protein production.

Potency–Term used to describe the ability or inability of a stem cell to differentiate into different cell types.

Primary lymphoid organs–The sites where the immune system's lymphocytes, specifically T-cells and B-cells, are created and mature into functional, antigen-ready cells. The two primary lymphoid organs are the thymus and bone marrow.

Primary response–Humoral immune response against an invader during the first encounter; takes seven to ten days to become effective.

Prion–Infectious protein that causes disease by causing changes in the three-dimensional structure of other proteins from α-helices to β-pleated sheets.

Prokaryote–Cell lacking a nuclear membrane and membrane-bound organelles, such as a bacterium.

Prophase–The stage of mitosis or meiosis during which the DNA strands condense to form visible chromosomes; during prophase I of meiosis, homologous chromosomes align.

Prostate–A gland in phenotypically male mammals that secretes alkaline seminal fluid.

Pulmonary embolism–The medical condition that occurs when an artery in the lungs becomes blocked by a substance, known as an embolus, that has traveled from another part of the body.

Pulmonary valve–One of the semilunar valves, separating the right ventricle from the pulmonary arteries.

Purkinje fibers–The terminal fibers of the heart's conduction system; located in the walls of ventricles.

Pyloric sphincter–The valve that regulates the flow of chyme from the stomach into the small intestine.

Recessive–An allele that requires two copies to be expressed.

Recombination–New gene combinations achieved by sexual reproduction or crossing over in eukaryotes and by transformation, transduction, or conjugation in prokaryotes.

Recombination frequency–Measurement of how often genes recombine in different combinations; genes that are closer together have lower recombination frequencies.

Rectum–Terminal portion of the large intestine, where feces is stored until defecation.

Reflex–An involuntary nervous pathway consisting of sensory neurons, interneurons, motor neurons, and effectors; it occurs in response to a specific stimulus.

Refractory period–The period of time following an action potential during which the neuron is incapable of depolarization.

Releasing hormones–Proteins synthesized and secreted by the hypothalamus that stimulate the pituitary to synthesize and release its hormones. Also known as tropic hormones.

Renal pelvis–The widest part of the ureter, located within the kidney; location into which all collecting ducts eventually empty.

Renin–angiotensin–aldosterone system–Hormonal pathway that, among other functions, raises blood pressure.

Repolarization–Restoration of the resting membrane potential in neurons from being depolarized by both active and passive processes.

Respiration–In biochemistry, the series of oxygen-requiring biochemical reactions that lead to ATP synthesis; in physiology, the inhalation and exhalation of gases and their exchange in the lungs.

Responder–Embryonic cell that is undergoing induction.

Resting potential–The electrical potential of a cell at rest, approximately -70 mV in most excitable cells.

Restriction point–A point in the cell cycle that prevents the cell from entering the next portion of the cell cycle unless certain criteria are met.

Reticular layer–Lower layer of the dermis, consisting of dense connective tissue.

Retrovirus–An RNA virus that contains the enzyme reverse transcriptase, which transcribes RNA into DNA.

Rh factor–An antigen on a red blood cell, the presence or absence of which is indicated by + or −, respectively, in blood type notation; may also be called the D allele.

Ribosome–Organelle composed of RNA and protein; it translates mRNA during protein synthesis.

RNA-dependent RNA polymerase (RdRp)–An enzyme that synthesizes a new, complementary RNA strand using an existing RNA molecule as a template; common in RNA viruses.

Rough endoplasmic reticulum–Portion of the endoplasmic reticulum that appears rough microscopically due to the presence of ribosomes attached to the outer surface; site of protein synthesis for proteins destined to be membrane-bound or secreted.

Saltatory conduction–Process by which an electrical signal jumps across the nodes of Ranvier to travel down the axon.

Sarcolemma–Muscle cell membrane capable of propagating action potentials.

Sarcomere–The functional contractile unit of striated muscle.

Sarcoplasmic reticulum–The endoplasmic reticulum of a muscle cell; it envelops myofibrils.

Scanning electron microscopy–A type of microscopy that uses a beam of electrons to create a topographical map of the cell surface.

Schwann cell–Myelin-producing cell in the peripheral nervous system.

Second messenger–Substance that is mobilized within a cell after the binding of a hormone to its receptor.

Secondary lymphoid organs–Including the spleen, lymph nodes, tonsils, and Peyer's patches, these are the strategically located sites where mature lymphocytes encounter antigens and initiate an adaptive immune response.

Secondary response–Humoral immune response against a previously encountered invader; results in activation of memory cells and an immediate response.

Semen–Fluid released during ejaculation consisting of sperm cells suspended in seminal fluid.

Seminal vesicle–A gland found in phenotypically male mammals that produces seminal fluid.

Sex factor–Plasmid containing genetic material for the formation of a sex pili, required for conjugation.

Sex pilus–Appendage extending from the donor male (+) bacterial cell to the recipient female (−), allowing for the formation of the cytoplasmic bridge and transfer of genetic material.

Sex-linked gene–A gene located only on a sex chromosome (almost always the X chromosome); such genes exhibit different inheritance patterns in genotypical males and genotypical females.

Sexual reproduction–Any reproductive process that involves the fusion of gametes, resulting in the passage of combined genetic information to offspring.

Silent mutation–Change of one nucleotide for another that does not result in a change in the protein due to the degenerative nature of the genetic code (multiple codons code for the same amino acid).

Small intestine–Long tube-like structure; longer, but narrower than the large intestine, largely responsible for chemical digestion of foodstuffs and absorption of nutrients; consists of the duodenum, jejunum, and ileum.

Smooth endoplasmic reticulum–Portion of the endoplasmic reticulum that lacks ribosomes on its surface; location of lipid synthesis and detoxification of drugs and poisons.

Somatic cells–All cells in the body except germ cells and gametes.

Somatic nervous system–Subdivision of the peripheral nervous system that governs all voluntary actions.

Species–The largest group of organisms capable of mating to produce viable, fertile offspring.

Specific immune response–An organism's targeted fight against a specific pathogen using both antibodies and cytotoxic immunity.

Sperm–The mature male gamete or sex cell.

Spermatids–Immature haploid sperm cells.

Spermatogenesis–Gametogenesis in the testes leading to sperm formation.

Spermatogonia–Diploid stem cells in males that eventually give rise to sperm cells.

Spermatozoa–Mature haploid sperm cells.

Sphincter–A ring-shaped muscle that closes and opens a tube (such as the pyloric sphincter).

Sphygmomanometer–Device used to measure blood pressure, consisting of an inflatable cuff and a gauge that measures pressure.

Spindle–A structure within dividing cells composed of microtubules; it is involved in the separation of chromosomes during mitosis and meiosis.

Spirilli–Spiral-shaped bacteria.

Spleen–Highly vascular organ in the left upper quadrant of the abdomen; serves as a location for disposal of aged red blood cells and the presentation of antigens to B-cells.

Stabilizing selection–Selective pressure resulting in the elimination of extremes.

Starling forces–A sum of the forces generated by hydrostatic and osmotic pressures; results in a greater attraction of fluid to one side of a membrane.

Stroke volume–Amount of blood ejected from a ventricle with each heartbeat.

Summation–Process that occurs when the postsynaptic neuron or target organ requires stimulation from multiple presynaptic neurons in order to respond to the stimulus; may be spatial or temporal.

Suppressor T-cells–Also known as regulatory T-cells (T_{reg}), these T-cells limit the immune response to prevent detrimental immune reactions, such as autoimmunity.

Surfactant–A detergent that lowers surface tension and prevents collapse of the alveoli.

Symbiote–Organism living closely with a host and engaging in a mutually beneficial relationship.

Sympathetic nervous system–The subdivision of the autonomic nervous system that produces the "fight-or-flight" response.

Synapse–The junction between two neurons into which neurotransmitters are released.

Synapsis–The pairing of homologous chromosomes during prophase I of meiosis.

Synovial capsule–Fluid-filled space between bones in a joint; enclosed by fibrous tissue; synovial fluid lubricates the joint.

Systole–The period of the cardiac cycle during which the ventricles contract and pump blood into the aorta and pulmonary arteries.

T-cells–Type of leukocyte that matures in the thymus and participates in adaptive immunity.

Telophase–The final stage of mitosis or meiosis during which the chromosomes uncoil, nuclear membranes reform, and cytokinesis occurs.

Tendon–A fibrous connective tissue that connects a bone to a muscle.

Test cross–A cross between an organism showing a dominant trait and an organism showing a recessive trait to determine whether the former organism is homozygous or heterozygous for that trait.

Testis–The sperm-producing organ; also secretes testosterone.

Tetanus–Sustained muscle contraction that results from continuous stimulation.

Tetrad–A pair of homologous chromosomes synapsing during prophase I of meiosis. Each chromosome consists of two sister chromatids; thus, each tetrad consists of four chromatids.

Thermoregulation–Process by which an organism regulates its internal temperature by using the respiratory, integumentary, and circulatory systems.

Thoracic duct–The main lymphatic vessel that empties lymph into the bloodstream.

Threshold–The lowest magnitude of stimulus strength that will induce a response.

Thrombin–An enzyme that participates in blood clotting; it converts fibrinogen into fibrin.

Thrombopoiesis–The complex process of producing platelets (thrombocytes), the small, colorless cell fragments essential for blood clotting.

Thymus–A ductless gland in the upper chest region of vertebrates; it functions in the development of the immune system.

Thyroid–A vertebrate endocrine gland located in the neck that synthesizes triiodothyronine, thyroxine, and calcitonin.

Tissue–A mass of similar cells and support structures organized into a functional unit.

Tonus–A continuous state of low-level muscle contraction.

Totipotent–Type of stem-cell potency describing cells that are able to differentiate into all cell types within an organism.

Trachea–The tube that connects the pharynx to the bronchi.

Transduction–The transposition of genetic material from one organism to another by a virus.

Transformation–Uptake and incorporation of DNA from the environment by a recipient bacterial cell.

Transformation efficiency–A measure of how effectively foreign DNA can be introduced into bacterial cells, calculated by dividing the number of colony-forming units by the mass of DNA used.

Transitional epithelium–A type of epithelial tissue that changes shape when stretched. Found in the urinary system, including the bladder, allowing for elasticity; also known as urothelium.

Transmission electron microscopy–A type of microscopy that uses electrons to visualize subcellular structures.

Transposon–Genetic element capable of inserting and removing itself from the genome.

Tricuspid valve–One of the atrioventricular valves, separating the right atrium from the right ventricle.

Trophoblast–Embryonic cells that line the blastocoel and give rise to the chorion and the placenta.

Tropic hormone–Hormone that is secreted and travels to a target cell or organ, where it triggers release of another hormone, which causes changes in the physiological activity of target cells.

Tubulin–Protein constituent of microtubules.

Universal donor–A person (O^- blood) whose blood is able to be given to all types without inducing an immune response.

Universal recipient–A person (AB^+ blood) who is able to receive all blood types without undergoing an immune response.

Urea–A nitrogenous waste product produced in the liver from ammonia.

Ureter–The tube that carries urine from the kidneys to the bladder.

Urethra–The tube that carries urine from the bladder to the exterior.

Urine–Liquid waste resulting from the filtration, reabsorption, and secretion of filtrate in the nephron.

Uterus–Organ in the mammalian female reproductive system that is the site of embryonic development.

Vaccine–A solution of fractionated, dead, or attenuated live pathogenic material that is introduced into an individual for the purpose of stimulating a primary immune response or "boosting" a previously produced anamnestic state.

Vagina–Passageway through which childbirth occurs; location into which sperm is deposited during sexual intercourse.

Vagus nerve–The tenth cranial nerve; it innervates the palate, pharynx, larynx, heart, lungs, and abdominal viscera; responsible for maintaining homeostatic activity through the parasympathetic response.

Vas deferens–The tube carrying sperm from the testis to the urethra in phenotypically male mammals.

Vasa recta–Second capillary bed within the kidney that removes substances from the interstitium of the kidney to be returned to the systemic circulation.

Vein–Thin-walled blood vessel that carries blood toward the heart.

Venae cavae–Two large veins (superior and inferior) that return deoxygenated blood from the periphery to the right atrium of the heart.

Ventilation center–Groups of neurons in the medulla oblongata that regulate respiration.

Ventricles–The chambers of the heart that pump blood into pulmonary and systemic circulation.

Venule–Small venous structure that links the capillaries to the veins.

Vestigial–Referring to an organ or limb that has no apparent function now, but was functional at some time in the organism's evolutionary past.

Villus–A small projection from the wall of the small intestine that increases the surface area for digestion and absorption.

Viroid–A small plant pathogen consisting of a very short, circular, single strand of RNA.

Virus–A tiny, organism-like particle composed of protein-encased nucleic acid; viruses are obligate parasites.

Vitamin–An organic nutrient that an organism cannot produce itself and that is required by the organism in small amounts to aid in proper metabolic functioning; vitamins often function as cofactors for enzymes.

White matter–The portion of the central nervous system consisting primarily of myelinated axons.

X-linked recessive–A pattern of inheritance in which the trait is encoded by a gene on the X chromosome and requires all X chromosomes present to contain the allele of interest for the trait to be expressed. This results in males with only one X chromosome being disproportionately affected.

Y-linked–An inheritance pattern in which a trait is carried on the Y chromosome, affecting only males.

Zona pellucida–One of two layers of cells surrounding an oocyte.

Zygote–The diploid ($2n$) cell that results from the fusion of two haploid (n) gametes.

Zymogen–An inactive enzyme precursor that is converted into an active enzyme.

INDEX

B

C

F

G

M

N

R

S

T

U

V

W

X

Y

Z

ART CREDITS

Chapter 1 Cover—Image credited to MichaelTaylor3d. From Shutterstock.

Figure 1.8—Image credited to Mopic. From Shutterstock.

Figure 1.14—Image credited to NANOCLUSTERING/SCIENCE PHOTO LIBRARY. From Getty Images. Modified from source.

Chapter 2 Cover—Image credited to Jose Luis Calvo. From Shutterstock.

Figure 3.3—Image credited to Science Photo Library - ZEPHYR. From Getty Images.

Figure 3.4—Image credited to Ed Reschke. From Getty Images.

Figure 3.11—Image credited to Callista Images. From Getty Images.

Chapter 4 Cover—Image credited to Juane Gaertner. From Shutterstock.

Figure 4.4—Image credited to Vitalii Dumma. From Getty Images. Modified from source.

Figure 4.17—Image credited to Alila Medical Media. From Shutterstock.

Figure 4.18—Image credited to Alila Medical Media. From Shutterstock.

Chapter 5 Cover—Image credited to Vitapix. From Getty Images.

Figure 5.15—Image credited to Alila Medical Media. From Shutterstock.

Chapter 6 Cover—Image credited to Guzel Studio. From Shutterstock.

Chapter 7 Cover—Image credited to decade3d. From Shutterstock.

Figure 7.21—Image credited to Stocktrek Images. From Getty Images.

Chapter 9 Cover—Image credited to Juan Gaertner. From Shutterstock.

Figure 9.9—Image credited to User: BruceBlaus. From Wikimedia Commons. Copyright © 2013. Used under license: CC-BY-3.0.

Figure 10.10—Image credited to Anton Nalivayko. From Shutterstock.

Figure 10.11—Image credited to User: Blamb. From Shutterstock. Modified from source.

Chapter 11 Cover—Image credited to SEBASTIAN KAULITZKI. From Getty Images.

Figure 11.19—Image credited to OpenStax College. In: Anatomy & Physiology, Connexions website. Copyright © 2013. Used under license: CC-BY-3.0.

Notes

Notes

Notes

Notes

Notes

Notes

Notes